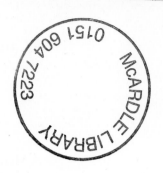
Lung Cancer

A Multidisciplinary Approach to Diagnosis and Management

Current Multidisciplinary Oncology Series

Charles R. Thomas, Jr., MD
Series Editor

Breast Cancer
A Multidisciplinary Approach to Diagnosis and Management
Alphonse G. Taghian, Barbara L. Smith, and John K. Erban

Lung Cancer
A Multidisciplinary Approach to Diagnosis and Management
Kemp H. Kernstine and Karen L. Reckamp

Current Multidisciplinary Oncology

Lung Cancer
A Multidisciplinary Approach to Diagnosis and Management

Kemp H. Kernstine, MD, PhD

Professor and Chief, Division of Thoracic Surgery
Director, Lung Cancer and Thoracic Oncology Program
City of Hope Comprehensive Cancer Center
Beckman Research Institute
Duarte, California

Karen L. Reckamp, MD, MS

Assistant Professor
Departments of Medical Oncology and Experimental
 Therapautics, and Hematology and Hematopoietic Cell Transpant
City of Hope Comprehensive Cancer Center
Beckman Research Institute
Duarte, California

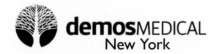
demosMEDICAL
New York

Acquisitions Editor: Richard Winters
Cover Design: Joe Tenerelli
Compositor: NewGen Imaging
Printer: Hamilton Printing Company

Visit our website at www.demosmedpub.com

Library of Congress Cataloging-in-Publication Data
Lung cancer : a multidisciplinary approach to diagnosis and management /
[edited by] Kemp H. Kernstine, Karen L. Reckamp.
    p. ; cm.— (Current multidisciplinary oncology)
  Includes bibliographical references and index.
  ISBN 978-1-936287-06-2
1. Lungs—Cancer. I. Kernstine, Kemp H. II. Reckamp, Karen L. III.
Series: Current multidisciplinary oncology.
[DNLM: 1. Lung Neoplasms—diagnosis. 2. Lung Neoplasms—therapy. WF 658]
RC280.L8L7672 2011
616.99′424—dc22   2010035586

Medicine is an ever-changing science. Research and clinical experience are continually expanding our knowledge, in particular our understanding of proper treatment and drug therapy. The authors, editors, and publisher have made every effort to ensure that all information in this book is in accordance with the state of knowledge at the time of production of the book. Nevertheless, the authors, editors, and publisher are not responsible for errors or omissions or for any consequences from application of the information in this book and make no warranty, express or implied, with respect to the contents of the publication. Every reader should examine carefully the package inserts accompanying each drug and should carefully check whether the dosage schedules mentioned therein or the contraindications stated by the manufacturer differ from the statements made in this book. Such examination is particularly important with drugs that are either rarely used or have been newly released on the market.

Special discounts on bulk quantities of Demos Medical Publishing books are available to corporations, professional associations, pharmaceutical companies, health care organizations, and other qualifying groups. For details, please contact:

Special Sales Department
Demos Medical Publishing
11 W. 42nd Street, 15th Floor
New York, NY 10036
Phone: 800-532-8663 or 212-683-0072
Fax: 212-941-7842
E-mail: rsantana@demosmedpub.com

Made in the United States of America
10 11 12 13 14   5 4 3 2 1

Contents

Series Foreword   vii
Preface   ix
Contributors   xi

1. Overview   1
   Kemp H. Kernstine and Karen L. Reckamp

2. Multidisciplinary Approach to the
   Evaluation of the Lung Cancer Patient   7
   Michael K. Gould

3. Pathology of Lung Cancer   19
   Heidi S. Erickson and Ignacio I. Wistuba

4. The New Lung Cancer Staging System   43
   *Ramon Rami-Porta, Dorothy J Giroux,
   and Peter Goldstraw*

5. Screening and Prevention of Lung Cancer   53
   V. Paul Doria-Rose and Eva Szabo

6. Imaging in Lung Cancer   73
   Eric Y. Chang and Paul Stark

Treatment According to Stage

7. Early Stage, Local Disease NSCLC,
   Surgical Therapy Options   91
   *Paul C. Y. Tang, Todd L. Demmy, and
   Sai Yendamuri*

8. Surgical Treatment of
   Small Cell Lung Cancer   105
   James E. Harris, Jr. and Malcolm V. Brock

9. Evaluation, Management, and Medical
   Therapy of Small Cell Lung Cancer   111
   *Randeep Sangha and
   Primo N. Lara, Jr.*

10. Stages IB to IIIA NSCLC: The Case for
    Induction versus Adjuvant Chemotherapy   123
    Stephanie L. Graff and Karen Kelly

11. Stage IIIA–N2 NSCLC: The Case Against Surgical
    Involvement   133
    I. K. Demedts and Jan P. Van Meerbeeckman

12. Stage IIIA NSCLC: The Case for
    Surgical Involvement   139
    *Justin D. Blasberg, Harvey I. Pass, and
    Jessica S. Donington*

13. Management of Unresectable Stage III NSCLC   151
    *Anjali Bharne, Lyudmila Bazhenova,
    and Barbara Gitlitz*

14. Surgery for T4 and N3 NSCLC, Additional
    Pulmonary Nodules, and Isolated Distant
    Metastases   161
    Anthony W. Kim and Frank C. Detterbeck

15. Stage IIIB and IV NSCLC:
    Primary Therapy   183
    Millie Das and Heather Wakelee

16. Stage IIIB and IV NSCLC:
    Recurrent Disease   197
    *Enriqueta Felip, Teresa Morán, Bartomeu Massuti,
    and Rafael Rosell*

17. Conformal Radiotherapy for Non–Small Cell
    and Small Cell Lung Cancer: Primary,
    Metastatic, and Recurrent Disease   205
    Charlotte Dai Kubicky and John M. Holland

18. Stereotactic Radiation Therapy for Primary, Metastatic, and Recurrent Disease 217
Simona S. Lo, Nina A. Mayr, and Robert D. Timmerman

Special Circumstances

19. Tracheobronchial Cancers: Nd:YAG Laser Resection, Brachytherapy, and Photodynamic Ablation 235
Henri G. Colt

20. Targeting Pathways in NSCLC and SCLC 243
Sumanta Kumar Pal and Karen Reckamp

21. Role of Personalized Medicine: Now and the Future 263
Nir Peled, Celine Mascaux, Murry W. Wynes, and Fred R. Hirsch

22. Lung Cancer in Older Adults 277
Sumanta Kumar Pal and Arti Hurria

23. Racial Disparities in Lung Cancer 293
Christopher Lathan

24. Immunological Approaches to the Treatment of Lung Cancer 299
Nick Levonyak, Mitchell Magee, and John Nemunaitis

25. Multidisciplinary Approach to Palliative and Symptom Management of Disease 313
Betty Ferrell and Marianna Koczywas

26. Psychologic Distress in Patients with Lung Cancer 323
Andrea A. Thornton

27. Multidisciplinary Management of Lung Cancer in the Community Setting 335
Jonathan W. Goldman

28. Future Directions in the Multidisciplinary Cancer of Patients with Lung Cancer 353
Paul A. Bunn , Robert C. Doebele, York E. Miller, Nir Peled, Ali Musani, Kavita Garg, Wilbur Franklin, Fred R. Hirsch, John D. Mitchell, Michael Weyant, D. Ross Camidge, Laurie Gaspar, Brian Kavanagh, T.J. Pugh, Jessica Flagiello, Ana B. Oton

Index 359

Series Foreword

This second volume in the Current Multidisciplinary Oncology series is devoted to lung cancer, and it brings me great pleasure to introduce the practicing clinician to a new resource that will aid in the multidisciplinary approach of solid tumors.

Drs. Kemp Kernstine and Karen Reckamp have put together a cadre of highly respected thought leaders as contributors on the multidisciplinary approach to lung cancer.

Over the past two decades, a myriad of advances in the diagnosis and treatment of lung cancer have occurred. Some of the advances include, but are not unlimited to, diagnostic molecular tools which may aid in predicting a response to certain treatment approaches and/or providing a guide of prognostic outcomes for certain patients.

Drs. Kernstine and Reckamp have compiled 28 chapters into three well-defined sections.

Lung cancer is one of the most common malignancies in the world and hence warrants intense efforts to find a cure. In recent years, investment of resources to help further understand the nature of this malignancy has increased.

It is clear that Drs. Kernstine and Reckamp are examples of the next generation of academic, forward-thinking oncologists who have committed their careers to eradicating lung cancer. Their collective vision and ability to assemble an outstanding group of investigators in the field has provided a very high quality product that will be a useful resource to the busy clinician as well as those along various stages of the learning spectrum. I'm sure that you will enjoy this innovative and easy to read text as you look for guidance in the multidisciplinary approach of your patients with lung cancer.

Charles R. Thomas, Jr., MD
Series Editor
Department of Radiation Medicine
Oregon Health and Science University
Knight Cancer Institute
Portland, Oregon

Preface

Lung cancer accounts for nearly a third of all cancer deaths and is the second most common cancer diagnosis in United States. Medical professionals, scientists and patients are fully aware of the complexities and encumbrances of the disease and the need for greater understanding of it. In the last decade, there have been tremendous advances in the diagnosis, biological assessment and the treatment. This is the second book in the series, *Current Multidisciplinary Oncology*, edited by Dr. Charles R. Thomas, Jr. with the overall purpose of providing a textbook that approaches the disease in an organized fashion, attempting to consolidate and integrate the many specialty approaches and discoveries that are involved in managing the disease.

This book is organized in similar fashion to the other books in the series, initially reviewing the more general aspects of lung cancer; the multidisciplinary evaluation of patients with known and suspicious disease, the pathological assessment, screening and prevention, the new lung cancer staging system and radiological imaging. The treatment is stage dependent and, thus, the remainder of the book is organized accordingly, initially reviewing surgical treatment options for early-stage disease as well as surgical treatment opportunities in small cell cancer, locally advanced disease as well is in systemic disease. The attempt to identify controversial points has provided chapters in a point-counterpoint fashion so that the reader may better understand the arguments and the research opportunities as well as potential future developments. For advanced disease, primary therapy and treatment of recurrent disease are presented and there is a review of the most recent developments in radiation therapy. There is a detailed review of the advances in the development and study of targeted agents, as well as personalizing the treatment of lung cancer and the development of vaccines and other immunological approaches. Newer endoscopic treatment opportunities are now available and the indications are reviewed. Special topics are presented such as the issues involved in the treatment of the elderly, minorities, palliation and the psychosocial issues involved with the diagnosis and management. In keeping with the series, Dr. Jonathan Goldman, a private practice oncologist, describes management of the disease in the community setting. Then, in the final chapter, one of the international leaders in lung cancer, Dr. Paul Bunn, describes the future directions of multidisciplinary management.

This book is written by international leaders in the field of lung cancer and we are indebted to them for their thorough review and detailed analysis, providing in each chapter an evidence-based approach to evaluation and management that has been extensively referenced. This book should be a uniquely valuable resource and serve as a handbook for physicians and medical specialists dealing with the disease; medical oncologists, radiation oncologists, thoracic surgeons, pulmonologists, radiologists, pathologists, pain experts, psychiatrists/psychologists, nurses and other allied health professionals, students, residents and fellows in-training, as well as patients and their families.

Kemp H. Kernstine, MD, PhD
Karen L. Reckamp, MD, MS

Contributors

Lyudmila Bazhenova, MD
Assistant Clinical Professor Medicine
Division of Hematology Oncology
University of California San Diego,
    Moores Cancer Center
San Diego, California

Anjali Bharne, MD
Physician
Department of Hematology/Oncology
Cedars-Sinai Medical Group
Beverly Hills, California

Justin D. Blasberg, MD
Surgical Resident
General Surgery
St. Luke's-Roosevelt Hospital Center
Columbia University College of Physicians
    and Surgeons
New York, New York

Malcolm V. Brock, MLitt, MD
Department of Surgery
Johns Hopkins University School of Medicine
Department of Environmental Health Sciences
Johns Hopkins Bloomberg School
Baltimore, Maryland

Paul A. Bunn, MD
James Dudley Chair in Cancer Research
Professor of Medicine
Department of Medical Oncology
University of Colorado Denver
Aurora, Colorado

D. Ross Camidge, MD, PhD
Department of Medicine
University of Colorado Denver
Aurora, Colorado

Eric Y. Chang, MD
Diagnostic Radiologist
Department of Radiology
University of California, San Diego Medical Center
San Diego, California

Henri G. Colt, MD
Professor of Medicine
Pulmonary and Critical Care Medicine
University of California, Irvine
Orange, California

Millie Das, MD
Hematology/Oncology Fellow
Department of Medicine
Division of Oncology
Stanford University Cancer Center
Stanford, California

I. K. Demedts, MD, PhD
Respiratory Medicine
Heilig Hart Ziekenhuis
Roeselare, Belgium

Todd L. Demmy, MD
Chairman
Department of Thoracic Surgery
Roswell Park Cancer Institute
Buffalo, New York

Frank C. Detterbeck, MD
Professor and Chief
Department of Thoracic Surgery
Yale University School of Medicine
New Haven, Connecticut

Robert C. Doebele, MD, PhD
Department of Medicine
University of Colorado Denver
Aurora, Colorado

Jessica S. Donington, MD
Assistant Professor
Cardiothoracic Surgery
New York University School of Medicine
New York, New York

V. Paul Doria-Rose, DVM, PhD
Epidemiologist
Division of Cancer Control and Population Sciences
National Cancer Institute
National Institutes of Health
Bethesda, Maryland

Heidi S. Erickson, PhD, MS
Assistant Professor
Department of Thoracic/Head and
    Neck Medical Oncology
The University of Texas M. D. Anderson Cancer Center
Houston, Texas

Enriqueta Felip, MD
Senior Medical Oncologist
Medical Oncology Service
Hospital Vall d'Hebron
Barcelona, Spain

Betty Ferrell, PhD, FAAN, MA, FPCN
Professor and Research Scientist
Nursing Research and Education/
    Population Sciences
City of Hope Comprehensive Cancer Center
Duarte, California

Jessica Flagiello, RN
Department of Medicine
University of Colorado Denver
Aurora, Colorado

Wilbur Franklin, MD
Department of Pathology
University of Colorado Denver
Aurora, Colorado

Kavita Garg, MD
Department of Radiology
University of Colorado Denver
Aurora, Colorado

Laurie Gaspar, MD
Department of Radiation Oncology
University of Colorado Denver
Aurora, Colorado

Dorothy J. Giroux, MS
Biostatistician
Cancer Research and Biostatistics
Seattle, Washington

Barbara Gitlitz, MD
Associate Professor of Clinical Medicine
Department of Medicine/Oncology
University of Southern California, Keck School of Medicine
Norris Comprehensive Cancer Center
Los Angeles, California

Jonathan W. Goldman, MD
Director, Premiere Oncology's Thoracic
Malignancy Research Program
Department of Medical Oncology
Santa Monica, California

Peter Goldstraw, MB, FRCS
Consultant and Professor of Thoracic Surgery
Department of Thoracic Surgery
Royal Brompton Hospital and Imperial College
London, United Kingdom

Michael K. Gould, MD, MS
Visiting Associate Professor
Departments of Medicine and Preventive Medicine
Keck School of Medicine of the University of
    Southern California
Los Angeles, California

Stephanie L. Graff, MD
Fellow in Hematology Oncology
Department of Internal Medicine
University of Kansas Medical Center
Kansas City, Kansas

James E. Harris, Jr., MD
Surgical Resident
Department of Surgery
Johns Hopkins Hospital
Baltimore, Maryland

Fred R. Hirsch, MD, PhD
Professor of Medicine and Pathology
Departments of Medical Oncology and Pathology
University of Colorado Denver
Aurora, Colorado

John M. Holland, MD
Associate Professor
Radiation Medicine
Oregon Health Science University
Portland, Oregon

Arti Hurria, MD
Associate Professor
Director, Cancer and Aging Research Program
Department of Medical Oncology and
    Experimental Therapeutics
City of Hope Comprehensive Cancer Center
Duarte, California

Brian Kavanagh, MD, PhD
Department of Radiation Oncology
University of Colorado Denver
Aurora, Colorado

Karen Kelly, MD
Professor
Department of Internal Medicine
University of Kansas Medical Center
Kansas City, Kansas

Kemp H. Kernstine, MD, PhD
Professor and Chief
Division of Thoracic Surgery
Director
Lung Cancer and Thoracic Oncology Program
City of Hope Comprehensive Cancer Center
Beckman Research Institute
Duarte, California

Anthony W. Kim, MD
Assistant Professor
Department of Thoracic Surgery
Yale University School of Medicine
New Haven, Connecticut

Marianna Koczywas, MD
Associate Professor of Medicine
Division of Medical Oncology and
    Therapeutic Research
Thoracic Oncology and Lung Cancer Program
City of Hope
Duarte, CA 91010

Charlotte Dai Kubicky, MD, PhD
Assistant Professor
Radiation Medicine
Oregon Health Science University
Portland, Oregon

Primo N. Lara, Jr., MD
Professor of Medicine
Department of Internal Medicine, Division of
    Hematology and Oncology
University of California Davis School of Medicine
Sacramento, California

Christopher Lathan, MD, MS, MPH
Faculty Director for Cancer Care Equity
Mcgraw/Patterson Center for Outcomes and
    Policy Research
Lowe Center for Thoracic Oncology
Dana-Farber Cancer Institute
Boston, Massachusetts

Nick Levonyak
Gradalis, Inc.
Dallas, Texas

Simon S. Lo, MD
Associate Professor of Radiation Oncology and
    Neurosurgery
Department of Radiation Oncology
Arthur G. James Cancer Hospital
Ohio State University
Columbus, Ohio

Mitchell Magee, MD
Director of Thoracic Surgical Oncology
Cardiovascular Specialty Associates of North Texas,
    P.A. (CSANT)
Dallas, Texas

Celine Mascaux, MD, PhD
Postdoctoral Fellow
Department of Medical Oncology
University of Colorado
Aurora, Colorado

Bartomeu Massuti, MD
Head, Medical Oncology Service
Hospital General de Alicante
Alicante, Spain

Nina A. Mayr, MD
Professor of Radiation Oncology
Department of Radiation Oncology
Arthur G. James Cancer Hospital
Ohio State University
Columbus, Ohio

Jan. P. van Meerbeeck, MD, PhD
Professor
Division of Blood, Respiration, and Digestion
Ghent University Hospital
Ghent, Belgium

York E. Miller, MD
Department of Medicine
VA Hospital
Denver, Colorado

John D. Mitchell, MD
Department of Surgery
University of Colorado Denver
Aurora, Colorado

Teresa Morán, MD
Senior Medical Oncologist
Medical Oncology Service
Catalan Institute of Oncology, Hospital Germans
    Trias i Pujol
Badalona, Spain

Ali Musani, MD, FACP, FCCP
Department of Medicine
National Jewish Health
Denver, Colorado

John Nemunaitis, MD
Executive Medical Director
Mary Crowley Cancer Research Center
Dallas, Texas

Ana B. Oton, MD
Department of Medicine
University of Colorado
Aurora, Colorado

Sumanta Kumar Pal, MD
Assistant Professor
Department of Medical Oncology and
    Experimental Therapeutics
City of Hope Comprehensive Cancer Center
Duarte, California

Harvey I. Pass, MD
Professor of Cardiothoracic Surgery
Chief, Division of Thoracic Surgery
Cardiothoracic Surgery
New York University School of Medicine
New York, New York

Nir Peled, MD, PhD
Visiting Professor
Department of Medical Oncology
University of Colorado Cancer Center
Denver, Colorado
Pulmonologist and Medical Oncologist
Davidoff Cancer Center
Rabin Medical Center, Tel Aviv University
Tel-Aviv, Israel

T. J. Pugh, MD
Department of Radiation Oncology
University of Colorado
Aurora, Colorado

Ramon Rami-Porta, MD
Attending Thoracic Surgeon
Thoracic Surgery Service
Hospital Universitari Mutua Terrassa
Terrassa, Spain

Karen L. Reckamp, MD, MS
Assistant Professor
Departments of Medical Oncology and
    Experimental Therapeutics, and Hematology and
    Hematopoietic Cell Transplant
City of Hope Comprehensive Cancer Center
Beckman Research Institute
Duarte, California

Rafael Rosell, MD, PhD
Head, Medical Oncology Service
Catalan Institute of Oncology
Hospital Germans Trias i Pujol
USP Dexeus University Institute
Badalona, Spain

Randeep Sangha, MD
Assistant Professor
Department of Medical Oncology
Cross Cancer Institute, University of Alberta
Edmonton, Alberta, Canada

Paul Stark, MD
Chief of Cardiothoracic Imaging
Department of Radiology
VA San Diego Healthcare System
San Diego, California

Eva Szabo, MD
Chief, Lung and Upper Aerodigestive
    Cancer Research Group
Division of Cancer Prevention
National Cancer Institute
National Institutes of Health
Bethesda, Maryland

Paul C. Y. Tang, MD, PhD
Resident
Department of Surgery
State University of New York
Buffalo, New York

Andrea A. Thornton, PhD
Attending Psychologist
Resnick Neuropsychiatric Hospital and Semel Institute
University of California, Los Angeles
Los Angeles, California

Robert D. Timmerman, MD
Professor of Radiation Oncology and Neurosurgery
Department of Radiation Oncology
University of Texas Southwestern
    Medical Center
Dallas, Texas

Heather Wakelee, MD
Assistant Professor of Medicine
Department of Medicine
Division of Oncology
Stanford University Cancer Center
Stanford, California

Michael Weyant, MD
Department of Surgery
University of Colorado Denver
Aurora, Colorado

Ignacio I. Wistuba, MD
Professor
Departments of Pathology and Thoracic/Head and
    Neck Medical Oncology
The University of Texas M. D. Anderson Cancer Center
Houston, Texas

Murry W. Wynes, PhD
Department of Medical Oncology
University of Colorado
Aurora, Colorado

Sai Yendamuri, MBBS
Assistant Professor
Department of Thoracic Surgery
Roswell Park Cancer Institute
Buffalo, New York

I Overview

KEMP H. KERNSTINE

KAREN L. RECKAMP

Lung cancer is responsible for more deaths each year than colon, breast, and prostate cancer combined. According to the American Cancer Society, for 2010, it is expected that there will be approximately 222,520 new cases of and 157,300 deaths from lung cancer. Despite modest improvements in survival in the last decade, new strategies for the prevention, screening, diagnosis, and treatment of lung cancer are clearly needed. There is increasing emphasis on tailoring selection of therapy to specific tumor biology to optimize treatment for individual patients with this disease, which supports a collaborative approach to therapy. The management of lung cancer in this era of rapidly evolving technologies requires a multidisciplinary team comprising pulmonologists, radiologists, pathologists, thoracic surgeons, radiation oncologists, medical oncologists, palliative care specialists, and mental health professionals who work together to define appropriate treatment strategies. The purpose of this textbook seeks to provide guidance from these specialists to form a framework for the treatment of lung cancer.

■ EVALUATION OF THE PATIENT SUSPICIOUS FOR LUNG CANCER

In patients with suspicious lung lesions, new imaging technologies have provided additional information to assign patients into a low-, moderate-, or high-risk category. The fluorodeoxyglucose-positron emission tomography (FDG-PET) is not diagnostic of malignancy, and cytologic or histologic confirmation must be obtained to confirm the presence of malignancy. Ultrasound-guided transesophageal and transbronchial biopsies offer both diagnostic as well as staging opportunities of the hilum and mediastinum and for, regional metastatic lesions in the liver and adrenal. New navigational bronchoscopy systems provide greater access to the peripheral bronchial tree, improving the diagnostic yield of very peripheral small lung lesions. A thorough

evaluation provides diagnostic tissue, determines the tumor stage, and assesses patient-related comorbidities.

Multidisciplinary tumor boards are more commonly utilized in major medical centers to assist in complex diagnostic cases and in treatment design. These forums provide opportunities for cross medical professional education and direct patient management. Some centers provide multidisciplinary clinics that allow immediate evaluation of complex patients.

■ LUNG CANCER PATHOLOGY

The International Union against Cancer (UICC) has improved the pathologic classification of lung cancer for the primary and metastatic lesions. The 2010 version of the staging system provides superior prognostic information. For small cell cancer, rather than the broad terms of "limited" and "extensive" or systemic disease, it can now be better classified using the new staging version with greater prognostic implications. Adenocarcinomas continue to comprise 40% of all lung cancers, and approximately 90% have mixed with two or more subtypes. Bronchioloalveolar cancer, a subtype of adenocarcinoma, is a noninvasive and rare tumor. Pathologists often over diagnose them. Squamous cell is estimated to be about 25% to 30% of the total number of lung cancers and is centrally located, tends to spread along airways and into regional lymphatics, and recur locally. A mixture of the two cell types, adenosquamous carcinomas are 10% of the total and have a particularly poor prognosis. Large cell carcinomas also comprise 10% of lung cancers and small cell carcinomas about 15%. Small cell is frequently centrally located with extensive perihilar and mediastinal lymphatic involvement. Immunohistochemistry stains assist in the differentiation of these subtypes. Chromosomal rearrangements, such as the *EML4-ALK* gene fusion, and point mutations, such as epidermal growth factor receptor (*EGFR*), *KRAS*, and *BRAF*, have been discovered that provide clues to the pathogenesis and offer treatment opportunities. Normal lung stem cells reside in specialized and protective environments termed niche. These too, the stem cells and the niche, appear to have a role in the development of a malignancy. Already available for patients, although with little to no validation, is molecular profiling to assist in determining prognosis and predicting response to therapy and even sites of potential metastasis. Epigenetic heritable factors have proven to provide even further prognostic information with the methylation of key genes regulating malignant characteristics, found to be significant in early-stage non–small cell lung cancer (NSCLC). High through-put methods to assess gene expression, miRNA arrays, and proteins have provided even more information about the biological processes involved in NSCLC. Expression panels of chemoresistant proteins are now commercially available, excision repair cross-complementation group 1 (*ERCC1*) overexpression is related to resistance to cisplatin; ribonucleotide reductase subunit M1 (*RRM1*) overexpression to gemcitabine resistance; thymidylate synthase (*TS*) overexpression to pemetrexed resistance; and *KRAS* mutation is correlated with paclitaxel and *EGFR*–tyrosine kinase inhibitors (*TKI*) resistance. There is great future in molecular analyses to determine prognosis and selecting treatment.

together with the fact that the radiation exposure itself may increase the probability of cancer development, the discovery of lung lesions that have no longterm risk to the patients and will require unnecessary invasive procedures and expense, and the lack of recommended radiologic screening in "low risk" individuals, make it a less viable option. Other screening methods have been developed using sputum, buccal smears, exhaled breath, blood and serum, but have yet been validated. To date, there is no recommendation for lung cancer screening.

Patients who are at risk for the development of lung cancer are those who have had significant exposure to tobacco smoke, radiation, prior lung cancers, and exposure to known carcinogens such as asbestos. The single most important preventative measure is smoking cessation, which has lead to a 55% reduction in lung cancer mortality in the treatment arm. Other interventions, such as vitamin A and its derivatives, isotretinoin, selenium, and other vitamins and micronutrients have been less promising. Smoking cessation is the only currently recommended intervention to reduce lung cancer mortality.

■ NEW LUNG CANCER STAGING SYSTEM

The beginning of 2010 marks major changes in lung cancer staging revised by the International Association for the Study of Lung Cancer and the UICC in its 7th edition. In contrast to the previous TNM system, the new system is based from data acquired from 20 countries and in more than 100,000 patients and is the result of significant effort by the authors and their team of investigators. Highlights of the new system include subclassification of T1 and T2 into a and b, and movement of lesions larger than 7 cm into the T3 category. Separate tumor nodules within the same lobe are now T3, rather than T4, and patients with separate nodules in a different ipsilateral lobe are T4, rather than M1. M1 is now divided into a and b, where M1a includes pleural or pericardial effusion, and separate nodules on the contralateral lung. The mediastinal map has changed slightly as well, providing greater clarification to that available in the 6th edition. Already externally validated assessment gives greater prognostic relevance to the new system.

■ LUNG CANCER SCREENING AND PREVENTION

Waiting for symptoms to develop from lung cancer does not appear to be a good strategy. To date, regular radiologic and sputum analyses have not appeared to improve lung cancer survival in the screened cohort and

■ IMAGING IN LUNG CANCER

In the early 1980s, computed tomography (CT) was clinically introduced into the evaluation of patients diagnosed or suspicious of having lung cancer. Since then, imaging quality and the radiation amount have improved. CT can provide greater diagnostic information for lung nodules and masses, and pick up two to four times more lung cancers than a chest radiograph, and it can provide greater detail for prognostication and treatment planning: lesion size determination, location to critical structures, evaluation of the pulmonary parenchymal health, presence of other lesions and effusions, and assessment of hilar and mediastinal adenopathy, as well as the airway and cardiovascular anatomy. Magnetic resonance imaging (MRI) provides additional information for the assessment of mediastinal, chest wall, great vessel, brachial plexus, and spinal invasion. PET using the glucose analog, FDG, provides even further prognostic information both in assessing the metabolic activity in the primary lesion and assessing for metastatic disease not readily discernible using other modalities. It is now considered standard-of-care in most circumstances. The combination of the PET and CT technologies provides further information, not readily available from either technology alone, but loses some of the fine detail available from the CT alone. Invasive radiologic techniques such as percutaneous needle biopsy and navigational bronchoscopy provide a nonsurgical highly accurate means of achieving a diagnosis of primary lung lesions. Brain MRI is indicated in patients who have neurologic symptoms and in patients with more advanced disease. PET should not be regarded as diagnostic of cancer in either the primary or any metastatic lesion, cytology or histology being necessary to confirm the diagnosis.

■ SURGICAL TREATMENT OF LUNG CANCER

Surgical resection provides the highest likelihood for lung cancer cure. A curative resection is defined as an anatomic resection of a lobe or two adjacent lobes or a pneumonectomy along with the en bloc resection of any adjacent nonvital structure involved to achieve a negative microscopic surgical margin and including regional lymph nodes in a sampling or complete dissection manner. Cure rates for stage I are reported to be between 65% and 85% with a 50% to 60% rate for stage II and 20% to 25% for stage III. Newer technologies are now available to perform minimally invasive lobectomy using either video-assisted thoracic surgery or with robotic technology. There appears to be less pain and debility with shorter hospital stays without compromising the oncological principles. Rather than pneumonectomy and again without violating basic principles of cancer surgery, most centers are attempting lung preserving procedures, in particular sleeve lobectomy, resecting hilar lesions along with the adjacent airway and possibly the adjacent pulmonary artery with regional nodes and then anastomosing the airway and pulmonary artery. These patients appear to have a superior survival and greater functional status. High-risk patients and the elderly may not be able to undergo a lobectomy and in some situations a sublobar resection either by segmentectomy or wedge resection may be performed, possibly using brachytherapy to reduce local recurrence.

■ SURGICAL ROLE IN SMALL CALL LUNG CANCER

Since the British Medical Council results of 1969, small cell lung cancer (SCLC) has primarily been treated nonsurgically, even for early-stage disease. Today, staging methods, surgical techniques, and the chemotherapy have all improved. Perhaps surgery has a role in early-stage disease to improve survival and quality of life (QOL). A prospective trial has been designed for this evaluation of surgical resection with platinum-based adjuvant therapy through the American College of Surgeons Oncology Group.

■ SURGICAL ROLE IN STAGE IIIA NSCLC

In 2007, the American College of Chest Physicians guidelines stated that surgical resection for patients with stage III A disease should be a part of a clinical trial and that the role of surgery for IIIA lung cancer is questionable. But, stage IIIA disease is heterogeneous and a statement about treating it as a single entity is likely not warranted, especially when there is significant information to justify surgical involvement. Patients who appear to have the greatest advantage with surgical resection are those who have micrometastatic and single lymph node station disease. Additionally, surgical resection of T3N1 disease has survival advantage, a nearly 40% 5-year survival with complete margin-negative surgical resection and with further advantage by providing adjuvant platinum-based chemotherapy. For those patients with positive surgical margins, postoperative radiation therapy appears to have survival advantage. For patients with N2 potentially resectable disease, the fairly recent results of the induction chemoradiotherapy trials European Organization for Research and Treatment of Cancer (EORTC) 08941 and INT 0139 are somewhat conflicting where the EORTC trial found no survival advantage in the surgery/trimodality arm compared with the chemoradiotherapy-alone treatment arm, but the INT trial demonstrated an improvement with the addition of non-pneumonectomy anatomic resection. Both trials agreed that the use of pneumonectomy in IIIA patients was less likely to provide longterm survival. The difference may be related to definitions of resectability and patient selection. Adjuvant therapy has been studied as well in these patients, and for completely resected patients with early disease, patients appear to have the greatest survival improvement as a group compared with earlier disease patients, stage I and II. Future research will help to define those patients who are more likely to benefit from combined therapies and assess response to treatment, as well as determine the best chemotherapy for treatment.

■ SURGERY FOR LOCALLY ADVANCED AND METASTATIC NSCLC

Although surgery is largely relegated to the earlier stage disease, there are situations where there is survival improvement in patients with more advanced disease. In general, resection of the carina, the superior vena cava, portion of the aorta (nonadvential) and left atrium, and the vertebral body, if the procedure is performed safely and if a lobectomy is performed rather than a pneumonectomy and there are no other organ or nodal involvement, appear to improve longterm survival. Knowledge and experience of the techniques utilized to perform these procedures safely is critical. Fifteen percent of potentially surgically resectable NSCLC patients have additional pulmonary nodules or lesions. For those pulmonary lesions/nodules less than 8 mm in diameter and especially those that are nonsolid density or centrally calcified, observation is a safe course of action—where more suspicious lesions should be evaluated prior to performing a more extensive resection either pre-operatively or at the time of surgery. When lung cancer is present in these additional lesions, it is more likely a new primary rather than metastatic according to the criteria of Martini and Melamed and should be surgically addressed according to the evaluation of comorbidities and stage of the most advanced lung cancer. Although there are some N3 patients who may benefit from surgery, it is not clear who they are and thus any N3 patient who undergoes surgery should be enrolled in a clinical trial. There are situations where there is an isolated metastasis that may be resected along with the primary lesion for survival advantage, such as those to the brain and adrenal gland.

■ RADIOTHERAPY FOR LUNG CANCER

Newer techniques of radiation therapy, such as intensity-modulated radiation therapy, and improved software for treatment planning can now offer greater possibilities of delivering higher radiation dosages yet minimizing collateral damage. External beam dosages of more than 60 to 70 Gy are now being provided with superior survival. Elective nodal irradiation has not been shown to improve either local control or survival. Radiation administered concurrently with chemotherapy appears to improve response to therapy, but increases toxicity. Altering dose and fractionation has yet to consistently demonstrate improved effectiveness. Palliation can be achieved by reirradiation for those patients with recurrence even after definitive doses of radiation have been given. For NSCLC, prophylactic cranial irradiation has reduced the incidence of brain metastasis, but has yet to consistently improve survival.

Initially used for brain lesions, stereotactic body radiotherapy delivers, through multiple focus beams, hypofractionated dosages over a short period of time to a confined region, maximizing tumor kill and further minimizing collateral toxicity. The results of Radiation Therapy Oncology Group 0236 for medically inoperable patients with early-stage peripheral NSCLC with maximum diameter less than 5 cm were treated in a phase II fashion with 18 Gy in three fractions over approximately 2 weeks. The 3-year primary tumor control rate was 97.6% with a disease-free and overall survival (OS) of 48.3% and 55.8%, respectively. The same technique has been used to treat isolated metastatic lesions to the lung, liver, and spine with significant tumor response and acceptable toxicity.

■ ENDOBRONCHIAL TREATMENT OF LUNG CANCER

Patients with obstructive and bleeding airway lesions may obtain significant palliation by local ablative therapies.

Under general anesthesia, rigid bronchoscopy is performed where visualized lesions can be manually removed, coagulated, frozen with cryospray, or resected with a contact or noncontact laser system. Where airways are weakened by the invading malignancy, temporary or permanent stents can be placed. Brachytherapy afterloading catheters can be placed to provide further treatment to slow the recurrence. Palliating patients in this manner can improve survival and QOL.

■ THE ROLE OF SYSTEMIC THERAPY IN LUNG CANCER

Although surgery is the most effective treatment for early-stage NSCLC, nearly half of all patients treated surgically, stages I–IIIA, will show recurrence within 5 years. Three randomized phase III trials demonstrated a survival benefit for adjuvant cisplatin-based chemotherapy in patients with stage I–IIIA NSCLC. The Lung Adjuvant Cisplatin Evaluation meta-analysis of 4,584 individual patient data from five trials confirmed the benefit of adjuvant chemotherapy and demonstrated potential harm for stage IA patients. Some controversial topics remain for adjuvant therapy in early-stage NSCLC, including the value of chemotherapy in selected patients with stage IB disease and the choice of chemotherapy drugs. Current research evaluating systemic therapy for lung cancer is focused on identifying and validating molecular markers to predict treatment efficacy and evaluating novel therapeutics.

In patients with locally advanced NSCLC, surgical resection after induction treatment can result in improved survival in a carefully selected subset. It remains unproven that this approach is superior to modern thoracic radiotherapy and chemotherapy. The optimal treatment in locally advanced NSCLC is widely debated, and a multimodality approach to stage III patients is essential to improve outcomes. Novel radiation techniques have been developed which may increase the local control through the delivery of higher radiation doses to smaller volumes, allowing for lesser toxicity. A combined modality approach with the use of concurrent chemoradiotherapy is the preferred treatment for patients with stage IIIB disease. A platinum-based doublet remains the chemotherapy treatment of choice, although the optimal regimen has not yet been defined. There is emphasis on tailoring chemotherapy and targeted therapy to optimize treatment for individual patients with this disease. The management of unresectable stage III disease continues to evolve and the participation of a multidisciplinary team is essential.

For patients with metastatic NSCLC, systemic therapy offers an improvement in survival and QOL. The addition of the anti–vascular endothelial growth factor (VEGF) antibody, bevacizumab, should be considered in selected patients . Oral EGFR-TKIs have demonstrated efficacy as a first-line option for patients with EGFR-activating mutations. The optimal duration of first-line chemotherapy remains unknown, and there is increasing data to suggest a role for sequential or maintenance chemotherapy to delay progression, and may impact OS. Special patient populations, including patients with poor performance status, those who are elderly, and women, have unique considerations that must be taken into account when deciding upon a treatment plan. In recent years, substantial progress has been made in the search for second- and third-line therapeutic options for advanced NSCLC. Incorporating targeted therapies and defining appropriate patient populations for treatment are under investigation.

Targeted therapy for NSCLC has made significant progress in the last decade. Improved survival has been demonstrated with VEGF inhibition by bevacizumab when combined with chemotherapy and with EGFR inhibition by erlotinib. Trials evaluating patients with activating EGFR mutations have demonstrated improved outcomes with the EGFR-TKI, gefitinib. Phase III trials examining platinum-based chemotherapy in combination with the EGFR-directed monoclonal antibody cetuximab have demonstrated a modest survival benefit in patients with advanced NSCLC, although a molecular marker to define a population with benefit has not been defined. Novel translocations involving the *ALK* gene defines a mechanism of lung cancer development, and ALK inhibition has shown significant efficacy in this subset of NSCLC. A rapidly growing pipeline of agents is being assessed in the setting of advanced NSCLC, including pan-HER inhibitors, met inhibitors, Akt/PI3K inhibitors, IGF-IR targeting antibodies, mTOR inhibitors, and COX-2 inhibitors.

As we evaluate novel, targeted agents, we must determine their appropriate use, and to this end, there are several biomarkers that may lead to better therapies for lung cancer. Tailoring therapy could ultimately lead to better responses and improved survival, particularly in lung cancer, where the OS is very low in advanced disease. The predictive biomarkers most extensively evaluated include ERCC1, RRM1, TS, *EGFR* mutations, *EGFR* gene copy number, KRAS mutations, and EML4-ALK translocations.

Immunotherapeutic approaches to the treatment of lung cancer have been evaluated, and novel therapies in both NSCLC and SCLC in the last 5 to 7 years have demonstrated promising results. Belagenpumatucel is a vaccine that has been engineered to silence transforming growth factor-β2 expression and is currently being investigated in a phase III trial in late-stage NSCLC. α-Galactosylceramide is a glycolipid-based vaccine that activates Vα24 NKT cells that produce immune-stimulating molecules such as interferon-γ. The L-BLP-25 vaccine targets the MUC-1 antigen on the surfaces of many epithelial cells and a phase III trial is now ongoing . IDM-2101 is a peptide-based vaccine designed to induce cytotoxic T lymphocytes against five tumor-associated antigens. The B7.1 vaccine is a molecule associated with the induction of a T cell and natural killer (NK) cell response. MAGE-3 vaccines target an antigen present in many NSCLC cell lines, and an adjuvant phase III trial is currently enrolling patients. Several immunological approaches have shown efficacy in a subset of lung cancer patients, and further investigation in phase III trials will determine their relevance in lung cancer.

In addition, the multidisciplinary evaluation and management of SCLC is described with emphasis on improving our understanding of the biology of the disease to improve outcomes. Although the treatment for SCLC has not significantly changed over the last 2 decades, collaborations to identify new targets and optimal treatment strategies are underway.

Community-based lung cancer care dramatically impacts national cancer outcomes, and care can be provided in a cohesive multidisciplinary setting. Community-based physicians, generalists, and specialists play the greatest role in supporting their patients to quit smoking. Community practices, with their large patient populations and leaner bureaucracies, are often ideal sites for clinical research. Multimodality care is crucial to elevating the level of clinical care and improving accrual to clinical trials in the community setting.

■ TREATMENT IN SELECT POPULATIONS

Since most patients diagnosed with lung cancer are older than 65 years, it is important to recognize the limitations of available data in an older population. Subset analyses of pivotal trials assessing adjuvant chemotherapy for NSCLC in older adults suggest similar benefit as compared with younger adults. Concurrent chemoradiation appears to yield benefit in older adults with unresectable, stage III NSCLC, although this approach may result in higher rates of hematologic toxicity as compared with younger adults. Patients aged 70 had improved survival with vinorelbine over best supportive care. It appears that combination chemotherapy offers an advantage in comparison with sequential, single-agent therapy in older adults with advanced NSCLC, but also results in greater toxicity. Data for the efficacy of targeted agents in older adults with NSCLC is emerging; pivotal studies of erlotinib and bevacizumab suggest that clinical benefit is largely maintained in this subset. Treatment of both limited- and extensive-stage SCLC in older adults must address toxicity considerations.

Differential approaches to lung cancer exist by race and socioeconomic status (SES). These disparities have an effect on survival in early-stage and advanced disease. As treatment makes advances in personalized medicine, these differences may become more apparent. Disparities in healthcare are multifactorial, and interventions must address all issues. Access to care, patient/provider interaction, and biology all interact to create multiple differences and it is important to realize that scientific advances in the treatment of lung cancer should extend to all patients and not exclude those who are most adversely affected—low SES and ethnic minorities.

■ PSYCHOSOCIAL AND PALLIATIVE CARE IN LUNG CANCER

It is well known that individuals diagnosed with lung cancer develop a significant symptom burden due to the disease and associated treatments. These symptoms can be debilitating and negatively affect the QOL of patients. Despite this knowledge, the optimal approach to symptom management and palliative care has not been defined. Improving the quality of palliative care will allow patients to maximize disease treatment benefit by reducing debilitating symptoms and enhancing QOL. Multidisciplinary symptom management is essential to improve QOL in lung cancer patients.

Lung cancer is also associated with significant psychologic distress, and is higher in patients who are more physically symptomatic, have pre-existing emotional distress, and use avoidance-based coping mechanisms. Rates of psychologic distress appear higher in patients with lung cancer compared with other cancers. Research aimed at developing, implementing, and testing psychosocial interventions in lung cancer patients is lacking and will be an important next step for psychosocial researchers working with this population.

2 Multidisciplinary Approach to the Evaluation of the Lung Cancer Patient

MICHAEL K. GOULD

This chapter discusses general issues related to the evaluation of the patient with known or suspected lung cancer. Each patient and practice setting is unique, so any generalizations should be applied carefully, whether referral patterns, diagnostic algorithms, goals for timely care, or treatment recommendations. That said, certain core principles apply in all patients: care should be safe, effective, and consistent with the patient's values and preferences (1). Recent advances in imaging, tissue sampling, molecular diagnosis, and targeted treatment hold promise for improving lung cancer outcomes, but the expanded menu of options makes it even more challenging to provide coordinated care that is both efficient and timely. Another important caveat is that relatively little research has addressed structures and processes of care and their effect on lung cancer outcomes. To a large extent, best practices for delivering coordinated lung cancer care are yet to be defined.

■ GENERAL PRINCIPLES OF LUNG CANCER DIAGNOSIS AND STAGING

The accuracy of noninvasive imaging tests and invasive tissue sampling procedures have been summarized in several recent systematic reviews (2–5), and guidelines for their use have been published by the National Comprehensive Cancer Network (6) and the American College of Chest Physicians (7). What follows is not an exhaustive review of these authoritative recommendations, but rather a summary of the most important principles that should guide the clinician during the evaluation process (Table 2.1). Because almost all patients with suspected lung cancer undergo chest computed tomography (CT), the following discussion defines subgroups according to the CT findings.

In patients who present with a solitary pulmonary nodule or a potentially resectable peripheral mass lesion on chest CT, the clinician should first estimate the probability of malignancy. If clinical judgment or a validated prediction model (8–10) suggests that the probability of lung cancer is low to moderate (<50%), then positron emission tomography (PET) may help to characterize the lesion further. In such patients, the posttest probability of malignancy following a negative PET scan is sufficiently low that the nodule can probably be followed safely by watchful waiting, provided that the patient is comfortable with this approach and its uncertain risks (11,12). In a patient without serious underlying comorbidity who is a good candidate for surgery, neither PET nor nonsurgical biopsy is necessary when the probability of malignancy is high. Such patients should be referred promptly for thoracic surgical evaluation. In contrast, in patients with severe comorbidity who are not surgical candidates, tissue biopsy should be obtained by the safest means possible to confirm the diagnosis of cancer, usually via CT-guided transthoracic needle biopsy. Subsequent treatment options for poor surgical candidates include traditional radiotherapy and experimental approaches such as stereotactic radiotherapy (13) and radiofrequency ablation. However, it has not been established that aggressive treatment in this situation clearly improves longevity or quality of life, and while most patients would elect treatment, it is not mandatory.

In patients who present with a large, central mass lesion, bronchoscopy is usually the procedure of choice for establishing the diagnosis. In addition, endobronchial biopsy of the primary tumor can be accompanied by either blind transbronchial needle aspiration biopsy (TBNA) or endobronchial ultrasound (EBUS)-guided biopsy of accessible mediastinal lymph nodes. Invasive mediastinal staging is usually required in these patients, even if there is no evidence of mediastinal lymph node enlargement on chest CT. The choice of sampling procedure should be determined by the location of the primary tumor and the presence and location of enlarged nodes. For example, large subcarinal nodes can often be sampled successfully by TBNA (14), while hilar nodes are better approached by EBUS-guided *fine-needle aspiration*, and prevascular or periaortic lymph nodes can only be sampled by anterior mediastinotomy. Tissue confirmation of unresectable mediastinal lymph node involvement

■ Table 2.1 General principles of evaluation and referral in the patient with suspected lung cancer

Imaging

Use imaging tests to help determine the extent of disease and provide a road map for invasive tissue sampling procedures

Unless there is overwhelming evidence of regional or distant metastasis, positive findings on imaging tests require cytological or histological confirmation before determining that an otherwise eligible patient is not a candidate for curative therapy with surgery or radiotherapy

Tissue Sampling

The plan for tissue sampling should strike the best possible balance between the following considerations:

1. Minimize risk by selecting the least invasive alternative
2. Perform diagnosis and staging in the same procedure, when possible (e.g., bronchoscopy with transbronchial needle aspiration of mediastinal lymph nodes)
3. Select an accessible site that will establish the highest possible disease stage (e.g., adrenal biopsy in a patient with suspicious adrenal enlargement)
4. Maximize diagnostic yield by using direct visualization (e.g., bronchoscopy) or radiographic guidance (e.g., computed tomography–guided needle biopsy)
5. Obtain core samples when possible to facilitate pathological interpretation and provide sufficient tissue for molecular profiling
6. Use symptoms, signs, and routine laboratory tests to determine the extent of the staging evaluation, e.g., reserve bone scanning for patients with bone pain or an elevated alkaline phosphatase

Negative results of a minimally invasive mediastinal sampling procedure (e.g., transbronchial needle aspiration biopsy (TBNA) or endobronchial ultrasound (EBUS)–guided needle aspiration) do not exclude the possibility of regional metastasis, unless the procedure included systematic sampling of lymph nodes at all accessible lymph node stations

Physiological Evaluation

Order pulmonary function tests, including spirometry and diffusing capacity, to help determine eligibility for curative therapy

Use more specialized tests (e.g., cardiopulmonary exercise testing, quantitative lung perfusion scan) in patients with borderline cardiopulmonary reserve

Referral to Pulmonary Medicine

Bronchoscopy: large, central lesion; postobstructive atelectasis; or pneumonia

Thoracentesis: moderate to large pleural effusion

Serial follow-up (watchful waiting): subcentimeter nodules and larger nodules when the probability of cancer is very low

Referral to Thoracic Surgery

Video-assisted thoracoscopy: solitary nodule when probability of malignancy is moderate to high

Mediastinoscopy or anterior mediastinotomy: enlarged mediastinal nodes not accessible to TBNA, *endoscopic ultrasound,* or EBUS; mediastinum prior to surgical resection

Thoracoscopy: large or recurrent malignant pleural effusion requiring pleurodesis

Referral to Medical Oncology

Chemotherapy: for regional, distant, or recurrent disease

Referral to Palliative Care or Hospice

Poor performance status

Progressive or recurrent disease despite treatment

Life expectancy <6 months

is mandatory before excluding the possibility of curative surgical resection (2).

In patients with a peripheral lung mass and no evidence of mediastinal lymph node enlargement or distant metastasis on chest CT, CT-guided transthoracic needle biopsy is usually performed, although recent interest has focused on electromagnetic navigational bronchoscopy-guided biopsy as another option (15). In surgical candidates, mediastinoscopy should be performed prior to resection.

Several recent randomized, controlled trials have examined whether preoperative staging with PET improves lung cancer outcomes (Table 2.2) (16–20). While study design and results have differed across studies, the weight of the evidence suggests that preoperative

staging with PET reduces the frequency of futile thoracotomy (generally defined as benign or unresectable disease at the time of operation or recurrence or death within 1 year of surgery), but this reduction has not been accompanied by improvements in survival. Some have questioned the validity of futile thoracotomy as an outcome.

In patients who present with evidence of extrathoracic disease on examination or chest CT, the initial tissue sampling procedure should target the most accessible site of suspected distant metastasis, whether a palpable supraclavicular lymph node, a peripheral liver lesion, or an enlarged adrenal gland. Biopsy of suspected brain or bone metastasis is more difficult but mandatory when there are

■ Table 2.2 Randomized, controlled trials of PET for preoperative staging in lung cancer

Author, Year	N	Population	Clinical Stage	Outcome	Results (Control vs. PET)
Van Tinteren, 2002 (19)	188	Known or suspected NSCLC	I or II: 70% III or IV: 30%	Futile thoracotomy	41% vs. 21% ($P = 0.003$)
Viney, 2004 (20)	184	Confirmed NSCLC	I or II: 100%	Thoracotomy avoided	2% vs. 4% ($P = 0.44$)
Herder, 2006 (17)	465	Suspected lung cancer	NS	Number of staging procedures	7.9 vs. 7.9 ($P = 0.90$)
Maziak, 2009 (18)	337	Confirmed NSCLC	I: 78% II: 12% IIIA: 10%	Correct upstaging	6.8% vs. 13.8% ($P = 0.046$)
Fischer, 2009 (16)	189	Known or suspected NSCLC	I or II: 34% III or IV: 66%	Futile thoracotomy	52% vs. 35% ($P = 0.05$)

NSCLC, non–small cell lung cancer; PET, positron emission tomography.

no other suitable targets unless there is overwhelming evidence of distant metastasis on CT (or PET). Because brain involvement is common in patients with clinical stage III or IV disease, brain imaging is indicated in these patients even when there are no symptoms or signs of nervous system disease (4).

Indications for referral to specialists are summarized in Table 2.1. Structures and processes of care that define the interactions between various specialists and the primary care clinician are discussed in the following sections.

■ CARE COORDINATION

Even a relatively straightforward case presents challenges for care coordination across the members of a formal or informal multidisciplinary team. For example, consider a 68-year-old smoker who presents to his primary care physician complaining of dyspnea and is incidentally found to have a spiculated lesion in the periphery of the right upper lobe on chest radiography. It would not be unusual for this patient to undergo chest CT, PET, pulmonary function testing, pulmonary medicine and thoracic surgical consultation, cervical mediastinoscopy, video-assisted thoracoscopic surgical (VATS) wedge resection, and lobectomy, either via VATS or thoracotomy, if the frozen section confirms a diagnosis of non–small cell lung cancer. Perioperative care would require the skills of a thoracic surgeon, anesthesiologist, intensivist, and pain management specialist, not to mention the many nurses, therapists, and technicians who are an integral part of the hospital team. Depending on the size of the tumor and the resection margins, the patient might be advised to consult with a medical oncologist about options for adjuvant chemotherapy (for pathological stage IB to IIIA tumors) or a radiation oncologist for consideration of radiation therapy

(for positive tumor margins). After completing adjuvant therapy, subsequent care and surveillance for recurrence might be provided by the primary care clinician, pulmonologist, surgeon, and/or oncologist. In the event of a local or distant recurrence, additional palliative treatment would be considered to relieve pain or dyspnea. At one or more times across the continuum of care, input from a formal multidisciplinary tumor board might be sought.

It should come as no surprise that coordinating the efforts of these professionals requires a heroic effort on the part of the patient, family, and one or more primary caregivers. There is little evidence to suggest that better care coordination is provided by one type of specialist over the others. In most U.S. practice settings, the primary care physician often initiates the evaluation by ordering a chest CT scan and referring the patient to pulmonary medicine for diagnostic bronchoscopy (for central lesions) or interventional radiology (for peripheral lesions), although in some cases, direct referral to a thoracic surgeon for lung resection may be appropriate. Given the increasing complexity of lung cancer care, many primary care physicians do not have the time, training, or experience to direct the evaluation and management. Hence, it is not uncommon for the pulmonologist to subsequently assume responsibility for diagnosis, staging, and preoperative evaluation (in those patients with potentially resectable disease). In one study from the United Kingdom, initial referral to a nonrespiratory physician was associated with a significantly longer time to surgery (21). Beyond the immediate postoperative period, care coordination is frequently resumed by the primary care physician, with or without additional oversight from the pulmonologist. For patients with advanced or recurrent disease, the medical oncologist commonly assumes the role of primary care physician, as care transitions from palliative chemotherapy and/or radiation therapy to symptom control, end-of-life planning, and hospice.

What seems obvious is that primary care and specialty physicians should communicate clearly with each other about their respective roles and responsibilities. In many medical groups, these roles evolve and are clarified implicitly over time. Unfortunately, this ad hoc approach sets the stage for occasional misunderstandings, potentially leading to avoidable delays in care. Clear, explicit, direct communication may help to minimize such lapses and facilitate care that is timely and efficient. Traditional roles and responsibilities of various involved specialists are outlined in Table 2.3.

■ THORACIC TUMOR BOARD

A multidisciplinary thoracic tumor board facilitates communication between members of the multidisciplinary team, with each contributing the unique perspective of his or her respective field. Depending on volume, lung cancer patients may be discussed at either a general oncology or thoracic specialty tumor board. While the American College of Surgeons' Commission on Cancer requires accredited programs to hold multidisciplinary cancer conferences, the frequency and format of conferences, attendance of particular specialists, and percentage of prospectively discussed cases vary by accreditation category (e.g., teaching hospital vs. community hospital). Even within accreditation categories, the percentage of cancer cases to be discussed is left to the discretion of the local cancer care committee (22).

Few studies have examined the effect of a tumor board on cancer outcomes, and none have specifically focused on lung cancer patients. In a systematic review of studies of multidisciplinary patient management (23), only one study attempted to measure an improvement in diagnosis and treatment planning. In this study of 459 gynecological oncology cases presented over a 3-year period at the University of Texas Medical Branch, case discussion at tumor board resulted in a change in tumor site, stage, or treatment in almost 7% of cases (24).

Although hard evidence of benefit is lacking, reasonable criteria for when a case should be discussed at a multidisciplinary tumor board include:

1. Regional (clinical stage IIIA) disease, for consideration of multimodality therapy including concurrent chemoradiation with or without surgery
2. Nondiagnostic biopsy for diagnosis or staging at one or more sites, with uncertainty about further tissue sampling
3. Medical comorbidity with uncertain ability to tolerate curative treatment with surgery or radiotherapy
4. Superior sulcus tumors, with or without Pancoast syndrome
5. Suspected recurrence following curative treatment with surgery or radiotherapy

■ MULTIDISCIPLINARY CLINIC

A somewhat larger body of literature has examined the effect of multidisciplinary lung cancer care, broadly defined as a clinic, meeting, or teleconference in which teams of providers discuss various aspects of patient evaluation and management. A systematic review performed in 2008 identified 16 studies of multidisciplinary lung cancer care, including one randomized trial, seven pre- and postintervention studies, and seven case series or audits (25). Interventions included a rapid assessment process (including a 1-day admission for imaging and biopsy, followed by a multidisciplinary meeting 3 days later), telemedicine meetings, and a multidisciplinary clinic. Several studies showed that multidisciplinary care resulted in higher rates of surgical resection (26–28), radical radiotherapy (29), and chemotherapy (30), and three studies found improvements in measures of the timeliness of care (27,31,32). However, of the five studies that examined survival, only two pre- and postimplementation studies showed modest improvements among those who received multidisciplinary care (29,30). Stronger, but still limited, evidence that multidisciplinary clinics improve survival comes from nonrandomized, retrospective studies of patients with ovarian cancer in Scotland and head and neck cancer in England (33,34).

■ LUNG NODULE CLINICS

Although population-based studies have not been performed, uncontrolled studies of CT screening in high-risk smokers suggest that pulmonary nodules are highly prevalent, and that most of them are benign (35–38). In response, some medical centers have developed specialty referral programs that provide "one-stop shopping" for patients with lung nodules. Ideally, such programs would minimize the number of patients who are lost to follow-up (with potentially dangerous consequences), facilitate discussion of the risks and benefits associated with different management approaches (including VATS biopsy, nonsurgical biopsy, and watchful waiting), and encourage participation in clinical trials. However, the potential benefits of formal lung nodule programs have not been evaluated in studies to date.

■ PHYSICIAN AND HOSPITAL VOLUME

The relationship between volume and outcome has been examined in many studies of lung cancer surgery (Table 2.4) (39–49), but surprisingly little is known about the volume-outcome relationship for lung cancer patients who are treated with chemotherapy or radiotherapy. Only one study has specifically looked at surgeon experience, finding a 1.1% absolute increase in in-hospital mortality

■ **Table 2.3** Possible roles and responsibilities of primary care and specialist physicians

Specialty	Roles and Responsibilities
All involved clinicians	Actively help patient to stop smoking Manage lung cancer symptoms, including dyspnea, pain, anxiety, and depression Identify and address psychosocial needs of patient and family members Participate in multidisciplinary tumor board Facilitate coordination of care across specialties
Primary care provider Family medicine Internal medicine Geriatrics	Recognize and evaluate symptoms and signs at the time of initial presentation Initiate evaluation by ordering CXR, chest CT, complete blood count, and metabolic panel Initiate referrals to appropriate specialists Coordinate care across specialists Manage comorbid conditions Monitor for recurrence
Pulmonary medicine Diagnostic Interventional	Coordinate diagnosis and staging evaluation in patients with potentially resectable disease Perform bronchoscopy with or without TBNA, EBUS, or electromagnetic navigation, when indicated Coordinate preoperative evaluation Manage comorbid respiratory disease Initiate referral to thoracic surgery or medical oncology Palliate symptoms of airway obstruction, hemoptysis, and dyspnea (interventional pulmonology) Monitor for recurrence
Radiology Diagnostic Interventional	Interpret results of imaging studies Help formulate plans for diagnosis and staging Perform percutaneous biopsy of primary tumor and/or accessible site of suspected metastasis, when indicated
Thoracic surgery	Perform invasive mediastinal staging, when indicated Determine medical operability and surgical resectability Discuss risks and benefits of major lung resection Perform major lung resection, when indicated Manage postoperative complications Palliate dyspnea from bronchial obstruction (rigid bronchoscopy with or without stenting) or pleural effusion (tube thoracostomy, VATS, pleurodesis) Monitor for recurrence
Medical oncology	Coordinate diagnosis and staging evaluation in patients with advanced disease Determine performance status Discuss risks and benefits of adjuvant or palliative chemotherapy Prescribe chemotherapy, when indicated Manage complications of chemotherapy Monitor for recurrence
Radiation oncology	Discuss risks and benefits of curative or palliative radiotherapy Determine performance status Plan and administer curative or palliative radiotherapy, when indicated Manage complications of radiotherapy
Palliative care	Manage symptoms of lung cancer, including pain, dyspnea, anxiety, and depression Identify and address psychosocial needs of patient and family members

CT, computed tomography; CXR, chest X-rays; EBUS, endobronchial ultrasound; TBNA, transbronchial needle aspiration biopsy; VATS, video-assisted thoracoscopic surgical.

for lung cancer patients who underwent lobectomy by a low-volume (1–22 procedures) versus high-volume (>22 procedures) surgeon (P = 0.08) (44). Most, but not all, of the studies that examined hospital volume have found worse perioperative survival for patients who underwent resection at low-volume hospitals. Several studies have shown better long-term survival for lung cancer patients who underwent surgery at a high-volume hospital, suggesting that volume may be a marker of better overall care (39,42,49). Another study showed that 30-day mortality for complicated surgical procedures was inversely associated with not only volume of the specific procedure but

■ Table 2.4 Studies of the relationship between volume and outcome in lung cancer

Author, Year (Data Collection Period)	Data Source	Hospital or Surgeon Volume (Number of Procedures)	Outcome	Procedure (n)	Results (95% CI or P Value)
Romano and Mark, 1992 (1983–1986) (48)	California hospitals (n = 499)	Hospital (quartiles): Low (<9) High (>24)	Postoperative mortality	Pneumonectomy (1,529) Lesser resection (10,908)	Adjusted OR 0.6 (0.4–1.0) for high vs. low Adjusted OR 0.6 (0.4–0.8)
Begg, 1998 (1984–1993) (40)	SEER-Medicare	Hospital (tertiles): Low (1–5) Medium (6–10) High (>11)	30-day mortality	Pneumonectomy (1,375)	13.8% (low) 14.1% (medium) 10.7% (high) (P = 0.19)
Khuri, 1999 (46)	VA hospitals (107)		30-day mortality	Lobectomy and pneumonectomy (4,890)	No association between procedure (P = 0.50) or specialty (0.71) volume and outcome
Bach, 2001 (1985–1996) (39)	SEER-Medicare, 76 hospitals from NIS	Hospital (tertiles): Low (1–8) High (67–100)	30-day mortality Comp 5YS	Lung resection (2,118)	Adjusted OR 0.48 for high vs. Low 44% (low) 20% (high) Adjusted HR 0.77 for high vs. Low
Hannan, 2002 (1994–1997) (44)	New York hospitals (178) New York surgeons (373)	Hospital (quartiles): Low (1–37) High (≥169) Surgeon (quartiles): Low (1–22) High (≥131)	In-hospital mortality	Lobectomy (6,954)	Absolute increase of 1.65% (P = 0.006) for low vs. high (adjusted) Absolute increase of 1.12% (P = 0.08) for low vs. high (adjusted)

Study	Data source	Volume	Outcome	Procedure (n)	Result
Birkmeyer, 2002 (1994–1999) (41)	Medicare, NIS (2,753 hospitals [a])	Hospital (quartiles): Low (<9) High (>46)	Operative mortality	Lobectomy (75,569)	Adjusted OR 0.70 (0.60–0.81) for high versus low
				Pneumonectomy (10,410)	Adjusted OR 0.62 (0.50–0.77) for high vs. Low
Finlayson, 2003 (1995–1997) (43)	NIS (674 hospitals)	Hospital (tertiles): Low (<19) Med (19–37) High (>37)	Operative mortality	Lobectomy	Adjusted OR 0.93 (0.59–1.46) for age <65
					Adjusted OR 0.82 (0.64–1.04) for age≥65
				Pneumonectomy	Adjusted OR 0.72 (0.40–1.30) for age <65
					Adjusted OR 0.91 (0.58–1.41) for age <65
Little, 2005 (2001) (47)	729 U.S. hospitals	Hospital: Low (<90) High (>90)	Perioperative mortality	Lung resection	Adjusted OR 0.82 (0.64–1.04) for age≥65
Simunovic, 2006 (1990–2000) (49)	Ontario Cancer Registry	Hospital: Low () High ()	Operative mortality	Lung resection (2,698)	NS
			Long-term survival		Adjusted HR 1.3 (1.1–1.6)
Birkmeyer, 2007 (1992–1999) (42)	SEER-Medicare (517 hospitals)	Hospital (tertiles): Low (0.3–11.4) Med (11.4–24.9) High (25.2–313.2)	Survival	Lung resection (12,967)	Adjusted HR 0.84 (0.79–0.90) for high vs. Low
Hollenbeck, 2007 (1993–2003) (45)	NIS	Hospital (deciles): Low (mean 3.6) High (mean 116.3)	Operative mortality	Pneumonectomy (90,088)	Adjusted OR 1.4 (1.2–1.7) for low vs. high

[a] Number of hospitals for lobectomy; fewer hospitals performed pneumonectomy (n = 1,877).

5YS, 5-year survival; Comp, operative complications; HR, hazard ratio; NIS, Nationwide inpatient sample; NS, not significant; OR, odds ratio; SEER, Survival, Epidemiology and End Results Tumor Registry.

volume of other procedures as well (50). Yet another study found that, despite low volumes, operative mortality at a small community hospital was very low when a thoracic surgeon from a high volume, tertiary center performed the operation (51), suggesting that the surgeon's experience may be more important than the hospital's experience. This conclusion is supported by multiple studies that showed better perioperative and/or long-term outcomes for patients who underwent operations performed by general thoracic surgeons compared with those whose operations were performed by general surgeons (52–54). In one of these studies, the association between specialty and outcome appeared to be at least partly mediated (explained) by physician volume (53).

The relationship between volume and outcome therefore appears to be complicated and influenced by multiple factors. While the idea of directing thoracic surgical care to high-volume centers holds considerable appeal, the potential benefits from the patient's perspective may be offset by inconvenience and discontinuity of care. In addition, it is not clear how one would implement a plan for regionalized care in the context of a typical noninte-grated U.S. health care setting, given the possible negative economic consequences for surgeons at low-volume centers.

■ TIMELINESS OF CARE

Timeliness of care is one of six dimensions of health care quality identified by the Institute of Medicine (1). Most studies of timeliness of care in lung cancer have been performed in Europe and Japan, limiting their relevance to health care settings in the United States. Of eight studies performed in the United States (Table 2.5), five examined timeliness in the VA Healthcare System (55–59), whereas the others examined practices in Hawaii (60), Texas (61), and Massachusetts (62). In three studies, the median time from diagnosis to treatment ranged between 21 and 31 days, with similar time intervals for Asians and non-Asians (62), native Hawaiians and non-Hawaiians (60), and those who were versus those who were not evaluated in a multidisciplinary clinic (61). In four studies, the median time from lung cancer suspicion to treatment ranged between 45 and 90 days (56,57,59,61), with shorter time intervals for patients with more advanced disease and those who received care in a private (vs. public) hospital (refs) (61).

Among international studies that examined patient characteristics and other factors associated with timeliness of care, several that examined the effect of age reported mixed results (63–65). In contrast, there is some evidence that atypical symptoms (66,67), less advanced disease stage (64), and the presence of at least one comorbidity are linked to receipt of less timely care (65). Other factors shown to be associated with less timely care include initial referral to a nonrespiratory clinician (21), need for multiple diagnostic tests (68,69), and care provided at a public hospital (61) or in a teaching hospital setting (63,65).

It has been difficult to determine the relationship between timeliness of care and lung cancer outcomes. In an uncontrolled study from Scotland, the median time between a diagnostic CT scan and a follow-up CT scan for radiotherapy planning was 54 days (range 18–131 days).

■ Table 2.5 U.S. studies of timeliness of care in lung cancer

Author, Year (Data Collection Period)	N	Setting	Cohort	Results
Finlay, 2002 (1992–1996) (62)	42	New England Medical Center	Lung cancer	Median days from diagnosis to treatment: 31 (Asian) vs. 26 (non-Asian)
Quarterman, 2003 (1989–1999) (57)	84	San Francisco VA	Surgery for NSCLC	Median days from suspicion to treatment: 82
Liu, 2004 (1995–2001) (60)	1,394	Hawaii	NSCLC cases in cancer registry	Median days from diagnosis to treatment: 27 (native Hawaiian) vs. 28 (non-Hawaiian)
Dransfield, 2006 (1999–2003) (55)	156	Birmingham VA	Surgery for NSCLC (n = 31)	Median days from surgical consultation to resection: 104
Riedel, 2006 (1999–2003) (58)	345	Durham VA	Lung cancer	Median days from diagnosis to treatment: 21 (multidisciplinary clinic) vs. 23 (conventional)
Gould, 2008 (2002–2003) (56)	129	Palo Alto VA	NSCLC	Median days from suspicion to treatment: 84
Schultz, 2009 (2002–2005) (59)	2,372	127 VA hospitals	Lung cancer	Median days from suspicion to treatment: 90 (stage I or II) vs. 52 (stage III or IV)
Yorio, 2009 (2000–2005) (61)	482	UT Southwestern	Stage I to III NSCLC	Median days from suspicion to treatment: 76 (public hospital) vs. 45 (private)

NSCLC, non–small cell lung cancer.

During this time interval, median tumor cross-sectional diameter increased by 19% (range 0–373%) (70).

However, several studies reported no association between timeliness of lung cancer care and survival, including four studies of patients with surgically treated lung cancer (57,71–73). For example, in a study of 83 veterans who underwent resection for stage I or II non–small cell lung cancer (NSCLC) at the San Francisco VA Hospital between 1989 and 1999, Quarterman et al. (57) found no difference in the hazard of death for patients who did and did not receive surgery within 90 days. These results might be confounded by the exclusion of patients who did not undergo surgery. It is possible that some patients were systematically excluded from the study because they had long delays in care and therefore had disease that progressed to a stage that was not surgically resectable. In addition, these studies in surgical patients did not control fully for other factors that might confound the relationship between timeliness and survival, such as tumor size and the presence of symptoms at the time of presentation.

Another study from Sweden examined timeliness of care and survival in a more heterogeneous sample of 432 patients with NSCLC (74). In this study, median time from symptom onset to treatment was 4.6 months, and median time from hospitalization to treatment was 1.6 months. Both before and after adjusting for age, gender, tumor histology, TNM stage, and surgical treatment, longer time to treatment was associated with a reduced hazard of death. Similar paradoxical results were reported in a smaller study of veterans with NSCLC (56). In these studies, the relationship between timeliness and survival was likely confounded by the biological aggressiveness of disease, such that the patients with the most aggressive disease were both more likely to receive more timely care and to die.

Future studies of timeliness and survival will need to rely on either natural experiments or sophisticated methods of statistical adjustment to answer to this question. In the meantime, clinicians should strive to provide timely care without compromising other dimensions of health care quality. Likewise, much additional research is needed to determine those structures and processes of multidisciplinary care that improve patient-centered outcomes in lung cancer.

■ REFERENCES

1. Institute of Medicine (Committee on Quality of Health Care in America). Crossing the Quality Chasm: A New Health System for the 21st Century. Washington, DC: National Academies Press; 2001.

2. Detterbeck FC, Jantz MA, Wallace M, Vansteenkiste J, Silvestri GA; American College of Chest Physicians. Invasive mediastinal staging of lung cancer: ACCP evidence-based clinical practice guidelines (2nd edition). Chest. 2007;132(3 suppl):202S–220S.

3. Rivera MP, Mehta AC; American College of Chest Physicians. Initial diagnosis of lung cancer: ACCP evidence-based clinical practice guidelines (2nd edition). Chest. 2007;132(3 suppl):131S–148S.

4. Silvestri GA, Gould MK, Margolis ML, et al.; American College of Chest Physicians. Noninvasive staging of non-small cell lung cancer: ACCP evidenced-based clinical practice guidelines (2nd edition). Chest. 2007;132(3 suppl):178S–201S.

5. Wahidi MM, Govert JA, Goudar RK, Gould MK, McCrory DC; American College of Chest Physicians. Evidence for the treatment of patients with pulmonary nodules: when is it lung cancer?: ACCP evidence-based clinical practice guidelines (2nd edition). Chest. 2007;132(3 suppl):94S–107S.

6. National Comprehensive Cancer Network, NCCN Clinical Practice Guidelines in Oncology: Non-Small Cell Lung Cancer. http://www.nccn.org/ Accessed July 29, 2010.

7. Alberts WM; American College of Chest Physicians. Introduction: Diagnosis and management of lung cancer: ACCP evidence-based clinical practice guidelines (2nd Edition). Chest. 2007;132(3 suppl):20S–22S.

8. Gould MK, Ananth L, Barnett PG; Veterans Affairs SNAP Cooperative Study Group. A clinical model to estimate the pretest probability of lung cancer in patients with solitary pulmonary nodules. Chest. 2007;131(2):383–388.

9. Schultz EM, Sanders GD, Trotter PR, et al. Validation of two models to estimate the probability of malignancy in patients with solitary pulmonary nodules. Thorax. 2008;63(4):335–341.

10. Swensen SJ, Silverstein MD, Ilstrup DM, Schleck CD, Edell ES. The probability of malignancy in solitary pulmonary nodules. Application to small radiologically indeterminate nodules. Arch Intern Med. 1997;157(8):849–855.

11. Gould MK, Fletcher J, Iannettoni MD, et al.; American College of Chest Physicians. Evaluation of patients with pulmonary nodules: when is it lung cancer?: ACCP evidence-based clinical practice guidelines (2nd edition). Chest. 2007;132(3 suppl):108S–130S.

12. Gould MK, Sanders GD, Barnett PG, et al. Cost-effectiveness of alternative management strategies for patients with solitary pulmonary nodules. Ann Intern Med. 2003;138(9):724–735.

13. Timmerman R, Paulus R, Galvin J, et al. Stereotactic body radiation therapy for inoperable early stage lung cancer. JAMA. 2010;303(11):1070–1076.

14. Holty JE, Kuschner WG, Gould MK. Accuracy of transbronchial needle aspiration for mediastinal staging of non-small cell lung cancer: a meta-analysis. Thorax. 2005;60(11):949–955.

15. Gildea TR, Mazzone PJ, Karnak D, Meziane M, Mehta AC. Electromagnetic navigation diagnostic bronchoscopy: a prospective study. Am J Respir Crit Care Med. 2006;174(9):982–989.

16. Fischer B, Lassen U, Mortensen J, et al. Preoperative staging of lung cancer with combined PET-CT. N Engl J Med. 2009;361(1):32–39.

17. Herder GJ, Kramer H, Hoekstra OS, et al.; POORT Study Group. Traditional versus up-front [18F] fluorodeoxyglucose-positron emission tomography staging of non-small-cell lung cancer: a Dutch cooperative randomized study. J Clin Oncol. 2006;24(12):1800–1806.

18. Maziak DE, Darling GE, Inculet RI, et al. Positron emission tomography in staging early lung cancer: a randomized trial. Ann Intern Med. 2009;151(4):221–228, W-48.

19. van Tinteren H, Hoekstra OS, Smit EF, et al. Effectiveness of positron emission tomography in the preoperative assessment of patients with suspected non-small-cell lung cancer: the PLUS multicentre randomised trial. Lancet. 2002;359(9315):1388–1393.

20. Viney RC, Boyer MJ, King MT, et al. Randomized controlled trial of the role of positron emission tomography in the management of stage I and II non-small-cell lung cancer. J Clin Oncol. 2004;22(12):2357–2362.

21. Kesson E, Bucknall CE, McAlpine LG, et al. Lung cancer–management and outcome in Glasgow, 1991–92. Br J Cancer. 1998;78(10):1391–1395.

22. Cancer (2009) Cancer Program Standards 2009, Revised Edition. Available at: www.facs.org/cancer/coc/publications.html. Accessed July 29, 2010.

23. Wright FC, De Vito C, Langer B, Hunter A; Expert Panel on Multidisciplinary Cancer Conference Standards. Multidisciplinary cancer conferences: a systematic review and development of practice standards. Eur J Cancer. 2007;43(6):1002–1010.

24. Santoso JT, Schwertner B, Coleman RL, Hannigan EV. Tumor board in gynecologic oncology. Int J Gynecol Cancer. 2004;14(2):206–209.

25. Commission on Coory M, Gkolia P, Yang IA, Bowman RV, Fong KM. Systematic review of multidisciplinary teams in the management of lung cancer. Lung Cancer. 2008;60(1):14–21.

26. Bowen EF, Anderson JR, Roddie ME. Improving surgical resection rates in lung cancer without a two stop service. Thorax. 2003;58(4):368.

27. Davison AG, Eraut CD, Haque AS, et al. Telemedicine for multidisciplinary lung cancer meetings. J Telemed Telecare. 2004;10(3):140–143.

28. Martin-Ucar AE, Waller DA, Atkins JL, Swinson D, O'Byrne KJ, Peake MD. The beneficial effects of specialist thoracic surgery on the resection rate for non-small-cell lung cancer. Lung Cancer. 2004;46(2):227–232.

29. Price A, Kerr G, Gregor A, Ironside J, Little F. The impact of multidisciplinary teams and site specialisation on the use of radiotherapy in elderly people with non-small cell lung cancer (NSCLC) [abstract]. Radiother Oncol. 2002;64(suppl 1):S80.

30. Forrest LM, McMillan DC, McArdle CS, Dunlop DJ. An evaluation of the impact of a multidisciplinary team, in a single centre, on treatment and survival in patients with inoperable non-small-cell lung cancer. Br J Cancer. 2005;93(9):977–978.

31. Murray PV, O'Brien ME, Sayer R, et al. The pathway study: results of a pilot feasibility study in patients suspected of having lung carcinoma investigated in a conventional chest clinic setting compared to a centralised two-stop pathway. Lung Cancer. 2003;42(3):283–290.

32. Seek A, Hogle WP. Modeling a better way: navigating the healthcare system for patients with lung cancer. Clin J Oncol Nurs. 2007;11(1):81–85.

33. Birchall M, Bailey D, King P; South West Cancer Intelligence Service Head and Neck Tumour Panel. Effect of process standards on survival of patients with head and neck cancer in the south and west of England. Br J Cancer. 2004;91(8):1477–1481.

34. Junor EJ, Hole DJ, Gillis CR. Management of ovarian cancer: referral to a multidisciplinary team matters. Br J Cancer. 1994;70(2):363–370.

35. Henschke CI, McCauley DI, Yankelevitz DF, et al. Early Lung Cancer Action Project: overall design and findings from baseline screening. Lancet. 1999;354(9173):99–105.

36. Henschke CI, Naidich DP, Yankelevitz DF, et al. Early lung cancer action project: initial findings on repeat screenings. Cancer. 2001;92(1):153–159.

37. Swensen SJ, Jett JR, Sloan JA, et al. Screening for lung cancer with low-dose spiral computed tomography. Am J Respir Crit Care Med. 2002;165(4):508–513.

38. Croswell JM, Baker SG, Marcus PM, Clapp JD, Kramer BS. Cumulative incidence of false-positive test results in lung cancer screening: a randomized trial. Ann Intern Med. 2010;152(8): 505–512, W176.

39. Bach PB, Cramer LD, Schrag D, Downey RJ, Gelfand SE, Begg CB. The influence of hospital volume on survival after resection for lung cancer. N Engl J Med. 2001;345(3):181–188.

40. Begg CB, Cramer LD, Hoskins WJ, Brennan MF. Impact of hospital volume on operative mortality for major cancer surgery. JAMA. 1998;280(20):1747–1751.

41. Birkmeyer JD, Siewers AE, Finlayson EV, et al. Hospital volume and surgical mortality in the United States. N Engl J Med. 2002;346(15):1128–1137.

42. Birkmeyer JD, Sun Y, Wong SL, Stukel TA. Hospital volume and late survival after cancer surgery. Ann Surg. 2007;245(5):777–783.

43. Finlayson, EV, Goodney, PP, Birkmeyer, JD. Hospital volume and operative mortality in cancer surgery: a national study. Arch Surg. 2003;138(7):721–725; discussion 726.

44. Hannan EL, Radzyner M, Rubin D, Dougherty J, Brennan MF. The influence of hospital and surgeon volume on in-hospital mortality for colectomy, gastrectomy, and lung lobectomy in patients with cancer. Surgery. 2002;131(1):6–15.

45. Hollenbeck BK, Dunn RL, Miller DC, Daignault S, Taub DA, Wei JT. Volume-based referral for cancer surgery: informing the debate. J Clin Oncol. 2007;25(1):91–96.

46. Khuri SF, Daley J, Henderson W, et al. Relation of surgical volume to outcome in eight common operations: results from the VA National Surgical Quality Improvement Program. Ann Surg. 1999;230(3):414–429; discussion 429.

47. Little AG, Rusch VW, Bonner JA, et al. Patterns of surgical care of lung cancer patients. Ann Thorac Surg. 2005;80(6):2051–2016; discussion 2056.

48. Romano PS, Mark DH. Patient and hospital characteristics related to in-hospital mortality after lung cancer resection. Chest. 1992;101(5):1332–1337.

49. Simunovic M, Rempel E, Thériault ME, et al. Influence of hospital characteristics on operative death and survival of patients after major cancer surgery in Ontario. Can J Surg. 2006;49(4):251–258.

50. Urbach DR, Baxter NN. Does it matter what a hospital is "high volume" for? Specificity of hospital volume-outcome associations for surgical procedures: analysis of administrative data. BMJ. 2004;328(7442):737–740.

51. Urschel JD, Urschel DM. The hospital volume-outcome relationship in general thoracic surgery. Is the surgeon the critical determinant? J Cardiovasc Surg (Torino). 2000;41(1):153–155.

52. Farjah F, Flum DR, Varghese TK Jr, Symons RG, Wood DE. Surgeon specialty and long-term survival after pulmonary resection for lung cancer. Ann Thorac Surg. 2009;87(4):995–1004; discussion 1005.

53. Schipper PH, Diggs BS, Ungerleider RM, Welke KF. The influence of surgeon specialty on outcomes in general thoracic surgery: a national sample 1996 to 2005. Ann Thorac Surg. 2009;88(5):1566–1572; discussion 1572–1573.

54. Silvestri GA, Handy J, Lackland D, Corley E, Reed CE. Specialists achieve better outcomes than generalists for lung cancer surgery. Chest. 1998;114(3):675–680.

55. Dransfield MT, Lock BJ, Garver RI Jr. Improving the lung cancer resection rate in the US Department of Veterans Affairs Health System. Clin Lung Cancer. 2006;7(4):268–272.

56. Gould MK, Ghaus SJ, Olsson JK, Schultz EM. Timeliness of care in veterans with non-small cell lung cancer. Chest. 2008;133(5):1167–1173.

57. Quarterman RL, McMillan A, Ratcliffe MB, Block MI. Effect of preoperative delay on prognosis for patients with early stage non-small cell lung cancer. J Thorac Cardiovasc Surg. 2003;125(1):108–113; discussion 113.

58. Riedel RF, Wang X, McCormack M, et al. Impact of a multidisciplinary thoracic oncology clinic on the timeliness of care. J Thorac Oncol. 2006;1(7):692–696.

59. Schultz EM, Powell AA, McMillan A, et al. Hospital characteristics associated with timeliness of care in veterans with lung cancer. Am J Respir Crit Care Med. 2009;179(7):595–600.

60. Liu DM, Kwee SA. Demographic, treatment, and survival patterns for Native Hawaiians with lung cancer treated at a community medical center from 1995 to 2001. Pac Health Dialog. 2004;11(2):139–145.

61. Yorio JT, Xie Y, Yan J, Gerber DE. Lung cancer diagnostic and treatment intervals in the United States: a health care disparity? J Thorac Oncol. 2009;4(11):1322–1330.

62. Finlay GA, Joseph B, Rodrigues CR, Griffith J, White AC. Advanced presentation of lung cancer in Asian immigrants: a case-control study. Chest. 2002;122(6):1938–1943.

63. Bardell T, Belliveau P, Kong W, Mackillop WJ. Waiting times for cancer surgery in Ontario: 1984–2000. Clin Oncol (R Coll Radiol). 2006;18(5):401–409.

64. Johnston GM, MacGarvie VL, Elliott D, Dewar RA, MacIntyre MM, Nolan MC. Radiotherapy wait times for patients with a diagnosis of invasive cancer, 1992–2000. Clin Invest Med. 2004;27(3):142–156.

65. Simunovic M, Thériault ME, Paszat L, et al. Using administrative databases to measure waiting times for patients undergoing major cancer surgery in Ontario, 1993-2000. Can J Surg. 2005;48(2):137–142.

66. Bjerager M, Palshof T, Dahl R, Vedsted P, Olesen F. Delay in diagnosis of lung cancer in general practice. Br J Gen Pract. 2006;56(532):863–868.

67. Strojan, P, Debevec, M, Kovac, V. Superior sulcus tumor (SST): management at the Institute of Oncology in Ljubljana, Slovenia, 1981–1994. Lung Cancer. 1997:17(2–3):249–259.

68. Devbhandari MP, Soon SY, Quennell P, et al. UK waiting time targets in lung cancer treatment: are they achievable? Results of a prospective tracking study. J Cardiothorac Surg. 2007;2:5.

69. Lim WS, Macfarlane JT, Deegan PC, Manhire A, Holmes WF, Baldwin DR. How do general practitioners respond to reports of ab chest X-rays? J R Soc Med. 1999;92(9):446–449.

70. O'Rourke N, Edwards R. Lung cancer treatment waiting times and tumour growth. Clin Oncol (R Coll Radiol). 2000;12(3):141–144.

71. Aragoneses FG, Moreno N, Leon P, Fontan EG, Folque E; Bronchogenic Carcinoma Cooperative Group of the Spanish Society of Pneumology and Thoracic Surgery (GCCB-S). Influence of delays on survival in the surgical treatment of bronchogenic carcinoma. Lung Cancer. 2002;36(1):59–63.

72. Billing JS, Wells FC. Delays in the diagnosis and surgical treatment of lung cancer. Thorax. 1996;51(9):903–906.

73. Pita-Fernández S, Montero-Martinez C, Pértega-Diaz S, Verea-Hernando H. Relationship between delayed diagnosis and the degree of invasion and survival in lung cancer. J Clin Epidemiol. 2003;56(9):820–825.

74. Myrdal G, Lambe M, Hillerdal G, Lamberg K, Agustsson T, Ståhle E. Effect of delays on prognosis in patients with non-small cell lung cancer. Thorax. 2004;59(1):45–49.

3 Pathology of Lung Cancer

HEIDI S. ERICKSON

IGNACIO I. WISTUBA

■ INTRODUCTION

In the United States and worldwide, lung cancer is the leading cause of cancer deaths (1) with the majority of lung cancers being diagnosed at advanced stages when treatment options are primarily palliative. In order for patients to receive suitable therapy, accurate pathologic classification of lung cancer is essential. Classification of the vast majority of lung cancers is straightforward; however, areas of controversy and diagnostic challenges still remain. Histologically and biologically, lung cancer is a highly complex neoplasm (2) with several histologic types and subtypes. The most frequently occurring types are small cell lung carcinoma (SCLC, 15%) and non–small cell lung carcinoma (NSCLC), with NSCLC consisting of squamous cell carcinoma (SCC) (30%), adenocarcinoma (45%), and large cell carcinoma (9%) subtypes (3).

Molecular technologic advances are providing insight into the biological processes involved in lung cancer pathogenesis. Data indicate that clinically evident lung cancers are due to the accumulation of various genetic and epigenetic changes, including but not limited to oncogene activation and tumor suppressor gene (TSG) inactivation (2). These molecular abnormalities comprise the "hallmarks of cancer": self-sufficiency of growth signals, insensitivity to antigrowth signals, sustained angiogenesis, evasion of apoptosis, limitless replicative potential, and tissue invasion and metastasis (4,5). Insight gleamed from molecular advances have also provided an opportunity to develop rational targeted therapies for lung cancer. These new targeted therapies have led to an emerging and exciting new area of lung cancer therapy by taking advantage of cancer-specific molecular defects that render the cancer cells more likely to respond to specific agents (6–8). In the lung cancer targeted therapy arena, the analysis of molecular changes is becoming increasingly important and presents an interesting challenge to

adequately integrate both routine pathologic and molecular examinations into the diagnosis, classification, and choice of therapy.

Even though clinically relevant lung cancer molecular abnormalities have been described, relatively little is known about the molecular events preceding lung carcinogenesis and its underlying genetic bias (9). Molecular characterization of preneoplastic changes involved in lung cancer pathogenesis have been reported, especially SCC and adenocarcinoma; however, not much has changed in the last decade since these early studies (9,10).

In this chapter, we will describe the most common histologic types of lung cancer with regard to their pathologic, molecular, and genetic characteristics. We will also review the current understanding of this cancer's early pathogenesis and progression. And finally, we will focus on the molecular profiling and predictive markers of NSCLC.

■ PATHOLOGY

Premalignant Lesions

Lung cancers are thought to occur as the culmination of a series of progressive pathologic changes (i.e., precursor lesions) in the respiratory mucosa. As histologically classified by the 2004 World Health Organization (WHO) International Association for the Study of Lung Cancer (IASLC), there are three main morphologic forms of preinvasive lesions of the lung (3): (a) squamous dysplasia and carcinoma in situ (CIS); (b) atypical adenomatous hyperplasia (AAH); and (c) diffuse idiopathic pulmonary neuroendocrine cell hyperplasia. Sequential preneoplastic changes have been characterized for centrally arising squamous carcinomas; however, they remain poorly documented for large cell carcinomas (LCC), adenocarcinomas, and SCLCs (Table 3.1) (11,12).

Squamous Dysplasia/Carcinoma In Situ

Hyperplasia, squamous metaplasia, squamous dysplasia, and CIS are large airway mucosal changes that may precede or accompany invasive SCC (Figure 3.1A–B) (11,12).

■ Table 3.1 Histopathologic and molecular abnormalities of lung cancer precursor lesions

Abnormality	NSCLC Adenocarcinoma	NSCLC SCC	SCLC
Histopathology			
Precursor	Probable	Known	Unknown
Lesion	AAH?	Squamous dysplasia and CIS	Normal epithelium and hyperplasia?
Molecular			
Gene abnormalities	*KRAS* mutation	*TP53* LOH and mutation	*MYC* overexpression
	EGFR mutation		*TP53* LOH and mutation
Genetic instability	Low	Intermediate	High
Frequency	13%	10%	68%
LOH	Low	Intermediate	High
Frequency	10%	54%	90%
Chromosomal regions	9p21, 17p/*TP53*	8p21–23, 9p21, 17p/*TP53*	5q21, 8p21–23, 9p21, 17p/*TP53*

CIS, carcinoma in situ; LOH, loss of heterozygosity; NSCLC, non–small cell lung carcinoma; SCC, squamous cell carcinoma; SCLC, small cell lung carcinoma. ?, hypothesized.

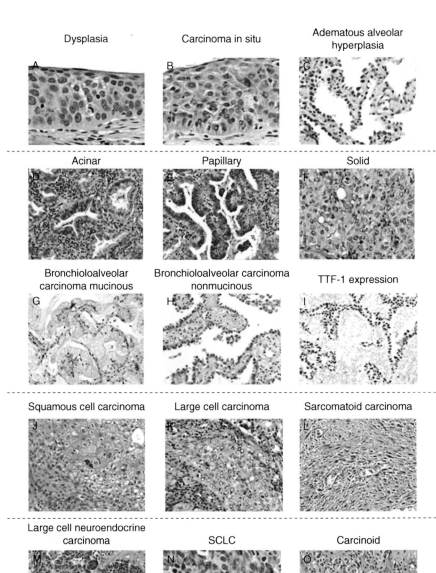

FIGURE 3.1 Histologic overview of lung epithelial precursor lesions and tumors. Major histological types of lung cancer precursor lesions: dysplasia (A), carcinoma in situ (B), and adenometous alveolar hyperplasia (C). Major histologic types of lung cancer malignant lesions: non–small cell lung carcinoma (NSCLC) histological subtypes of adenocarcinoma (D, E, F, G, H), TTF-1 IHC of adenocarcinoma (I), squamous cell carcinoma (J), large-cell carcinoma (K), and sarcomatoid carcinoma (L); neuroendocrine histologic subtypes: large cell neuroendocrine carcinoma (M), small-cell lung carcinoma (N), and typical carcinoid (O).

Dysplastic squamous lesions (mild, moderate, and severe) represent a continuum of cytologic and histologic atypical changes that demonstrate plasticity between categories. Rate and risks of progression of squamous dysplasia to CIS and, ultimately, to invasive SCC, remain relatively unknown.

Despite this progress, neither histologic features nor molecular changes of SCC precursor lesions have been shown to be useful to predict their progression to invasive carcinoma (13,14).

Atypical Adenomatous Hyperplasia

AAH in peripheral airway cells is considered a putative precursor of adenocarcinoma (10,11); however, the origin of most lung adenocarcinomas, including respiratory structures and specific epithelia cell types, remain unknown. AAH arises in the alveoli near respiratory and terminal bronchioles as a discrete parenchymal lesion. AAH lesions can be detected grossly if they are 0.5 cm or larger, but are usually incidental histologic findings due to their typical small size. These lesions have an alveolar structure lined by low columnar, cuboidal, or rounded cells and are called "ground glass opacities" (Figure 3.1C). AAH is an important differential diagnosis of air-filled peripheral lesions and its awareness has been improved due to increased use of high-resolution computed tomography (CT). Increasing atypical morphology gives evidence to the putative progression of AAH to adenocarcinoma with bronchioloalveolar carcinoma (BAC) features and is supported by cytofluorometric, morphometric, and molecular analysis (10,12). Despite these data, the origin of AAH is still unknown. However, immunohistochemical and ultrastructural analysis has provided a differentiation phenotype which suggests origination from peripheral airway progenitor cells, such as Clara cells and type II pneumocytes (15,16).

Diffuse Idiopathic Pulmonary Neuroendocrine Cell Hyperplasia

A rare lesion known as diffuse idiopathic pulmonary neuroendocrine cell hyperplasia (DIPENECH) has been associated with lung neuroendocrine tumor development, including typical and atypical carcinoids (11,17,18). DIPENECH lesions comprise local extraluminal neuroendocrine proliferations as tumorlets of less than 0.5 cm; whereas, carcinoid tumors are lesions with neuroendocrine proliferation of 0.5 cm or greater.

Precursor lesions of SCLC, the most common neuroendocrine lung carcinoma, remain unknown (11,12) despite widespread and extensive genetic damage in normal and hyperplastic bronchial epithelium suggesting that SCLC may arise directly from histologically normal or mildly abnormal epithelium without passing through a more complex histologic sequence (19).

Malignant Tumors

Lung cancer pathologic diagnosis is established by examining cytologic or surgical pathology specimens. Histologic specimens are acquired from bronchoscopic and needle biopsies (fine needle aspirates [FNA] and core needle biopsies [CNB]) or open biopsy procedures such as thoracoscopy, excisional wedge biopsy, lobectomy, or pneumonectomy. Malignant lung tumor lesions can be classified into two main groups: NSCLC and SCLC.

Pathologic disease stage, as classified by the internationally accepted TNM staging system (20), is an important basis for prognosis and treatment decisions. NSCLC staging is based on characteristics of tumor tissue samples (tumor size, distance from the invasion to the main bronchus carina, pleural invasion, atelectasis or obstructive pneumonitis, mediastinal organs or chest wall invasion, malignant pleural effusion, and separate tumor nodule in the same lobe), status of lymph nodes, and presence of distant metastases. However, the staging system for lung cancers is always evolving (21). In 2010, a new staging system developed by the IASLC will go into effect (22–24).

Previously, SCLC was not classified according to the TNM staging system because the tendency toward widespread dissemination at presentation has led to the staging of SCLCs as limited or extensive disease (25). Limited SCLC disease is defined as disease constrained to one hemithorax with regional lymph node metastases, including ipsilateral pleural effusion and hilar, mediastinal, supraclavicular ipsilateral, and contralateral lymph node involvement. Extensive SCLC includes all the disease sites beyond those defined as limited SCLC disease. However, it has been proposed that SCLC can now be classified according to the new IASLC TNM staging system (26).

Non–Small Cell Lung Carcinoma

The classification of NSCLC consists of five subclassifications: adenocarcinoma, SCC, adenosquamous carcinoma, large cell carcinoma, and sarcomatoid carcinomas, with the predominant subclassifications of NSCLC being adenocarcinoma and SCC (Table 3.1). Each of the NSCLC subclassifications may also have major subtypes. The NSCLC subclassifications and subtypes are identified by histologic characteristics, localization in the lung, and route of dissemination (Table 3.2).

Adenocarcinoma. Nearly 40% of all lung cancers are adenocarcinomas. The WHO classifies adenocarcinoma into five major subtypes: acinar, papillary, solid with mucin production, BAC, and mixed adenocarcinomas (Figure 3.1D–H) (3). Most adenocarcinomas (~90%) are categorized as mixed because they consist of two or more of the histologic subtypes (27). Adenocarcinomas occur as single or multiple foci, have a wide range of sizes, most commonly present a macroscopic pattern of peripheral

■ **Table 3.2** Pathologic and molecular characteristics of adenocarcinoma and SCC of the lung

Abnormality	Adenocarcinoma	SCC
Frequency of lesion type	~40%	~30%
Pathogenesis	Smoking and nonsmoking	Smoking
Pathology		
Location	Mostly peripheral	Mostly central
Gross features	Tendency to scar	Tendency to cavitation
Histology	Heterogeneous	Subtypes infrequent
Subtypes	Acinar, papillary, solid with mucin, BAC	Basaloid, clear cell and small cell
Molecular abnormalities		
KRAS mutation	10–20%[a]	Very rare
EGFR mutation	10–30%[a]	Very rare
HER2 mutation	10–20%[a]	Very rare
LKB1 changes	34%	19%
Deletions (LOH)	3p discrete deletions	3p extensive deletion
Methylation	*APC, CDH13, RARß*	

[a] With variations based in patients' smoking history and ethnicity.

BAC, bronchioloalveolar; LOH, loss of heterozygosity; SCC, squamous cell carcinoma.

lung localization with pleural invasion (28), and spread primarily by lymphatic and hematogenous routes. Mixed-subtype adenocarcinomas with a BAC component and BAC have been recognized to have several gross pathologies in the lung, including a solitary peripheral nodule, multiple nodules, and lobar consolidation (29).

BAC is traditionally defined as a true noninvasive tumor with purely lepidic growth and no evidence of invasion (29). Unfortunately, there has been considerable confusion regarding BAC terminology, as pathologists frequently do not adhere to this strict definition by often labeling mixed tumors with varying degrees of lepidic growth as BAC or adenocarcinoma with BAC features. Conversely to the lymphatic and hematogenous routes of adenocarcinoma dissemination, BAC often undergoes aerogenous dissemination away from the main mass by the spread of tumor cells through the airways (30). Even though a BAC-like pattern of spread often occurs at the edge of conventional adenocarcinomas, histologically pure BAC rarely occurs (only 3% of all lung cancers) (29). BAC consists of three subtypes: nonmucinous, mucinous, and mixed.

Squamous Cell Carcinoma. Approximately 30% of lung cancers are SCC. SCC is characterized by intercellular bridges, squamous pearl formation, and individual cell keratinization (Figure 3.1J). These features are obvious in well-differentiated SCC, but they are difficult to find in poorly differentiated SCC. About 70% of SCC present as central lung tumors (31). As these tumors grow, they may become large cavitating masses, and subsequently, most cavitating lung cancers are SCC (32). Similar to adenocarcinomas, SCC disseminates primarily by lymphatic and hematogenous routes. SCC is also able to spread by extending through periobronchial tubes which allow them to directly invade mediastinal lymph nodes and other mediastinal structures

(31). Thus, locoregional recurrence after surgical resection is more common for SCC than for other cell types (33).

Adenosquamous Carcinoma. Adenosquamous carcinomas are a mixed histologic type of NSCLC characterized by the presence of both SCC and adenocarcinoma, with each histologic type making up at least 10% of the tumor (34). Adenosquamous carcinomas are usually located in the periphery of the lung and disseminate by similar mechanisms to those of other NSCLC types.

Large Cell Carcinoma. Approximately 9% of all lung cancers are LCC. LCC are a diagnosis of exclusion as they are undifferentiated carcinomas lacking features of adenocarcinoma, SCC, or SCLC (Figure 3.1K) (35). LCC have a spectrum of morphologies, but most LCC consist of large cells with abundant cytoplasm and large nuclei with prominent nucleoli (32). Variants of LCC include large cell neuroendocrine carcinomas (LCNEC), lymphoepithelioma-like carcinomas, clear cell carcinomas, basaloid carcinomas, and LCC with rabdoid component (35). The LCC variants can be identified by the major histologic characteristics that give rise to their names: (a) LCNEC exhibit neuroendocrine differentiation (Figure 3.1L) (36); (b) lymphoepithelioma-like carcinomas are characterized by dense lymphocytic infiltration and the presence of Epstein-Barr virus viral sequences (37,38); and (c) for the most part, LCC are large, peripheral masses (35). LCC dissemination patterns are usually similar to that of other NSCLC.

Sarcomatoid Carcinomas. The least common of lung cancers (0.3–1.3%) are sarcomatoid carcinomas (27,39). Sarcomatoid carcinomas comprise a group of poorly differentiated NSCLC variants that contain a component of sarcoma or sarcoma-like (spindle and/or giant cell)

differentiation (Figure 3.1M) (39). To date, five sarcomatoid carcinoma variants have been identified: spindle cell carcinoma; pleomorphic carcinoma; giant cell carcinoma; carcinosarcoma; and pulmonary blastoma (39,40). They can arise in the central or peripheral lung. Sarcomatoid tumors are usually large masses which arise in the central or peripheral lung and disseminate to the chest wall (41).

Small Cell Lung Carcinoma

Approximately 15% of all lung cancers are SCLCs (42). SCLC is characterized by small epithelial tumor cell, roughly no larger than the diameter of two or three small mature lymphocytes (43), with finely granular chromatin and absent or inconspicuous nucleoli (Figure 3.1N; Table 3.1) (42). Mitotic figure count is high and the presence of necrosis is frequent and extensive. Less than 10% of SCLCs demonstrate a mixture of NSCLC histologic types. But when they do occur, these "combined SCLCs" usually consist of adenocarcinoma, SCC, or large cell carcinoma (42). Most SCLCs present as large perihilar masses with extensive necrosis and extensive lymph node metastases (44). These tumors are typically situated in a peribronchial location with infiltration of the bronchial submucosa and peribronchial tissue (42). SCLC is classified as limited or extensive disease due to the tendency toward widespread dissemination at presentation.

Carcinoid Tumors

Less than 5% of all lung cancers are carcinoid tumors. Carcinoid tumors are differentiated neuroendocrine tumors derived from neuroendocrine cells existing in normal airways (45). In contrast to most other lung cancers, they have no relationship to smoke exposure (45). An organoid growth pattern, uniform cytologic features,

and immunohistochemical expression of neuroendocrine markers (e.g., chromogranin and synatophysin) are characteristic of carcinoid tumors (Figure 3.1O) (46). Based on pathologic features and clinical behavior, carcinoid tumors are classified as typical or atypical (47). Histologically, typical carcinoids lack necrosis and demonstrate less than 2 mitoses per 2 mm^2, whereas atypical carcinoids demonstrate foci(s) of necrosis and/or 2 to 10 mitosis per 2 mm^2 (46). Compared with typical carcinoids, atypical carcinoids have more histologic and clinical features of malignancy. Atypical carcinoids generally have larger metastases and a higher rate of metastases. Overall survival of patients with atypical carcinoids is significantly reduced (48).

Ancillary Diagnostic Immunohistochemistry

SCLC is routinely diagnosed by examination of histologic and cytologic specimens. In rare instances, it is necessary to perform immunohistochemistry (IHC) analysis of synathopysin and chromagrannin neuroendocrine markers. In addition to SCLC, the other two histologic neuroendocrine subtypes often require IHC expression of the neuroendocrine markers to confirm LCNEC and carcinoid tumor neuroendocrine lineages. Diagnosis of lung cancer and subtyping of NSCLC is typically accomplished by careful morphologic examination of hematoxylin and eosin (H&E)-stained biopsy samples or Papanicolaou-stained cytology samples (49). However, in approximately 20% to 30% of NSCLCs, IHC analysis is necessary to determine adenocarcinoma or SCC tumor cell lineages (49). NSCLC can usually be subtyped by using a small panel of IHC markers, including *TTF-1*, cytokeratin 7 (*CK7*), *p63*, and high-molecular-weight cytokeratins (e.g., *CK5* and *CK6*) (Table 3.3) (50). Positive *TTF-1* IHC expression usually confirms lung adenocarcinoma, can differentiate lung primary tumors from

■ **Table 3.3** Diagnostic IHC of primary lung cancer specific biomarkers

Marker	NSCLC Adenocarcinoma	SCC	SCLC
CK 5/6	Negative	Positive	Negative
p63	Negative	Positive	Negative
TTF-1	Positive (77%)	Negative (11%)	Positive (87%)
CK7	Positive (97%)		Negative
CK20[a]	Negative (9%)		Negative
CK8	Positive (72%)	Negative	Positive (75%)
CEACAM6	Positive[b] (33%—those that do not stain well with *TTF-1*)		Negative
Napsin A	Positive[b] (90%)		Negative
TIMP-2	Negative[b]		Positive (87%)

[a] CK20 is frequently positive (67%) in subtype BAC adenocarcinoma.

[b] NSCLC—no distinction made as to histologic subtype.

CEACAM6, carcinoembryonic antigen-related cell adhesion molecule 6; *CK*, cytokeratin; IHC, immunohistochemistry; *Napsin A*, Napsin A aspartic peptidase (NAPSA); NSCLC, non–small cell lung carcinoma; SCC, squamous cell carcinoma; SCLC, small cell lung cancer; *TIMP-2*, tissue inhibitor of metalloproteinases (TIMP) metallopeptidase inhibitor 2; *TTF1*, thyroid transcription factor 1.

metastatic tumors to the lung (Figure 3.1I) (51), and mostly rules out SCC. Whereas, a diffuse strong *p63* and *CK5/6* IHC expression is essentially restricted to SCC.

■ MOLECULAR CHARACTERISTICS OF TUMORS

Clinically evident lung cancers arise from multiple genetic changes which involve several dominant and putative recessive oncogenes known as TSGs (2). Cancer cells and adjacent "normal" cells overexpress numerous regulatory or growth factor proteins and their receptors, which impart a series of paracrine and autocrine growth stimulatory loops in lung cancer (52). There are as many as 15 known and putative recessive oncogenes involved in lung cancer (2). Recessive oncogenes are believed to be inactivated according to Knudson's two-hit hypothesis in which the first "hit" frequently is a point mutation, and the second "hit" is subsequent inactivation of the second allele due to chromosomal deletion, translocation, or other events (e.g., methylation) (53,54).

Chromosomal rearrangements have historically been linked primarily to nonsolid tumors (i.e., blood-related) and rarely to solid tumors (i.e., tissue-related). However, recently, chromosomal rearrangements resulting in fusion genes (e.g., *EML4-ALK*: echinoderm microtubule-associated protein-like 4 gene and anaplastic lymphoma kinase gene) have been discovered in NSCLC cells (55,56), leading to the belief that chromosomal rearrangements and activated fusion genes are likely common and play an important role in lung cancer.

Different patterns of molecular changes have been shown between the two major lung cancer groups (SCLC and NSCLC) (Table 3.4) (2) and amid the two major histologic types of NSCLC (adenocarcinoma and SCC; Table 3.2) (56–61).

Non–Small Cell Lung Cancer

Adenocarcinoma

Lung adenocarcinoma genetic changes include point mutations of dominant oncogenes (e.g., *KRAS, BRAF*, and *EGFR*) and TSGs (e.g., *TP53* and *p16^{Ink4}*) (Figure 3.2) (2,8,62–66). Two different molecular pathways have been identified in the pathogenesis of lung adenocarcinoma, a smoking-associated activation of *KRAS*-signaling, and non–smoking-associated activation of *EGFR* signaling, the latter of which is detected in histologically normal bronchial and bronchiolar epithelium (Figure 3.3) (67).

Lung adenocarcinomas in never-smokers are characterized by significantly higher frequencies of *EGFR* and *HER2* tyrosine kinase domain mutations, *EML4-ALK* fusion gene abnormalities in smokers and never-smokers (55,68,69), and

higher expression of *KRAS* mutations (70) and expression of the estrogen receptor in smokers (71). Of note, the *KRAS*-mutation profile differs between lung adenocarcinomas in smokers (mostly G-to-T or G-to-C transversions) and never-smokers (G-to-A transition) (70). *Tp53* is frequently mutated in lung cancer (66), and the differing pattern of *Tp53* point mutations in smokers (G-to-T transversions and A-to-G transitions) and never-smokers (G-to-A transitions) with lung cancer is similar to that of *KRAS* (Table 3.5). MiRNAs have also been found to be differentially expressed in never-smokers, including miR-21 and miR-38 (72). Of interest, miR expression, including miR-21, was more remarkable in adenocarcinomas with *EGFR* mutations and results demonstrated that *EGFR* signaling pathway was positively regulated by miR-21 (72).

Activating *KRAS* mutations preferentially target adenocarcinomas (20–30%) (2,66,70) and are smoking-related mutations of G-to-T or G-to-C transversions, affecting exons 12 (~90% of the mutations), 13, and 61 (65,66,73,74). Activating *BRAF* mutations have also been found in adenocarcinoma primary tumors (3%) (65) and lung adenocarcinoma cell lines 11% (64).

Recently, a body of evidence has indicated that *EGFR* mutations affecting the tyrosine kinase domain of the gene (exons 18–21) are present in approximately 10% to 55% of adenocarcinomas and that they are almost entirely absent in other types of lung carcinomas (62). *EGFR* mutations are somatic in origin, and they occur significantly more frequently in adenocarcinomas of patients who have never smoked (51–68%), women (42–62%), and patients from countries in East Asia (30–50%) compared with Western countries (~10%) (62,75–80). These *EGFR* mutations are clinically relevant because most of them have been associated with sensitivity of lung adenocarcinoma to small molecule tyrosine kinase inhibitors (TKIs; gefitinib and erlotinib) (75–77,81). More than 80% of the mutations detected in *EGFR* are in-frame deletions in exon 19 or a single missense mutation in exon 21 (L858R) (62,75–80). It has been proposed that lung cancer cells with mutant *EGFR* might become physiologically dependent on the continued activity of the gene for the maintenance of their malignant phenotype, leading to an accelerated development of lung adenocarcinoma (82).

An increase in the number of *EGFR* copies, including high polysomy and gene amplification shown by fluorescent in situ hybridization (FISH), has been detected in 22% of patients with surgically resected (stages I–IIIA) NSCLC and correlated with *EGFR* protein overexpression (83). Higher frequencies (40–50%) of a high number of *EGFR* copies have been reported in patients with advanced NSCLC (84–89). Recent studies have demonstrated that tumor cells' high number of *EGFR* copies, identified using FISH, may also be a predictor for response to *EGFR* TKIs (84–89).

In addition, *HER2* gene mutations, although infrequent (3%), have been detected in lung cancer, predominantly

■ Table 3.4 Summary of molecular differences between NSCLC and SCLC

Feature	NSCLC	SCLC
Frequency of lung cancer type	80–85%	20–25%
Neuroendocrine cells	No	Yes
Putative autocrine loop	HGM/MET	GRP/GRP receptor
	NDF/ERBB	SCF/KIT
DMBT1 abnormal expression	43%	100%
EGFR TK domain mutations	10–40%	No
EGFR gain copy number	25–50%	No
HER2 mutations	4%	Not studied
HER2 gain copy number	10%	No
LKB1 mutation or deletion	26%	Not studied
MYC amplification	8–20%	18–31%
NKX2-1 (*TITF-1*) amplification	14%	Not studied
RAS mutations	15–20%	<1%
RB LOH	31%	67%
TP53 LOH	65%	90%
TP53 Mutation	~50%	75%
p16^{Ink4} LOH	66%	53%
p16^{Ink4} Mutation	10–40%	<1%
PTEN/MMAC1 loci LOH	41%	91%
TSG101 abnormal transcripts	0%	~100%
3p LOH various regions	>80%	>90%
4p LOH various regions	~20%	50%
4q LOH various regions	30%	80%
8p21–23 LOH	80–100%	80–90%
Other specific LOH regions	13q11, Xq22.1	1q23, 9q22–32, 10p15, 13q34
Microsatellite instability	22%	35%
Promoter hypermethylation		
RASSF1 gene	~40%	>90%
RARβ gene	41%	72%
Other genes	10–40% various genes*	Not studied

ERBB, neuregulin receptor; GRP, gastrin-releasing peptide; KIT, KIT proto-oncogene; LOH, loss of heterozygosity; MET, MET proto-oncogene; NDF, neu differentiation factor; NSCLC, non–small cell lung carcinoma; SCF, stem cell factor; SCLC, small cell lung cancer.

in lung adenocarcinomas and patients with an East Asian ethnic background (63). The remarkable similarities of mutations in *EGFR* and *HER2* genes involving adenocarcinoma histologic type, mutation type, gene location (tyrosine kinase domain), and specific patient subpopulations targeted are unprecedented and suggest similar etiologic factors. Of great interest, *EGFR*, *HER2*, and *KRAS* mutations are mutually exclusive, suggesting different pathways to lung cancer in smokers and never-smokers.

Using high-resolution gene copy analysis of a large number of lung adenocarcinomas, it was shown that the most common focal event in this tumor type was amplification of the *NKX2-1* gene (also known as *TITF1*) located at the 14.q13.3 region (90,91). *NKX2-1* is a transcription factor that plays an essential role in the formation of type II pneumocytes, the cell type that lines lung alveoli (92). The protein coded by *NKX2-1* has been called (*TTF-1*) thyroid transcription factor 1 and is considered to be a reliable marker for primary adenocarcinoma of the lung.

On the basis of findings of higher levels of protein expression of nuclear *TTF-1* in *EGFR*-mutant lung adenocarcinomas than in wild-type tumors, it has been suggested that *EGFR*-mutant lung adenocarcinoma originates from the terminal respiratory unit (93).

TP53 mutations are frequent in lung adenocarcinomas, with different patterns detected by sex and smoking status (94). *p16^{Ink4}* inactivation by multiple mechanisms occurs frequently in adenocarcinomas and may be related to smoking (2). In addition, gene methylation studies have shown that methylation rates of *APC*, *CDH13*, and *RARβ* genes are significantly higher in adenocarcinomas than in SCC (95,96). Among other chromosomal abnormalities, localized chromosome 3p deletions are also frequently detected in lung adenocarcinomas (57).

Recently, a major breakthrough in the understanding of key pathways affected by somatic mutations in lung adenocarcinoma was discovered by a large collaborative study (97). Over 1,000 somatic mutations,

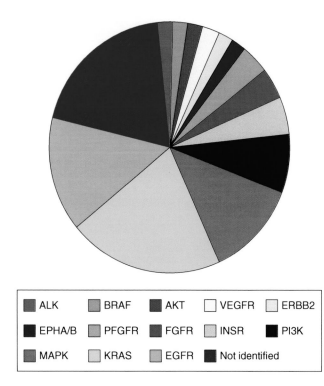

ALK	BRAF	AKT	VEGFR	ERBB2
EPHA/B	PFGFR	FGFR	INSR	PI3K
MAPK	KRAS	EGFR	Not identified	

FIGURE 3.2 Lung adenocarcinoma mutated molecular pathways/ genes percentages. Summary of mutated pathways/genes in adenocarcinoma. *KRAS, EGFR, MAPK,* and *PI3K* make up the majority of known mutations. However, a proportion of adenocarcinomas do not present any of the known mutations.

representing 623 genes related to cancer, were analyzed from 188 lung adenocarcinomas, and data was integrated with single-nucleotide polymorphism (SNP) profiling and gene-expression arrays for validation. Twenty-six genes were found to be significantly mutated at high frequencies, including, from highest to lowest number of mutations, *TP53, KRAS, STK11, EGFR, LRP1B, NF1, ATM, APC, EPHA3, PTPRD, CDKN2A, ERBB4, KDR, FGFR4, NTRK1, RB1, NTRK3, EPHA5, PDGFRA, GNAS, LTK, INHBA, PAK3, ZMYND10, NRAS,* and *XLC38A3* (97). Somatic mutations in lung adenocarcinoma that are also seen in other cancers included TSGs (*NF1, APC, RB1, ATM*) and sequence changes in *PTPRD* and the often deleted *LRP1B* (97). The key pathways containing genetic alterations in lung adenocarcinoma were MAPK, *p53,* Wnt signaling, cell cycle, and mTOR (97).

Squamous Cell Carcinoma

SCC demonstrate most of the genetic abnormalities commonly present in lung NSCLCs, except for *KRAS* and *EGFR* gene mutations, which are more frequent in adenocarcinomas (2,62). Disruption of the *TP53* and *RB* gene pathways is frequent in SCC (2). Most tumors demonstrate large segments of chromosome 3p deletions (57). Recently, it is has been shown that the inactivation of the TSG *LKB1* by mutation and deletion is a relatively

frequent event in both SCC (19%) and adenocarcinomas (34%) of the lung (98). In addition, genomic amplification of SOX-2 transcription factor gene has been shown to be a lineage-survival oncogene of lung SCC (99).

Other Histologic Subtypes

Few molecular studies have focused on LCC, mostly because the diagnosis is usually one of exclusion. LCC share the molecular and genetic abnormalities commonly seen in NSCLCs, including *TP53* and *RB* pathway disruptions (100,101). There are no specific studies that have reported molecular abnormalities in adenosquamous and sarcomatoid carcinomas of the lung, although they have been included in NSCLC studies.

Small Cell Lung Cancer

The etiology of SCLC is strongly tied to cigarette smoking, and now there is considerable information concerning molecular abnormalities involved in its pathogenesis (2,59,102). Autocrine growth factors such as neuroendocrine regulatory peptides (e.g., bombesin/gastrin-releasing peptide) are prominent in SCLC (59). Dominant oncogenes of the *MYC* family are frequently overexpressed (and may be amplified) in both SCLC and NSCLC, whereas the *KRAS* oncogene is never mutated in SCLC. *TP53* is mutated in more than 90% of SCLCs, and the *RB* gene is inactivated in more than 90% of SCLCs. In contrast to NSCLC, $p16^{INK4a}$, the other component of the retinoblastoma/p16 pathway, is almost never abnormal in SCLC. A genome-wide allelotyping study of approximately 400 polymorphic markers distributed at around 10 cM resolution across the human genome found that, on average, 17 loci showed loss of heterozygosity (LOH) in individual SCLCs and 22 for NSCLC, with an average size of loss of 50 to 60 cM and an average frequency of microsatellite abnormalities of five per tumor (103). There were 22 different "hot spots" for LOH, 13 with a preference for SCLC, 7 with a preference for NSCLC, and 2 affecting both. This provides clear evidence on a genome-wide scale that SCLC and NSCLC differ significantly in the TSGs that are inactivated during their pathogenesis. In addition, differences in gene methylation profiles have been detected between SCLC and NSCLC tumors (58).

■ PATHOGENESIS OF NSCLC

Lung premalignant lesions of the central airway are frequent in smokers and rare in never-smokers (9,11,104). Although the quantity of tobacco exposure needed to cause these premalignant lesions is not known, there is consensus that increasing tobacco exposure is related to increasing frequency and severity of the lesions (105).

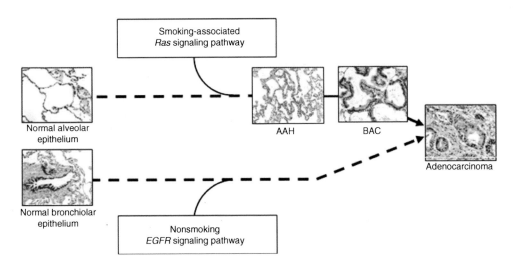

FIGURE 3.3 Comparison of adenocarcinoma pathogenesis of smokers and never-smokers. Even though the mechanisms of lung adenocarcinoma are relatively unknown, distinct smoking- and non–smoking-related molecular pathways have been identified in lung adenocarcinoma pathogenesis. Both smoking and never-smoking pathways lead to the development of invasive adenocarcinoma, with or without the intermediate BAC tumor. The smoking pathway comprises discrete molecular mechanisms, including inactivation of tumor suppressor genes (TSG), inflammation, angiogenesis, and activation of numerous signaling pathways. The smoking pathway includes smokers with and without chronic obstructive pulmonary disease (COPD).

■ **Table 3.5** Lung cancer molecular characteristics comparison of never-smokers and smokers

Feature	Never-smokers	Smokers
EGFR mutations	~25–60%[a]	~10%
ERBB2 mutations	~3%[a]	~1%
EML4-ALK fusion protein	~6%[a]	Rare
KRAS mutations	~5–15%	20–30%[b]
KRAS mutation signature	G→A transitions	G→T or G→C transversions[b]
TP53 mutations	~50%	70%[b]
TP53 mutation signature	G→A transitions	G→T transversions[b]
STK11 mutations	Rare	Frequent
Genes methylated	Relatively low	Relatively high, e.g., p16 and RASSF1A
Allelic loss	Relatively low	Relatively high
Allelic loss pattern	9p, 12p, 19q	3p, 6q, 9p, 16p, 17p, 19p
15q25 susceptibility locus	Disputed	Lung cancer risk associated
Intracellular nitrotyrosine (chronic inflammation marker)	Higher levels	Low levels

[a] Driving mutations in never-smokers.
[b] Driving mutations in smokers.

Currently, research methods have not elucidated the characteristics to identify the subpopulation of smokers at high risk for developing lung cancer. To better characterize this high-risk population, an improved understanding of the biology and molecular pathology of lung cancer early pathogenesis, including premalignancy, is still needed.

Adenocarcinoma Pathogenesis

AAH frequently presents molecular changes often found in lung adenocarcinomas, providing evidence to the hypothesis that AAH is a precursor of some of the major subtypes of adenocarcinoma and that AAH might be true preneoplastic lesions (15). Most importantly, *KRAS* mutations (codon 12) are present in 39% of AAH lesions, and these mutations are often found in smoking-associated adenocarcinomas (Figure 3.3) (10,67,106). In addition, overexpression of the cyclin D1 (~70%), *TP53* (10–58%), survivin (48%), and HER2/neu (7%) protein are also found in AAH (10,107,108).

The role of *EGFR* mutation in the pathogenesis of lung adenocarcinomas is becoming better understood (Figure 3.3). *EGFR* mutations have been detected in normal appearing peripheral respiratory epithelium in 9 (44%) of 21 adenocarcinoma patients but not in patients without mutations in the tumors (109). Also, *EGFR* mutations have been found more frequently in normal epithelium within the tumor (43%) than in adjacent sites (24%) suggesting a localized field effect phenomenon in respiratory epithelium. Even though the cell type(s) having *EGFR* mutations is unknown, it is hypothesized that stem or progenitor cells of the bronchial and bronchiolar epithelium are the cell type bearing the *EGFR* mutations. The finding of relatively infrequent *EGFR* mutations in AAH lesions (3 of 40 examined) (93,110) and the finding of no mutation (62) or relatively low frequency of mutation in true BACs of the lung support the concept that genetic abnormalities of *EGFR* are not relevant in the pathogenesis of alveolar-type lung neoplasia. However, further studies are needed to clarify the association between *EGFR* mutation and pathogenesis of AAH and BAC lesions.

SCC Pathogenesis

Squamous dysplasia and CIS are thought to progress to invasive SCC; however, not much is known about the risks and rate of progression. The current squamous cell lung carcinoma pathogenesis molecular abnormalities working model (Figure 3.4) indicates the following: (a) Genetic abnormalities originate in histologically normal epithelium and increase with escalating severity of histologic changes (111). (b) Mutations are sequential, with progressive allelic losses at multiple 3p (3p21, 3p14, 3p22–24, and 3p12) and 9p21 (*p16^{INK4a}*) chromosome sites as the earliest detected changes, followed by 8p21–23, 13q14 (*RB*), and 17p13 (*TP53*) (57,111,112). In addition to mutation, *p16^{INK4a}* methylation occurs in early-stage squamous preinvasive lesions

and increases in frequency with histologic disease progression (24% in squamous metaplasia and 50% in CIS) (113). (c) Respiratory epithelium of smokers and lung cancer patients presents extensive and multifocal molecular changes indicative of a field effect (field cancerization) (57,111,114–116). This field effect is presumably due to tobacco-related carcinogen exposure and results in widespread mutagenesis of the respiratory epithelium. (d) Multiple clonal and subclonal patches of molecular abnormalities (e.g., genomic instability and allelic losses) can be detected in the normal and slightly abnormal bronchial epithelium of patients with lung cancer from specimens obtained by fluorescent bronchoscopy (estimated to be ~40,000–360,000 cells) (117). Despite this progress, neither SCC precursor lesion histologic features nor molecular changes are yet to prove useful in predicting progression to invasive carcinoma (13,14).

Progenitors and Stem Cells

Classically, stem cells are located in a specialized niche and are preserved from overuse in maintaining tissue homeostatis for their conservation throughout the organism's life. As such, stem cells undergo infrequent cycling and stem cell compartments are identified based upon this characteristic. Progenitor cell compartments located near the stem cells are responsible for the majority of proliferation via "transient amplification" (118). Currently it is believed that four stem cell niches are present in adult airway pseudostratified epithelium (118). The four putative stem cell niches as one travels distally are (a) gland duct basal cells; (b) intercartilaginous zone surface basal

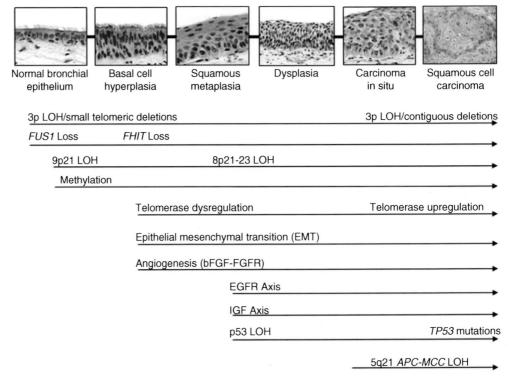

FIGURE 3.4 Sequential biomarkers and pathway changes in the stages of squamous cell carcinoma (SCC) progression. Summary of histopathologic and molecular alterations involved in lung SCC pathogenesis. Molecular changes begin at histologically normal epithelium. LOH, loss of heterozygosity.

cells; (c) bronchiolar Clara cells associated with pulmonary neuroendocrine cell (PNEC) bodies; and (d) broncholoalveolar duct junction variant Clara cells (118).

Of interest recently has been the latter niche, specifically bronchioloalveolar stems cells (BASCs). From mouse model studies, it has been shown that BASCs are putative stem cell initiators of *KRAS*-induced NSCLC adenocarcinoma (119). Regulators of BASCs include *PI3K*, (120), *PTEN* (121), *Bmil* (122), and miRNAs (123). In addition to the identification of BASCs, several stem cell markers in tumors have been identified. A rare population of cancer stem-like cells expressing *CD133* has been shown in SCLC and NSCLCs (124,125). These *CD133* positive cells also share expression of human stem cell markers including *CD24, CD29, CD31, CD34, CD44, CD326, CD34, BCRP1,* and *Oct4* (119,124–126). Of interest, each of these molecular biomarkers represents potential pathway targets in the treatment of NSCLC. For example, miR-34a has been shown to be a prognostic marker of NSCLC following surgical resection (127) and *CD133* positive tumors have been shown to be resistant to cisplatin therapy (128).

■ PROGRESSION TO METASTASIS

More than 70% of patients with NSCLC are diagnosed with incurable disease metastatic to lungs, liver, bone, and/or brain, with the incidence of brain and lymph node metastases as high as 65% (129,130). Brain metastases carry a particularly poor prognosis for NSCLC patients, and are associated with a 1-year survival rate of only 10% despite therapy (129,130). Patients with NSCLC brain metastases that become resistant or are not amenable to radiotherapy and surgery need effective drug therapies, but standard chemotherapy is only minimally and transiently effective. Mediastinal lymph node is the most frequent metastasis site for NSCLC, and their tumor involvement is a key criterion for NSCLC clinical and pathologic staging (131,132). Identifying tumor involvement of mediastinal lymph nodes is of great importance because its presence significantly affects outcomes and potential treatment adjuvant or neoadjuvant strategies (132).

There is currently a lack of clinical or biologic markers that can reliably predict the development of distant metastases in patients treated for NSCLC, as well as a lack of effective interventions once metastasis occurs. Although there have been several studies focused on identifying biomarkers that predict early recurrence and death in patients with NSCLC, only a handful of studies have focused on metastasis prediction, and these limited results have not yet identified reliable markers. The identification of markers to predict risk of metastases in patients may guide more aggressive and/or more personalized therapeutic or preventive strategies for those patients, and, thus, significantly improve outcomes.

D'Amico et al. (133) demonstrated that NSCLC patients with isolated brain relapse had significantly higher immunohistochemical expression of *TP53* and urokinase plasminogen activator. It was also shown that high levels of immunohistochemical expression of *EphA2* receptor kinase in primary NSCLC predict brain metastasis (134). Recently, *p-S6* has been shown to be overexpressed in metastases and that primary tumors exhibiting high *p-S6* expression were related to shorter metastatic-free survival (135).

In an attempt to elucidate the pattern of expression of targeted therapy-related biomarkers comparing lung cancer primary tumor and metastasis, studies have recently examined *EGFR* molecular biomarkers in NSCLC (136–140) primary tumors and corresponding lymph node and brain metastasis sites ((141–144)). Of interest, recent data showed that lymph node and brain metastasis sites demonstrate a different pattern of *EGFR* abnormalities including the immunhistochemical expression of *EGFR* protein and gene copy number changes (144). For brain metastasis, the active form of *EGFR* (phosphorylated, *p-EGFR*) was significantly overexpressed in metastasis sites compared with matched primary tumors (144). Primary tumors in patients that developed brain metastasis exhibited a significantly higher frequency (72%) of *EGFR*-increased copy number by FISH compared with tumors without metastasis (50%) (144). The brain metastasis sites demonstrated similar frequency of *EGFR*-increased copy number compared with primary tumors; however, the frequency of gene amplification was significantly higher in brain sites. For lymph node metastasis, total *EGFR* and p-*EGFR* demonstrated significantly higher levels in 20 metastasis sites compared with corresponding primary tumors, as well as higher levels of increased copy number by FISH (142). Recent data also suggest that the *EGFR* mutation precedes an increase in the number of copies of the gene in the pathogenesis of lung adenocarcinoma (142) and that the increase in the number of copies of *EGFR* is a phenomenon associated with tumor progression and metastasis. These data suggest that molecular abnormalities and the corresponding biomarkers express differently in tumor and metastasis, and to better utilize predictive biomarkers in advanced NSCLC they must be characterized in both settings.

■ MOLECULAR PROFILING OF NSCLC

As stated, the classification of lung cancers has traditionally been based primarily on histologic findings. However, it is clear that each histologic type can harbor distinct molecular characteristics that may determine the tumors' biological behavior. A large effort has been made to study multiple individual molecular abnormalities to identify unique characteristics of histologic subtypes of lung cancers that might have clinical relevance (2). Unfortunately, besides *EGFR* and *KRAS* mutations in adenocarcinoma, none of these individual candidates has proved to be unique for each histologic type of lung cancer. Molecular profiling studies that began with single or relatively small groups of genes or proteins have now progressed to large-scale and high-throughput methods using DNA-, RNA-, and protein-based approaches (Figure 3.5). These large-scale methods analyze thousands of genes at one time and have led to a better understanding of the complexity of gene abnormality patterns of lung cancer, and they have

accelerated the uncovering of novel genes involved in cancer pathogenesis.

Tissue Considerations

Clinical tissue specimens allow for the analysis of both histologic and molecular characteristics of lung cancer. Tumor tissue samples can be studied comparatively with metastases, different histologic subtypes, or matched normal tissues, and matched clinical data. The two main issues encountered using human tissue samples are fixation and tissue sample size/method of collection.

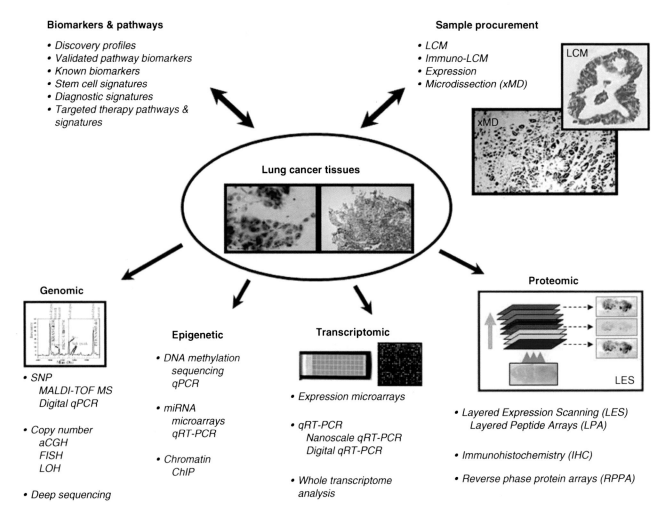

FIGURE 3.5 Molecular profiling of lung cancer. Lung cancer tissues in the form of resected specimens, core needle biopsies, and fine needle aspirates coupled with high-throughput molecular analysis methodologies can be used to elucidate the molecular characteristics of lung cancer. Sample procurement methods such as laser capture microdissection (LCM) (145), immuno-LCM (146), and expression microdissection (xMD) (147) are used to enrich tissue samples for pure cell populations by selectively procuring cell types of interest (e.g., tumor epithelial cells) from among the heterogeneous tissue sample. These tissues are then used for various molecular profiling analyses. Genetic analysis includes SNP analysis by matrix-assisted desorption/ionization time-of-flight mass spectrometry (MALDI-TOF MS) and quantitative PCR (qPCR), copy number variation analysis by array comparative genomic hybridization (aCGH), fluorescence in situ hybridization (FISH) and loss of heterozygosity, and deep sequencing. Epigenetic analysis includes DNA methylation analysis by sequencing and qPCR, micro RNA (miRNA) analysis by microarray and quantitative reverse transcription PCR (qRT-PCR), and chromatin analysis by chromatin immunoprecipitation (ChIP). Transcriptomic (gene expression) analysis by expression microarrays, qRT-PCR (both digital and nanoscale), and whole transcriptome analysis. Protein analysis by layered expression scanning (LES) (148), layered peptide arrays (LPA) (149,150), immunohistochemistry (IHC), and reverse phase protein arrays (151). Each of these molecular analysis techniques can be used with known biomarker profiles to screen lung cancer tissues, but they are also vital tools used to generate discovery profiles, validate pathway biomarkers, identify stem cell signatures, improve and expand diagnostic signatures, and identify targeted therapy-related pathways and signatures for use in patient care.

Formalin-fixed paraffin embedded (FFPE) tissues are the gold standard for making histologic diagnoses; however, molecular analysis is limited due to the inability to recover molecular analytes, particularly RNA and proteins, due to crosslinking and heat degradation (152–156). DNA, and to some extent RNA, can still be retrieved (152,154,155), and many new nucleic acid extraction and isolation kits have improved the recovery of RNA from FFPE (156). Alternative fixatives such as ethanol fixation with or without paraffin embedding are still being assessed for biomolecule preservation, but morphology is not as well preserved as with FFPE (157).

Snap-freezing of fresh tissue is optimal for downstream molecular analysis in terms of quantity and quality of biomolecules preserved and recovered. However, only recently have snap-frozen tissues been collected by pathology laboratories for clinical and research purposes (158,159). Unfortunately, tissue morphology is not retained by snap-freezing and extensive freeze-artifact is introduced. It is possible to discern tumor cells from normal and stroma, but pathologic diagnoses cannot be made using snap-frozen tissues. A matched FFPE tissue sample is used to make the diagnosis, and this diagnosis is recorded for the other matched tissue samples, regardless of fixative.

Tissue sample size must also be taken into consideration for downstream molecular analysis. Tissues range in size from resected specimens yielding bulk tissue samples and small chunks of tissues to smaller sizes such as CNB and finally to the smallest FNA. Resected specimens generally yield adequate tissue (i.e., millions of cells) to perform a multitude of molecular analysis techniques; however, CNBs and FNAs are limited in the amounts of cells recovered (i.e., 1,000 cells and often <2,000 cells of interest), making molecular analysis challenging.

In addition to the tissue sample size, it is important to take into consideration the heterogeneous cell populations (i.e., epithelial cells, neural cells, fibroblasts, lymphocytes, blood, endothelial cells, cartilage, etc.) contained within the sample size, and clinical samples often contain normal and tumor tissues of various disease grades. This heterogeneity in tissue sample components must be considered when performing molecular analysis of said tissue samples. For example, a recent study comparing microdissected tissue samples to matched whole tissue samples identified >1,000 gene-expression changes between primary tumor and corresponding metastasis using laser capture microdissection (LCM), but less than 1% of these changes were identifiable in nonmicrodissected material of the same samples (160). Moreover, tumor microenvironment studies demonstrate the significance of using microdissection techniques with tissue samples. For example, a study of GSTP1 methylation of microdissected tissues identified an epigenetically unique tumor-associated stroma microenvironment (161).

In addition, the use of microdissected tissues has demonstrated diverse gene-expression profiles between tumor-associated stroma and normal stroma (162). As important as microdissection has been shown to be and even with the advent of methods specifically for analysis of small microdissected tissue samples (163,164), it is often not possible to obtain enough cells of interest from a clinical tissue specimen to perform certain downstream molecular analysis techniques that require several micrograms of a specific analyte (e.g., DNA, RNA, miRNA, protein).

This is more of challenge with CNBs and FNAs, which generally do not yield micrograms of analytes, even without procuring a pure cell population from the tissue sample. However, a technical revolution has occurred in our ability to examine multiple molecular targets in tissue specimens at DNA, RNA, and protein levels (90,165,166), which have been recently extended to small archival diagnostic FNAs and CNBs (167,168). A current major obstacle is to be able to obtain tumor tissue from patients to perform these biomarker analyses. However, most NSCLC patients treated with standard or experimental therapies already have FNAs and/or CNBs available. Unfortunately, clinical and translational investigators are not taking advantage of those specimens. From 2003 to 2006, 30% of advanced NSCLC were diagnosed by FNA alone at The University of Texas M.D. Anderson Cancer Center (personal communication from Dr Daniel Karp, 2008). Approximately 40% of all cell blocks prepared from FNAs are usable for downstream analysis, with ~ 50% of this being tumor cells. Each cell block can be sectioned into 50 to 100 tissue sections with ~ 500 cells per section (personal communication from Dr Neda Kalhor, 2008). Also, combination of FNA and CNB substantially improves the rate of malignancy diagnosis (95.2%) compared with FNA or CNB alone (85.1% or 86.7%, respectively) (169).

In summary, tissue specimen size and tissue fixation play a large role in the ability to perform downstream molecular analysis. Each of these issues must be thoroughly considered and planned for, as the tissue size (with or without microdissection) and fixation type determines what type of molecular analysis can be performed.

DNA Copy Number Profiles

Chromosomal regions harboring TSG and oncogenes are often deleted or amplified. Deletions have been analyzed mostly by LOH studies using microsatellites (57,103). Amplifications have been investigated by comparative genomic hybridization (CGH) and SNP arrays (90,170,171). Although lung cancers have been profiled using CGH (171), few high-throughput and comprehensive whole genome efforts examining lung cancer tissue specimens are available (90,170). Recently, Weir et al. (90) reported a large-scale characterization of copy number alterations in a large set (n = 371) of lung adenocarcinomas using dense SNP arrays. Twenty-six of 39 autosomal chromosome arms showed consistent large-scale copy number gains or losses, of which only a handful were linked to a specific gene. The most common event, amplification of chromosome 14q13.3, was found in approximately 12% of tumors. On the basis of genomic and functional analyses, it was demonstrated that *NKX2–1* (NK2 homeobox 1, also called *TITF1*), which lies in the minimal 14q13.3 amplification interval and encodes a lineage-specific transcription factor (known as *TTF-1*), is a novel candidate oncogene involved in a significant subset of lung adenocarcinomas. In addition, other genes were shown to have an increased number of copies in adenocarcinoma, including *MDM2*, *MYC*, *CDK4*, *KRAS*, *TERT*, and *VGFA*. However, the results of the study indicated that many of the genes that are involved in lung adenocarcinoma remain to be discovered.

Epigenetics

The term "epigenetic" refers to a heritable change in the pattern of gene expression that is mediated by mechanisms other than alterations in the primary nucleotide sequence of a gene (172). This process controls the packaging and function of the human genome and plays an important role in normal development and disease, including cancer (173). This change in gene expression involves the methylation of DNA in promoter regions of genes, the sites where the transcription of DNA into RNA begins (172). Using high-throughput approaches, multiple known and putative TSGs have been described as inactivated by hypermethylation in lung cancer (174). Shames et al. (174) performed a genome-wide screen using a high-throughput global expression profiling approach in NSCLC cell lines and identified 132 genes induced from undetectable levels by 5′-aza-2′-deoxycytidine. Methylation analysis of a subset of these promoter regions in primary lung tumors and adjacent nonmalignant tissues showed that 31 genes were methylated in tumors and were not methylated in normal lung tissue or peripheral blood cells. Tsou et al. (175) identified 13 loci showing significant differential DNA methylation levels between tumor and nontumor lung tissue, and 8 of these showed highly significant hypermethylation in lung adenocarcinoma histology.

Different patterns of gene methylation have been found in the major histologic types of NSCLCs, with the methylation of *APC*, *CDH13*, and *RARβ* being significantly higher in adenocarcinomas than in SCC (95). In lung cancer, the most frequently hypermethylated gene seems to be the *RAS* association domain family 1 gene (*RASSF1*). Recently, it has been shown that methylation of three genes—*RASSF1A*, *RUNX3*, and *CDH13*—correlated with worse prognosis in patients with surgically resected NSCLC (176). Interestingly, *RUNX3* methylation

correlated with a worse prognosis in adenocarcinoma, whereas methylation of *RASSF1A* was associated with a worse prognosis in SCC. In multivariate analysis, both genes have been found to be independent prognostic factors of worse outcome (176). Recently, it has been shown that methylation of *p16^{Ink4}*, *CDH13*, *RASSF1A*, and *APC* in NSCLC stage I tumors and in histologically tumor-negative lymph nodes was associated with disease recurrence, independent of other clinical and pathologic factors (177). These findings suggest that methylation of four genes in patients with stage I NSCLC treated with curative intent by means of surgery is associated with early recurrence.

Gene-Expression (mRNA) Profiles

Among RNA-based methods, cDNA microarray is a powerful technique for the global analysis of gene expression. cDNA microarray technology has become a standard tool in molecular biology and has succeeded in identifying multiple crucial genes that are up- or down-regulated in a variety of tumors, including lung (60,178–185). Several groups have reported cDNA microarray-based molecular classification (60,178,179), prognosis (182–184), and response to treatment (185) of lung cancer. Most studies focusing on molecular classification have shown that cDNA microarray profiles recapitulate the morphologic classification of lung cancer (60,178). Recently, Potti et al. (183) developed a genomic strategy to refine prognosis in early-stage NSCLC by identifying a gene-expression profile that predicted the risk of recurrence in a cohort of 89 patients with stage I and II tumors. Then, they evaluated the predictor profile in two independent cohorts to find an overall predictive accuracy of 72% and 79%, respectively. In addition, a subgroup of patients with stage IA disease who were at high risk for recurrence and who might be best treated by adjuvant chemotherapy was identified. Recently, using cDNA microarray strategy coupled with quantitative polymerase chain reaction (PCR) analysis, Chen et al. (184) developed a five-gene signature (*DUSP6*, *MMD*, *STAT1*, *ERBB3*, and *LCK*) that correlated with clinical outcome in stages I and II NSCLC. This five-gene signature model was validated in two independent cohorts, and they closely associated with relapse-free and overall survival.

The only study of cDNA microarray associated with treatment response was performed by Oshita et al. (185) and determined that the gene-expression profile in peripheral blood obtained from 31 patients before chemotherapy (with paclitaxel and irinotecan) correlated with the outcome of treatment in patients with advanced NSCLC. Multivariate analysis revealed that genes encoding protein phosphatase, IL-1α, and IgA were independent predictive factors for chemosensitivity. On the basis of these findings, it was concluded that the expression of certain genes was able to predict the benefits of chemotherapy. Using in vitro drug sensitivity data coupled with cDNA microarray data, Potti et al. (186) developed gene-expression signatures that predicted sensitivity to individual chemotherapeutic drugs for several solid human tumors, including lung tumors. Each signature was validated with response data from an independent set of cell line studies. Of interest, signatures developed to predict response to individual agents, when combined, could also predict response to multidrug regimens. In summary, genomic profiles are providing a framework to move forward in the understanding of the complex gene-expression patterns of lung cancer and to pave the way of taking gene-expression profiling to the clinic.

miRNA Profiles

miRNAs are a recently discovered class of small (~18 to 24 mer) nucleic acids that negatively regulate gene expression (187). This novel class of molecules modulates a wide array of growth and differentiation processes in human cancers (187). An emerging number of studies have shown that miRNAs can act as oncogenes, as TSGs, or sometimes as both (188). High-throughput analyses have demonstrated that miRNA expression is commonly dysregulated in human cancer (187), including lung cancer (189–191). However, considerable disagreement remains with respect to the miRNA signature for specific cancer cell types, which appears to depend largely on the analytic platform (187). In lung cancer, miRNA profiles have been shown to correlate with disease outcome (189,191). Using real-time reverse transcription PCR, Yu et al. (191) identified a five-miRNA signature in NSCLC that predicts treatment outcome. In that study, patients with high-risk scores in their miRNA signatures showed poor overall and disease-free survivals compared with patients with low risk scores (191). In addition, it has been shown that miRNAs regulate several important pathways in lung cancer. Weiss et al. (192) showed that loss of miRNA-128b, located on chromosome 3p and a putative regulator of *EGFR*, correlated with response to targeted *EGFR* inhibition. Interestingly, loss of expression of microRNA-128b correlated with response to *EGFR* TKI in primary NSCLC. miRNA is an area of very active research that will have an impact on lung cancer pathogenesis and therapy.

Proteomic Profiles

Recently, it has been suggested that proteomics-based approaches complement the genomics initiatives and represent the next step in attempts to understand the biology of cancer. Because mRNA expression is not always correlated with levels of protein expression, cDNA-based gene-expression analysis cannot always indicate which proteins are expressed or how their activity might be modulated after translation (193). Accordingly, a comprehensive analysis of protein expression patterns in tissues might improve our ability to understand the molecular complexities of tumor cells. Among others, matrix-assisted laser desorption/ionization time-of-flight mass spectrometry (MALDI-TOF MS) can profile proteins in tissues (194). This technology can not only address peptides and proteins in sections of tumor tissues but also be used for high-resolution imaging of individual biomolecules present in tissue sections (194). Proteomic pattern analysis, using MALDI-TOF MS directly on small amounts of frozen lung tumor tissues, has been used to accurately classify and predict histologic groups as well as nodal involvement and patient survival in resected NSCLCs (195). Recently, reverse phase protein arrays (RPPA) have contributed to the characterization of NSCLC. Identification of *c-Src* and *STAT3*'s role in NSCLC by RPPA provided rationale to combine inhibition of these genes to improve clinical response (196). In addition, RPPA analysis of microdissected NSCLC tumors demonstrated that *EGFR*-mutant NSCLC cells putatively exhibit activation of the AKT/mTOR pathway (197). If these proteomic data are confirmed in larger series, the resulting analysis could have great prognostic and therapeutic implications for patients with NSCLC.

■ PREDICTIVE MARKERS OF NSCLC

Traditionally, the strongest predictor for NSCLC survival had been according to the tumor staging classification. Recently in NSCLC the number of metastatic organ sites has been shown to be a strong predictor of overall survival (198). But tumor stage and tumor load alone have not been sufficient predictive characteristics. Recent advances have taken place in the molecular classification of lung carcinomas and the identification of genetic and epigenetic aberrations in these cancers. Several studies have focused on the identification of biologic markers that predict early recurrence and death in patients with NSCLC. For example, molecular biologic substaging had been applied in the development of a prognostic model of recurrence in stage I NSCLC patients (133,199–201).

Chemotherapy Resistance Markers

Currently, platinum-based doublet combination chemotherapy (e.g., paclitaxel + carboplatin, Cisplatin + vinorelbine tartrate) is the standard of care for metastatic lung cancer (202). Chemotherapy triplet combination (gemcitabine hydrochloride + cisplatin + vinorelbine tartrate) has also been shown to be safe and effective in patients with advanced NSCLC (202). Recently, NSCLC subtype specific therapies have been approved: bevacizumab for nonsquamous NSCLC (203) (overall response rate = 35%) (204), and pemetrexed for adenocarcinoma and large cell carcinoma (205). However, not all patients are responsive to chemotherapy treatment. Molecular biomarker analysis studies have revealed a subset of markers that are putative predictors of chemotherapy resistance: *ERCC1*, *RRM1*, *TP53*, and *KRAS*.

ERCC1 is believed to be important in cisplatin-induced DNA damage repair (206), and overexpression of *ERCC1* protein is present in about 40% to 46% of NSCLC patients (207–209). Chemosensitivity assays of resected NSCLC tissue have demonstrated *ERCC1* expression correlation with cisplatin resistance (210). Cisplatin resistance appears to be the only chemotherapy treatment associated with *ERCC1* overexpression (210), as other studies have not correlated sensitivity to other chemotherapies such as paclitaxel, vinorelbine, etoposide, irinotecan, 5-fluorouracil, or gemcitabine (211–215). As such, assigning advanced NSCLC patients with high *ERCC1* mRNA expression to docetaxel plus gemcitabine chemotherapy instead of to docetaxel plus cisplatin has significantly improved the response rate by 39.3% in a phase III trial (216).

ERCC1-negative tumors tend to respond better to chemotherapy treatment than tumors overexpressing *ERCC1*. Some studies have shown *ERCC1*-negative tumors to be correlated with a trend toward or a significantly higher response rate (208,217–219). Patients with *ERCC1*-negative or low expressing tumors have also demonstrated a trend toward or a statistically significant longer overall survival or median progression-free survival (207–209,211–214), and improved chemotherapy survival benefit has been shown in patients with resection of *ERCC1*-negative tumors (207).

RRM1 encodes the ribonucleotide reductase regulatory subunit and thus is important in DNA repair. This regulatory subunit is molecular target of gemcitabine (219). In vitro association between *RRM1* and gemcitabine resistance has been substantially demonstrated (219–223). In similar studies, the addition of agents to prevent or reverse *RRM1* gene amplification (i.e., bexarotene) and siRNA have been shown to reduce gemcitabine resistance in cell lines overexpressing *RRM1* (which prevents or reverses *RRM1* gene amplification (222,224). Advanced NSCLC tissue studies have also demonstrated a strong correlation between *ERCC1* and *RRM1* expression levels (213,225,226) with several studies suggesting a connection to gemcitabine efficacy.

TP53 mutations are present in 40% to 90% of resected NSCLC tumors (227–229). The type of *Tp53* mutation and sensitivity to chemotherapy agents has not been identified (228,230), but the ability of *Tp53* mutations to produce chemotherapy resistance has been associated with mutation type (231). Several NSCLC clinical studies have also assessed the relationship between tumor *Tp53* mutations or IHC expression and outcome, and findings have been inconsistent across studies. In many of these studies, platinum agents were combined with one or more other agents, and in studies using more than one combination, there was generally no breakdown with respect to interaction (if any) of *Tp53* abnormality and individual agent added to the platinum. Hence, it remains possible that some of the inconsistency is due to differences between different agents with respect to impact of the *Tp53* abnormality. In patients receiving preoperative neoadjuvant cisplatin plus etoposide and radiation (232) or in patients receiving cisplatin-based combinations for advanced disease (233), presence of mutant *Tp53* in tumor (defined by DNA sequencing) was associated with significantly lower response rates and shorter overall survival compared with patients with wild-type *Tp53*, while there was no significant association between response and tumor *Tp53* mutation status in patients with locally advanced NSCLC treated with radiotherapy and a taxane (without a platinum) (229). In studies analyzing NSCLC response to neoadjuvant or locally advanced treatment, presence of *Tp53* by IHC has been associated with shorter survival, lower probability of response, and lower response rates (212,234–247).

KRAS mutations have been shown in 26% of lung adenocarcinomas and specifically 21% of NSCLCs (248,249) which are associated with significantly worse (250). *KRAS* mutation has been correlated with resistance to paclitaxel in NSCLC (251), but has not been correlated with resistance or improved survival with other treatments (248,249,252). Of interest, taxane-refractory NSCLC patients receiving lonafarnib (inhibits mutant *KRAS* function) with paclitaxel have demonstrated a 10% response rate and 38% stable disease (253), suggesting lonafarnib putatively augments paclitaxel efficacy.

Targeted Therapy

Advances in understanding the molecular pathogenesis of lung cancer have provided a unique opportunity to attack advanced lung cancer by targeted therapy (254). Examination of molecular abnormalities in tumors is becoming increasingly important and requires adequate integration of routine pathologic and molecular examinations to achieve more accurate diagnoses and classifications. Likewise the development of biomarker "signatures" (such as mRNA expression profiles) from tumors that provide information on the prognosis and predict the response of individual patient's tumors to specified therapy would be major steps forward. In addition, an effective targeted therapy also needs biomarkers to precisely predict or monitor tumor response or resistance to cytotoxic and targeted agents (5).

Currently, there are no good clinical or biologic markers to predict outcomes of targeted therapy. Several studies have focused on the identification of biologic markers that predict early recurrence and death in patients with NSCLC; however, few studies have focused on indicators of success for targeted therapy. Never-smokers frequently have *EGFR* mutations, respond to TKI drugs (e.g., gefitinib, erlotinib), and develop resistance to TKI drugs (137–139). On the other hand, ever-smokers are generally resistant to *EGFR* TKIs but more commonly have *KRAS* mutations (77,255).

EGFR was the first receptor tyrosine kinase to be discovered (136). Constitutive activation of mutated *EGFR* leads to receptor dimerization and intracellular autophosphorylation of the activation loop of the protein tyrosine kinase domain, leading to a cascade of intracellular events that cause cellular proliferation and tumor invasion (136). *EGFR* TKIs are the first two targeted agents recently approved for the treatment of NSCLC in the United States. These *EGFR* TKIs produce responses in approximately 10% of patients with NSCLC that has progressed with prior chemotherapy (137–139). In patients with NSCLC who benefit from gefitinib or erlotinib, the responses can be dramatic and may last for longer than a year (137–139,256). Several markers have been identified that predict response to the *EGFR*-specific TKIs in patients with NSCLC. Activating mutations in the *EGFR* tyrosine kinase domain (exons 18–21), increased gene copy number, and increased protein expression have been associated with favorable response to *EGFR* TKIs (137–139,256). Recently, in addition to *EGFR*, 25 other gene somatic mutations in seven significantly mutated pathways (*EGFR*, *FGFR*, *PDGFR*, *BEGFR*, *NTRK*, *EPhA/B*, and *INSR*) have been identified from 188 human lung adenocarcinomas at significantly high frequencies and are thus thought to be involved in lung carcinogenesis (97).

Although targeting *EGFR* mutated (exon 19 deletions or L858R mutation) NSCLCs with TKIs (gefitinib/erlotinib) has been effective, the majority of these patients acquire resistance to the *EGFR* TKI therapy (257,258) in an average of 6 to 12 months (259). A secondary *EGFR* T790M mutation has been shown to occur in 50% of *EGFR* TKI resistant patients; representing one of two hypothesized resistance mechanisms (259). The other putative resistance mechanism which is present in 20% of TKI resistant NSCLCs is an "oncogene kinase switch" system represented by amplification of MET oncogene. However, half of cases with MET amplification also have the *EGFR* T790M mutation (259) and it has been demonstrated that *MET* amplification is not a suitable marker for identifying *EGFR* TKI resistance (260). Researchers have been working to identify ways to counteract these resistance mechanisms. Currently,

in vitro analysis has shown that TKI resistant NSCLCs can be treated by administering *PI3K-mTOR* and *MEK* signaling inhibitors simultaneously with *EGFR* TKIs (261); but, to date this has not been tested in patient populations.

■ CONCLUSION

In contrast to most other organs, the lungs demonstrate a very wide range of epithelial tumors that vary in their location and histology. These tumors show varying degrees of relationship to smoke exposure, with the central carcinomas showing the greatest relationship. The molecular lesions found in the tumors share certain common elements and have characteristic changes. Their precursor lesions also differ, with some being well defined, whereas others are poorly understood because of the difficulty of identifying them before surgical resection of an existing tumor. Thus, their natural history is also poorly understood.

During the last decade, encouraged by the development of methodologies for isolation of cells from small histologic lesions, such as laser microdissection, combined with techniques to perform genomic studies from minute amount of DNA, RNA, and protein, several groups have made substantial progress in unveiling the molecular and genetic abnormalities of lung cancer precursor lesions, including those evolving to centrally located SCC and peripheral adenocarcinoma. The recent development of a panel of human normal bronchial epithelial cells immortalized with telomerase and CdK4-mediated *p16^{INK4a}* bypass which can be modified with a combination of oncogenes activation and TSG knockdowns for in vitro discovery work (262), coupled with the development of more relevant lung cancer animal models (263) and new high-throughput genomic (255) and proteomic (195,264) profiling techniques that can be applied to small amount of microdissected tissues may stimulate the scientific community to perform innovative investigations in the fields of molecular and pathologic research to understand the molecular malignant potential of respiratory epithelium even before histologic changes occur. The advent of newer molecular genetic methods to examine lung tumor and preneoplastic lesion tissue specimens will help delineate all the significant molecular abnormalities responsible for lung cancer development and progression.

The ultimate goal is to be able to identify all molecular changes present in any one patient's tumor and to use this information for early molecular detection, prediction of biological/clinical behavior and prognosis, and selection or rational development of therapeutics.

■ ACKNOWLEDGMENTS

The authors thank Dr. David Stewart for discussions regarding chemotherapy resistance.

■ REFERENCES

1. Jemal A, Siegel R, Ward E, et al. Cancer statistics, 2008. *CA Cancer J Clin.* 2008;58(2):71–96.

2. Minna JD, Roth JA, Gazdar AF. Focus on lung cancer. *Cancer Cell.* 2002;1(1):49–52.

3. Travis WD, Brambilla E, Muller-Hermelink HK, et al., Tumours of the lung. In: Travis WD, Brambilla E, Muller-Hermelink HK, et al., eds. Pathology and Genetics: Tumours of the Lung, Pleura,Thymus And Heart. Lyon: International Agency for Research on Cancer (IARC); 2004:9–124.

4. Hanahan D, Weinberg RA. The hallmarks of cancer. *Cell.* 2000;100(1):57–70.

5. Fong KM, Sekido Y, Gazdar AF, Minna JD. Lung cancer. 9: Molecular biology of lung cancer: clinical implications. *Thorax.* 2003;58(10):892–900.

6. Herbst RS, Sandler AB. Overview of the current status of human epidermal growth factor receptor inhibitors in lung cancer. *Clin Lung Cancer.* 2004;6(suppl 1):S7–S19.

7. Herbst RS, Onn A, Sandler A. Angiogenesis and lung cancer: prognostic and therapeutic implications. *J Clin Oncol.* 2005;23(14):3243–3256.

8. Herbst RS, Heymach JV, Lippman SM. Lung cancer. *N Engl J Med.* 2008;359(13):1367–1380.

9. Wistuba II, Mao L, Gazdar AF. Smoking molecular damage in bronchial epithelium. *Oncogene.* 2002;21(48):7298–7306.

10. Westra WH. Early glandular neoplasia of the lung. *Respir Res.* 2000;1(3):163–169.

11. Colby TV, Wistuba II, Gazdar A. Precursors to pulmonary neoplasia. *Adv Anat Pathol.* 1998;5(4):205–215.

12. Kerr KM. Pulmonary preinvasive neoplasia. *J Clin Pathol.* 2001;54(4):257–271.

13. Wistuba II. Histologic evaluation of bronchial squamous lesions: any role in lung cancer risk assessment? *Clin Cancer Res.* 2005;11(4):1358–1360.

14. Wistuba II. Genetics of preneoplasia: lessons from lung cancer. *Curr Mol Med.* 2007;7(1):3–14.

15. Kitamura H, Kameda Y, Ito T, Hayashi H. Atypical adenomatous hyperplasia of the lung. Implications for the pathogenesis of peripheral lung adenocarcinoma. *Am J Clin Pathol.* 1999;111(5):610–622.

16. Osanai M, Igarashi T, Yoshida Y. Unique cellular features in atypical adenomatous hyperplasia of the lung: ultrastructural evidence of its cytodifferentiation. *Ultrastruct Pathol.* 2001;25(5):367–373.

17. Aguayo SM, Miller YE, Waldron JA Jr, et al. Brief report: idiopathic diffuse hyperplasia of pulmonary neuroendocrine cells and airways disease. *N Engl J Med.* 1992;327(18):1285–1288.

18. Armas OA, White DA, Erlanson RA, et al. Diffuse idiopathic pulmonary neuroendocrine cell proliferation presenting as interstitial lung disease. *Am J Surg Pathol.* 1995;19:963–970.

19. Wistuba II, Berry J, Behrens C, et al. Molecular changes in the bronchial epithelium of patients with small cell lung cancer. *Clin Cancer Res.* 2000;6(7):2604–2610.

20. Mountain CF. Revisions in the International System for Staging Lung Cancer. *Chest.* 1997;111(6):1710–1717.

21. Berghmans T. [News for lung cancer care]. *Rev Med Brux.* 2009;30(4):287–291.

22. Goldstraw P. The 7th Edition of TNM in Lung Cancer: what now? *J Thorac Oncol.* 2009;4(6):671–673.

23. Kassis ES, Vaporciyan AA, Swisher SG, et al. Application of the revised lung cancer staging system (IASLC Staging Project) to a cancer center population. *J Thorac Cardiovasc Surg.* 2009;138(2):412–418.e1.

24. Goldstraw P, Crowley J, Chansky K, et al.; International Association for the Study of Lung Cancer International Staging Committee; Participating Institutions. The IASLC Lung Cancer Staging Project: proposals for the revision of the TNM stage groupings in the forthcoming (seventh) edition of the TNM Classification of malignant tumours. *J Thorac Oncol.* 2007;2(8):706–714.

25. Argiris A, Murren JR. Staging and clinical prognostic factors for small-cell lung cancer. *Cancer J.* 2001;7(5):437–447.

26. Vallières E, Shepherd FA, Crowley J, et al.; International Association for the Study of Lung Cancer International Staging Committee and Participating Institutions. The IASLC Lung Cancer Staging Project: proposals regarding the relevance of TNM in the pathologic staging of small cell lung cancer in the forthcoming (seventh) edition of the TNM classification for lung cancer. *J Thorac Oncol.* 2009;4(9):1049–1059.

27. Brambilla E, Travis WD, Colby TV, Corrin B, Shimosato Y. The new World Health Organization classification of lung tumours. *Eur Respir J.* 2001;18(6):1059–1068.

28. Shimosato Y, Suzuki A, Hashimoto T, et al. Prognostic implications of fibrotic focus (scar) in small peripheral lung cancers. *Am J Surg Pathol.* 1980;4(4):365–373.

29. Travis WD, Garg K, Franklin WA, et al. Evolving concepts in the pathology and computed tomography imaging of lung adenocarcinoma and bronchioloalveolar carcinoma. *J Clin Oncol.* 2005;23(14):3279–3287.

30. Colby TV, Noguchi M, Henschke C, et al. Tumours of the lung. Adenocarcinoma. In: Travis WD, Brambilla E, Muller-Hermelink HK, et al., eds. *Pathology and Genetics: Tumours of the Lung, Pleura, Thymus And Heart.* Lyon: IARC Press, 2004:35–44.

31. Hammar SP, Brambilla C, Pugatch B, et al. Tumours of the lung. Squamous cell carcinoma. In: Travis WD, Brambilla E, Muller-Hermelink HK, et al., eds. *Pathology and Genetics: Tumours of the Lung, Pleura, Thymus And Heart.* Lyon: IARC Press; 2004:26–34.

32. Colby TV, Koss MN, Travis WD. Tumors of the lower respiratory tract, 3rd. Series, fascicle 13. In: Rosai J, Sobin LH, eds. *Atlas of Tumor Pathology.* Washington, DC: Armed Forces Institute of Pathology; 1995:1–554.

33. Jang KM, Lee KS, Shim YM, et al. The rates and CT patterns of locoregional recurrence after resection surgery of lung cancer: correlation with histopathology and tumor staging. *J Thorac Imaging.* 2003;18(4):225–230.

34. Brambilla C, Travis WD. Tumours of the lung. Adenosquamous carcinoma. In: Travis WD, Brambilla E, Muller-Hermelink HK, et al., eds. *Pathology and Genetics: Tumours of the Lung, Pleura, Thymus And Heart.* Lyon: IARC Press; 2004:51–52.

35. Brambilla C, Pugatch B, Geisinger K et al., Tumours of the lung. Large cell carcinoma. In: Travis WD, Brambilla E, Muller-Hermelink HK, et al., eds. *Pathology and Genetics: Tumours of the Lung, Pleura, Thymus and Heart.* Lyon: IARC Press, 2004:45–50 p

36. Takei H, Asamura H, Maeshima A, et al. Large cell neuroendocrine carcinoma of the lung: a clinicopathologic study of eighty-seven cases. *J Thorac Cardiovasc Surg.* 2002;124(2):285–292.

37. Pittaluga S, Wong MP, Chung LP, Loke SL. Clonal Epstein-Barr virus in lymphoepithelioma-like carcinoma of the lung. *Am J Surg Pathol.* 1993;17(7):678–682.

38. Kobayashi M, Ito M, Sano K, Honda T, Nakayama J. Pulmonary lymphoepithelioma-like carcinoma: predominant infiltration of tumor-associated cytotoxic T lymphocytes might represent the enhanced tumor immunity. *Intern Med.* 2004;43(4):323–326.

39. Corrin B, Chang YL, Rossi G, et al. Tumors of the lung. Sarcomatoid carcinoma. In: Travis WD, Brambilla E, Muller-Hermelink HK, et al., eds. Pathology and genetics: Tumours of the lung, pleura, thymus and heart. Lyon, IARC Press, 2004: 53–58 p

40. Rossi G, Cavazza A, Sturm N, et al. Pulmonary carcinomas with pleomorphic, sarcomatoid, or sarcomatous elements: a clinicopathologic and immunohistochemical study of 75 cases. *Am J Surg Pathol*. 2003;27(3):311–324.

41. Wick MR, Ritter JH, Humphrey PA. Sarcomatoid carcinomas of the lung: a clinicopathologic review. *Am J Clin Pathol*. 1997;108(1):40–53.

42. Travis WD, Nicholson S, Hirsch F, et al., Tumours of the lung. Small cell carcinoma. In: Travis WD, Brambilla E, Muller-Hermelink HK, et al., eds. Pathology and genetics: Tumours of the lung, pleura, thymus and heart. Lyon, IARC Press, 2004: 31–34 p

43. Nicholson SA, Beasley MB, Brambilla E, et al. Small cell lung carcinoma (SCLC): a clinicopathologic study of 100 cases with surgical specimens. *Am J Surg Pathol*. 2002;26(9):1184–1197.

44. Abrams J, Doyle LA, Aisner J. Staging, prognostic factors, and special considerations in small cell lung cancer. *Semin Oncol*. 1988;15(3):261–277.

45. Flieder DB. Neuroendocrine tumors of the lung: recent developments in histopathology. *Curr Opin Pulm Med*. 2002;8(4):275–280.

46. Beasley MB, Thunissen FB, Hasleton PS, et al., Tumours of the lung. Carcinoid tumor. In: Travis WD, Brambilla E, Muller-Hermelink HK, et al., eds. Pathology and genetics: Tumours of the lung, pleura, thymus and heart. Lyon, IARC Press, 2004: 59–62 p

47. Travis WD, Rush W, Flieder DB, et al. Survival analysis of 200 pulmonary neuroendocrine tumors with clarification of criteria for atypical carcinoid and its separation from typical carcinoid. *Am J Surg Pathol*. 1998;22(8):934–944.

48. Beasley MB, Thunnissen FB, Brambilla E, et al. Pulmonary atypical carcinoid: predictors of survival in 106 cases. *Hum Pathol*. 2000;31(10):1255–1265.

49. Rossi G, Pelosi G, Graziano P, Barbareschi M, Papotti M. A reevaluation of the clinical significance of histological subtyping of non–small-cell lung carcinoma: diagnostic algorithms in the era of personalized treatments. *Int J Surg Pathol*. 2009;17(3):206–218.

50. Capelozzi VL. Role of immunohistochemistry in the diagnosis of lung cancer. *J Bras Pneumol*. 2009;35(4):375–382.

51. Jagirdar J. Application of immunohistochemistry to the diagnosis of primary and metastatic carcinoma to the lung. *Arch Pathol Lab Med*. 2008;132(3):384–396.

52. Fong KM, Minna JD. Molecular biology of lung cancer: clinical implications. *Clin Chest Med*. 2002;23(1):83–101.

53. Knudson AG Jr. Mutation and cancer: statistical study of retinoblastoma. *Proc Natl Acad Sci USA*. 1971;68(4):820–823.

54. Knudson AG Jr. The ninth Gordon Hamilton-Fairley memorial lecture. Hereditary cancers: clues to mechanisms of carcinogenesis. *Br J Cancer*. 1989;59(5):661–666.

55. Soda M, Choi YL, Enomoto M, et al. Identification of the transforming EML4-ALK fusion gene in non-small-cell lung cancer. *Nature*. 2007;448(7153):561–566.

56. Inamura K, Takeuchi K, Togashi Y, et al. EML4-ALK fusion is linked to histological characteristics in a subset of lung cancers. *J Thorac Oncol*. 2008;3(1):13–17.

57. Wistuba II, Behrens C, Virmani AK, et al. High resolution chromosome 3p allelotyping of human lung cancer and preneoplastic/preinvasive bronchial epithelium reveals multiple, discontinuous sites of 3p allele loss and three regions of frequent breakpoints. *Cancer Res*. 2000;60(7):1949–1960.

58. Toyooka S, Toyooka KO, Maruyama R, et al. DNA methylation profiles of lung tumors. *Mol Cancer Ther*. 2001;1(1):61–67.

59. Wistuba II, Gazdar AF, Minna JD. Molecular genetics of small cell lung carcinoma. *Semin Oncol*. 2001;28(2 suppl 4):3–13.

60. Bhattacharjee A, Richards WG, Staunton J, et al. Classification of human lung carcinomas by mRNA expression profiling reveals distinct adenocarcinoma subclasses. *Proc Natl Acad Sci USA*. 2001;98(24):13790–13795.

61. Garber AC, Shu MA, Hu J, Renne R. DNA binding and modulation of gene expression by the latency-associated nuclear antigen of Kaposi's sarcoma-associated herpesvirus. *J Virol*. 2001;75(17):7882–7892.

62. Shigematsu H, Lin L, Takahashi T, et al. Clinical and biological features associated with epidermal growth factor receptor gene mutations in lung cancers. *J Natl Cancer Inst*. 2005;97(5):339–346.

63. Shigematsu H, Takahashi T, Nomura M, et al. Somatic mutations of the her2 kinase domain in lung adenocarcinomas. *Cancer Res*. 2005;65(5):1642–1646.

64. Davies H, Bignell GR, Cox C, et al. Mutations of the braf gene in human cancer. *Nature*. 2002;417(6892):949–954.

65. Brose MS, Volpe P, Feldman M, et al. Braf and ras mutations in human lung cancer and melanoma. *Cancer Res*. 2002;62(23):6997–7000.

66. Sun S, Schiller JH, Gazdar AF. Lung cancer in never smokers—a different disease. *Nat Rev Cancer*. 2007;7(10):778–790.

67. Wistuba I, Gazdar A. Lung cancer prenoplasia. *Annu Rev Pathol Mech Dis*. 2006;1:331–348.

68. Shaw AT, Yeap BY, Mino-Kenudson M, et al. Clinical features and outcome of patients with non-small-cell lung cancer who harbor eml4-alk. *J Clin Oncol*. 2009;27(26):4247–4253.

69. Koivunen JP, Mermel C, Zejnullahu K, et al. Eml4-alk fusion gene and efficacy of an alk kinase inhibitor in lung cancer. *Clin Cancer Res*. 2008;14(13):4275–4283.

70. Riely GJ, Kris MG, Rosenbaum D, et al. Frequency and distinctive spectrum of kras mutations in never smokers with lung adenocarcinoma. *Clin Cancer Res*. 2008;14(18):5731–5734.

71. Raso MG, Behrens C, Herynk MH, et al. Immunohistochemical expression of estrogen and progesterone receptors identifies a subset of nsclcs and correlates with egfr mutation. *Clin Cancer Res*. 2009;15(17):5359–5368.

72. Seike M, Yanaihara N, Bowman ED, et al. Use of a cytokine gene expression signature in lung adenocarcinoma and the surrounding tissue as a prognostic classifier. *J Natl Cancer Inst*. 2007;99(16):1257–1269.

73. Slebos RJ, Rodenhuis S. The ras gene family in human non-small-cell lung cancer. *J Natl Cancer Inst Monographs*. 1992;13:23–29.

74. Zudaire I, Lozano MD, Vazquez MF, et al. Molecular characterization of small peripheral lung tumors based on the analysis of fine needle aspirates. *Histol Histopathol*. 2008;23(1):33–40.

75. Paez JG, Jänne PA, Lee JC, et al. EGFR mutations in lung cancer: correlation with clinical response to gefitinib therapy. *Science*. 2004;304(5676):1497–1500.

76. Lynch TJ, Bell DW, Sordella R, et al. Activating mutations in the epidermal growth factor receptor underlying responsiveness of non-small-cell lung cancer to gefitinib. *N Engl J Med*. 2004;350(21):2129–2139.

77. Pao W, Miller V, Zakowski M, et al. EGF receptor gene mutations are common in lung cancers from "never smokers" and are associated with sensitivity of tumors to gefitinib and erlotinib. *Proc Natl Acad Sci USA*. 2004;101(36):13306–13311.

78. Huang SF, Liu HP, Li LH, et al. High frequency of epidermal growth factor receptor mutations with complex patterns in non-small cell lung cancers related to gefitinib responsiveness in Taiwan. *Clin Cancer Res*. 2004;10(24):8195–8203.

79. Kosaka T, Yatabe Y, Endoh H, Kuwano H, Takahashi T, Mitsudomi T. Mutations of the epidermal growth factor receptor gene in lung cancer: biological and clinical implications. *Cancer Res*. 2004;64(24):8919–8923.

80. Tokumo M, Toyooka S, Kiura K, et al. The relationship between epidermal growth factor receptor mutations and clinicopathologic features in non-small cell lung cancers. *Clin Cancer Res*. 2005;11(3):1167–1173.

81. Amann J, Kalyankrishna S, Massion PP, et al. Aberrant epidermal growth factor receptor signaling and enhanced sensitivity to EGFR inhibitors in lung cancer. *Cancer Res*. 2005;65(1):226–235.

82. Gazdar AF, Shigematsu H, Herz J, Minna JD. Mutations and addiction to EGFR: the Achilles 'heal' of lung cancers? *Trends Mol Med*. 2004;10(10):481–486.

83. Hirsch FR, Varella-Garcia M, Bunn PA Jr, et al. Epidermal growth factor receptor in non-small-cell lung carcinomas: correlation between gene copy number and protein expression and impact on prognosis. *J Clin Oncol.* 2003;21(20):3798–3807.

84. Cappuzzo F, Hirsch FR, Rossi E, et al. Epidermal growth factor receptor gene and protein and gefitinib sensitivity in non-small-cell lung cancer. *J Natl Cancer Inst.* 2005;97(9):643–655.

85. Tsao MS, Sakurada A, Cutz JC, et al. Erlotinib in lung cancer - molecular and clinical predictors of outcome. *N Engl J Med.* 2005;353(2):133–144.

86. Hirsch FR, Varella-Garcia M, McCoy J, et al.; Southwest Oncology Group. Increased epidermal growth factor receptor gene copy number detected by fluorescence in situ hybridization associates with increased sensitivity to gefitinib in patients with bronchioloalveolar carcinoma subtypes: a Southwest Oncology Group Study. *J Clin Oncol.* 2005;23(28):6838–6845.

87. Jackman DM, Holmes AJ, Lindeman N, et al. Response and resistance in a non-small-cell lung cancer patient with an epidermal growth factor receptor mutation and leptomeningeal metastases treated with high-dose gefitinib. *J Clin Oncol.* 2006;24(27):4517–4520.

88. Massarelli E, Varella-Garcia M, Tang X, et al. KRAS mutation is an important predictor of resistance to therapy with epidermal growth factor receptor tyrosine kinase inhibitors in non-small-cell lung cancer. *Clin Cancer Res.* 2007;13(10):2890–2896.

89. Bunn PA Jr, Dziadziuszko R, Varella-Garcia M, et al. Biological markers for non-small cell lung cancer patient selection for epidermal growth factor receptor tyrosine kinase inhibitor therapy. *Clin Cancer Res.* 2006;12(12):3652–3656.

90. Weir BA, Woo MS, Getz G, et al. Characterizing the cancer genome in lung adenocarcinoma. *Nature.* 2007;450(7171):893–898.

91. Tanaka H, Matsumura A, Ohta M, Ikeda N, Kitahara N, Iuchi K. Late sequelae of lobectomy for primary lung cancer: fibrobullous changes in ipsilateral residual lobes. *Eur J Cardiothorac Surg.* 2007;32(6):859–862.

92. Ikeda N, Takahashi H, Hiyoshi T, et al. [Resection of recurrent lung cancer]. *Kyobu Geka.* 1995;48(1):43–46.

93. Yatabe Y, Kosaka T, Takahashi T, Mitsudomi T. EGFR mutation is specific for terminal respiratory unit type adenocarcinoma. *Am J Surg Pathol.* 2005;29(5):633–639.

94. Toyooka S, Tsuda T, Gazdar AF. The TP53 gene, tobacco exposure, and lung cancer. *Hum Mutat.* 2003;21(3):229–239.

95. Toyooka S, Maruyama R, Toyooka KO, et al. Smoke exposure, histologic type and geography-related differences in the methylation profiles of non-small cell lung cancer. *Int J Cancer.* 2003;103(2):153–160.

96. Toyooka S, Suzuki M, Maruyama R, et al. The relationship between aberrant methylation and survival in non-small-cell lung cancers. *Br J Cancer.* 2004;91(4):771–774.

97. Ding L, Getz G, Wheeler DA, et al. Somatic mutations affect key pathways in lung adenocarcinoma. *Nature.* 2008;455(7216):1069–1075.

98. Ji H, Ramsey MR, Hayes DN, et al. LKB1 modulates lung cancer differentiation and metastasis. *Nature.* 2007;448(7155):807–810.

99. Bass AJ, Watanabe H, Mermel CH, et al. SOX2 is an amplified lineage-survival oncogene in lung and esophageal squamous cell carcinomas. *Nat Genet.* 2009;41(11):1238–1242.

100. Przygodzki RM, Finkelstein SD, Langer JC, et al. Analysis of p53, K-ras-2, and C-raf-1 in pulmonary neuroendocrine tumors. Correlation with histological subtype and clinical outcome. *Am J Pathol.* 1996;148(5):1531–1541.

101. Onuki N, Wistuba II, Travis WD, et al. Genetic changes in the spectrum of neuroendocrine lung tumors. *Cancer.* 1999;85(3):600–607.

102. Wistuba II, Gazdar AF. Molecular pathology of lung cancer. *Verh Dtsch Ges Pathol.* 2000;84:96–105.

103. Girard L, Zöchbauer-Müller S, Virmani AK, Gazdar AF, Minna JD. Genome-wide allelotyping of lung cancer identifies new regions of allelic loss, differences between small cell lung cancer and non-small cell lung cancer, and loci clustering. *Cancer Res.* 2000;60(17):4894–4906.

104. Franklin W, Wistuba I, Geisinger K et al., Squamous dysplasia and carcinoma in situ. In: Travis W, Brambilla E, Muller-Hermelink HK, et al., eds. *Pathology and Genetics. Tumors of the Lung, Pleura, Thymus and Heart.* Lyon, International Agency for Research on Cancer (IARC); 2004:68–72.

105. Lam S, leRiche JC, Zheng Y, et al. Sex-related differences in bronchial epithelial changes associated with tobacco smoking. *J Natl Cancer Inst.* 1999;91(8):691–696.

106. Westra WH, Baas IO, Hruban RH, et al. K-ras oncogene activation in atypical alveolar hyperplasias of the human lung. *Cancer Res.* 1996;56(9):2224–2228.

107. Tominaga M, Sueoka N, Irie K, et al. Detection and discrimination of preneoplastic and early stages of lung adenocarcinoma using hnRNP B1 combined with the cell cycle-related markers p16, cyclin D1, and Ki-67. *Lung Cancer.* 2003;40(1):45–53.

108. Nakanishi K, Kawai T, Kumaki F, Hiroi S, Mukai M, Ikeda E. Survivin expression in atypical adenomatous hyperplasia of the lung. *Am J Clin Pathol.* 2003;120(5):712–719.

109. Tang X, Shigematsu H, Bekele BN, et al. EGFR tyrosine kinase domain mutations are detected in histologically normal respiratory epithelium in lung cancer patients. *Cancer Res.* 2005;65(17):7568–7572.

110. Yoshida Y, Shibata T, Kokubu A, et al. Mutations of the epidermal growth factor receptor gene in atypical adenomatous hyperplasia and bronchioloalveolar carcinoma of the lung. *Lung Cancer.* 2005;50(1):1–8.

111. Wistuba II, Behrens C, Milchgrub S, et al. Sequential molecular abnormalities are involved in the multistage development of squamous cell lung carcinoma. *Oncogene.* 1999;18(3):643–650.

112. Wistuba II, Behrens C, Virmani AK, et al. Allelic losses at chromosome 8p21–23 are early and frequent events in the pathogenesis of lung cancer. *Cancer Res.* 1999;59(8):1973–1979.

113. Belinsky SA, Nikula KJ, Palmisano WA, et al. Aberrant methylation of p16(INK4a) is an early event in lung cancer and a potential biomarker for early diagnosis. *Proc Natl Acad Sci USA.* 1998;95(20):11891–11896.

114. Wistuba II, Lam S, Behrens C, et al. Molecular damage in the bronchial epithelium of current and former smokers. *J Natl Cancer Inst.* 1997;89(18):1366–1373.

115. Mao L, Lee JS, Kurie JM, et al. Clonal genetic alterations in the lungs of current and former smokers. *J Natl Cancer Inst.* 1997;89:857–862.

116. Wistuba II, Meyerson M. Chromosomal deletions and progression of premalignant lesions: less is more. *Cancer Prev Res (Phila Pa).* 2008;1(6):404–408.

117. Park IW, Wistuba II, Maitra A, et al. Multiple clonal abnormalities in the bronchial epithelium of patients with lung cancer. *J Natl Cancer Inst.* 1999;91(21):1863–1868.

118. Randell SH. Airway epithelial stem cells and the pathophysiology of chronic obstructive pulmonary disease. *Proc Am Thorac Soc.* 2006;3(8):718–725.

119. Kim CF, Jackson EL, Woolfenden AE, et al. Identification of bronchioalveolar stem cells in normal lung and lung cancer. *Cell.* 2005;121(6):823–835.

120. Yang Y, Iwanaga K, Raso MG, et al. Phosphatidylinositol 3-kinase mediates bronchioalveolar stem cell expansion in mouse models of oncogenic K-ras-induced lung cancer. *PLoS ONE.* 2008;3(5):e2220.

121. Yanagi S, Kishimoto H, Kawahara K, et al. Pten controls lung morphogenesis, bronchioalveolar stem cells, and onset of lung adenocarcinomas in mice. *J Clin Invest.* 2007;117(10):2929–2940.

122. Dovey JS, Zacharek SJ, Kim CF, Lees JA. Bmi1 is critical for lung tumorigenesis and bronchioalveolar stem cell expansion. *Proc Natl Acad Sci USA.* 2008;105(33):11857–11862.

123. Qian S, Ding JY, Xie R, et al. MicroRNA expression profile of bronchioalveolar stem cells from mouse lung. *Biochem Biophys Res Commun.* 2008;377(2):668–673.

124. Eramo A, Lotti F, Sette G, et al. Identification and expansion of the tumorigenic lung cancer stem cell population. *Cell Death Differ.* 2008;15(3):504–514.

125. Tirino V, Camerlingo R, Franco R, et al. The role of CD133 in the identification and characterisation of tumour-initiating cells in non-small-cell lung cancer. *Eur J Cardiothorac Surg.* 2009;36(3):446–453.

126. Lin DM, Ma Y, Zheng S, Liu XY, Zou SM, Wei WQ. Prognostic value of bronchioloalveolar carcinoma component in lung adenocarcinoma. *Histol Histopathol.* 2006;21(6):627–632.

127. Gallardo E, Navarro A, Viñolas N, et al. miR-34a as a prognostic marker of relapse in surgically resected non-small-cell lung cancer. *Carcinogenesis.* 2009;30(11):1903–1909.

128. Bertolini G, Roz L, Perego P, et al. Highly tumorigenic lung cancer CD133+ cells display stem-like features and are spared by cisplatin treatment. *Proc Natl Acad Sci USA.* 2009;106(38):16281–16286.

129. Komaki R, Cox JD, Stark R. Frequency of brain metastasis in adenocarcinoma and large cell carcinoma of the lung: correlation with survival. *Int J Radiat Oncol Biol Phys.* 1983;9(10):1467–1470.

130. Lagerwaard FJ, Levendag PC, Nowak PJ, Eijkenboom WM, Hanssens PE, Schmitz PI. Identification of prognostic factors in patients with brain metastases: a review of 1292 patients. *Int J Radiat Oncol Biol Phys.* 1999;43(4):795–803.

131. Mountain CF. Value of the new tnm staging system for lung cancer [published erratum appears in chest 1990 mar;97(3):768]. *Chest.* 1989;96:47S–49S.

132. Kim ES, Bosquée L. The importance of accurate lymph node staging in early and locally advanced non-small cell lung cancer: an update on available techniques. *J Thorac Oncol.* 2007;2 (suppl 2):S59–S67.

133. D'Amico TA, Massey M, Herndon JE 2nd, Moore MB, Harpole DH Jr. A biologic risk model for stage I lung cancer: immunohistochemical analysis of 408 patients with the use of ten molecular markers. *J Thorac Cardiovasc Surg.* 1999;117(4):736–743.

134. Kinch MS, Moore MB, Harpole DH Jr. Predictive value of the EphA2 receptor tyrosine kinase in lung cancer recurrence and survival. *Clin Cancer Res.* 2003;9(2):613–618.

135. McDonald JM, Pelloski CE, Ledoux A, et al. Elevated phospho-S6 expression is associated with metastasis in adenocarcinoma of the lung. *Clin Cancer Res.* 2008;14(23):7832–7837.

136. Herbst RS. Review of epidermal growth factor receptor biology. *Int J Radiat Oncol Biol Phys.* 2004;59(2 suppl):21–26.

137. Shepherd FA, Rosell R. Weighing tumor biology in treatment decisions for patients with non-small cell lung cancer. *J Thorac Oncol.* 2007;2(suppl 2):S68–S76.

138. Sequist LV, Lynch TJ. Egfr tyrosine kinase inhibitors in lung cancer: An evolving story. *Annu Rev Med.* 2008;59:429–442.

139. Sequist LV, Bell DW, Lynch TJ, Haber DA. Molecular predictors of response to epidermal growth factor receptor antagonists in non-small-cell lung cancer. *J Clin Oncol.* 2007;25(5):587–595.

140. Gibbons DL, Lin W, Creighton CJ, et al. Expression signatures of metastatic capacity in a genetic mouse model of lung adenocarcinoma. *PLoS ONE.* 2009;4(4):e5401.

141. Akita K, Inagaki H, Sato S, et al. p185(HER-2/neu) and p21(CIP1/WAF1) expression in primary tumors and lymph node metastases in non-small cell lung cancer. *Jpn J Cancer Res.* 2002;93(9):1007–1011.

142. Tang X, Varella-Garcia M, Xavier AC, et al. Egfr abnormalities in the pathogenesis and progression of lung adenocarcinomas. *Cancer Prev Res.* 2008;1:404–408.

143. Yang G, Truong LD, Timme TL, et al. Elevated expression of caveolin is associated with prostate and breast cancer. *Clin Cancer Res.* 1998;4(8):1873–1880.

144. Sun M, Behrens C, Feng L, et al. HER family receptor abnormalities in lung cancer brain metastases and corresponding primary tumors. *Clin Cancer Res.* 2009;15(15):4829–4837.

145. Emmert-Buck MR, Bonner RF, Smith PD, et al. Laser capture microdissection. *Science.* 1996;274(5289):998–1001.

146. Fend F, Emmert-Buck MR, Chuaqui R, et al. Immuno-LCM: laser capture microdissection of immunostained frozen sections for mRNA analysis. *Am J Pathol.* 1999;154(1):61–66.

147. Tangrea MA, Chuaqui RF, Gillespie JW, et al. Expression microdissection: operator-independent retrieval of cells for molecular profiling. *Diagn Mol Pathol.* 2004;13(4):207–212.

148. Englert CR, Baibakov GV, Emmert-Buck MR. Layered expression scanning: rapid molecular profiling of tumor samples. *Cancer Res.* 2000;60(6):1526–1530.

149. Gannot G, Tangrea MA, Gillespie JW, et al. Layered peptide arrays: high-throughput antibody screening of clinical samples. *J Mol Diagn.* 2005;7(4):427–436.

150. Gannot G, Tangrea MA, Richardson AM, et al. Layered expression scanning: multiplex molecular analysis of diverse life science platforms. *Clin Chim Acta.* 2007;376(1–2):9–16.

151. Tibes R, Qiu Y, Lu Y, et al. Reverse phase protein array: validation of a novel proteomic technology and utility for analysis of primary leukemia specimens and hematopoietic stem cells. *Mol Cancer Ther.* 2006;5(10):2512–2521.

152. Gannot G, Gillespie JW, Chuaqui RF, Tangrea MA, Linehan WM, Emmert-Buck MR. Histomathematical analysis of clinical specimens: challenges and progress. *J Histochem Cytochem.* 2005;53(2):177–185.

153. Perlmutter MA, Best CJ, Gillespie JW, et al. Comparison of snap freezing versus ethanol fixation for gene expression profiling of tissue specimens. *J Mol Diagn.* 2004;6(4):371–377.

154. Gillespie JW, Best CJ, Bichsel VE, et al. Evaluation of non-formalin tissue fixation for molecular profiling studies. *Am J Pathol.* 2002;160(2):449–457.

155. Stanta G, Mucelli SP, Petrera F, Bonin S, Bussolati G. A novel fixative improves opportunities of nucleic acids and proteomic analysis in human archive's tissues. *Diagn Mol Pathol.* 2006;15(2):115–123.

156. Gilbert MT, Haselkorn T, Bunce M, et al. The isolation of nucleic acids from fixed, paraffin-embedded tissues-which methods are useful when? *PLoS ONE.* 2007;2(6):e537.

157. Olert J, Wiedorn KH, Goldmann T, et al. HOPE fixation: a novel fixing method and paraffin-embedding technique for human soft tissues. *Pathol Res Pract.* 2001;197(12):823–826.

158. Naber SP, Smith LL Jr, Wolfe HJ. Role of the frozen tissue bank in molecular pathology. *Diagn Mol Pathol.* 1992;1(1):73–79.

159. Naber SP. Continuing role of a frozen-tissue bank in molecular pathology. *Diagn Mol Pathol.* 1996;5(4):253–259.

160. Harrell JC, Dye WW, Harvell DM, Sartorius CA, Horwitz KB. Contaminating cells alter gene signatures in whole organ versus laser capture microdissected tumors: a comparison of experimental breast cancers and their lymph node metastases. *Clin Exp Metastasis.* 2008;25(1):81–88.

161. Rodriguez-Canales J, Hanson JC, Tangrea MA, et al. Identification of a unique epigenetic sub-microenvironment in prostate cancer. *J Pathol.* 2007;211(4):410–419.

162. Richardson AM, Woodson K, Wang Y, et al. Global expression analysis of prostate cancer-associated stroma and epithelia. *Diagn Mol Pathol.* 2007;16(4):189–197.

163. Erickson HS, Albert PS, Gillespie JW, et al. Assessment of normalization strategies for quantitative RT-PCR using microdissected tissue samples. *Lab Invest.* 2007;87(9):951–962.

164. Erickson HS, Albert PS, Gillespie JW, et al. Quantitative RT-PCR gene expression analysis of laser microdissected tissue samples. *Nat Protoc.* 2009;4(6):902–922.

165. Meyerson M, Carbone D. Genomic and proteomic profiling of lung cancers: lung cancer classification in the age of targeted therapy. *J Clin Oncol.* 2005;23(14):3219–3226.

166. Speer R, Wulfkuhle J, Espina V, et al. Development of reverse phase protein microarrays for clinical applications and patient-tailored therapy. *Cancer Genomics Proteomics.* 2007;4(3):157–164.

167. Amann JM, Chaurand P, Gonzalez A, et al. Selective profiling of proteins in lung cancer cells from fine-needle aspirates by

matrix-assisted laser desorption ionization time-of-flight mass spectrometry. *Clin Cancer Res.* 2006;12(17):5142–5150.

168. Krishnamurthy S. Applications of molecular techniques to fine-needle aspiration biopsy. *Cancer.* 2007;111(2):106–122.

169. Gong Y, Sneige N, Guo M, Hicks ME, Moran CA. Transthoracic fine-needle aspiration vs concurrent core needle biopsy in diagnosis of intrathoracic lesions: a retrospective comparison of diagnostic accuracy. *Am J Clin Pathol.* 2006;125(3): 438–444.

170. Jiang F, Yin Z, Caraway NP, Li R, Katz RL. Genomic profiles in stage I primary non small cell lung cancer using comparative genomic hybridization analysis of cDNA microarrays. *Neoplasia.* 2004;6(5):623–635.

171. Garnis C, Lockwood WW, Vucic E, et al. High resolution analysis of non-small cell lung cancer cell lines by whole genome tiling path array CGH. *Int J Cancer.* 2006;118(6):1556–1564.

172. Callinan PA, Feinberg AP. The emerging science of epigenomics. *Hum Mol Genet.* 2006;15(Spec No 1):R95–101.

173. Herman JG, Baylin SB. Gene silencing in cancer in association with promoter hypermethylation. *N Engl J Med.* 2003;349(21):2042–2054.

174. Shames DS, Girard L, Gao B, et al. A genome-wide screen for promoter methylation in lung cancer identifies novel methylation markers for multiple malignancies. *PLoS Med.* 2006;3(12):e486.

175. Tsou JA, Galler JS, Siegmund KD, et al. Identification of a panel of sensitive and specific DNA methylation markers for lung adenocarcinoma. *Mol Cancer.* 2007;6:70.

176. Yanagawa N, Tamura G, Oizumi H, et al. Promoter hypermethylation of RASSF1A and RUNX3 genes as an independent prognostic prediction marker in surgically resected non-small cell lung cancers. *Lung Cancer.* 2007;58(1):131–138.

177. Brock MV, Hooker CM, Ota-Machida E, et al. DNA methylation markers and early recurrence in stage I lung cancer. *N Engl J Med.* 2008;358(11):1118–1128.

178. Garber ME, Troyanskaya OG, Schluens K, et al. Diversity of gene expression in adenocarcinoma of the lung. *Proc Natl Acad Sci USA.* 2001;98(24):13784–13789.

179. Beer DG, Kardia SL, Huang CC, et al. Gene-expression profiles predict survival of patients with lung adenocarcinoma. *Nat Med.* 2002;8(8):816–824.

180. Larsen JE, Fong KM, Hayward NK. Refining prognosis in non-small-cell lung cancer. *N Engl J Med.* 2007;356(2):190; author reply 190–190; author reply 191.

181. Larsen JE, Pavey SJ, Bowman R, et al. Gene expression of lung squamous cell carcinoma reflects mode of lymph node involvement. *Eur Respir J.* 2007;30(1):21–25.

182. Larsen JE, Pavey SJ, Passmore LH, Bowman RV, Hayward NK, Fong KM. Gene expression signature predicts recurrence in lung adenocarcinoma. *Clin Cancer Res.* 2007;13(10):2946–2954.

183. Potti A, Mukherjee S, Petersen R, et al. A genomic strategy to refine prognosis in early-stage non-small-cell lung cancer. *N Engl J Med.* 2006;355(6):570–580.

184. Chen HY, Yu SL, Chen CH, et al. A five-gene signature and clinical outcome in non-small-cell lung cancer. *N Engl J Med.* 2007;356(1):11–20.

185. Oshita F, Sekiyama A, Saito H, Yamada K, Noda K, Miyagi Y. Genome-wide cDNA microarray screening of genes related to the benefits of paclitaxel and irinotecan chemotherapy in patients with advanced non-small cell lung cancer. *J Exp Ther Oncol.* 2006;6(1):49–53.

186. Potti A, Dressman HK, Bild A, et al. Genomic signatures to guide the use of chemotherapeutics. *Nat Med.* 2006;12(11): 1294–1300.

187. Jay C, Nemunaitis J, Chen P, Fulgham P, Tong AW. miRNA profiling for diagnosis and prognosis of human cancer. *DNA Cell Biol.* 2007;26(5):293–300.

188. Fabbri M. MicroRNAs and cancer epigenetics. *Curr Opin Investig Drugs.* 2008;9(6):583–590.

189. Yanaihara N, Caplen N, Bowman E, et al. Unique microRNA molecular profiles in lung cancer diagnosis and prognosis. *Cancer Cell.* 2006;9(3):189–198.

190. Volinia S, Calin GA, Liu CG, et al. A microRNA expression signature of human solid tumors defines cancer gene targets. *Proc Natl Acad Sci USA.* 2006;103(7):2257–2261.

191. Yu SL, Chen HY, Chang GC, et al. MicroRNA signature predicts survival and relapse in lung cancer. *Cancer Cell.* 2008;13(1):48–57.

192. Weiss GJ, Bemis LT, Nakajima E, et al. EGFR regulation by microRNA in lung cancer: correlation with clinical response and survival to gefitinib and EGFR expression in cell lines. *Ann Oncol.* 2008;19(6):1053–1059.

193. Wilkins-Haug L. The emerging genetic theories of unstable DNA, uniparental disomy, and imprinting. *Curr Opin Obstet Gynecol.* 1993;5(2):179–185.

194. Caprioli RM, Farmer TB, Gile J. Molecular imaging of biological samples: localization of peptides and proteins using MALDI-TOF MS. *Anal Chem.* 1997;69(23):4751–4760.

195. Yanagisawa K, Shyr Y, Xu BJ, et al. Proteomic patterns of tumour subsets in non-small-cell lung cancer. *Lancet.* 2003;362(9382):433–439.

196. Byers LA, Sen B, Saigal B, et al. Reciprocal regulation of c-Src and STAT3 in non-small cell lung cancer. *Clin Cancer Res.* 2009;15(22):6852–6861.

197. VanMeter AJ, Rodriguez AS, Bowman ED, et al. Laser capture microdissection and protein microarray analysis of human non-small cell lung cancer: differential epidermal growth factor receptor (EGPR) phosphorylation events associated with mutated EGFR compared with wild type. *Mol Cell Proteomics.* 2008;7(10):1902–1924.

198. Oh Y, Taylor S, Bekele BN, et al. Number of metastatic sites is a strong predictor of survival in patients with nonsmall cell lung cancer with or without brain metastases. *Cancer.* 2009;115(13):2930–2938.

199. D'Amico TA. Molecular biologic staging of lung cancer. *Ann Thorac Surg.* 2008;85(2):S737–S742.

200. Harpole DH Jr, Richards WG, Herndon JE 2nd, Sugarbaker DJ. Angiogenesis and molecular biologic substaging in patients with stage I non-small cell lung cancer. *Ann Thorac Surg.* 1996;61(5):1470–1476.

201. Kwiatkowski DJ, Harpole DH Jr, Godleski J, et al. Molecular pathologic substaging in 244 stage I non-small-cell lung cancer patients: clinical implications. *J Clin Oncol.* 1998;16(7):2468–2477.

202. Stewart DJ. Tumor and host factors that may limit efficacy of chemotherapy in non-small cell and small cell lung cancer. *Crit Rev Oncol Hematol.* 2010;<Volume>:</Pa>.

203. Sandler A, Gray R, Perry MC, et al. Paclitaxel-carboplatin alone or with bevacizumab for non-small-cell lung cancer. *N Engl J Med.* 2006;355(24):2542–2550.

204. Schiller JH, Harrington D, Belani CP, et al.; Eastern Cooperative Oncology Group. Comparison of four chemotherapy regimens for advanced non-small-cell lung cancer. *N Engl J Med.* 2002;346(2):92–98.

205. Scagliotti GV, Parikh P, von Pawel J, et al. Phase III study comparing cisplatin plus gemcitabine with cisplatin plus pemetrexed in chemotherapy-naive patients with advanced-stage non-small-cell lung cancer. *J Clin Oncol.* 2008;26(21):3543–3551.

206. Stewart DJ, Chiritescu G, Dahrouge S, Banerjee S, Tomiak EM. Chemotherapy dose–response relationships in non-small cell lung cancer and implied resistance mechanisms. *Cancer Treat Rev.* 2007;33(2):101–137.

207. Olaussen KA, Dunant A, Fouret P, et al.; IALT Bio Investigators. DNA repair by ERCC1 in non-small-cell lung cancer and cisplatin-based adjuvant chemotherapy. *N Engl J Med.* 2006;355(10):983–991.

208. Huang PY, Liang XM, Lin SX, Luo RZ, Hou JH, Zhang L. [Correlation analysis among expression of ERCC-1,

metallothionein, p53 and platinum resistance and prognosis in advanced non-small cell lung cancer]. *Ai Zheng*. 2004;23(7): 845–850.

209. Hwang IG, Ahn MJ, Park BB, et al. ERCC1 expression as a prognostic marker in N2(+) nonsmall-cell lung cancer patients treated with platinum-based neoadjuvant concurrent chemoradiotherapy. *Cancer*. 2008;113(6):1379–1386.

210. Takenaka T, Yoshino I, Kouso H, et al. Combined evaluation of Rad51 and ERCC1 expressions for sensitivity to platinum agents in non-small cell lung cancer. *Int J Cancer*. 2007;121(4):895–900.

211. Lord RV, Brabender J, Gandara D, et al. Low ERCC1 expression correlates with prolonged survival after cisplatin plus gemcitabine chemotherapy in non-small cell lung cancer. *Clin Cancer Res*. 2002;8(7):2286–2291.

212. Azuma K, Komohara Y, Sasada T, et al. Excision repair cross-complementation group 1 predicts progression-free and over-all survival in non-small cell lung cancer patients treated with platinum-based chemotherapy. *Cancer Sci*. 2007;98(9):1336–1343.

213. Ceppi P, Volante M, Novello S, et al. ERCC1 and RRM1 gene expressions but not EGFR are predictive of shorter survival in advanced non-small-cell lung cancer treated with cisplatin and gemcitabine. *Ann Oncol*. 2006;17(12):1818–1825.

214. Booton R, Ward T, Ashcroft L, Morris J, Heighway J, Thatcher N. ERCC1 mRNA expression is not associated with response and survival after platinum-based chemotherapy regimens in advanced non-small cell lung cancer. *J Thorac Oncol*. 2007;2(10):902–906.

215. Wachters FM, Wong LS, Timens W, Kampinga HH, Groen HJ. ERCC1, hRad51, and BRCA1 protein expression in relation to tumour response and survival of stage III/IV NSCLC patients treated with chemotherapy. *Lung Cancer*. 2005;50(2):211–219.

216. Cobo M, Isla D, Massuti B, et al. Customizing cisplatin based on quantitative excision repair cross-complementing 1 mRNA expression: a phase III trial in non-small-cell lung cancer. *J Clin Oncol*. 2007;25(19):2747–2754.

217. Fujii T, Toyooka S, Ichimura K, et al. ERCC1 protein expression predicts the response of cisplatin-based neoadjuvant chemotherapy in non-small-cell lung cancer. *Lung Cancer*. 2008;59(3):377–384.

218. Lee HW, Choi YW, Han JH, et al. Expression of excision repair cross-complementation group 1 protein predicts poor outcome in advanced non-small cell lung cancer patients treated with platinum-based doublet chemotherapy. *Lung Cancer*. 2009;65(3):377–382.

219. Bepler G, Kusmartseva I, Sharma S, et al. RRM1 modulated *in vitro* and *in vivo* efficacy of gemcitabine and platinum in non-small-cell lung cancer. *J Clin Oncol*. 2006;24(29):4731–4737.

220. Shimizu J, Horio Y, Osada H, et al. mRNA expression of RRM1, ERCC1 and ERCC2 is not associated with chemosensitivity to cisplatin, carboplatin and gemcitabine in human lung cancer cell lines. *Respirology*. 2008;13(4):510–517.

221. Kwon WS, Rha SY, Choi YH, et al. Ribonucleotide reductase M1 (RRM1) 2464G>A polymorphism shows an association with gemcitabine chemosensitivity in cancer cell lines. *Pharmacogenet Genomics*. 2006;16(6):429–438.

222. Tooker P, Yen WC, Ng SC, Negro-Vilar A, Hermann TW. Bexarotene (LGD1069, Targretin), a selective retinoid X receptor agonist, prevents and reverses gemcitabine resistance in NSCLC cells by modulating gene amplification. *Cancer Res*. 2007;67(9):4425–4433.

223. Davidson JD, Ma L, Flagella M, Geeganage S, Gelbert LM, Slapak CA. An increase in the expression of ribonucleotide reductase large subunit 1 is associated with gemcitabine resistance in non-small cell lung cancer cell lines. *Cancer Res*. 2004;64(11):3761–3766.

224. Oguri T, Achiwa H, Sato S, et al. The determinants of sensitivity and acquired resistance to gemcitabine differ in non-small cell lung cancer: a role of ABCC5 in gemcitabine sensitivity. *Mol Cancer Ther*. 2006;5(7):1800–1806.

225. Rosell R, Danenberg KD, Alberola V, et al.; Spanish Lung Cancer Group. Ribonucleotide reductase messenger RNA expression and survival in gemcitabine/cisplatin-treated advanced non-small cell lung cancer patients. *Clin Cancer Res*. 2004;10(4):1318–1325.

226. Simon GR, Ismail-Khan R, Bepler G. Nuclear excision repair-based personalized therapy for non-small cell lung cancer: from hypothesis to reality. *Int J Biochem Cell Biol*. 2007;39(7–8): 1318–1328.

227. Brattström D, Bergqvist M, Lamberg K, et al. Complete sequence of p53 gene in 20 patients with lung cancer: comparison with chemosensitivity and immunohistochemistry. *Med Oncol*. 1998;15(4):255–261.

228. Tsai CM, Chang KT, Wu LH, et al. Correlations between intrinsic chemoresistance and HER-2/neu gene expression, p53 gene mutations, and cell proliferation characteristics in non-small cell lung cancer cell lines. *Cancer Res*. 1996;56(1):206–209.

229. Safran H, King T, Choy H, et al. p53 mutations do not predict response to paclitaxel/radiation for nonsmall cell lung carcinoma. *Cancer*. 1996;78(6):1203–1210.

230. Bergqvist M, Brattström D, Gullbo J, Hesselius P, Brodin O, Wagenius G. p53 status and its *in vitro* relationship to radiosensitivity and chemosensitivity in lung cancer. *Anticancer Res*. 2003;23(2B):1207–1212.

231. Blandino G, Levine AJ, Oren M. Mutant p53 gain of function: differential effects of different p53 mutants on resistance of cultured cells to chemotherapy. *Oncogene*. 1999;18(2): 477–485.

232. Kandioler D, Stamatis G, Eberhardt W, et al. Growing clinical evidence for the interaction of the p53 genotype and response to induction chemotherapy in advanced non-small cell lung cancer. *J Thorac Cardiovasc Surg*. 2008;135(5):1036–1041.

233. Kandioler-Eckersberger D, Kappel S, Mittlböck M, et al. The TP53 genotype but not immunohistochemical result is predictive of response to cisplatin-based neoadjuvant therapy in stage III non-small cell lung cancer. *J Thorac Cardiovasc Surg*. 1999;117(4):744–750.

234. Fijolek J, Wiatr E, Rowinska-Zakrzewska E, et al. p53 and HER2/neu expression in relation to chemotherapy response in patients with non-small cell lung cancer. *Int J Biol Markers*. 2006;21(2):81–87.

235. Johnson EA, Klimstra DS, Herndon JE, 2nd, et al. Aberrant p53 staining does not predict cisplatin resistance in locally advanced non-small cell lung cancer. *Cancer Invest*. 2002;20(5–6):686–692.

236. Brooks KR, To K, Joshi MB, et al. Measurement of chemoresistance markers in patients with stage III non-small cell lung cancer: a novel approach for patient selection. *Ann Thorac Surg*. 2003;76(1):187–93; discussion 193.

237. Graziano SL, Tatum A, Herndon JE 2nd, et al. Use of neuroendocrine markers, p53, and HER2 to predict response to chemotherapy in patients with stage III non-small cell lung cancer: a Cancer and Leukemia Group B study. *Lung Cancer*. 2001;33(2–3):115–123.

238. Rusch V, Klimstra D, Venkatraman E, et al. Aberrant p53 expression predicts clinical resistance to cisplatin-based chemotherapy in locally advanced non-small cell lung cancer. *Cancer Res*. 1995;55(21):5038–5042.

239. Gajra A, Tatum AH, Newman N, et al. The predictive value of neuroendocrine markers and p53 for response to chemotherapy and survival in patients with advanced non-small cell lung cancer. *Lung Cancer*. 2002;36(2):159–165.

240. Ludovini V, Gregorc V, Pistola L, et al. Vascular endothelial growth factor, p53, Rb, Bcl-2 expression and response to chemotherapy in advanced non-small cell lung cancer. *Lung Cancer*. 2004;46(1):77–85.

241. Kawasaki M, Nakanishi Y, Kuwano K, Takayama K, Kiyohara C, Hara N. Immunohistochemically detected p53 and P-glycoprotein predict the response to chemotherapy in lung cancer. *Eur J Cancer*. 1998;34(9):1352–1357.

242. Miyatake K, Gemba K, Ueoka H, et al. Prognostic significance of mutant p53 protein, P-glycoprotein and glutathione S-transferase-pi in patients with unresectable non-small cell lung cancer. *Anticancer Res.* 2003;23(3C):2829–2836.

243. Berrieman HK, Cawkwell L, O'Kane SL, Smith L, Lind MJ. Hsp27 may allow prediction of the response to single-agent vinorelbine chemotherapy in non-small cell lung cancer. *Oncol Rep.* 2006;15(1):283–286.

244. Gregorc V, Ludovini V, Pistola L, et al. Relevance of p53, bcl-2 and Rb expression on resistance to cisplatin-based chemotherapy in advanced non-small cell lung cancer. *Lung Cancer.* 2003;39(1):41–48.

245. Harada T, Ogura S, Yamazaki K, et al. Predictive value of expression of P53, Bcl-2 and lung resistance-related protein for response to chemotherapy in non-small cell lung cancers. *Cancer Sci.* 2003;94(4):394–399.

246. Oshita F, Nishio K, Kameda Y, et al. Increased expression levels of p53 correlate with good response to cisplatin-based chemotherapy in non-small cell lung cancer. *Oncol Rep.* 2000;7(6):1225–1228.

247. Higashiyama M, Miyoshi Y, Kodama K, et al. p53-regulated GML gene expression in non-small cell lung cancer. a promising relationship to cisplatin chemosensitivity. *Eur J Cancer.* 2000;36(4):489–495.

248. Eberhard DA, Johnson BE, Amler LC, et al. Mutations in the epidermal growth factor receptor and in KRAS are predictive and prognostic indicators in patients with non-small-cell lung cancer treated with chemotherapy alone and in combination with erlotinib. *J Clin Oncol.* 2005;23(25):5900–5909.

249. Rodenhuis S, Boerrigter L, Top B, et al. Mutational activation of the K-ras oncogene and the effect of chemotherapy in advanced adenocarcinoma of the lung: a prospective study. *J Clin Oncol.* 1997;15(1):285–291.

250. Mascaux C, Martin B, Verdebout JM, Ninane V, Sculier JP. COX-2 expression during early lung squamous cell carcinoma oncogenesis. *Eur Respir J.* 2005;26(2):198–203.

251. Rosell R, Molina F, Moreno I, et al. Mutated K-ras gene analysis in a randomized trial of preoperative chemotherapy plus surgery versus surgery in stage IIIA non-small cell lung cancer. *Lung Cancer.* 1995;12(suppl 1):S59–S70.

252. Schiller JH, Adak S, Feins RH, et al. Lack of prognostic significance of p53 and K-ras mutations in primary resected non-small-cell lung cancer on E4592: a Laboratory Ancillary Study on an Eastern Cooperative Oncology Group Prospective Randomized Trial of Postoperative Adjuvant Therapy. *J Clin Oncol.* 2001;19(2):448–457.

253. Kim KS, Jeong JY, Kim YC, et al. Predictors of the response to gefitinib in refractory non-small cell lung cancer. *Clin Cancer Res.* 2005;11(6):2244–2251.

254. Lynch TJ, Bonomi PD, Butts C, et al. Novel agents in the treatment of lung cancer: Fourth Cambridge Conference. *Clin Cancer Res.* 2007;13(15 Pt 2):s4583–s4588.

255. Kobayashi K, Nishioka M, Kohno T, et al. Identification of genes whose expression is upregulated in lung adenocarcinoma cells in comparison with type II alveolar cells and bronchiolar epithelial cells in vivo. *Oncogene.* 2004;23(17):3089–3096.

256. John T, Liu G, Tsao MS. Overview of molecular testing in non-small-cell lung cancer: mutational analysis, gene copy number, protein expression and other biomarkers of EGFR for the prediction of response to tyrosine kinase inhibitors. *Oncogene.* 2009;28(suppl 1):S14–S23.

257. Jackman D, Pao W, Riely GJ, et al. Clinical definition of acquired resistance to epidermal growth factor receptor tyrosine kinase inhibitors in non-small-cell lung cancer. *J Clin Oncol.* 2010;28(2):191–192.

258. Linardou H, Dahabreh IJ, Bafaloukos D, Kosmidis P, Murray S. Somatic EGFR mutations and efficacy of tyrosine kinase inhibitors in NSCLC. *Nat Rev Clin Oncol.* 2009;6(6):352–366.

259. Nguyen KS, Kobayashi S, Costa DB. Acquired resistance to epidermal growth factor receptor tyrosine kinase inhibitors in non-small-cell lung cancers dependent on the epidermal growth factor receptor pathway. *Clin Lung Cancer.* 2009;10(4):281–289.

260. Rho JK, Choi YJ, Lee JK, et al. The role of MET activation in determining the sensitivity to epidermal growth factor receptor tyrosine kinase inhibitors. *Mol Cancer Res.* 2009;7(10):1736–1743.

261. Faber AC, Li D, Song Y, et al. Differential induction of apoptosis in HER2 and EGFR addicted cancers following PI3K inhibition. *Proc Natl Acad Sci USA.* 2009;106(46):19503–19508.

262. Sato M, Vaughan MB, Girard L, et al. Multiple oncogenic changes (K-RAS(V12), p53 knockdown, mutant EGFRs, p16 bypass, telomerase) are not sufficient to confer a full malignant phenotype on human bronchial epithelial cells. *Cancer Res.* 2006;66(4):2116–2128.

263. Kwak I, Tsai SY, DeMayo FJ. Genetically engineered mouse models for lung cancer. *Annu Rev Physiol.* 2004;66:647–663.

264. Rahman SM, Shyr Y, Yildiz PB, et al. Proteomic patterns of preinvasive bronchial lesions. *Am J Respir Crit Care Med.* 2005;172(12):1556–1562.

4 | *The New Lung Cancer Staging System*

RAMON RAMI-PORTA

DOROTHY J. GIROUX

PETER GOLDSTRAW

■ INTRODUCTION

The lung cancer staging system is based on the anatomic extent of the primary tumor (T), the regional lymph nodes (N), and the distant metastasis (M). Since its development in the mid-20th century, it has been periodically revised by the International Union Against Cancer (UICC) and the American Joint Committee on Cancer (AJCC). Their latest edition, the 6th, of the tumor, node, and metastasis (TNM) classification (TNM6) for lung cancer was published in 2002 (1,2), and the modifications included in the previous edition of 1997 remained unchanged: separate tumor nodule(s) in the same lobe were classified as T4; separate tumor nodule(s) in a different ipsilateral or contralateral lobe were classified as M1; T3N0M0 tumors were downstaged from stage IIIA to IIB; stage I was divided into stage IA (T1N0M0) and stage IB (T2N0M0); and stage II was divided into stage IIA (T1N1M0) and stage IIB (T2N1M0 and T3N0M0).

In 1998, the International Association for the Study of Lung Cancer (IASLC) organized an International Staging Committee (ISC) with the objective to collect a large population of patients with lung cancer from around the world to create an international database (3). The results of the analyses of this database served to support the recommendations for changes in the 7th edition of the TNM classification (TNM7) for lung cancer (4–7) (Table 4.1), published in 2009 by the UICC, the AJCC, and the IASLC (8).

■ THE IASLC DATABASE, METHODOLOGY, AND LIMITATIONS

More than 100,000 patients from 20 countries in four large geographic areas of the world were submitted to the IASLC database (Table 4.2). The cases originated in 46 databases designed to address varying research objectives, and included registries, series of surgically treated patients, clinical trials, series of patients treated by all therapeutic modalities, consortia, and institutional registries. The inclusion criteria were (a) diagnosis of bronchogenic carcinoma in the period from 1990 to 2000 and (b) adequate staging and follow-up information (3). After excluding those cases diagnosed outside of the established time period, those with incomplete staging or follow-up information, those with no known histological type, those with other tumors, such as carcinoids or sarcomas, and those with recurrent tumors, 81,015 cases remained for analysis—13,290 with small cell lung cancer and 67,725 with non–small cell lung cancer. The IASLC database is stored, managed, and analyzed by Cancer Research and Biostatistics (9).

The findings leading to recommendations to modify the TNM classification were validated to confirm the consistency of results: first internally, analyzing the data by geographic area and type of database and then by applying the recommendations to the Surveillance, Epidemiology, and End Results (SEER) registries for the same period. When the number of cases allowed, the population under study was randomly divided into a training set (two thirds of the population) and a validation set (the remaining one third), thus providing an additional internal validation of findings (9).

All databases that contributed cases to the IASLC database did not have the objective to assess the TNM classification, and many cases lacked specific information on the TNM descriptors. This limited the analyses of the T descriptors to tumor size, additional nodule(s) in the same lobe or in another ipsilateral or contralateral lobe, and pleural dissemination (malignant pleural effusion or separated pleural nodules) (4). The four N categories could be validated both clinically and pathologically, but no further subclassification could be recommended because of lack of validation (5). Subclassification of M1 into M1a and M1b could be recommended with the available data on metastatic disease, but no further recommendation could be made based on site or number of metastases (6).

■ Table 4.1 Proposed definitions for T, N, and M descriptors based on the recommendations of the IASLC for the 7th edition of the TNM classification of lung cancer

TNM Component and Categories	Definitions
T: Primary tumor	
TX	Primary tumor cannot be assessed; or tumor proven by the presence of malignant cells in sputum or bronchial washings but not visualized by imaging or bronchoscopy
T0	No evidence of primary tumor
Tis	Carcinoma in situ
T1	Tumor ≤3 cm in greatest dimension, surrounded by lung or visceral pleura, without bronchoscopic evidence of invasion more proximal than the lobar bronchus (i.e., not the main bronchus) [a]
T1a	**Tumor ≤2 cm in greatest dimension**
T1b	**Tumor >2 cm but ≤3 cm in greatest dimension**
T2	Tumor >3 cm **but ≤7 cm** or tumor with any of the following features (**T2 tumors with these features are classified T2a if ≤5 cm**): Involves main bronchus, ≥2 cm distal to the carina Invades visceral pleura Associated with atelectasis or obstructive pneumonitis that extends to the hilar region but does not involve the entire lung
T2a	**Tumor >3 cm but ≤5 cm in greatest dimension**
T2b	**Tumor >5 cm but ≤7 cm in greatest dimension**
T3	**Tumor >7 cm** or one that directly invades any of the following: chest wall (including superior sulcus tumors), diaphragm, phrenic nerve, mediastinal pleura, parietal pericardium; or tumor in the main bronchus <2 cm distal to the carina [a] but without involvement of the carina; or associated atelectasis or obstructive pneumonitis of the entire lung; **or separate tumor nodule(s) in the same lobe**
T4	Tumor of any size that invades any of the following: mediastinum, heart, great vessels, trachea, recurrent laryngeal nerve, esophagus, vertebral body, carina; **separate tumor nodule(s) in a different ipsilateral lobe**
N: Regional lymph nodes	
NX	Regional lymph nodes cannot be assessed
N0	No regional lymph node metastasis
N1	Metastasis in ipsilateral peribronchial and/or ipsilateral hilar lymph nodes and intrapulmonary nodes, including involvement by direct extension
N2	Metastasis in ipsilateral mediastinal and/or subcarinal lymph nodes
N3	Metastasis in contralateral mediastinal, contralateral hilar, ipsilateral or contralateral scalene, or supraclavicular lymph node(s)
M: Distant metastasis	
M0	No distant metastasis
M1	Distant metastasis
M1a	**Separate tumor nodule(s) in a contralateral lobe; tumor with pleural nodules or malignant pleural (or pericardial) effusion[b]**
M1b	**Distant metastasis**

Innovations in the 7th edition of the classification are in bold letters.

[a] The uncommon superficial spreading tumor of any size with its invasive component limited to the bronchial wall, which may extend proximal to the main bronchus, is classified as T1; [b] Most pleural (**and pericardial**) effusions with lung cancer are due to tumor. In a few patients, however, multiple cytopathologic examinations of the pleural (**pericardial**) fluid are negative for tumor, and the fluid is nonbloody and is not an exudate. Where these elements and clinical judgment dictate that the effusion is not related to the tumor, the effusion should be excluded as a staging element and the patient should be classified as M0.

IASLC, International Association for the Study of Lung Cancer.

■ **Table 4.2** Number of cases submitted by geographic area

Geographic Area	Number of Cases
Australia	9,416
Asia	11,622
North America	21,130
Europe	58,701
Total	100,869

■ RESULTS SUPPORTING THE RECOMMENDED CHANGES

The analysis of the TNM descriptors was performed in the population of patients with non–small cell lung cancer (Table 4.3).

T Descriptors

Tumor Size

Tumor size was first analyzed in the population of patients with pathologic (p) T1-T2N0M0 completely resected (R0) tumors who had not received induction therapy. Multiple comparisons of different tumor sizes showed that the best cutpoints separating populations of patients with tumors of different prognosis were at 2 cm, in patients with pT1N0M0 tumors, and at 5 and 7 cm, in patients with pT2N0M0 tumors. These three cutpoints and the classic 3-cm landmark that separates T1 from T2 tumors generated five tumor size groups with significantly different 5-year survival rates: ≤2 cm, 77%; >2–3 cm, 71%; >3–5 cm, 58%; >5–7 cm, 49%; and >7 cm, 35%. The survival of the largest pT2 tumors (>7 cm) was not significantly different from that of pT3 tumors. The analyses of the populations of patients with any type of resection or with nodal disease, and that of patients with clinically staged tumors, revealed similar findings. Therefore, the ISC proposed to subclassify T1 and T2 tumors around these cutpoints, into T1a and T1b and T2a and T2b, respectively, and to reclassify T2 tumors larger than 7 cm as T3 (4) (Table 4.1).

Additional Tumor Nodule(s) and Pleural Dissemination

Additional tumor nodule(s) in another ipsilateral lobe was formerly an M1 descriptor according to TNM6, and pleural dissemination was a T4 descriptor according to TNM6. However, based initially on completely resected, node negative patients, but with support from less selected populations, the ISC recommended to reclassify tumors with additional nodule(s) in the same lobe as T3, to reclassify tumors with additional nodules(s) in another ipsilateral lobe as T4, and to reclassify pleural dissemination as metastatic disease (4) (Table 4.1). Survival comparisons among patients with R0 pN0 pT3 tumors, pT4 by additional nodule(s) in the same lobe, pT4 by other T4 descriptor, pM1 by additional

■ **Table 4.3** Number of patients with non–small cell lung cancer registered in the IASLC database used for the analysis of the TNM descriptors

Type of TNM Descriptor Information	Number of Patients
Sufficient cT descriptor information (M0)	5,760
Sufficient pT descriptor information (M0)	15,234
Sufficient cN descriptor information (M0)	38,265
Sufficient pN descriptor information (M0)	28,371
Sufficient pN descriptor information for the analyses of the nodal stations (R0 without induction therapy)	2,876
Sufficient c and/or pM information	6,596

c, clinical; IASLC, International Association for the Study of Lung Cancer; M, distant metastases; M0, no distant metastases; p, pathologic; R0, complete resection; T, primary tumor.

nodule(s) in another ipsilateral lobe, and pT4 by pleural dissemination revealed that pT3 and pT4 tumors by additional nodule(s) in the same lobe had similar 5-year survival rates: 41% and 45%, respectively ($P = 0.6488$). Pathologic M1 tumors by additional nodule(s) in another ipsilateral lobe and pT4 tumors by other T4 descriptors also had similar prognosis. Five-year survival rates were 48% and 35%, respectively ($P = 0.1090$). Similar results were found when the less selected population of patients who underwent any type of resection and whose tumors had nodal disease was studied. Pleural dissemination had the worst survival compared with that of the other groups. This difference was especially apparent when survival of patients with cT4 tumors by pleural dissemination was compared with that of patients with cT4 tumors by other T4 descriptors. Five-year survival rates were 2% and 14%, respectively, when tumors with any N category were included, and 2% and 25%, respectively, when only those cN0 were considered ($P < 0.0001$).

N Descriptors

Although no changes were derived from the analyses of cases with information on the nodal status, the prognostic relevance of the four present N categories was validated both clinically and pathologically for the first time in a large, international database of cases treated by all modalities of care. In both circumstances, the expected reduction in 5-year survival rates was observed: cN0, 42%; cN1, 29%; cN2, 16%; and cN3, 7%; pN0, 56%; pN1, 38%; pN2, 22%; and pN3, 6%. No significant differences in survival were found when the individual N1 and N2 stations were compared, although the subcarinal nodal station tended to have the worst prognosis, and the subaortic, the best. When neighboring nodal stations of the Mountain and Dressler map (10) were amalgamated into nodal zones, the extent of nodal involvement was found to have prognostic impact. In a group of 1992 patients whose tumors had sufficiently detailed patho-logic information on N status, single zone pN1 disease was found to have the best prognosis, with a 5-year sur-vival rate of 48%; multiple pN1 and single pN2 disease had similar survival, with 5-year survival rates of 35% and 34%, respectively; finally, multiple pN2 disease had the worst survival, with a 5-year survival rate of 20% (5). This clinically relevant information could not be used to modify the N descriptors because the sample size precluded validation in the clinically staged, cTNM, population or by geographic region, type of database or T categories.

M Descriptors

Based on the results discussed earlier and additional comparisons of T4 and M1 subgroups as characterized by "best" TNM (clinical or pathologic, as was available), the ISC recommended to reclassify pleural dissemina-tion and contralateral lung nodules as M1a, and distant metastases as M1b (6) (Table 4.1). Survival was com-pared among the following cohorts as defined by best stage: T4M0 any N tumors, pleural dissemination (T4 in TNM6), contralateral lung nodules (M1 in TNM6), and distant metastases (M1 in TNM6). Survival was best for T4M0 tumors with any nodal disease: 5-year survival rate was 16%. Pleural dissemination and con-tralateral nodules had similar survival: 5-year survival rates were 6% and 3%, respectively ($P = 0.3816$). Distant

metastases had significantly worse survival than both pleural dissemination and contralateral nodules, with a 5-year survival rate of 1%.

Stage Grouping

The modifications in the T and the M descriptors generated changes in the stage grouping. Many combinations were tested, but the one that showed the strongest impact of sur-vival with increasing tumor stage was the one that included T2bN0M0 tumors in stage IIA; T2aN1M0 tumors in stage IIA; and T4N0-N1M0 tumors in stage IIIA (Table 4.4). Five-year survival rates for clinical and pathologic stages, respectively, proposed by the IASLC are 50% and 73% for stage IA; 43% and 58% for IB; 36% and 46% for IIA; 25% and 36% for IIB; 19% and 24% for IIIA; 7% and 9% for IIIB; and 2% and 13% for stage IV (7).

■ OTHER RESULTS AND RECOMMENDATIONS

Small Cell Lung Cancer

Of the 13,290 patients with small cell lung cancer, 8,088 had clinical (7,745 patients) and/or pathologic (343 patients) TNM information. The patients with clinically staged tumors were used to apply the TNM6 stages, and those whose tumor information allowed reclassification were used to test the new stages proposed in the TNM7. The same analysis was done in the population of patients with small cell lung cancer in the SEER registries. These analyses consistently showed that the TNM staging sys-tem is relevant in small cell lung cancer: the greater the stage, the worse the survival, with statistically significant differences, with exception of stage IIA that has better survival than expected. However, this paradoxical finding disappeared in the analysis of the SEER database in which there were more patients with tumors in this stage. Five-year survival rates for the patients in the IASLC database were 38% for stage IA; 21% for IB; 38% for IIA; 18% for IIB; 13% for IIIA; 9% for IIIB; and 1% for stage IV. In the light of these findings, the ISC recommended that the TNM classification and staging system should be favored over the classic dichotomous staging system (limited and extensive disease), and that stage stratification should be done in future clinical trials in limited disease, because there clearly are groups of tumors with significantly dif-ferent prognosis (11).

Bronchopulmonary Carcinoids

The recommendation of the ISC was that the TNM clas-sification and staging system be used to stage bronchopul-monary carcinoids. In the IASLC database there were 513 bronchopulmonary carcinoids that were excluded

■ Table 4.4 Stage grouping proposed by the IASLC

Stage	T Category	N Category	N Category
Occult carcinoma	Tx	N0	M0
Stage 0	Tis	N0	M0
Stage IA	**T1a**	N0	M0
	T1b	N0	M0
Stage IB	**T2a**	N0	M0
Stage IIA	**T1a**	N1	M0
	T1b	N1	M0
	T2a	**N1**	M0
	T2b	N0	M0
Stage IIB	**T2b**	N1	M0
	T3	N0	M0
Stage IIIA	T1	N2	M0
	T2	N2	M0
	T3	N1	M0
	T3	N2	M0
	T4	**N0**	M0
	T4	**N1**	M0
Stage IIIB	T4	N2	M0
	Any T	N3	M0
Stage IV	Any T	Any N	**M1a**
	Any T	Any N	**M1b**

Innovations are highlighted in bold.
IASLC, International Association for the Study of Lung Cancer.

from the general analyses of the TNM descriptors, but, together with 1,619 bronchopulmonary carcinoids of the SEER registries, were used to test the TNM classification in this type of tumor, traditionally excluded from the TNM classification and staging system. Although there are important differences between bronchopulmonary carcinoids and non–small cell lung cancer (e.g., 82% of the IASLC database carcinoids were in stage I, and there were few tumors larger than 3 cm), the TNM classification predicted prognosis for bronchopulmonary carcinoids. Although differences are not so clear as for non–small cell lung cancer, T and N have prognostic impact, but differences are very small among T1 and T2 tumors. Five-year survival rates in the population of surgically treated patients of the SEER registries were 93% for T1a; 92% for T1b; 90% for T2a; 90% for T2b; 65% for T3 >3 cm; 74% for other T3; and 79% for T3 with same lobe additional nodules. Regarding the N category, 5-year survival rates were 92% for N0; 81% for N1; 74% for N2; and 67% for N3. Five-year survival rates for M0 and M1 disease were 91% and 57%, respectively. The stage grouping proposed by the IASLC also separated tumors with different prognosis, but this was more apparent when the A and B substages were combined (12).

Visceral Pleura Invasion

A review of the pertinent literature showed that invasion of the visceral pleura (a T2 descriptor) is an adverse prognostic factor. The ISC recommended to define the invasion of the visceral pleura as invasion beyond the elastic layer and to use elastic stains when this layer is not clearly seen on hematoxylin-eosin preparations. It also recommended to use the abbreviation PL for pleura and, following Hammar classification (13) (Figure 4.1), to use numeric codes to describe the absence of invasion or its presence and extent as follows:

- PL0: tumor within the subpleural lung parenchyma or invading superficially into the pleural connective tissue beneath the elastic layer. It is not regarded as a T descriptor and the T category should be assigned on other features.
- PL1: tumor invades beyond the elastic layer. It indicates visceral pleura invasion and is a T2 descriptor.
- PL2: tumor invades the pleural surface. It indicates visceral pleura invasion and is a T2 descriptor.
- PL3: tumor invades any component of the parietal pleura. It indicates invasion of the parietal pleura and is a T3 descriptor.

The IASLC Lymph Node Map

The IASLC has designed a new lymph node map that reconciles the differences between the Naruke-Japan Lung Cancer Society (14,15) and the Mountain and Dressler

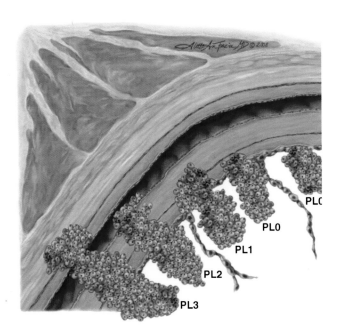

FIGURE 4.1 Modified Hammar classification of visceral pleural invasion for lung cancer. See text for the definitions of the different pleura (PL) categories. From Ref. 13 with permission. © 2008 Aletta Ann Frazier, MD.

(10) maps. In this lymph node map (Figure 4.2), nodal stations have clear anatomic boundaries (Table 4.5) and are grouped in nodal zones to facilitate nodal staging especially in those patients who will not undergo resection (16). This new map incorporates an extrathoracic station 1 that coincides with the new supraclavicular zone. It includes the low cervical, the supraclavicular, and the sternal notch nodes. All these nodes, if involved, are N3 regardless of the side of the tumor. Another innovation is the shift of the "oncologic midline" to the left paratracheal border. This implies that any involved nodes that are on the left of the anatomic midline, but on the right of this left paratracheal line, will be N2 for right-sided tumors, but N3 for left-sided ones. This line shift is based on the fact that the right paratracheal and pretracheal nodes are contained in fatty tissue that can be removed en bloc, while the left paratracheal nodes are along the posterior margin of the trachea along the left laryngeal recurrent nerve, and are independent from the other peritracheal nodes. Finally, the subcarinal space is larger in the new IASLC map and includes the nodes at the tracheal bifurcation and those along the inferior aspects of both main bronchi down to the lower border of the bronchus intermedius on the right and to the upper border of the lower lobe bronchus on the left. The enlargement of the subcarinal space implies that there will be more N2 tumors in detriment of N1 and N3 tumors, because the nodes along the inferior aspects of the main bronchi were considered hilar in the Japanese map and, therefore, if involved, would be classified as N3 if contralateral to the tumor side, and N1 if ipsilateral.

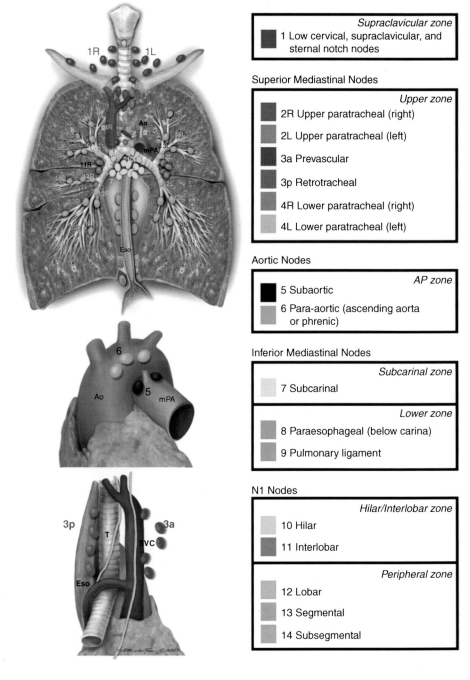

FIGURE 4.2 The International Association for the Study of Lung Cancer lymph node map, including the proposed grouping of lymph node stations into "zones" for the purposes of prognostic analyses. From Ref. 16 with permission. © 2009 Aletta Ann Frazier, MD.

	Supraclavicular zone
	1 Low cervical, supraclavicular, and sternal notch nodes

Superior Mediastinal Nodes

	Upper zone
	2R Upper paratracheal (right)
	2L Upper paratracheal (left)
	3a Prevascular
	3p Retrotracheal
	4R Lower paratracheal (right)
	4L Lower paratracheal (left)

Aortic Nodes

	AP zone
	5 Subaortic
	6 Para-aortic (ascending aorta or phrenic)

Inferior Mediastinal Nodes

	Subcarinal zone
	7 Subcarinal
	Lower zone
	8 Paraesophageal (below carina)
	9 Pulmonary ligament

N1 Nodes

	Hilar/Interlobar zone
	10 Hilar
	11 Interlobar
	Peripheral zone
	12 Lobar
	13 Segmental
	14 Subsegmental

■ ADDITIONAL EXTERNAL VALIDATION OF THE IASLC RECOMMENDATIONS

Since the publication of the main recommendations (4,5,6,7,11), independent groups have tried to validate them based on their own data or on data from registries. The proposed revisions better reflected survival for advanced bronchioloalveolar carcinoma (17) and small cell lung cancer (18). The proposals for reclassification of additional tumor nodule(s) (19,20,21,22) and the modifications in the M descriptors (22) have been validated and allow better prognostication. Finally, the prognostic relevance of the T descriptors, the extent of nodal involvement, and the overall validity of the revised

TNM classification and staging system also have been validated (23,24,25).

■ REMAINING CONTROVERSIAL POINTS

With the analyses of the retrospective data, the T2 descriptors, except for tumor size, the T3 descriptors, and the T4 descriptors, other than additional tumor nodule(s) in the same lobe and pleural dissemination, could not be validated because of lack of specific data. A possible subclassification of the N categories, based on the extent of nodal disease, could not be recommended because of

■ **Table 4.5** Anatomic definitions for each lymph node station in the map proposed by the IASLC

Lymph Node Station	Anatomic Limits
#1: Low cervical, supraclavicular, and sternal notch nodes.	Upper border: lower margin of cricoid cartilage. Lower border: clavicles bilaterally and, in the midline, the upper border of the manubrium. 1R designates right-sided nodes, 1L left-sided nodes in this region. For lymph node station 1, the midline of the trachea serves as the border between 1R and 1L.
#2: Upper paratracheal nodes.	2R: Upper border: apex of the right lung and pleural space, and, in the midline, the upper border of the manubrium. Lower border: intersection of caudal margin of innominate vein with the trachea. As for lymph node station 4R, 2R includes nodes extending to the left lateral border of the trachea. 2L: Upper border: apex of the lung and pleural space, and, in the midline, the upper border of the manubrium. Lower border: superior border of the aortic arch.
#3 Prevascular and retrotracheal nodes.	3a: Prevascular. On the right: Upper border: apex of chest. Lower border: level of carina. Anterior border: posterior aspect of sternum. Posterior border: anterior border of superior vena cava. On the left: Upper border: apex of chest. Lower border: level of carina. Anterior border: posterior aspect of sternum. Posterior border: left carotid artery. 3p: Retrotracheal. Upper border: apex of chest. Lower border: carina.
#4: Lower paratracheal nodes.	4R: includes right paratracheal nodes, and pretracheal nodes extending to the left lateral border of the tracheal. Upper border: intersection of caudal margin of innominate vein with the trachea. Lower border: lower border of the azygos vein. 4L: includes nodes to the left of the left lateral border of the trachea, medial to the ligamentum arteriosum. Upper border: upper margin of the aortic arch. Lower border: upper rim of the left main pulmonary artery.
#5: Subaortic (aortopulmonary window).	Subaortic lymph nodes lateral to the ligamentum arteriosum. Upper border: the lower border of the aortic arch. Lower border: upper rim of the left main pulmonary artery.
#6: Para-aortic nodes (ascending aorta or phrenic).	Lymph nodes anterior and lateral to the ascending aorta and aortic arch. Upper border: a line tangential to the upper border of the aortic arch. Lower border: the lower border of the aortic arch.
#7: Subcarinal nodes.	Upper border: the carina of the trachea. Lower border: the upper border of the lower lobe bronchus on the left; the lower border of the bronchus intermedius on the right.
#8: Paraesophageal nodes (below carina).	Nodes lying adjacent to the wall of the esophagus and to the right or the left of the midline, excluding subcarinal nodes. Upper border: the upper border of the lower lobe bronchus on the left; the lower border of the bronchus intermedius on the right. Lower border: the diaphragm.
#9: Pulmonary ligament nodes.	Nodes lying within the pulmonary ligament. Upper border: the inferior pulmonary vein. Lower border: the diaphragm.
#10: Hilar nodes.	Includes nodes immediately adjacent to the mainstem bronchus and hilar vessels including the proximal portions of the pulmonary veins and main pulmonary artery. Upper border: the lower rim of the azygos vein in the right; upper rim of the pulmonary artery on the left. Lower border: interlobar region bilaterally.
#11: Interlobar nodes.	Between the origin of the lobar bronchi. [a] #11s: between the upper lobe bronchus and bronchus intermedius on the right. [a] #11i: between the middle and lower bronchi on the right.
#12: Lobar nodes.	Adjacent to the lobar bronchi.
#13: Segmental nodes.	Adjacent to the segmental bronchi.
#14: Subsegmental nodes.	Adjacent to the subsegmental bronchi.

#, nodal station number; IASLC, International Association for the Study of Lung Cancer.

[a] Optional notations for subcategories of station.

From Ref. 16 with permission.

lack of validation. Lack of data did not allow further refinement of the M descriptors. All these shortcomings will hopefully be solved by the prospective phase of the IASLC staging project, started in 2009 (26,27). The collection of detailed staging data will be essential to revise the 7th edition of the TNM classification and prepare the 8th edition of 2016.

The TNM classification and staging system for lung cancer is still a strictly anatomic classification. Nonanatomic factors, such as performance status, age, and gender, are important, too, and should be integrated with the TNM classification to evaluate the prognosis of a tumor in a given patient. All these, together with biological, molecular, and genetic factors, will have to be integrated into a prognostic index to improve our present capacity to prognosticate. However, at present, staging remains the most important prognostic factor (28,29).

■ KEY POINTS

- The innovations in the 7th edition of the tumor, node, metastasis (TNM) classification for lung cancer are based on a large international database and have been extensively validated.
- T1 is subclassified as T1a (≤2 cm) and T1b (>2 cm but ≤3 cm).
- T2 is subclassified as T2a (>3 cm but ≤5 cm) and T2b (>5 cm but ≤7 cm).
- T2 >7 cm is reclassified as T3.
- T4 by additional nodule(s) in the same lobe of the primary tumor is reclassified as T3.
- M1 by additional nodule(s) in another ipsilateral lobe is reclassified as T4.
- T4 by pleural or pericardial dissemination (malignant pleural or pericardial effusion or nodules) is reclassified as M1a.
- Contralateral tumor nodules are reclassified as M1a.
- Distant metastases are reclassified as M1b.
- T2bN0M0 tumors are upstaged from stage IB to stage IIA.
- T2aN1M0 tumors are downstaged from stage IIB to stage IIA.
- T4N0–N1M0 tumors are downstaged from stage IIIB to stage IIIA.
- The use of the TNM classification and staging system is emphasized for small cell lung cancer, and stratification by tumor stage recommended in future clinical trials on early small cell lung cancer.
- The TNM classification and staging system are recommended for bronchopulmonary carcinoid tumors for the first time.
- Visceral pleura invasion is defined as tumor involvement beyond the elastic layer, and elastic stains are recommended to confirm or rule out visceral pleura invasion if it is not clear with hematoxylin and eosin stains.
- A new nodal map is proposed for prospective evaluation.

■ REFERENCES

1. Sobin LH, Wittekind C, eds. *International Union Against Cancer (UICC), TNM Classification of Malignant Tumours*. 6th ed. New York: Wiley-Liss; 2002:99–103.

2. Greene FL, Page DL, Fleming ID, et al., eds. *American Joint Committee on Cancer (AJCC), Cancer Staging Handbook*. 6th ed. New York: Springer; 2002:191–203.

3. Goldstraw P, Crowley JJ. The International Association for the Study of Lung Cancer international staging project on lung cancer. *J Thorac Oncol*. 2006;1(4):281–286.

4. Rami-Porta R, Ball D, Crowley J, et al.; International Staging Committee; Cancer Research and Biostatistics; Observers to the Committee; Participating Institutions. The IASLC Lung Cancer Staging Project: proposals for the revision of the T descriptors in the forthcoming (seventh) edition of the TNM classification for lung cancer. *J Thorac Oncol*. 2007;2(7):593–602.

5. Rusch VW, Crowley J, Giroux DJ, et al.; International Staging Committee; Cancer Research and Biostatistics; Observers to the Committee; Participating Institutions. The IASLC Lung Cancer Staging Project: proposals for the revision of the N descriptors in the forthcoming seventh edition of the TNM classification for lung cancer. *J Thorac Oncol*. 2007;2(7):603–612.

6. Postmus PE, Brambilla E, Chansky K, et al.; International Association for the Study of Lung Cancer International Staging Committee; Cancer Research and Biostatistics; Observers to the Committee; Participating Institutions. The IASLC Lung Cancer Staging Project: proposals for revision of the M descriptors in the forthcoming (seventh) edition of the TNM classification of lung cancer. *J Thorac Oncol*. 2007;2(8):686–693.

7. Goldstraw P, Crowley J, Chansky K, et al.; International Association for the Study of Lung Cancer International Staging Committee; Participating Institutions. The IASLC Lung Cancer Staging Project: proposals for the revision of the TNM stage groupings in the forthcoming (seventh) edition of the TNM classification of malignant tumours. *J Thorac Oncol*. 2007;2(8):706–714.

8. Goldstraw P. *International Association for the Study of Lung Cancer Staging Handbook in Thoracic Oncology*. Orange Park, FL: Editorial Rx Press; 2009.

9. Groome PA, Bolejack V, Crowley JJ, et al.; IASLC International Staging Committee; Cancer Research and Biostatistics; Observers to the Committee; Participating Institutions. The IASLC LungCancer Staging Project: validation of the proposals for revision of the T, N, and M descriptors and consequent stage groupings in the forthcoming (seventh) edition of the TNM classification of malignant tumours. *J Thorac Oncol*. 2007;2(8):694–705.

10. Mountain CF, Dresler CM. Regional lymph node classification for lung cancer staging. *Chest*. 1997;111(6):1718–1723.

11. Shepherd FA, Crowley J, Van Houtte P, et al.; International Association for the Study of Lung Cancer International Staging Committee and Participating Institutions. The International Association for the Study of Lung Cancer lung cancer staging project: proposals regarding the clinical staging of small cell lung cancer in the forthcoming (seventh) edition of the tumor, node, metastasis classification for lung cancer. *J Thorac Oncol*. 2007;2(12):1067–1077.

12. Travis WD, Giroux DJ, Chansky K, et al.; International Staging Committee and Participating Institutions. The IASLC Lung

Cancer Staging Project: proposals for the inclusion of broncho-pulmonary carcinoid tumors in the forthcoming (seventh) edition of the TNM classification for lung cancer. *J Thorac Oncol.* 2008;3(11):1213–1223.

13. Travis WD, Brambilla E, Rami-Porta R, et al.; International Staging Committee. Visceral pleural invasion: pathologic criteria and use of elastic stains: proposal for the 7th edition of the TNM classification for lung cancer. *J Thorac Oncol.* 2008;3(12):1384–1390.

14. Naruke T, Suemasu K, Ishikawa S. Lymph node mapping and curability at various levels of metastasis in resected lung cancer. *J Thorac Cardiovasc Surg.* 1978;76(6):832–839.

15. The Japan Lung Cancer Society. *Classification of Lung Cancer.* First English Edition. Tokyo, Japan: Kanehara & Co Ltd; 2000.

16. Rusch VW, Asamura H, Watanabe H, Giroux DJ, Rami-Porta R, Goldstraw P; Members of IASLC Staging Committee. The IASLC lung cancer staging project: a proposal for a new international lymph node map in the forthcoming seventh edition of the TNM classification for lung cancer. *J Thorac Oncol.* 2009;4(5):568–577.

17. Zell JA, Ignatius Ou SH, Ziogas A, Anton-Culver H. Validation of the proposed International Association for the Study of Lung Cancer non-small cell lung cancer staging system revisions for advanced bronchioloalveolar carcinoma using data from the California Cancer Registry. *J Thorac Oncol.* 2007;2(12):1078–1085.

18. Ignatius Ou SH, Zell JA. The applicability of the proposed IASLC staging revisions to small cell lung cancer (SCLC) with comparison to the current UICC 6th TNM Edition. *J Thorac Oncol.* 2009;4(3):300–310.

19. Oliaro A, Filosso PL, Cavallo A, et al. The significance of intrapulmonary metastasis in non-small cell lung cancer: upstaging or downstaging? A re-appraisal for the next TNM staging system. *Eur J Cardiothorac Surg.* 2008;34(2):438–43; discussion 443.

20. Lee JG, Lee CY, Kim DJ, Chung KY, Park IK. Non-small cell lung cancer with ipsilateral pulmonary metastases: prognosis analysis and staging assessment. *Eur J Cardiothorac Surg.* 2008;33(3):480–484.

21. Filosso PL, Ruffini E, Pizzato E, Lyberis P, Giobbe R, Oliaro A. Multifocal (MF) T4 non-small cell lung cancer: a subset with favourable prognosis. *Interac Cardiovasc Thorac Surg.* 2008;7(suppl 3):227.

22. Ou SH, Zell JA. Validation study of the proposed IASLC staging revisions of the T4 and M non-small cell lung cancer descriptors using data from 23,583 patients in the California Cancer Registry. *J Thorac Oncol.* 2008;3(3):216–227.

23. Ruffini E, Filosso PL, Molinatti M, et al. Recommended changes for T and N descriptors proposed by the IASLC Lung Cancer Staging Project: a validation study from a single centre. *Interac Cardiovas Thorac Surg.* 2008;7(suppl 3):226–227.

24. Lee JG, Lee CY, Bae MK, et al. Validity of International Association for the Study of Lung Cancer proposals for the revision of N descriptors in lung cancer. *J Thorac Oncol.* 2008;3(12):1421–1426.

25. Fukui T, Mori S, Hatooka S, Shinoda M, Mitsudomi T. Prognostic evaluation based on a new TNM staging system proposed by the International Association for the Study of Lung Cancer for resected non-small cell lung cancers. *J Thorac Cardiovasc Surg.* 2008;136(5):1343–1348.

26. Giroux DJ, Rami-Porta R, Chansky K, et al.; International Association for the Study of Lung Cancer International Staging Committee. The IASLC Lung Cancer Staging Project: data elements for the prospective project. *J Thorac Oncol.* 2009;4(6):679–683.

27. Goldstraw P. The 7th edition of TNM in Lung Cancer: what now? *J Thorac Oncol.* 2009;4(6):671–673.

28. Sculier JP, Chansky K, Crowley JJ, Van Meerbeeck J, Goldstraw P; International Staging Committee and Participating Institutions. The impact of additional prognostic factors on survival and their relationship with the anatomical extent of disease expressed by the 6th Edition of the TNM Classification of Malignant Tumors and the proposals for the 7th Edition. *J Thorac Oncol.* 2008;3(5):457–466.

29. Chansky K, Sculier JP, Crowley JJ, Giroux D, Van Meerbeeck J, Goldstraw P; International Staging Committee and Participating Institutions. The International Association for the Study of Lung Cancer Staging Project: prognostic factors and pathologic TNM stage in surgically managed non-small cell lung cancer. *J Thorac Oncol.* 2009;4(7):792–801.

5 | Screening and Prevention of Lung Cancer

V. PAUL DORIA-ROSE

EVA SZABO

■ INTRODUCTION

Despite recent advances in the understanding of the biology of lung cancer and improvements in cancer therapeutics, the overall 5-year survival after the diagnosis of lung cancer remains a disappointing 15% (1). The majority of lung cancers continue to be diagnosed in advanced stages; long-term cure remains elusive despite recent modest gains in prolongation of survival with targeted therapeutic approaches. Thus, additional strategies are needed to reduce the burden of lung cancer. This chapter will focus on screening and prevention of lung cancer as two promising strategies to alter the natural history of the carcinogenic process.

■ LUNG CANCER SCREENING

Theoretically, lung cancer is an excellent candidate for screening. It is typically diagnosed at advanced stages, when survival is very poor. Data from the Surveillance, Epidemiology, and End Results (SEER) tumor registry in the United States from 1996 to 2004 indicate overall 5-year survival among all lung cancer cases is only 15% (1). Conversely, when detected at a localized stage, survival is much better, with SEER reporting a 5-year survival (among both screen- and clinically detected cases) of 50% (1). Survival is even greater for those with smaller, screen-detected cancers that undergo resection. For example, among stage I non-small cell lung cancers (NSCLC) detected by chest x-ray as part of three U.S. randomized controlled trials of lung cancer screening conducted in the 1970s and 1980s, 5-year survival among surgically resected cancers was 70% (2). More recently, among stage I resected cancers detected by computed tomography (CT) as part of the International Early Lung Cancer Action Program (I-ELCAP), 10-year survival was estimated to be 92% (3).

Unfortunately, these promising survival figures conflict with mortality results from completed randomized trials of lung cancer screening. Of five prior trials of lung cancer screening, all of which evaluated some combination of chest x-ray and/or sputum cytology (4–21), none found a mortality benefit associated with screening, even though case survival was quite high. This highlights the fact that improved survival among cancer cases alone does not imply a screening test's efficacy, due to biases such as lead time, length-biased sampling, and overdiagnosis (22). In this section, we highlight the findings from randomized trials of chest x-ray and sputum cytology screening, as well as more recent studies of low-dose helical CT, including ongoing randomized controlled trials. Further, we examine some of the controversies that have surrounded lung cancer screening, with particular emphasis on overdiagnosis. Finally, we consider other newer technologies which have not yet been evaluated in large-scale population studies, but may hold promise for the future.

Randomized Controlled Trials of Chest X-ray and Sputum Cytology

The five previous randomized controlled trials of lung cancer screening by chest x-ray and/or sputum cytology (4–21) were initiated in the 1960s and 1970s. All enrolled male smokers only. Three of the trials (the North London study (4,5), the Mayo Lung Project (6–10), and the Czech study (11–13)) examined the impact of offering more versus less frequent chest x-ray (with or without sputum cytology screening), while the other two (the Johns Hopkins Lung Project [14–17,20] and the Memorial Sloan-Kettering Lung Study [18–20]) addressed the value of adding 4-monthly sputum cytology to a chest x-ray screening regimen. A summary of the trials' designs and findings is shown in Table 5.1.

None of the five trials showed a statistically significant benefit of more versus less intensive screening in preventing lung cancer deaths. Further, the three trials that examined different frequencies of chest x-ray screening provided some suggestion of a net harm, with all reporting higher lung cancer mortality in the more intensively screened arm (Table 5.1). In a meta-analysis that included

■ **Table 5.1** RR and 95% CI for lung cancer mortality in the intervention as compared with the control arm among completed randomized controlled trials of chest x-ray and sputum cytology

Trial (Refs.)	Years	n	Screening Offered		RR	95% CI
			Intervention Arm	**Control Arm**		
Trials comparing more to less frequent chest x-ray (with or without sputum cytology)						
North London (4,5)	1960–1964	55,034	6-monthly chest x-ray × 3 years	Chest x-ray at baseline and 3 years	1.03	0.74, 1.42
Mayo Lung Project[a] (6–10)	1971–1983	9,211	4-monthly chest x-ray × 6 years	Chest x-ray at baseline only	1.11[d]	0.95, 1.28
			4-monthly sputum cytology × 6 years	Sputum cytology at baseline only[c]		
Czech Study[b] (11–13)	1976–1986	6,364	Semiannual chest x-ray × 3 years	Chest x-ray at baseline and 3 years	1.27[d]	0.93, 1.74
			Semiannual sputum cytology × 3 years	Sputum cytology at baseline and 3 years		
			Annual chest x-ray in years 4–6	Annual chest x-ray in years 4–6		
Trials comparing chest x-ray plus sputum cytology to chest x-ray alone						
Johns Hopkins Lung Project (14–17,20)	1973–1983	10,386	Annual chest x-ray × 5–7 years	Annual chest x-ray × 5–7 years	0.83	0.67, 1.04
			4-monthly sputum cytology × 5–7 years			
Memorial Sloan-Kettering Lung Study (18–20)	1974–1984	10,040	Annual chest x-ray × 5–8 years	Annual chest x-ray × 5–8 years	0.95	0.73, 1.25
			4-monthly sputum cytology × 5–8 years			

[a] Subjects with positive screening exams by either chest x-ray or sputum cytology at baseline were not randomized; [b] Subjects with prevalent cancers diagnosed at baseline by chest x-ray and/or sputum cytology were not randomized; [c] Control arm subjects were advised at baseline to receive subsequent screens by both chest x-ray and sputum cytology annually (the Mayo Clinic recommendation at the time), but no screening was formally offered as part of the trial; [d] Considers only the initially specified follow-up period. Results from longer-term passive follow-up are discussed separately.

CI, confidence interval; RR, relative risk.

data from these three trials (as well as from an additional trial examining the impact of multiphasic health examinations including chest x-ray (23,24)), this net increase in lung cancer death in the intervention arm was statistically significant (relative risk [RR] 1.11, 95% confidence interval [CI] 1.00–1.23) (21).

Despite this finding, some have contended that weaknesses in the London, Czech, and Mayo Lung Project trials may have obscured a true benefit of lung cancer screening by chest x-ray. Several key criticisms have included (a) a lack of an unscreened comparison group (since both arms of all trials involved some degree of chest x-ray screening), which was further compounded by some degree of noncompliance with the invited screening invitations in the intervention arm and contamination (i.e., receiving additional screening outside of the study protocol) in the control arm (25); and (b) noncomparability of the intervention and control populations, based on the fact that a greater number of lung cancer cases were diagnosed in the intervention than in the control arm (26). The latter criticism implies that there was a failure to create balanced groups in the randomization

process. In order to view the imbalance in the number of lung cancer cases as evidence of noncomparability between the trial arms, which is highly unlikely based on chance alone, one must reject the possibility of overdiagnosis (see discussion in the Lead-time Bias, Length-biased Sampling, and Overdiagnosis section).

The former criticism is being addressed in an ongoing randomized controlled trial, the Prostate, Lung, Colorectal, and Ovarian Cancer Screening Trial (27), in which chest x-ray screening in the intervention arm is being compared with a usual care control arm, among male and female smokers and nonsmokers. Over 150,000 subjects between 55 and 74 years of age were enrolled into the trial between 1993 and 2001 in 10 screening centers throughout the United States. Forty-seven percent of subjects were never-smokers, 43% were former smokers, and 11% were current smokers. Those in the intervention arm were offered either three (never-smokers) or four (former or current smokers) annual chest x-rays, with active follow-up expected to continue for a total of at least 13 years in all subjects. At the baseline screening examination, 44% of the 126 lung cancers diagnosed in the intervention arm were stage I non–small cell cancers (28). Between-arm comparisons of lung cancer incidence and mortality will not be available for several years.

As opposed to the randomized trials examining differing frequencies of chest x-ray, in both trials which explored the value of adding 4-monthly sputum cytology to annual chest x-ray (the Johns Hopkins Lung Project and the Memorial Sloan-Kettering Lung Study) lung cancer mortality was slightly lower in the intervention group. Because these trials had very similar designs and data collection procedures, a recent reanalysis combined data from both for the purposes of calculating a joint estimate of screening effectiveness (20). Even with the added power obtained by combining the data, a statistically significant reduction in lung cancer mortality was not demonstrated, though the results suggested a small benefit (RR 0.88, 95% CI 0.74–1.05). Further, reductions in lung cancer mortality seemed to be greatest (~20%) where they were expected to be so—for squamous cell cancers, which are most likely to be centrally located and therefore to exfoliate cells into sputum (29), and in the heaviest smokers (with a 50 or more pack-year history).

Even if there is a small benefit associated with the use of sputum cytology, it seems unlikely that the magnitude of mortality reduction is sufficient to justify its widespread use as a screening tool. Thus, completed randomized trials of lung cancer screening jointly provide little evidence of benefit, and some evidence of harm. This is reflected in current screening guidelines, none of which advocate lung cancer screening by any modality (30). More recent efforts in the study of lung cancer screening have therefore focused on other screening modalities, with low-dose CT receiving the most attention.

Low-Dose Helical CT Screening

Single-Arm Studies of Helical CT

Until the 1990s, CT was not considered to be a viable option for lung cancer screening. While it was used as a diagnostic procedure, the dose of radiation delivered to the patient (~50 times the radiation exposure as from posterioanterior and lateral chest x-rays (31)) was considered to be too large for its use in asymptomatic individuals. This changed with the publication of a study by Naidich et al. (32), which demonstrated that a low-dose helical CT technique could be used which allowed for sufficient resolution to detect lung nodules while minimizing patient radiation dose (with an exposure approximately five times that of chest x-ray (31)). Naidich (32) further speculated that low-dose CT may have applications for lung cancer screening in high-risk populations.

Subsequently, a number of single-arm studies (i.e., all members of a cohort offered screening) ranging in size from several hundred to several thousand participants have investigated the ability of low-dose helical CT to detect early-stage lung cancers (3,33–54) (summarized in Table 5.2). Most restricted their study populations to smokers and/or those occupationally exposed to lung carcinogens (3,36–40,43,45–47,49–54), though several Asian studies also included a reasonably large proportion of nonsmokers with no occupational exposure (33–35,41,42,44,48). The Early Lung Cancer Action Project (ELCAP), which published its initial results in 1999, was the first to demonstrate the increased ability of low-dose spiral CT to detect lung cancers, as compared with chest x-ray; at a baseline screening of 1,000 individuals by both tests, the prevalence of lung cancer detected by CT was almost fourfold that of lung cancer detected by chest x-ray (27 vs. 7 cases), with no cases identified by chest x-ray that were not visible on CT (36). This finding has been replicated by another single-arm study in Japan, the Anti-Lung Cancer Association (ALCA) study (35). While other single-arm studies have not screened their subjects with both CT and chest x-ray, several randomized controlled trials which employed both modalities as part of their protocols have also noted similar increases in lung cancer detection rates by CT as compared with chest x-ray (55,57). Further, while there has been some variability in results, on the whole, these single-arm studies have shown that a high proportion of screen-detected lung cancers are non–small cell, stage I cancers which have a good prognosis with surgical resection. To date, only one study, the International Early Lung Cancer Action Project (I-ELCAP) has reported survival in a reasonably large number of lung cancer cases detected by CT (n = 484); I-ELCAP investigators reported 10-year survival of 80% (95% CI 74–85) for all detected lung cancers, and 88% (95% CI 84–91) for those with clinical stage I cancer (3). While these Kaplan-Meier survival estimates are based on a relatively small fraction of subjects followed for 10 years (median follow-up of 40 months (3)), and further follow-up of these and other cohorts is required to confirm these results, they nonetheless stand in stark contrast to survival in clinically detected cases.

Other Issues in Low-Dose Helical CT Screening

While the existing studies of CT screening have provided much-needed information regarding the ability of CT to detect early-stage lung cancers, they have also generated a number of other questions that need to be resolved, including who to screen, at what age to start, how to define a positive examination and how to follow it up, and what the appropriate interval for screening should be. Most importantly, despite the promising survival data coming from single-arm studies, it will be critical to definitively demonstrate a benefit of screening (through a cancer mortality outcome) which outweighs screening harms. Finally, assuming a net benefit of screening is demonstrated, it will also be important to examine the issue of

■ Table 5.2 Single-arm studies and randomized controlled trials of low-dose helical CT

Study (Refs.)	Year Initiated	Location	Age	% Male	Smoking	Prevalence or Repeat	N	% of Screens Positive	% With Lung Cancer	% of LC Stage I
Single-Arm Studies										
ALCA (33–35)	1993	Tokyo, Japan	40–79	88	62% Current 25% Former 14% Nonsmokers	Prevalence Repeat	1,611 1,180	12 9	0.8 1.6	77 79
ELCAP (36,37)	1993	New York, NY, USA	60+	54	10+ Pack-years	Prevalence Repeat	1,000 841	23 5	2.7 0.8	85 71
I-ELCAP (3)	1993	USA Japan Europe Israel China	40–86	NR	83% Smokers 17% Nonsmokers[a]	Prevalence Repeat	31,567 27,456	13 5	1.3 0.3	85
University of Munster (38–40)	1995	Germany	40–78	72	20+ Pack-years	Prevalence Repeat	817 668	46 13	2.0 0.4	63 33
Matsumoto Research Center (41,42)	1996	Nagano, Japan	40–74	54	46% >1 Pack-years 54% Nonsmokers	Prevalence Repeat	5,483 4,781	5 4	0.4 0.8	100 86
Finnish Asbestos Workers (43)	1997	Helsinki, Finland	38–81	98	≥10 years 97% Current/Former[b]	Prevalence	602	18	0.8	0
Hitachi (44)	1998	Japan	50–69	79	62% Smokers 38% Nonsmokers	Prevalence Repeat	7,956 5,568	7 3	0.5 0.1	86 100
Mayo Clinic (45–47)	1999	Rochester, MN, USA	50–85	52	20+ Pack-years 61% Current 39% Former	Prevalence Repeat	1,520 1,478	51 12	1.7 0.7	69 60
Samsung Medical Center (48)	1999	Seoul, Korea	46–85	86	52% 20+ Pack-years 25% < 20 Pack-years 23% Nonsmokers	Combined	6,406	35	0.4	57
University of Milan (49)	2000	Lombardy, Italy	50–84	71	20+ Pack-years 86% Current 14% Former	Prevalence Repeat	1,035 996	6 3	1.1 1.1	55 100

Study	Year	Location	Age	%	Smoking eligibility	Round	N			
PALCAD (50,51)	2000	Dublin, Ireland	50–74	50	10+ Pack-years 68% Current 32% Former	Prevalence	449	24	0.4	50
						Repeat	413	1	0.7	33
Nuclear Fuel Workers (52)	2000	Kentucky, Ohio, Tennessee, USA	45+	89	15% Current 51% Former 34% Nonsmokers	Combined	3,598	32	0.6	45
NY-ELCAP (53)	2000	New York State, USA	60+	49	10+ Pack-years 33% Current 67% Former	Prevalence	6,295	14	1.6	67
						Repeat	5,134	6	0.4	
PLuSS (54)	2002	Pittsburgh, PA, USA	50–79	51	0.5+ packs/day for 25+ years 60% Current 40% Former	Prevalence	3,642	41	1.5	58
						Repeat	3,423	42	0.7	33
Randomized Controlled Trials										
LSS (55,56)	2000	USA	55–74	58	30+ Pack-years 58% Current 42% Former	Prevalence	1,586[c]	20	1.9	53
						Repeat	1,398[c]	26	0.6	25
DANTE (57,58)	2001	Italy	60–74	100	20+ Pack-years 55% Current 45% Former	Prevalence	1,276	16	1.1	71
DLCST (59)	2004	Denmark	50–70	56	20+ Pack-years 75% Current 25% Former	Prevalence	2,052	9	0.8	53
ITALUNG (60)	2004	Tuscany, Italy	55–69	64	20+ Pack-years 66% Current 34% Former	Prevalence	1,406[c]	30	1.4	50

[a] Eligible nonsmokers had occupational exposure to asbestos, beryllium, uranium, or radon, or had been exposed to secondhand smoke; [b] Nonsmokers with asbestosis were eligible for inclusion; [c] # receiving the test, not number randomized.

ALCA, Anti-Lung Cancer Association; CT, computed tomography; DANTE, Detection and Screening of Early Lung Cancer by Novel Imaging Technology and Molecular Assays; DLCST, Danish Lung Cancer Screening Trial; ELCAP, Early Lung Cancer Action Project; I-ELCAP, International Early Lung Cancer Action Project; LSS, Lung Screening Study; NY-ELCAP, New York Early Lung Cancer Action Project; PALCAD, ProActive Lung Cancer Detection; PLuSS, Pittsburgh Lung Screening Study. LC, lung cancer; NR, not reported.

cost-effectiveness; several analyses have already attempted to address this issue (61–66).

Regarding which group(s) to target for CT screening, the single-arm studies have appropriately focused on high-risk populations, defined either on the basis of smoking history or occupational exposure to asbestos or radiation. Restriction to these groups maximizes the chances of identifying clinically important lung cancers. Generally, studies of smokers have required at least a 10-to-20 pack-year history (Table 5.2). Studies have also included subjects of varying ages, with different investigators specifying a lower age limit somewhere between 40 and 60 years (Table 5.2). Of the studies which have included younger individuals, two have presented the age-specific prevalence of CT-detected cancer. The ALCA group reported lung cancer prevalence of 0% in those aged 40 to 49, 0.38% in those aged 50 to 59, 1.43% in those aged 60 to 69, and 1.49% in those aged 70 to 79 (35); corresponding prevalences in I-ELCAP were 0.20%, 0.67%, 1.69%, and 2.40%, respectively (3). These figures are consistent with trends in the general population; for example, data from the SEER registry show low incidence rates of lung cancer in individuals under age 50, with rates increasing more rapidly during the sixth and especially seventh decades of life (67). With few cancers detected in those under age 50, it seems unlikely that this group should be targeted for screening. Consequently, ongoing randomized trials of CT screening have included only those aged 50 and older (55–60,68,69), with several only enrolling subjects at least 55 (55,56,60) or 60 (57,58) years old (Table 5.3).

Another important issue in CT screening concerns the definition of a positive examination, and the appropriate follow-up of small lung nodules identified at CT. Many of the single-arm studies classified only noncalcified nodules exceeding a certain size (commonly 5 or 10 mm) as a positive examination (3,33–35,43,48,49,54), while others considered noncalcified nodules of any size a positive screen (36–40). There are advantages and disadvantages to either approach. Further investigation of all noncalcified nodules is labor- and cost-intensive, and results in performing a larger number of invasive tests with the potential for adverse effects. Further, it creates worry among patients being worked up. However, it may also identify more cancers. For the extreme case, in the Mayo Clinic study, over 50% of subjects were screen positive at baseline (45), and almost 70% had experienced at least one positive test after three rounds of annual screening (46). Conversely, delaying further imaging or other tests for the smaller nodules may miss some cancers, but will not expose patients to the harms of additional diagnostics. Regardless of the approach used, most studies have reserved biopsy as an option only for the largest lesions and for those exhibiting growth. Nodules smaller than a certain size (usually 1 or 2 cm) have generally been followed with sequential CT (often with thin-section CT of the nodule(s) and/or standard dose CT) (3,33–54), and/or positron emission

tomography scanning (3,45–47,49,53,54). For example, in ELCAP those with noncalcified nodules 5 mm or less were recommended to undergo repeat high-resolution CT at 3, 6, 12, and 24 months, with biopsy if any growth occurs (36). However, a retrospective analysis by the ELCAP investigators found that, among nodules smaller than 5 mm discovered at screening CT, no malignancies were detected on the basis of surveillance examinations occurring less than 1 year after nodule detection (70). Consequently, more recent guidelines from the Fleischner Society have recommended that high-risk patients undergo only a 1-year follow-up CT for nodules that are 4 mm or less (71). Another option that has been used upon initial detection of a nodule is treatment with a course of broad-spectrum antibiotics, followed by repeat CT to determine whether the lesion has resolved (3,36,37,50,51,53).

The appropriate interval for screening has not yet been determined. All but one of the single-arm CT studies (ALCA (33–35)) offered screening examinations annually; ALCA offered CT every 6 months. For those with nodules identified, surveillance with CT was often more frequent, either every 3 months or every 6 months depending on study and nodule size (3,36–40,43–48,50–54). It seems unlikely that screening more often than annually is justified (with additional surveillance in those with nodules), based on very few interval cancers occurring in these cohorts (3,36–40,45–47,49–51,53); however, no study has evaluated the impact of a longer screening interval.

It is also important to consider possible harms associated with CT screening. The identification of lung nodules results in additional interventions which can include further low- or conventional-dose CT, percutaneous, endoscopic, or open biopsy, and potentially wedge resection, lobectomy, or pneumonectomy. Exposure to x-rays either as part of initial screening or follow-up can lead to radiation-induced lung (or other) cancers. Using cancer incidence data from atomic bomb survivors, it has been estimated that annual low-dose CT screening of 50% of current and former smokers aged 50 to 75 years in the United States would result in approximately 36,000 radiation-induced lung cancer cases (72). Biopsy of lung lesions is also associated with harms. Pneumothorax has been identified as a frequent complication, occurring in approximately 20% to 70% of biopsies, with chest tube placement required in about 5% to 40% of those biopsied (73–76). Finally, there are risks associated with surgery to resect lung cancers. Within single-arm studies, postoperative mortality was low (I-ELCAP reported 30-day mortality as 0.5% (3)). However, this is unlikely to be representative of mortality rates in the general population. An analysis of Medicare data found that the overall 30-day mortality following lobectomy was 5%, and increased with age (77). Another analysis of SEER data reported 3% to 6% 30-day mortality following lobectomy, with hospitals performing more lobectomies having lower mortality

Trial (Refs.)	Year Initiated	Location	Age	Smoking	n	Screening Offered	
						Intervention Arm	Control Arm
DANTE (57,58)	2001	Italy	60–74	20+ Pack-years	2,472	Annual LDCT × 5 years Chest x-ray at baseline Sputum cytology at baseline	Annual clinical exam × 5 years Chest x-ray at baseline Sputum cytology at baseline
NLST (55,56)	2002	USA	55–74	30+ Pack-years	53,364	Annual LDCT × 3 years	Annual chest x-ray × 3 years
NELSON (68)	2003	The Netherlands Belgium	50–75	>15 cigs/day × >25 years OR >10 cigs/day × >30 years	~16,000[a]	LDCT years 1, 2, 4	Usual care
DLCST (59)	2004	Denmark	50–70	20+ Pack-years	4,104	Annual LDCT × 5 years	Usual care
ITALUNG (60)	2004	Tuscany, Italy	55–69	20+ Pack-years	3,206	Annual LDCT × 4 years	Usual care
LUSI (69)	2007	Germany	50–69	Heavy smokers Pack-years unspecified	~4,000[a]	Annual LDCT × 5 years	Usual care

[a] Has not yet published results detailing the number of subjects randomized.

DANTE, Detection of Screening of Early Lunch Cancer by Novel Imaging Technology and Molecular Assays; DLCST, Danish Lung Cancer Screening Trial; LDCT, low-dose helical CT screening; NELSON, Dutch-Belgian Lung Cancer Screening Trial; NLST, National Lung Screening Trial.

rates (78). Others have posited a more long-term effects of lobectomy on mortality, as the resulting decreased lung volume could result in excess deaths due to respiratory failure, pneumonia, or heart disease (79). Because this last potential adverse consequence of lobectomy would occur at a time far removed from surgery, it is unlikely that these deaths would be directly linked to lobectomy.

All of the above risks associated with lung cancer screening and treatment might be acceptable, if the benefit associated with screening is reasonably large. And while survival following the diagnosis of CT-detected lung cancer has been estimated to be 80% (3), it is critical to recognize that increased survival does not necessarily equate to decreased mortality, due to biases inherent to using survival as a measure of screening efficacy, which are discussed as follows.

Lead-time Bias, Length-biased Sampling, and Overdiagnosis

There are three major biases impacting studies of screening: lead-time bias; length-biased sampling; and overdiagnosis. Lead-time bias occurs because screen-detected cancers are, by definition, diagnosed earlier than they otherwise would have been in the absence of screening. Therefore, even if treatment is completely ineffective (i.e., death occurs on the same date regardless of whether an individual is screened), screened individuals will survive for a longer time period following cancer diagnosis. Length-biased sampling is a phenomenon causing screening to preferentially identify cancers with a more indolent course. Because less aggressive cancers are present for a longer period of time before causing symptoms, they are more likely to be identified at a screening examination. Conversely, the most aggressive cancers, with a short preclinical natural history, are more likely to develop and progress to being symptomatic during the interval between screens. Finally, overdiagnosis can be considered to be an extreme form of lead-time bias, in which death occurs due to other causes prior to the cancer becoming clinically apparent. More detailed descriptions of these biases can be found elsewhere (80–82). Within the context of lung cancer screening, overdiagnosis has been extraordinarily controversial (31). For this reason, we focus our attention here on overdiagnosis, with examples from the lung cancer screening literature.

Evidence in Support of Overdiagnosis.   Several lines of evidence have been used in support of a considerable amount of overdiagnosis associated with lung cancer screening. First, all three randomized controlled trials comparing more versus less frequent chest x-ray screening (North London, Czech, Mayo Lung Project) found considerably more cases in the intensely screened arm. For example, in the Mayo Lung Project, during active follow-up there were 206 cases

of lung cancer detected in the arm offered screening every 4 months and only 160 cases in the usual care arm (in which subjects were advised to receive annual screening) (8). To address the question of whether initial follow-up was too short, such that there were asymptomatic, undetected cancers in the less-screened group that accounted for this difference, follow-up in the Mayo Lung Project was extended to 20 years; even with extended follow-up, the excess of cases in the 4-monthly screened group persisted (10). Further, the excess of cases in the more frequently screened arms of the three trials was entirely due to early-stage cancers; the number of advanced cancers detected between both arms of each trial was essentially identical. If there had been a true stage shift, one would have expected a smaller number of advanced cancers in the frequently screened arm. This suggests that there were a number of more indolent cancers detected by screening that would otherwise never have been diagnosed. Early results from the Detection and Screening of Early Lung Cancer by Novel Imaging Technology and Molecular Assays (DANTE) randomized controlled trial, which is comparing annual CT screening to usual care, have noted the same patterns, with 60 lung cancers diagnosed in the screening arm and 34 in the control arm, again with very similar numbers of advanced cancers in the two arms (after a median follow-up of 34 months) (58).

Additional evidence of overdiagnosis comes from autopsy studies. Based on a series of almost 16,000 autopsies conducted between 1953 and 1982, investigators at Yale-New Haven Hospital identified 525 lung cancers among those dying of natural causes. Sixty-eight of these (13%) were classified as not having been diagnosed during life, and were referred to as "necropsy surprises" (83). Similar findings were reported from a series of almost 25,000 autopsies in Victoria, Australia, with 47 out of 167 lung cancers (28%) classified as incidental (i.e., not diagnosed or symptomatic prior to death, and judged not to have been the underlying, or a contributing cause, of death based on autopsy review) (84).

Finally, overdiagnosis is suggested by the fact that the epidemiology of screen-detected cancers is very different from that of clinically detected cancers. For example, the Hitachi study of CT reported a higher prevalence of lung cancer in nonsmokers (0.76%) than in smokers (0.34%) (our calculations based on numbers presented in the manuscript) (44). Furthermore, the Matsumoto Research Center study found a similar prevalence of lung cancer in smokers (0.40%) and nonsmokers (0.44%) screened with CT (41). While men were highly overrepresented among smokers in these studies, confounding alone is not sufficient to explain the high prevalence of lung cancer observed in nonsmokers, based on what is known about (clinically detected) lung cancer epidemiology. Similarly, CT studies have found a much higher proportion of adenocarcinomas (and especially bronchioalveolar carcinomas) than would be expected; bronchioalveolar adenocarcinomas, in particular, may be more likely to be slow-growing, and thus overdiagnosed (31).

Evidence Against Overdiagnosis.   The most compelling evidence against a large degree of overdiagnosis comes from studies which have examined the clinical course of surgically treated versus untreated early-stage lung cancers. In an analysis of 336 cases of stage I NSCLC diagnosed as part of the Mayo Lung Project, Johns Hopkins Lung Project, and Memorial Sloan-Kettering Lung Study trials of chest x-ray and sputum cytology, lung cancer-specific 5-year survival was 70% among those who underwent surgical resection (n = 291), and only 10% among those not having surgery (n = 45) (2). Similar 10-year survival numbers (90% of all 407 stage I cases but 0% of three stage I cases not surgically treated) were seen in I-ELCAP (85).

There are several problems with this type of comparison, however, which should be considered. First, in the absence of resection, tumors are often clinically rather than pathologically staged; in this way, a number of untreated, clinical stage I cancers may well have been found to be of a higher pathologic stage, had the patient gone to surgery. Second, those who do not undergo surgery are an unusual (and further in the case of I-ELCAP, very small) group, one which may have a much worse prognosis due to, for example, serious comorbidities which make them poor candidates for surgery (86). Despite these problems, the differences in survival between resected and unresected stage I lung cancers are so striking that it would be tempting to conclude that these results could not be entirely due to bias. However, in light of the evidence in favor of overdiagnosis, particularly the increased number of lung cancer cases that have been consistently observed in the more intensely screened arms of randomized controlled trials, the preponderance of the evidence suggests that there may be a considerable degree of overdiagnosis, which makes the use of high survival estimates to infer screening efficacy unreliable.

Lung Cancer Mortality and Randomized Controlled Trials of CT

Because of the inherent limitations of a survival endpoint, as described above, a cancer mortality endpoint, which is calculated as the total number of cancer deaths divided by the total number of person-years at risk, is preferred. Cancer mortality is not subject to lead time, length, and overdiagnosis biases, since mortality is calculated for an entire screened cohort starting at date of enrollment (as opposed to survival, which is calculated in cancer cases only from the date of diagnosis). Consequently, randomized controlled trials with a cancer mortality endpoint are considered the gold standard in evaluating screening efficacy.

Because of this, several randomized controlled trials of CT have been initiated (Table 5.3). The largest,

the National Lung Screening Trial (NLST) in the United States, is comparing low-dose CT screening to chest x-ray. A feasibility study for the NLST, the Lung Screening Study (LSS), has reported findings from the baseline and repeat screens (55,56) (Table 5.2). The other trials, in Europe, are comparing CT to usual care (57–60,68,69). Several have reported baseline findings (57–60) (Table 5.2), and one, DANTE, has reported lung cancer mortality over a median follow-up period of approximately 3 years, with 20 deaths reported in each arm (58). However, it is far too early in follow-up to conclude that these early results from DANTE are suggestive of no mortality benefit associated with CT screening.

While there are no long-term mortality results available from randomized controlled trials of CT screening, there has been an attempt, using a risk prediction model which incorporates age, gender, and smoking history, to estimate the efficacy of CT screening (87). The basic approach was to compare observed rates of lung cancer in three different single-arm studies of CT (Mayo Clinic, Moffitt Cancer Center, and University of Milan) with rates predicted by the model. Observed rates of cancer were threefold higher than those expected, and surgical removal of early-stage lung cancer was 10-fold higher than expected. Unfortunately, the number of advanced lung cancer cases observed was not smaller than predicted, and the number of lung cancer deaths observed was essentially identical to that predicted by the model (RR 1.0, 95% CI 0.7–1.3). Yet despite this, observed 4-year survival was 94%. While these findings are based on only a short follow-up period (4 years), and are subject to the accuracy of the prediction model, they are remarkably consistent with findings from prior trials of chest x-ray screening. Specifically, they suggest no evidence of screening efficacy as measured by lung cancer mortality, but highly increased survival.

Other Screening Tests

In addition to the imaging and sputum cytology techniques described above, several other tests have been considered for lung cancer screening, including methods for the analysis of sputum, breath, blood, buccal smears, and urine. While randomized trials failed to demonstrate a significant reduction in lung cancer mortality associated with the examination of sputum by conventional light microscopy, other sputum analysis techniques have more recently been developed which have greater accuracy in identifying lung cancer, including automated quantitative image cytometry (88), detection of the overexpression of heterogeneous nuclear ribonucleoprotein (hnRNP) A2 B1 (89), and the identification of p53 and ras mutations (90) or promoter hypermethylation (91). Breath analysis has concentrated on the ability to distinguish differences in volatile organic compounds between lung cancer cases and control patients. Several studies have utilized gas chromatography–mass spectrometry (GC-MS) (92–94); however, these systems are expensive and results need to be interpreted by those with specialized training. Other types of breath analysis have utilized arrays of chemical sensors ("electronic noses") (95–97), which are much simpler to use and therefore have a broader appeal for mass screening, and nonvolatile biomarkers have also been measured in exhaled breath condensate (EBC) (98). A large number of biomarkers in blood have also been considered, including the total amount of free DNA, DNA hypermethylation and microsatellite alterations, gene mutations, and protein markers (99,100). With the idea that the alterations in the easily accessible oral epithelium can serve as a surrogate marker for malignancy in the lungs, examination of the cells of the buccal mucosa has also been considered as a screening tool (101,102). Finally, discriminating between lung cancer cases and noncases using analysis of urine for concentrations of trace elements (103) or the tobacco-specific nitrosamine metabolite NNAL (104) has also been assessed. While all of these alternate approaches to lung cancer screening hold promise, it should be noted that in their current form none are accurate enough to be considered for use in the general population, and consequently, none are being evaluated in large-scale trials.

Summary of Lung Cancer Screening

Despite decades of research, the search for a lung cancer screening modality with the ability to prevent lung cancer mortality continues. In the 1960s through 1980s, randomized controlled trials of chest x-ray and sputum cytology failed to demonstrate a mortality benefit. Currently, trials of low-dose CT screening are ongoing, with the NLST of CT screening expected to report its mortality results in 2011. While a reduction in the number of lung cancer deaths is of critical importance to public health, lung cancer screening also has the potential to result in harms. Therefore, only a test of proven benefit should be considered as a screening tool. Consequently, current guidelines do not recommend lung cancer screening by any modality (30).

■ PREVENTION OF LUNG CANCER

The rationale for prevention (or chemoprevention, as it is typically called) of lung cancer is based on the concepts that carcinogenesis evolves through various stages over a lengthy period of time in individuals exposed to carcinogens, and that the entire exposed epithelial surface is subject to damage from carcinogens (105,106). The genetic and epigenetic insults from carcinogen exposure (e.g., tobacco smoke) accumulate over time across the entire exposed field, leading to an accumulation of histologic and molecular changes that continue to evolve independently. Identification of multiple histologic changes at varying stages of progression in

the lungs of smokers with or without lung cancer (107,108) and the high incidence of second primary lung cancers after an initial diagnosis strongly support this view of lung carcinogenesis (109). Two major corollaries follow from these concepts. First, the lengthy nature of the carcinogenic process theoretically provides ample opportunities for intervention, if individuals undergoing carcinogenic evolution can be appropriately identified. Second, to adequately reduce all risk of subsequent cancer development, the entire exposed field needs to be treated. In this section, we provide a historical perspective on lung chemoprevention clinical trials and discuss current concepts as well as new directions in preventive agent development.

A Historical Perspective
Phase III Clinical Trials

Not only does smoking account for 80% to 90% of lung cancer and more than half of lung cancers occur in former smokers, but the risk of lung cancer in former smokers remains elevated (in relation to never-smokers) for years after smoking cessation (110). Unlike cardiovascular disease, where smoking cessation leads to relatively rapid return to baseline risk, the genetic injury to the bronchial epithelium is demonstrable for years after smoking cessation (108) and it takes years before risk of lung cancer begins to diminish in comparison to ongoing smoking (110). Nevertheless, smoking cessation is the only strategy that has been shown to reduce the risk of subsequent lung cancer. The Lung Health Study, which randomized smokers to smoking cessation intervention programs versus no intervention, demonstrated a 55% reduction in lung cancer mortality in successful sustained quitters after extended (14.5 years) follow-up (111). Of note, earlier follow-up (5 years) did not show a similar (or lesser) effect, emphasizing the need for long-term cessation to observe the benefits.

With regard to pharmacologic interventions, the phase III definitive efficacy lung cancer prevention trials performed to date have focused primarily on vitamins and micronutrients. A number of these large lung chemoprevention studies have studied β-carotene, vitamin A, and vitamin A derivatives. The results of these studies are summarized in Table 5.4. The rationale for this approach (summarized in (112)) was based primarily on epidemiologic associations between the increased incidence of lung cancer and a diet deficient in fruit and vegetable containing β-carotene, a provitamin A.

The Alpha-Tocopherol, Beta-Carotene Cancer Prevention Study (ATBC) investigated the effectiveness of β-carotene (20 mg per day) and α-tocopherol (50 mg per day), alone or in combination, in reducing lung cancer incidence in 29,133 Finnish male smokers (113). With a follow-up period ranging from 5 to 8 years, the treatment did not reduce lung cancer incidence. Moreover, subjects receiving β-carotene, alone or in combination with

■ **Table 5.4** Phase III lung chemoprevention trials

Trial	Cohort	Intervention	Outcome
ATBC, 1994	29,133 smokers	β-carotene, vitamin E, both, or placebo	18% increase in lung cancer
CARET, 1996	18,314 smokers or asbestos exposed	β-carotene + retinol vs. placebo	Increased lung cancer, RR = 1.36
EUROSCAN, 2000	2,592 lung or head & neck ca. patients	Retinyl palmitate, NAC, both, or placebo	No benefit
Intergroup, 2001	1,166 stage-I NSCLC patients	Isotretinoin	No benefit (increased recurrence current smokers)
Intergroup Selenium Trial, 2010	1,960 Stage I NSCLC patients (projected enrollment)	Selenium	Stopped early for futility

ATBC, Alpha-Tocopherol, Beta-Carotene Cancer Prevention Study; CARET, Beta-Carotene and Retinol Efficacy Trial; EUROSCAN, European study on chemoprevention with vitamin A and N-acetylcysteine; NAC, N-acetyl-l-cysteine; NSCLC, non–small cell lung cancer; RR, relative risk.

α-tocopherol, showed an 18% higher incidence of lung cancer compared with the placebo group. Similarly, the CARET study (Beta-Carotene and Retinol Efficacy Trial) was a randomized double-blinded placebo-controlled chemoprevention trial which recruited 18,314 participants to evaluate the efficacy of the β-carotene and retinol in a population at high risk for developing lung cancer (114). Current smokers, former smokers, and individuals exposed to asbestos were treated with 30 mg β-carotene and 25,000 IU retinyl palmitate (vitamin A) or placebo. The primary endpoint of the study was lung cancer incidence. After results of the Finnish ATBC study became available, the CARET trial was stopped 21 months early and the data showed that study participants receiving the active combination had an adverse outcome compared with the placebo group, with an RR of 1.36 (95% CI = 1.07–1.73, $P = 0.01$) for lung cancer incidence and an RR of 1.59 (95% CI = 1.13–2.23, $P = 0.01$) for lung cancer mortality. Subgroup analysis showed that the harm was restricted to current smokers, similar to the results of the ATBC trial. These results differ somewhat from the results of the Physicians' Health Study, which randomized 22,071 male physicians to β-carotene and/or aspirin or placebo for an average of 12 years and showed neither benefit nor harm (115). In this trial, however, only 11% of participants were current smokers while 39% were former smokers, consistent with the hypothesis that β-carotene's negative effects are limited to current smokers.

In contrast to the primary prevention studies exemplified by the ATBC and CARET, the EUROSCAN study (European study on chemoprevention with vitamin A and N-acetylcysteine) was a tertiary prevention study designed to assess whether a combination of retinyl palmitate and the antioxidant N-acetylcysteine could prevent second primary tumors in 2,592 patients with curatively treated head and neck or lung cancers (116). Intervention consisted of daily administration of retinyl palmitate, 300,000 IU

daily for 1 year, followed by 150,000 IU daily throughout the second year versus 600 mg of N-acetylcysteine versus both agents versus neither agent. No statistically significant improvement in overall survival or tumor-free survival was observed in treated individuals. These results failed to confirm a previous smaller study of 307 patients with stage I lung cancer who received high-dose vitamin A, 300,000 IU, or placebo daily for 12 months, which showed a statistically significant increase in time to second primary tumors in vitamin A–treated patients (117).

Clinical trials with isotretinoin (13-cis-retinoic acid, 13cRA) have demonstrated efficacy in treating oral leukoplakia, a precursor to cancer of the oral cavity (118,119) as well as prevention of second primary tumors in patients previously treated for head and neck cancers (120). However, trials of retinoids for lung chemoprevention have not been successful. The Phase III Intergroup Trial randomized 1,166 patients with resected stage I NSCLC to low-dose isotretinoin (30 mg/day) or placebo for 3 years (121). Treatment did not improve the rates of second primary tumors, recurrence, or mortality. Subset analysis suggested that isotretinoin was harmful in current smokers, with a higher recurrence rate than never-smokers or former smokers.

The most recent phase III prevention trial was a study of selenium in curatively treated stage I NSCLC patients. This trial was based on a secondary endpoint observation of significantly decreased lung cancer incidence in participants in a prior skin cancer prevention involving 1,312 patients with a history of skin cancer who were treated with selenium supplementation (200 μg/day) (122). While no significant decrease in skin cancer was noted, selenium supplementation resulted in 17 cases of lung cancer compared with 31 cases in the placebo group (RR = 0.54, 95% CI =0.30–0.98, $P = 0.04$). Based on this observation, a randomized phase III trial prospectively assessing whether selenium supplementation can prevent second primary tumors after curative resection of stage I NSCLC was established. Unfortunately, this trial was recently closed for futility after an interim analysis.

Lessons Learned

A number of important lessons have emerged from the lung cancer (and other organ) phase III clinical trials performed to date. One of the main lessons from the β-carotene experience concerns the levels of evidence required before embarking on large clinical trials. The basis for these trials was primarily epidemiologic in nature, without the benefit of animal carcinogenesis modeling studies or more mechanistic understanding of β-carotene actions that have subsequently become available (123,124). There are inherent limitations to translating epidemiologic observations based on complex foods to successful clinical trials using a single nutrient given for a finite amount of time during a defined phase during the lengthy process of carcinogenesis (125). Epidemiologic studies are unable to accurately assess the effect of replacing a single micronutrient because they cannot adequately describe the entire complex biologic milieu within which the micronutrient functions. The β-carotene studies thus underscore the need for assessing multiple types of evidence when selecting a particular prevention strategy, even if this calls for additional work to be done.

The second important lesson pertains to the all-important balance between risk and benefit, which is a critical consideration for all medical interventions but is particularly important in reference to individuals who appear to be healthy but are at risk for a future event such as lung cancer. Food constituents and vitamins are often considered to be safe by the public and by the medical establishment, even though pharmacologic doses are frequently considerably higher than the amounts obtained through ordinary diet. The ATBC and CARET studies required >29,000 and >18,000 participants, respectively, to definitely establish an 18% to 36% increased risk of lung cancer, which was not known at the time and would not have been identified in smaller trials. Despite the relatively small increased lung cancer risk with β-carotene supplementation, the existence of a large number of smoking individuals at any given time means that such risks are of considerable public health importance. Although the results of these trials were disappointing for failing to identify effective preventive interventions, they had important ramifications and led to recommendations against the use of β-carotene supplementation. Similar lessons were learned from studies of prevention of colorectal adenomas with selective cyclooxygenase (COX-2) inhibitors rofecoxib and celecoxib. Although associated with a 24% decrease in colorectal adenoma recurrence, extended use of 25 mg daily of rofecoxib was found to increase the RR of thrombotic events to 1.92 (95% CI, 1.19–3.11; $P = 0.008$), primarily due to cardiac events (hazard ratio [HR]

= 2.80, 95% CI, 1.44–5.45) and cerebrovascular events (HR = 2.32, 95% CI, 0.89–6.74) (126,127). Rofecoxib was subsequently withdrawn from the market. Extended celecoxib use was also associated with increased cardiovascular events, with an HR of 2.3 (95% CI, 0.9–5.5) for 200 mg twice daily and an HR of 3.4 (95% CI, 1.4–7.8) for 400 mg twice daily (128). Two celecoxib trials demonstrated a 33% to 45% reduction in adenoma number (129,130), but celecoxib cannot be recommended for colorectal polyp prevention due to the associated cardiovascular risk. It is important to note that the cardiovascular risks of these blockbuster drugs were not identified in the original relatively short registration studies that led to their primary Food and Drug Administration approvals.

Current Approaches to the Development of Agents for Lung Cancer Prevention

Given the necessity for thoroughly understanding the efficacy as well as the potential risks associated with any preventive interventional strategy, the selection of a target for intervention, and, consequently, a specific agent, needs to take into consideration a variety of attributes of the target, the available agents, and the cohorts to be treated. Since many agents studied for cancer prevention are already in clinical use or are nutritional in nature, there has been considerable temptation to avoid the tedious early drug development work and to proceed directly to definitive efficacy phase III trials. However, the experience obtained from a number of cancer prevention trials in a variety of organs, with negative or harmful outcomes (131,132), has suggested that considerably more attention needs to be focused on the early development of preventive agents, including preliminary efficacy phase II clinical trials. The following discussion summarizes the key concepts that need to be taken into consideration during the development of strategies for lung cancer prevention.

Target Identification

Identifying efficacy is the most critical component of the process of selection of agents for clinical development for cancer prevention or treatment. Indications of effectiveness fall into several major categories—knowledge of mechanisms, in vitro and animal in vivo experimental data, epidemiologic case-control and cohort studies, and data from clinical trials (reviewed in (131)). During each stage of drug development, but particularly at the juncture between preclinical and early clinical trials and then again at the juncture between early-phase and definitive phase III clinical trials, it is necessary to review all the available data and to examine it for consistency. The quality and consistency of the available data help determine whether additional data needs to be obtained prior to clinical trials, or if sufficient knowledge is available to make a "go-no go" decision.

The better one understands the process of lung carcinogenesis and the molecular basis for the evolution of the neoplastic phenotype, the more likely will one be able to develop interventions to abrogate neoplastic progression. Understanding the molecular events responsible for the various phases of lung carcinogenesis, and the results of their simultaneous versus sequential occurrence, is a complex task. The different histologic types of lung cancer arise from different progenitor cells and even a single histologic subtype, such as adenocarcinoma, is composed of many molecular subtypes with different prognoses and responses to treatment (133). Nevertheless, defining the events and their temporal occurrence is critical if progress in identifying appropriate lung cancer prevention targets is to occur.

The efficacy of an agent in preventing cancer will depend on how critical its target is to carcinogenesis, whether the agent can be delivered at the time that its target drives the carcinogenic process, and the potency of the intervention. Because different aspects of carcinogenic progression may depend on different molecular abnormalities or signaling pathways, it is important to determine when specific abnormalities should be targeted. For instance, targeting the initial DNA damage from tobacco-derived carcinogen exposure by blocking carcinogen metabolism may be very effective prior to the acquisition of much DNA damage, but is not likely to be effective once the damage already exists and cells have acquired multiple genetic lesions (after years of smoking). Furthermore, the effectiveness of an intervention depends not just on the presence of its target, but also on the importance of its target in determining the progression to cancer. A priori, there is no reason to theorize that interventions that are effective during some phases of carcinogenesis will be effective during other stages, unless the target has a critical biologic role during multiple stages of carcinogenesis. Finally, it is important to remember that phase III cancer prevention trials with tumor incidence endpoints generally test interventions for only a small number of years, so these trials are, by design, testing intervention efficacy on relatively advanced stages of premalignancy. Consequently, an intervention that blocks early events in carcinogenesis, such as initiating DNA damage events, is highly unlikely to prevent cancer in a trial where the duration of the intervention is 3 to 5 years. In selecting targets for cancer prevention, the ability to design the appropriate clinical trials to demonstrate efficacy must be considered—if one cannot demonstrate preventive ability within the context of our currently available clinical trial resources (for instance, if the intervention must be delivered prior to all carcinogen exposure), the drug development is not likely to be effective.

Identification of High-Risk Cohorts

Since almost all interventions are likely to have some side effects, it is critical to identify the most appropriate high-risk cohorts who stand to gain the most from interventions. The difficulty lies in the fact that current risk assessment tools are very imprecise for most cancer types. More than 80% of lung cancer is attributable to tobacco exposure, yet only a minority of smokers develop lung cancer during their lifetime. Peto et al. (110) estimated the cumulative risk of lung cancer at age 75 to be 15.9% for men and 9.5% for women. Identifying the smokers who are most likely to develop cancer has proven to be quite challenging. The history of a prior lung cancer is associated with a 1% to 2% yearly risk of a new cancer (109). The presence of chronic obstructive pulmonary disease (COPD) adds independent risk beyond tobacco exposure alone (134,135). Bach et al. (136) have developed a risk assessment tool to identify lung cancer risk in current and former smokers, based on the information available from the CARET trial of over 18,000 participants. While this tool is useful for individuals who fit the enrollment criteria for CARET, it is not applicable to individuals with different characteristics (e.g., those younger than 50 years or with less smoking exposure). Spitz et al. (137) have further expanded on lung cancer risk assessment to incorporate multiple exposures and family history as well as to assess risk in never-smokers. However, both of these models rely primarily on demographic information rather than on the specific molecular characteristics of a given individual and consequently have substantial limitations.

A variety of additional factors helps to identify individuals at high risk for lung cancer. Cytologic atypia in exfoliated cells in the sputum of smokers with COPD is further associated with increased lung cancer risk, with an HR of 2.8 (138). Varella-Garcia (139) recently reported that the presence of chromosomal aneusomy in sputum cells was associated with an adjusted odds ratio of lung cancer of 29.9. If confirmed in future studies, such a sputum-based approach to risk assessment offers tremendous potential to truly identify those who might most benefit from preventive interventions.

Intermediate Endpoints

Identification of appropriate study endpoints is a critical aspect of cancer prevention drug development. Although phase III randomized placebo-controlled trials are the gold standard for demonstrating effective cancer prevention, the sizable resources and lengthy time frame required for such trials require that preliminary efficacy be first demonstrated in smaller phase II (see discussion in Lessons Learned section). Whereas phase III cancer prevention trials aim to demonstrate changes in cancer incidence, phase II preliminary efficacy cancer prevention trials rely on short-term, or intermediate, endpoints that are theoretically predictive of patient outcomes such as cancer incidence. In contrast to phase II cancer treatment trials, which use tumor measurements to assess agent efficacy, phase II cancer prevention trials do not have easily measured primary trial endpoints established for indicating preventive efficacy. Therefore, early-phase cancer prevention trials generally assess surrogate efficacy measures that are even more distantly related to the definitive endpoint of cancer incidence than tumor shrinkage is related to survival.

To be useful, an intermediate marker should meet several major criteria (140–142). (a) It should be integrally involved in the process of carcinogenesis, such that its expression correlates with the disease course. (b) Its expression should differ between normal and at-risk epithelium, and it should be easily and reproducibly measurable in specimens likely to be obtained in clinical trials. (c) The expression of the marker should be modulated by effective interventions, and there should be minimal spontaneous fluctuations and no modulation by ineffective agents. A marker that satisfies these criteria then needs to be validated in prospective clinical trials (141).

To date, no intermediate endpoint marker has passed these rigorous validation requirements. However, it is becoming clear that the complex molecular mechanisms that regulate tumor development involve a number of molecules and regulatory pathways controlling various cellular processes, including proliferation, differentiation, apoptosis, invasion through the basement membrane, and angiogenesis (143). Classes of molecules found to be altered in lung cancer and precancerous lesions include oncogenes, tumor suppressor genes, growth factors or their receptors, and molecules regulating cellular immortality, immune defense, and tumor-associated angiogenesis. Improved understanding of aberrantly functioning molecules associated with lung cancer development provides the opportunity to develop biomarkers which can be used in risk assessment as well as in monitoring response to chemopreventive or therapeutic interventions. Biomarkers associated with early stages of carcinogenesis could be of great value for early detection of lung cancer and precancerous lesions. In addition, biomarkers that regulate molecular pathways critically important in lung carcinogenesis may also serve as targets for novel therapies.

Nevertheless, even the currently available intermediate endpoints can significantly inform early-phase drug development and can demonstrate effects of agents on the target epithelium. The most commonly used intermediate endpoint in phase II lung cancer prevention trials is bronchial dysplasia, the precursor to squamous carcinoma (144). Histologic precursors to invasive cancer are typically referred to as "intraepithelial neoplasia" (IEN). The presence of sequential changes in the bronchial epithelium of smokers, as elegantly demonstrated nearly 50 years ago by Auerbach and colleagues, provides an opportunity to assess the effects of interventions on IEN in tissues obtained via serial bronchoscopies. The incidence of mild, moderate, and severe bronchial dysplasia documented by fluorescence bronchoscopy in current and

former smokers with a ≥30 pack-year smoking history is 44%, 14%, 4.3%, and 1.2%, respectively (145). The natural history of these lesions is difficult to assess since some are completely removed during bronchoscopy, but studies using serial autofluorescence bronchoscopic biopsies suggest that approximately 3.5% of low or moderate dysplasias progress to severe dysplasia, 37% of severe dysplasias remain or progress, and approximately 50% of carcinomas in situ progress to invasive carcinoma within a 2 to 3 year follow-up period (146,147). Thus, these lesions identify a cohort at high risk for progression to cancer and also provide an opportunity to intervene in the pathway leading to the development of squamous carcinoma. A variety of other biomarkers, including the Ki-67 proliferation index, have also been used, although the direct correlation between such biomarkers and cancer incidence is even more remote than the relationship between bronchial dysplasia and cancer (142).

Early-Phase Clinical Trial Designs

Given that the majority of lung cancer develops in current or former smokers, phase II lung cancer prevention trial designs have primarily focused on individuals with heavy smoking exposure or on curatively treated aerodigestive cancer patients, frequently using these cohorts to further facilitate the identification of individuals who have dysplastic bronchial lesions at higher risk for progression to overt cancer, as discussed earlier. A typical trial design would be to identify smokers with bronchoscopically confirmed bronchial dysplasia, treat for 3 to 6 months (preferably in a placebo-controlled setting given the spontaneous resolution of some lesions and the removal of others during bronchoscopy), and repeat bronchoscopy with biopsy of known areas of abnormality as well as any new suspicious areas. Such a strategy is quite labor-intensive, requiring considerable screening (often with sputum cytology first, followed by bronchoscopy) to identify the higher risk individuals who actually have bronchial lesions that can then be followed with serial biopsies. Since bronchial dysplasia is a known precursor to cancer, as discussed earlier, it is felt to be an informative endpoint with regard to subsequent cancer incidence. The prototype of this kind of trial is the phase IIb study of the inhaled steroid budesonide performed by Lam et al. (148). Intermediate endpoint trials that focus on molecular abnormalities rather than IEN have the disadvantage of potentially using a less high-risk cohort (without IEN) and a less informative endpoint since the obligate association between lung cancer incidence and specific molecular markers has not been clearly established. The prototype of this trial is the phase IIb trial by Kurie et al. (149) using 9-cis-retinoic acid alone or with α-tocopherol to reverse the loss of retinoic acid receptor-β expression that occurs so frequently during lung carcinogenesis.

The bronchial dysplasia clinical trial model described above selects participants with central airway abnormalities within the reach of a bronchoscope, thus enriching for populations at risk for squamous carcinomas. It is not intuitively clear that the same strategies should be effective for the prevention of adenocarcinomas as well as squamous cell carcinomas, given that these tumors appear to have different molecular pathogenesis and likely arise from different progenitor cells. The availability of helical CT to follow peripheral nodules that may represent precursors to adenocarcinoma allows for the first time the assessment of interventions for peripheral lung carcinogenesis. A new trial design, focusing on high-risk smokers with lung nodules identified by helical CT that are not clearly malignant or benign, thus becomes possible. One such trial, using the inhaled steroid, budesonide, has thus far been completed, with publication of results pending. The disadvantage of this design is that such nodules are generally too small to biopsy and thus their histology cannot be determined. Most nodules are likely to be benign or inflammatory rather than premalignant. However, nonsolid nodules described as ground-glass opacities on helical CT are much more likely to represent adenocarcinomas or their precursor lesions, atypical adenomatous hyperplasia. Accumulating data further suggest that such ground-glass nodules are more likely to be malignant (59–73% of cases) than solid nodules (7–9% of cases) (150). Long-term follow-up of these nodules is needed to determine if they should be the focus of future trials.

As less toxic targeted agents are being developed for lung cancer treatment, another opportunity arises to simultaneously address their potential for prevention in the bronchial epithelium assessed via bronchoscopy. If there is a biologic rationale for expecting efficacy during early stages of carcinogenesis and the toxicity profile is favorable, when such agents are late in development for metastatic disease or in the adjuvant setting, pre- and post-treatment bronchoscopies could address their effect on bronchial dysplasia.

This would considerably speed up new prevention agent development by giving an early indication of effectiveness, which may or may not need to be followed by dose titration to establish the optimal dose for prevention indications.

Ongoing Studies and New Directions

Recent research directions in lung chemoprevention have focused on the identification of molecular targets for intervention and optimization of clinical trial design. The ability to rapidly identify efficacious agents using a relatively small number of participants prior to large phase III cancer prevention trials is the appeal of an intermediate endpoint-driven phase II trial design. Therefore, the emphasis has been on early-phase (primarily phase II) trials and on the molecular characterization of specimens obtained prior to and after intervention. Table 5.5 shows currently ongoing and recently closed phase II lung cancer prevention clinical trials. The following discussion is not meant to be exhaustive, but rather is meant to highlight some of the current areas of investigation.

A large body of evidence suggests that inflammation plays a critical role in the genesis of lung cancer and that various anti-inflammatory compounds can prevent cancer development. Wattenberg et al. (151,152) have demonstrated that both systemic and inhaled steroids, which inhibit the generation of arachidonic acid from membrane phospholipids by phospholipase A2, can inhibit the development of lung adenomas and carcinomas in mice treated with a variety of carcinogens. Based on this rationale, Lam et al. (148) conducted a phase IIb randomized placebo-controlled trial of inhaled budesonide in persons with bronchial dysplasia. Participants were selected on the basis of central airway pathology (bronchial dysplasia) but underwent monitoring of both their central and peripheral lung via autofluorescence bronchoscopy and helical CT, respectively. Although the 6-month treatment did not result in regression of the central airway dysplasia (the primary study endpoint), there

■ Table 5.5	Ongoing and recently closed early-phase clinical trials			
Agent	**Drug Class**	**Cohort**	**Endpoint**	**Status**
Myo-inositol	PI3K inhibitor	Smokers with dysplasia	Dysplasia	Open to accrual
Polyphenon E	Green tea constituent	Smokers with dysplasia	Dysplasia	Open to accrual
Phenylethyl isothiocyanate	Isothiocyanate (inhibit NNK metabolism)	Smokers	Carcinogen (NNK) metabolism	Open to accrual
Enzastaurin	PKC inhibitor	Former smokers	Ki-67	Open to accrual
Erlotinib	EGFR inhibitor	Smokers with history prior cancer	EGFR phosphorylation	Open to accrual
Celecoxib	COX-2 inhibitor	Former smokers	Ki-67	Closed, results pending
Sulindac	COX-1/COX-2 inhibitor	Smokers with dysplasia	Dysplasia	Closed, results pending
Zileuton	5-Lipoxygenase inhibitor	Smokers with dysplasia	Dysplasia	Closed, results pending
Budesonide	Corticosteroid	Smokers with lung nodules	CT-detected lung nodules	Closed, results pending

CT, computed tomography.

was an increased rate of resolution of CT-detected peripheral nodules (a secondary endpoint). Therefore, Veronesi and colleagues in Italy conducted a phase IIb chemoprevention trial with budesonide in persons with persistent peripheral lung nodules identified during helical CT screening. The results are pending publication. This is the first phase II lung cancer prevention trial to focus on the peripheral lung, where the majority of cancers arise (as discussed earlier). The results of this first study will inform the development of clinical trial models for adenocarcinoma prevention, which are critically needed.

Similar to inhaled steroids, animal data showing inhibition of carcinogen-induced lung tumorigenesis exist for inhibitors of arachidonic acid metabolism by the enzymes 5-lipoxygenase (5-LO) and cyclooxygenase (both the COX-1 and COX-2 isoforms), which give rise to multiple downstream products that have been implicated in various aspects of lung carcinogenesis (153,154). A number of phase IIb clinical trials using inhibitors of these enzymes (zileuton (5-LO), celecoxib (COX-2), and sulindac (COX-1 and COX-2)) have been initiated, with endpoints ranging from effects on proliferative indices to effects on bronchial dysplasia. Kim et al. (155) reported that high-dose celecoxib, 400 mg twice daily, significantly decreased proliferation in the bronchial epithelium, although a lower dose, 200 mg twice daily, was not effective. The results of the other trials (including a second trial of celecoxib with Ki-67 as an endpoint in former smokers) are pending publication.

Data also implicate another downstream product of the COX-2 pathway, prostacyclin (PGI$_2$), in carcinogenesis in that mice overexpressing prostacyclin synthase, which catalyzes prostacyclin formation, have a lower incidence and tumor multiplicity than wild-type littermates upon tobacco smoke exposure (156). The results of a recently completed phase IIb clinical trial assessing the chemopreventive potential of iloprost, a prostacyclin analogue, have been reported in abstract form, demonstrating that iloprost reversed bronchial dysplasia and metaplasia in former smokers, but not in current smokers (157). This is the first phase II trial to report regression of dysplasia, albeit in a preplanned secondary analysis of the former smoker subgroup. How this data should be translated into the next clinical trial remains to be determined.

Perhaps the most exciting recent new direction for lung cancer prevention was reported by Gustafson et al. (158), who showed that the phosphatidylinositol 3-kinase (PI3K) signaling pathway is activated early during lung cancer development and that the agent myo-inositol, a precursor of phosphatidylinositol, reverses this activation. These investigators studied gene expression signatures in normal bronchial epithelial brushings from smokers with and without lung cancer or bronchial dysplasia, showing that the PI3K pathway is activated in smokers with lung cancer or dysplasia, but not in smokers without dysplasia. A prior phase I study performed to determine the highest tolerable dose

of myo-inositol showed a very high rate of regression of bronchial dysplasia, although only a very small number of subjects was studied in this trial designed for dose-finding rather than efficacy determination (159). Gene expression analysis of samples from this intervention trial identified PI3K signaling as the mechanism of action of myo-inositol. The novel approach by Gustafson et al. is highly significant for several reasons. First, if early activation of PI3K during lung carcinogenesis is confirmed by subsequent studies and is shown to be critical to lung carcinogenesis, this could become an excellent biomarker to identify the truly high-risk smoker who needs intervention as well as to identify a potential target for intervention. Second, if myo-inositol is confirmed to effectively inhibit PI3K activity, it provides a cheap and nontoxic intervention to reverse this critical step in the development of lung cancer. A larger phase IIb study of myo-inositol is currently ongoing, with planned collection of bronchial brushings for gene expression analysis to confirm the current findings. However, since the phase II trial has dysplasia as an endpoint, a definitive phase III cancer incidence trial will still need to be performed. Finally, the use of gene expression analysis to study a small number of subjects treated with an intervention offers a faster and more efficient way to evaluate mechanisms of action of the intervention and to provide evidence of efficacy. Such an approach may eventually replace the relatively large phase IIb trials that study 100 or more participants with interventions lasting 3 to 6 months.

Summary of Lung Cancer Prevention

The past two decades have witnessed an explosion of knowledge regarding the development of lung cancer. Nevertheless, prevention of lung cancer has proven to be more complicated and elusive than initially anticipated. Several important research areas that require significant investment for progress to occur have been identified. There is no substitute for understanding the biology of the carcinogenic process to allow rational selection of targets for intervention. One must also keep in mind that carcinogenesis occurs over time, potentially with different mechanisms assuming primary importance during different stages of cancer development. Equally important is the identification of the appropriate high-risk cohort that should be targeted for intervention. The proper risk-benefit balance can only be reached when the cohort's cancer risk is high enough to justify the potential toxicities from the intervention. Finally, there is a tremendous need to develop new models of clinical trials that can efficiently identify promising agents for cancer prevention. This requires identification of biomarkers that reflect clinical benefit and, eventually, validation of these markers if they are to be used as surrogates. Novel technologies, including imaging modalities as well as molecular analyses of tissues and body fluids, will be needed to reach these goals. In the meantime, just as is the case with lung cancer screening, current guidelines do not recommend any chemopreventive interventions to reduce an individual's risk of lung cancer (160).

■ REFERENCES

1. Jemal A, Siegel R, Ward E, Hao Y, Xu J, Thun MJ. Cancer statistics, 2009. *CA Cancer J Clin.* 2009;59(4):225–249.

2. Flehinger BJ, Kimmel M, Melamed MR. The effect of surgical treatment on survival from early lung cancer. Implications for screening. *Chest.* 1992;101(4):1013–1018.

3. Henschke CI, Yankelevitz DF, Libby DM, Pasmantier MW, Smith JP, Miettinen OS; International Early Lung Cancer Action Program Investigators. Survival of patients with stage I lung cancer detected on CT screening. *N Engl J Med.* 2006;355(17): 1763–1771.

4. Brett GZ. The value of lung cancer detection by six-monthly chest radiographs. *Thorax.* 1968;23(4):414–420.

5. Brett GZ. Earlier diagnosis and survival in lung cancer. *Br Med J.* 1969;4(5678):260–262.

6. Fontana RS, Sanderson DR, Taylor WF, et al. Early lung cancer detection: results of the initial (prevalence) radiologic and cytologic screening in the Mayo Clinic study. *Am Rev Respir Dis.* 1984;130(4):561–565.

7. Fontana RS, Sanderson DR, Woolner LB, Taylor WF, Miller WE, Muhm JR. Lung cancer screening: the Mayo program. *J Occup Med.* 1986;28(8):746–750.

8. Fontana RS, Sanderson DR, Woolner LB, et al. Screening for lung cancer. A critique of the Mayo Lung Project. *Cancer.* 1991;67(4 suppl):1155–1164.

9. Marcus PM, Bergstralh EJ, Fagerstrom RM, et al. Lung cancer mortality in the Mayo Lung Project: impact of extended follow-up. *J Natl Cancer Inst.* 2000;92(16):1308–1316.

10. Marcus PM, Bergstralh EJ, Zweig MH, Harris A, Offord KP, Fontana RS. Extended lung cancer incidence follow-up in the Mayo Lung Project and overdiagnosis. *J Natl Cancer Inst.* 2006;98(11):748–756.

11. Kubík A, Polák J. Lung cancer detection. Results of a randomized prospective study in Czechoslovakia. *Cancer.* 1986;57(12):2427–2437.

12. Kubik A, Parkin DM, Khlat M, Erban J, Polak J, Adamec M. Lack of benefit from semi-annual screening for cancer of the lung: follow-up report of a randomized controlled trial on a population of high-risk males in Czechoslovakia. *Int J Cancer.* 1990;45(1):26–33.

13. Kubík AK, Parkin DM, Zatloukal P. Czech Study on Lung Cancer Screening: post-trial follow-up of lung cancer deaths up to year 15 since enrollment. *Cancer.* 2000;89(11 suppl):2363–2368.

14. Levin ML, Tockman MS, Frost JK, Ball WC Jr. Lung cancer mortality in males screened by chest X-ray and cytologic sputum examination: a preliminary report. *Recent Results Cancer Res.* 1982;82:138–146.

15. Frost JK, Ball WC Jr, Levin ML, et al. Early lung cancer detection: results of the initial (prevalence) radiologic and cytologic screening in the Johns Hopkins study. *Am Rev Respir Dis.* 1984;130(4):549–554.

16. Tockman MS, Frost JK, Stitik FP, et al. Screening and detection of lung cancer. In: Aisner J, ed. *Lung Cancer.* New York: Churchill Livingstone; 1985.

17. Tockman MS. Survival and mortality from lung cancer in a screened population: the Johns Hopkins study. *Chest.* 1986;89(4 suppl), 324S–325S.

18. Melamed M, Flehinger B, Miller D, et al. Preliminary report of the lung cancer detection program in New York. *Cancer.* 1977;39(2):369–382.

19. Melamed MR, Flehinger BJ, Zaman MB, Heelan RT, Perchick WA, Martini N. Screening for early lung cancer. Results of the Memorial Sloan-Kettering study in New York. *Chest.* 1984;86(1):44–53.

20. Doria-Rose VP, Marcus PM, Szabo E, Tockman MS, Melamed MR, Prorok PC. Randomized controlled trials of the efficacy of lung cancer screening by sputum cytology revisited: a combined mortality analysis from the Johns Hopkins Lung Project and the Memorial Sloan-Kettering Lung Study. *Cancer.* 2009;115(21):5007–5017.

21. Manser RL, Irving LB, Byrnes G, Abramson MJ, Stone CA, Campbell DA. Screening for lung cancer: a systematic review and meta-analysis of controlled trials. *Thorax.* 2003;58(9):784–789.

22. Patz EF Jr, Goodman PC, Bepler G. Screening for lung cancer. *N Engl J Med.* 2000;343(22):1627–1633.

23. Dales LG, Friedman GD, Collen MF. Evaluating periodic multiphasic health checkups: a controlled trial. *J Chronic Dis.* 1979;32(5):385–404.

24. Friedman GD, Collen MF, Fireman BH. Multiphasic Health Checkup Evaluation: a 16-year follow-up. *J Chronic Dis.* 1986;39(6):453–463.

25. Miettinen OS. Screening for lung cancer. *Radiol Clin North Am.* 2000;38(3):479–486.

26. Strauss GM, Gleason RE, Sugarbaker DJ. Screening for lung cancer. Another look; a different view. *Chest.* 1997;111(3):754–768.

27. Prorok PC, Andriole GL, Bresalier RS, et al.; Prostate, Lung, Colorectal and Ovarian Cancer Screening Trial Project Team. Design of the Prostate, Lung, Colorectal and Ovarian (PLCO) Cancer Screening Trial. *Control Clin Trials.* 2000;21(6 suppl):273S–309S.

28. Oken MM, Marcus PM, Hu P, et al.; PLCO Project Team. Baseline chest radiograph for lung cancer detection in the randomized Prostate, Lung, Colorectal and Ovarian Cancer Screening Trial. *J Natl Cancer Inst.* 2005;97(24):1832–1839.

29 Petty TL, Miller YE. Early diagnosis and intervention in lung cancer: clinical studies. In: Pass HI, Mitchell JB, Johnson DH, et al., eds. *Lung Cancer: Principles and Practice.* Philadelphia, PA: Lippincott Williams & Wilkins; 2000.

30. Bach PB, Silvestri GA, Hanger M, Jett JR; American College of Chest Physicians. Screening for lung cancer: ACCP evidence-based clinical practice guidelines (2nd edition). *Chest.* 2007;132(3 suppl):69S–77S.

31. Reich JM. A critical appraisal of overdiagnosis: estimates of its magnitude and implications for lung cancer screening. *Thorax.* 2008;63(4):377–383.

32. Naidich DP, Marshall CH, Gribbin C, Arams RS, McCauley DI. Low-dose CT of the lungs: preliminary observations. *Radiology.* 1990;175(3):729–731.

33. Kaneko M, Eguchi K, Ohmatsu H, et al. Peripheral lung cancer: screening and detection with low-dose spiral CT versus radiography. *Radiology.* 1996;201(3):798–802.

34. Kakinuma R, Ohmatsu H, Kaneko M, et al. Detection failures in spiral CT screening for lung cancer: analysis of CT findings. *Radiology.* 1999;212(1):61–66.

35. Sobue T, Moriyama N, Kaneko M, et al. Screening for lung cancer with low-dose helical computed tomography: anti-lung cancer association project. *J Clin Oncol.* 2002;20(4):911–920.

36. Henschke CI, McCauley DI, Yankelevitz DF, et al. Early Lung Cancer Action Project: overall design and findings from baseline screening. *Lancet.* 1999;354(9173):99–105.

37. Henschke CI, Naidich DP, Yankelevitz DF, et al. Early lung cancer action project: initial findings on repeat screenings. *Cancer.* 2001;92(1):153–159.

38. Diederich S, Wormanns D, Lenzen H, Semik M, Thomas M, Peters PE. Screening for asymptomatic early bronchogenic carcinoma with low dose CT of the chest. *Cancer.* 2000;89(11 suppl):2483–2484.

39. Diederich S, Wormanns D, Semik M, et al. Screening for early lung cancer with low-dose spiral CT: prevalence in 817 asymptomatic smokers. *Radiology.* 2002;222(3):773–781.

40. Diederich S, Thomas M, Semik M, et al. Screening for early lung cancer with low-dose spiral computed tomography: results of annual follow-up examinations in asymptomatic smokers. *Eur Radiol.* 2004;14(4):691–702.

41. Sone S, Li F, Yang ZG, et al. Results of three-year mass screening programme for lung cancer using mobile low-dose spiral computed tomography scanner. *Br J Cancer.* 2001;84(1):25–32.

42. Sone S, Takashima S, Li F, et al. Mass screening for lung cancer with mobile spiral computed tomography scanner. *Lancet.* 1998;351(9111):1242–1245.

43. Tiitola M, Kivisaari L, Huuskonen MS, et al. Computed tomography screening for lung cancer in asbestos-exposed workers. *Lung Cancer.* 2002;35(1):17–22.

44. Nawa T, Nakagawa T, Kusano S, Kawasaki Y, Sugawara Y, Nakata H. Lung cancer screening using low-dose spiral CT: results of baseline and 1-year follow-up studies. *Chest.* 2002;122(1):15–20.

45. Swensen SJ, Jett JR, Sloan JA, et al. Screening for lung cancer with low-dose spiral computed tomography. *Am J Respir Crit Care Med.* 2002;165(4):508–513.

46. Swensen SJ, Jett JR, Hartman TE, et al. Lung cancer screening with CT: Mayo Clinic experience. *Radiology.* 2003;226(3):756–761.

47. Swensen SJ, Jett JR, Hartman TE, et al. CT screening for lung cancer: five-year prospective experience. *Radiology.* 2005;235(1):259–265.

48. Chong S, Lee KS, Chung MJ, et al. Lung cancer screening with low-dose helical CT in Korea: experiences at the Samsung Medical Center. *J Korean Med Sci.* 2005;20(3):402–408.

49. Pastorino U, Bellomi M, Landoni C, et al. Early lung-cancer detection with spiral CT and positron emission tomography in heavy smokers: 2-year results. *Lancet.* 2003;362(9384):593–597.

50. MacRedmond R, Logan PM, Lee M, Kenny D, Foley C, Costello RW. Screening for lung cancer using low dose CT scanning. *Thorax.* 2004;59(3):237–241.

51. MacRedmond R, McVey G, Lee M, et al. Screening for lung cancer using low dose CT scanning: results of 2 year follow up. *Thorax.* 2006;61(1):54–56.

52. Miller A, Markowitz S, Manowitz A, Miller JA. Lung cancer screening using low-dose high-resolution CT scanning in a high-risk workforce: 3500 nuclear fuel workers in three US states. *Chest.* 2004;125(5 suppl):152S–153S.

53 New York Early Lung Cancer Action Project Investigators. CT Screening for lung cancer: diagnoses resulting from the New York Early Lung Cancer Action Project. *Radiology.* 2007;243(1):239–249.

54. Wilson DO, Weissfeld JL, Fuhrman CR, et al. The Pittsburgh Lung Screening Study (PLuSS): outcomes within 3 years of a first computed tomography scan. *Am J Respir Crit Care Med.* 2008;178(9):956–961.

55. Gohagan J, Marcus P, Fagerstrom R, Pinsky P, Kramer B, Prorok P; Writing Committee, Lung Screening Study Research Group. Baseline findings of a randomized feasibility trial of lung cancer screening with spiral CT scan vs chest radiograph: the Lung Screening Study of the National Cancer Institute. *Chest.* 2004;126(1):114–121.

56. Gohagan JK, Marcus PM, Fagerstrom RM, et al.; Lung Screening Study Research Group. Final results of the Lung Screening Study, a randomized feasibility study of spiral CT versus chest X-ray screening for lung cancer. *Lung Cancer.* 2005;47(1):9–15.

57. Infante M, Lutman FR, Cavuto S, et al.; DANTE Study Group. Lung cancer screening with spiral CT: baseline results of the randomized DANTE trial. *Lung Cancer.* 2008;59(3):355–363.

58. Infante M, Cavuto S, Lutman FR, et al.; DANTE Study Group. A randomized study of lung cancer screening with spiral computed tomography: three-year results from the DANTE trial. *Am J Respir Crit Care Med.* 2009;180(5):445–453.

59. Pedersen JH, Ashraf H, Dirksen A, et al. The Danish randomized lung cancer CT screening trial–overall design and results of the prevalence round. *J Thorac Oncol.* 2009;4(5):608–614.

60. Lopes Pegna A, Picozzi G, Mascalchi M, et al.; ITALUNG Study Research Group. Design, recruitment and baseline results of the ITALUNG trial for lung cancer screening with low-dose CT. *Lung Cancer.* 2009;64(1):34–40.

61. Chirikos TN, Hazelton T, Tockman M, Clark R. Screening for lung cancer with CT: a preliminary cost-effectiveness analysis. *Chest.* 2002;121(5):1507–1514.

62. Mahadevia PJ, Fleisher LA, Frick KD, Eng J, Goodman SN, Powe NR. Lung cancer screening with helical computed tomography in older adult smokers: a decision and cost-effectiveness analysis. *JAMA.* 2003;289(3):313–322.

63. Manser R, Dalton A, Carter R, Byrnes G, Elwood M, Campbell DA. Cost-effectiveness analysis of screening for lung cancer with low dose spiral CT (computed tomography) in the Australian setting. *Lung Cancer.* 2005;48(2):171–185.

64. Marshall D, Simpson KN, Earle CC, Chu C. Potential cost-effectiveness of one-time screening for lung cancer (LC) in a high risk cohort. *Lung Cancer.* 2001;32(3):227–236.

65. Marshall D, Simpson KN, Earle CC, Chu CW. Economic decision analysis model of screening for lung cancer. *Eur J Cancer.* 2001;37(14):1759–1767.

66. Wisnivesky JP, Mushlin AI, Sicherman N, Henschke C. The cost-effectiveness of low-dose CT screening for lung cancer: preliminary results of baseline screening. *Chest.* 2003;124(2):614–621.

67 Horner MJ, Ries LAG, Krapcho M, et al., eds. *SEER Cancer Statistics Review, 1975–2006.* Bethesda, MD: National Cancer Institute. http://seer.cancer.gov/csr/1975_2006/, based on November 2008 SEER data submission, posted to the SEER web site, 2009.

68. van Iersel CA, de Koning HJ, Draisma G, et al. Risk-based selection from the general population in a screening trial: selection criteria, recruitment and power for the Dutch-Belgian randomised lung cancer multi-slice CT screening trial (NELSON). *Int J Cancer.* 2007;120(4):868–874.

69 Becker N, Delorme S, Kauczor H-U. LUSI: The German component of the European trial on the efficacy of multislice-CT for the early detection of lung cancer. *Onkologie,* 2008; 31(suppl 1), PO320.

70. Henschke CI, Yankelevitz DF, Naidich DP, et al. CT screening for lung cancer: suspiciousness of nodules according to size on baseline scans. *Radiology.* 2004;231(1):164–168.

71. MacMahon H, Austin JH, Gamsu G, et al.; Fleischner Society. Guidelines for management of small pulmonary nodules detected on CT scans: a statement from the Fleischner Society. *Radiology.* 2005;237(2):395–400.

72. Brenner DJ. Radiation risks potentially associated with low-dose CT screening of adult smokers for lung cancer. *Radiology.* 2004;231(2):440–445.

73. Brown KT, Brody LA, Getrajdman GI, Napp TE. Outpatient treatment of iatrogenic pneumothorax after needle biopsy. *Radiology.* 1997;205(1):249–252.

74. Cox JE, Chiles C, McManus CM, Aquino SL, Choplin RH. Transthoracic needle aspiration biopsy: variables that affect risk of pneumothorax. *Radiology.* 1999;212(1):165–168.

75. Geraghty PR, Kee ST, McFarlane G, Razavi MK, Sze DY, Dake MD. CT-guided transthoracic needle aspiration biopsy of pulmonary nodules: needle size and pneumothorax rate. *Radiology.* 2003;229(2):475–481.

76. Gupta S, Krishnamurthy S, Broemeling LD, et al. Small (</=2-cm) subpleural pulmonary lesions: short- versus long-needle-path CT-guided Biopsy–comparison of diagnostic yields and complications. *Radiology.* 2005;234(2):631–637.

77. Finlayson EV, Birkmeyer JD. Operative mortality with elective surgery in older adults. *Eff Clin Pract.* 2001;4(4):172–177.

78. Bach PB, Cramer LD, Schrag D, Downey RJ, Gelfand SE, Begg CB. The influence of hospital volume on survival after resection for lung cancer. *N Engl J Med.* 2001;345(3):181–188.

79. Reich JM. Improved survival and higher mortality: the conundrum of lung cancer screening. *Chest.* 2002;122(1):329–337.

80 Morrison AS. *Screening in Chronic Disease.* New York: Oxford University Press; 1992.

81 Prorok PC, Kramer BS, Gohagan JK. Screening theory and study design: the basics. In: Kramer BS, ed. *Cancer Screening: Theory and Practice.* New York: Marcel Dekker, Inc.; 1999.

82 Welch HG, Woloshin S, Schwartz LM, et al. Overstating the evidence for lung cancer screening: the International Early Lung Cancer Action Program (I-ELCAP) study. *Arch Intern Med.* 2007;167(21):2289–2295.

83 Chan CK, Wells CK, McFarlane MJ, Feinstein AR. More lung cancer but better survival. Implications of secular trends in "necropsy surprise" rates. *Chest.* 1989;96(2):291–296.

84 Manser RL, Dodd M, Byrnes G, Irving LB, Campbell DA. Incidental lung cancers identified at coronial autopsy: implications for overdiagnosis of lung cancer by screening. *Respir Med.* 2005;99(4):501–507.

85 Henschke CI. Clarifying enrollment procedures in the trial of CT screening for lung cancer. *N Engl J Med.* 2008;359(8):871–873.

86 Bach PB. Overdiagnosis in lung cancer: different perspectives, definitions, implications. *Thorax.* 2008;63(4):298–300.

87 Bach PB, Jett JR, Pastorino U, Tockman MS, Swensen SJ, Begg CB. Computed tomography screening and lung cancer outcomes. *JAMA.* 2007;297(9):953–961.

88 McWilliams A, Mayo J, MacDonald S, et al. Lung cancer screening: a different paradigm. *Am J Respir Crit Care Med.* 2003;168(10):1167–1173.

89 Tockman MS, Mulshine JL, Piantadosi S, et al. Prospective detection of preclinical lung cancer: results from two studies of heterogeneous nuclear ribonucleoprotein A2/B1 overexpression. *Clin Cancer Res.* 1997;3(12 Pt 1):2237–2246.

90 Mao L, Hruban RH, Boyle JO, Tockman M, Sidransky D. Detection of oncogene mutations in sputum precedes diagnosis of lung cancer. *Cancer Res.* 1994;54(7):1634–1637.

91 Belinsky SA, Liechty KC, Gentry FD, et al. Promoter hypermethylation of multiple genes in sputum precedes lung cancer incidence in a high-risk cohort. *Cancer Res.* 2006;66(6):3338–3344.

92 Phillips M, Altorki N, Austin JH, et al. Prediction of lung cancer using volatile biomarkers in breath. *Cancer Biomark.* 2007;3(2):95–109.

93 Phillips M, Gleeson K, Hughes JM, et al. Volatile organic compounds in breath as markers of lung cancer: a cross-sectional study. *Lancet.* 1999;353(9168):1930–1933.

94 Poli D, Carbognani P, Corradi M, et al. Exhaled volatile organic compounds in patients with non-small cell lung cancer: cross sectional and nested short-term follow-up study. *Respir Res.* 2005;6:71.

95 Di Natale C, Macagnano A, Martinelli E, et al. Lung cancer identification by the analysis of breath by means of an array of non-selective gas sensors. *Biosens Bioelectron.* 2003;18(10):1209–1218.

96 Dragonieri S, Annema JT, Schot R, et al. An electronic nose in the discrimination of patients with non-small cell lung cancer and COPD. *Lung Cancer.* 2009;64(2):166–170.

97 Machado RF, Laskowski D, Deffenderfer O, et al. Detection of lung cancer by sensor array analyses of exhaled breath. *Am J Respir Crit Care Med.* 2005;171(11):1286–1291.

98 Kullmann T, Barta I, Csiszér E, Antus B, Horváth I. Differential cytokine pattern in the exhaled breath of patients with lung cancer. *Pathol Oncol Res.* 2008;14(4):481–483.

99 Cho JY, Sung HJ. Proteomic approaches in lung cancer biomarker development. *Expert Rev Proteomics.* 2009;6(1):27–42.

100 Chorostowska-Wynimko J, Szpechcinski A. The impact of genetic markers on the diagnosis of lung cancer: a current perspective. *J Thorac Oncol.* 2007;2(11):1044–1051.

101 Us-Krasovec M, Erzen J, Zganec M, et al. Malignancy associated changes in epithelial cells of buccal mucosa: a potential cancer detection test. *Anal Quant Cytol Histol.* 2005;27(5):254–262.

102 Xiong Z, Xiong G, Man Y, Wang L, Jing W. Detection of lung cancer by oral examination. *Med Hypotheses.* 2010;74(2):346–347.

103 Tan C, Chen H, Xia C. Early prediction of lung cancer based on the combination of trace element analysis in urine and an Adaboost algorithm. *J Pharm Biomed Anal.* 2009;49(3):746–752.

104 Yuan JM, Koh WP, Murphy SE, et al. Urinary levels of tobacco-specific nitrosamine metabolites in relation to lung cancer development in two prospective cohorts of cigarette smokers. *Cancer Res.* 2009;69(7):2990–2995.

105 Lippman SM, Benner SE, Hong WK. Cancer chemoprevention. *J Clin Oncol.* 1994;12(4):851–873.

106 Saccomanno G, Archer VE, Auerbach O, Saunders RP, Brennan LM. Development of carcinoma of the lung as reflected in exfoliated cells. *Cancer.* 1974;33(1):256–270.

107 Auerbach O, Stout AP, Hammond EC, Garfinkel L. Changes in bronchial epithelium in relation to cigarette smoking and in relation to lung cancer. *N Engl J Med.* 1961;265:253–267.

108 Mao L, Lee JS, Kurie JM, et al. Clonal genetic alterations in the lungs of current and former smokers. *J Natl Cancer Inst.* 1997;89(12):857–862.

109 Johnson BE. Second lung cancers in patients after treatment for an initial lung cancer. *J Natl Cancer Inst.* 1998;90(18):1335–1345.

110 Peto R, Darby S, Deo H, Silcocks P, Whitley E, Doll R. Smoking, smoking cessation, and lung cancer in the UK since 1950: combination of national statistics with two case-control studies. *BMJ.* 2000;321(7257):323–329.

111 Anthonisen NR, Skeans MA, Wise RA, Manfreda J, Kanner RE, Connett JE; Lung Health Study Research Group. The effects of a smoking cessation intervention on 14.5-year mortality: a randomized clinical trial. *Ann Intern Med.* 2005;142(4):233–239.

112 Omenn GS. Chemoprevention of lung cancer: the rise and demise of beta-carotene. *Annu Rev Public Health.* 1998;19:73–99.

113 The effect of vitamin E and beta carotene on the incidence of lung cancer and other cancers in male smokers. The Alpha-Tocopherol, Beta Carotene Cancer Prevention Study Group. *N Engl J Med.* 1994;330(15):1029–1035.

114 Omenn GS, Goodman GE, Thornquist MD, et al. Effects of a combination of beta carotene and vitamin A on lung cancer and cardiovascular disease. *N Engl J Med.* 1996;334(18):1150–1155.

115 Hennekens CH, Buring JE, Manson JE, et al. Lack of effect of long-term supplementation with beta carotene on the incidence of malignant neoplasms and cardiovascular disease. *N Engl J Med.* 1996;334(18):1145–1149.

116 van Zandwijk N, Dalesio O, Pastorino U, de Vries N, van Tinteren H. EUROSCAN, a randomized trial of vitamin A and N-acetylcysteine in patients with head and neck cancer or lung cancer. For the EUropean Organization for Research and Treatment of Cancer Head and Neck and Lung Cancer Cooperative Groups. *J Natl Cancer Inst.* 2000;92(12):977–986.

117 Pastorino U, Infante M, Maioli M, et al. Adjuvant treatment of stage I lung cancer with high-dose vitamin A. *J Clin Oncol.* 1993;11(7):1216–1222.

118 Hong WK, Endicott J, Itri LM, et al. 13-cis-retinoic acid in the treatment of oral leukoplakia. *N Engl J Med.* 1986;315(24):1501–1505.

119 Lippman SM, Batsakis JG, Toth BB, et al. Comparison of low-dose isotretinoin with beta carotene to prevent oral carcinogenesis. *N Engl J Med.* 1993;328(1):15–20.

120 Hong WK, Lippman SM, Itri LM, et al. Prevention of second primary tumors with isotretinoin in squamous-cell carcinoma of the head and neck. *N Engl J Med.* 1990;323(12):795–801.

121 Lippman SM, Lee JJ, Karp DD, et al. Randomized phase III intergroup trial of isotretinoin to prevent second primary tumors in stage I non-small-cell lung cancer. *J Natl Cancer Inst.* 2001;93(8):605–618.

122 Clark LC, Combs GF Jr, Turnbull BW, et al. Effects of selenium supplementation for cancer prevention in patients with carcinoma of the skin. A randomized controlled trial. Nutritional Prevention of Cancer Study Group. *JAMA.* 1996;276(24):1957–1963.

123 De Luca LM, Ross SA. Beta-carotene increases lung cancer incidence in cigarette smokers. *Nutr Rev.* 1996;54(6):178–180.

124. Greenwald P. Beta-carotene and lung cancer: a lesson for future chemoprevention investigations? *J Natl Cancer Inst.* 2003;95(1):E1.

125. Meyskens FL Jr, Szabo E. Diet and cancer: the disconnect between epidemiology and randomized clinical trials. *Cancer Epidemiol Biomarkers Prev.* 2005;14(6):1366–1369.

126. Baron JA, Sandler RS, Bresalier RS, et al.; APPROVe Trial Investigators. A randomized trial of rofecoxib for the chemoprevention of colorectal adenomas. *Gastroenterology.* 2006;131(6):1674–1682.

127. Bresalier RS, Sandler RS, Quan H, et al.; Adenomatous Polyp Prevention on Vioxx (APPROVe) Trial Investigators. Cardiovascular events associated with rofecoxib in a colorectal adenoma chemoprevention trial. *N Engl J Med.* 2005;352(11):1092–1102.

128. Solomon SD, McMurray JJ, Pfeffer MA, et al.; Adenoma Prevention with Celecoxib (APC) Study Investigators. Cardiovascular risk associated with celecoxib in a clinical trial for colorectal adenoma prevention. *N Engl J Med.* 2005;352(11):1071–1080.

129. Arber N, Eagle CJ, Spicak J, et al.; PreSAP Trial Investigators. Celecoxib for the prevention of colorectal adenomatous polyps. *N Engl J Med.* 2006;355(9):885–895.

130. Bertagnolli MM, Eagle CJ, Zauber AG, et al.; APC Study Investigators. Celecoxib for the prevention of sporadic colorectal adenomas. *N Engl J Med.* 2006;355(9):873–884.

131. Szabo E. Selecting targets for cancer prevention: where do we go from here? *Nat Rev Cancer.* 2006;6(11):867–874.

132. Szabo E. Primer: first do no harm–when is it appropriate to plan a cancer prevention clinical trial? *Nat Clin Pract Oncol.* 2008;5(6):348–356.

133. Ding L, Getz G, Wheeler DA, et al. Somatic mutations affect key pathways in lung adenocarcinoma. *Nature.* 2008;455(7216):1069–1075.

134. Punturieri A, Szabo E, Croxton TL, Shapiro SD, Dubinett SM. Lung cancer and chronic obstructive pulmonary disease: needs and opportunities for integrated research. *J Natl Cancer Inst.* 2009;101(8):554–559.

135. Tockman MS, Anthonisen NR, Wright EC, Donithan MG. Airways obstruction and the risk for lung cancer. *Ann Intern Med.* 1987;106(4):512–518.

136. Bach PB, Kattan MW, Thornquist MD, et al. Variations in lung cancer risk among smokers. *J Natl Cancer Inst.* 2003;95(6):470–478.

137. Spitz MR, Hong WK, Amos CI, et al. A risk model for prediction of lung cancer. *J Natl Cancer Inst.* 2007;99(9):715–726.

138. Prindiville SA, Byers T, Hirsch FR, et al. Sputum cytological atypia as a predictor of incident lung cancer in a cohort of heavy smokers with airflow obstruction. *Cancer Epidemiol Biomarkers Prev.* 2003;12(10):987–993.

139. Varella-Garcia M, Schulte AP, Wolf HJ, et al. The detection of chromosomal aneusomy by fluorescence in situ hybridization in sputum predicts lung cancer incidence. *Cancer Prev Res (Phila Pa).* 2010;3(4):447–453.

140. Lippman SM, Lee JS, Lotan R, Hittelman W, Wargovich MJ, Hong WK. Biomarkers as intermediate end points in chemoprevention trials. *J Natl Cancer Inst.* 1990;82(7):555–560.

141. Schatzkin A, Gail M. The promise and peril of surrogate end points in cancer research. *Nat Rev Cancer.* 2002;2(1):19–27.

142. Szabo E. Assessing efficacy in early-phase cancer prevention clinical trials: the case of ki-67 in the lung. *Cancer Prev Res (Phila Pa).* 2010;3(2):128–131.

143. Hanahan D, Weinberg RA. The hallmarks of cancer. *Cell.* 2000;100(1):57–70.

144. Kelloff GJ, Lippman SM, Dannenberg AJ, et al.; AACR Task Force on Cancer Prevention. Progress in chemoprevention drug development: the promise of molecular biomarkers for prevention of intraepithelial neoplasia and cancer–a plan to move forward. *Clin Cancer Res.* 2006;12(12):3661–3697.

145. Lam S, MacAulay C, leRiche JC, Palcic B. Detection and localization of early lung cancer by fluorescence bronchoscopy. *Cancer.* 2000;89(11 suppl):2468–2473.

146. Bota S, Auliac JB, Paris C, et al. Follow-up of bronchial precancerous lesions and carcinoma in situ using fluorescence endoscopy. *Am J Respir Crit Care Med.* 2001;164(9):1688–1693.

147. Venmans BJ, van Boxem TJ, Smit EF, Postmus PE, Sutedja TG. Outcome of bronchial carcinoma in situ. *Chest.* 2000;117(6):1572–1576.

148. Lam S, leRiche JC, McWilliams A, et al. A randomized phase IIb trial of pulmicort turbuhaler (budesonide) in people with dysplasia of the bronchial epithelium. *Clin Cancer Res.* 2004;10(19):6502–6511.

149. Kurie JM, Lotan R, Lee JJ, et al. Treatment of former smokers with 9-cis-retinoic acid reverses loss of retinoic acid receptor-beta expression in the bronchial epithelium: results from a randomized placebo-controlled trial. *J Natl Cancer Inst.* 2003;95(3):206–214.

150. Wahidi MM, Govert JA, Goudar RK, Gould MK, McCrory DC; American College of Chest Physicians. Evidence for the treatment of patients with pulmonary nodules: when is it lung cancer?: ACCP evidence-based clinical practice guidelines (2nd edition). *Chest.* 2007;132(3 suppl):94S–107S.

151. Pereira MA, Li Y, Gunning WT, et al. Prevention of mouse lung tumors by budesonide and its modulation of biomarkers. *Carcinogenesis.* 2002;23(7):1185–1192.

152. Wattenberg LW, Wiedmann TS, Estensen RD, et al. Chemoprevention of pulmonary carcinogenesis by brief exposures to aerosolized budesonide or beclomethasone dipropionate and by the combination of aerosolized budesonide and dietary myo-inositol. *Carcinogenesis.* 2000;21(2):179–182.

153. Gunning WT, Kramer PM, Steele VE, Pereira MA. Chemoprevention by lipoxygenase and leukotriene pathway inhibitors of vinyl carbamate-induced lung tumors in mice. *Cancer Res.* 2002;62(15):4199–4201.

154. Pepin P, Bouchard L, Nicole P, Castonguay A. Effects of sulindac and oltipraz on the tumorigenicity of 4-(methylnitrosamino)1-(3-pyridyl)-1-butanone in A/J mouse lung. *Carcinogenesis.* 1992;13(3):341–348.

155. Kim ES, Hong WK, Lee JJ, et al. Biological activity of celecoxib in the bronchial epithelium of current and former smokers. *Cancer Prev Res (Phila Pa).* 2010;3(2):148–159.

156. Keith RL, Miller YE, Hudish TM, et al. Pulmonary prostacyclin synthase overexpression chemoprevents tobacco smoke lung carcinogenesis in mice. *Cancer Res.* 2004;64(16):5897–5904.

157 Keith R, Blatchford P, Kittelson J, et al. Oral iloprost for the chemoprevention of lung cancer. IASLC 13th World Conference on Lung Cancer. San Francisco, CA. p.49.

158. Gustafson AM, Soldi R, Anderlind C, et al. Airway PI3K pathway activation is an early and reversible event in lung cancer development. *Sci Transl Med.* 2010;2(26):26ra25.

159. Lam S, McWilliams A, LeRiche J, MacAulay C, Wattenberg L, Szabo E. A phase I study of myo-inositol for lung cancer chemoprevention. *Cancer Epidemiol Biomarkers Prev.* 2006;15(8): 1526–1531.

160. Gray J, Mao JT, Szabo E, Kelley M, Kurie J, Bepler G; American College of Chest Physicians. Lung cancer chemoprevention: ACCP evidence-based clinical practice guidelines (2nd Edition). *Chest.* 2007;132(3 suppl):56S–68S.

6 Imaging in Lung Cancer

ERIC Y. CHANG

PAUL STARK

■ INTRODUCTION

Imaging plays a vital role in the detection, diagnosis, staging, and monitoring of lung cancer. The radiologist encounters patients with lung cancer under a variety of circumstances: for instance, lung cancer can be incidentally detected on a routine chest radiograph performed for unrelated reasons. Alternatively, the patient with a known lung cancer can be referred to the radiologist for staging or for planning of a percutaneous biopsy or bronchoscopy. Finally, imaging is utilized to follow the evolution of the tumor during and after therapy and to assess for complications of radiation or chemotherapy.

Staging for non–small cell lung cancers (NSCLC) applied in the figures and text of this chapter will be based on the seventh edition of the tumor, node, and metastasis (TNM) classification for NSCLC as proposed by the International Association for the Study of Lung Cancer (IASLC). The rational and data for this staging system is presented in Chapter 4.

■ IMAGING TECHNIQUES

Chest Radiography

Due to its widespread availability, low radiation dose, and low cost, chest radiography is frequently the first modality to suggest the diagnosis of lung cancer. Most malignant nodules are identified on chest radiography by the time they are 0.6 to 1 cm in diameter, although rarely nodules as small as 0.4 cm can be seen (1). Chest radiographs are useful because they are frequently obtained for other reasons throughout life. If a comparison examination is available, determination of lesion growth rate may aid in assessing probability of malignancy. However, numerous studies have shown that chest radiography lacks sensitivity to detect mediastinal lymph node

metastasis and chest wall and mediastinal invasion (2). For this reason, additional imaging is almost always performed.

Computed Tomography

Computed tomography (CT) should be performed in all patients with suspected lung cancer. In screening studies, CT can diagnose up to eight times more pulmonary nodules and two to four times more lung cancers than the chest radiograph, though for each detected lung cancer, 100 false alarms are triggered (3–8). CT can detect space-occupying lesions due to nonneoplastic entities, including hamartomas, arteriovenous fistulae, rounded atelectasis, rounded pneumonia, granulomas, fungus balls, mucoid impaction, and pulmonary infarcts. Overall, CT allows for earlier detection, more accurate size measurements and better tissue characterization than conventional chest radiographs (Figure 6.1). Utilizing multislice helical CT scanners and Picture Archive and Communications System workstations, nodules less than 5 mm in diameter can be detected (9).

With improved precision of size assessment, determination of growth on follow-up examinations has significantly improved. CT allows accurate lesion characterization including properties such as attenuation, edge characteristics, cavitation, and contrast enhancement determination (10). This will be discussed further in The Solitary Pulmonary Nodule section.

CT has limited accuracy in detecting lymph node metastasis. CT segregates normal from abnormal lymph nodes based on their size in short axis (11,12). Utilizing standard guidelines (discussed further in Evaluation of Nodal Metastasis section), however, sensitivities are reported to be 79% and specificities to be 78% or lower owing to the fact that normal-sized lymph nodes can harbor metastatic disease and enlarged lymph nodes result from lymph node hyperplasia (13,14). This is the predominant reason why CT staging of non–small cell carcinoma agrees in only approximately 50% with operative staging, leading to either over- or understaging (15,16). This emphasizes the need for further characterization of mediastinal lymph nodes during staging of bronchogenic carcinoma.

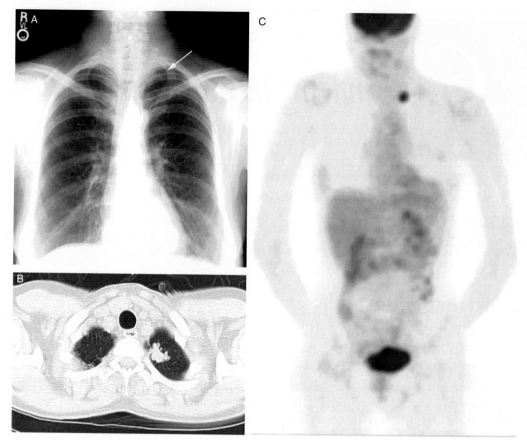

FIGURE 6.1 Extremely subtle lesion (pathology proven non–small cell lung cancer; T1a N0 M0, stage Ia). (A) PA chest radiograph shows a 2-cm lesion overlying the left posterior 4th rib (arrow). (B) and (C) Axial computed tomography and frontal maximum intensity projection *positron emission tomography* confirm 2 cm metabolically active left upper lobe nodule.

Initial CT scanning for diagnosing and staging lung cancer should preferably be performed with intravenous iodinated contrast medium. With iodinated contrast, some authors have found no increased benefit in detecting malignant lymph nodes, while others have demonstrated an 11% higher detection rate, particularly at the right upper paratracheal region (2R nodal station) (17,18). In addition, intravenous contrast material will facilitate potential detection of tumor invasion of cardiac and vascular structures as well as tumor embolization. However, use of intravenous iodinated contrast comes with a finite risk of anaphylactic reaction, renal failure, and death (19) . Adverse events with radiographic contrast agents: results of the SCVIR Contrast Agent Registry. **Radiology** 1997; 203:611–620.]

Magnetic Resonance Imaging

Magnetic resonance imaging (MRI) is an adjunct modality to CT in regards to lung cancer. Generally, MRI is slower, more elaborate, more expensive, and more prone to artifacts, and it demonstrates poorer spatial resolution than CT. Patient selection is also more difficult because the modality is contraindicated in those with indwelling electromagnetic devices and some prosthetic mechanical heart valves (20). In addition, MRI examinations are poorly tolerated by claustrophobic patients although MRI technology is constantly improving in regards to central bore size and length.

For characterization of lung parenchymal disease, MRI is limited due to artifact from respiratory motion, paucity of protons in the aerated lung parenchyma, and magnetic susceptibility from air-tissue interfaces. MRI is inferior to CT in detection of calcium content within lung lesions. Literature prior to the widespread use of multislice CT had suggested that the direct multiplanar imaging capabilities of MRI could be more accurate than CT in evaluation of superior sulcus (Pancoast) tumors or tumors abutting the diaphragm (Figure 6.2) (21,22). However, multidetector row CT, and in particular 64-, 256- and 320-slice scanners achieve superior multiplanar reformatted images with isotropic resolution (23,24,25).

MRI still plays a role due to its superior soft tissue contrast resolution. Theoretically, this is useful in evaluating invasion of compartments by carefully scrutinizing soft tissue planes. This may explain why MRI slightly outperforms CT in detection of mediastinal and, possibly, chest wall invasion (26,27). In addition, MRI exquisitely delineates the brachial plexus, spinal canal, and subclavian vessels and may be more accurate than CT for detection of invasion (27).

In the evaluation of CT-discovered adrenal lesions, MRI is complementary to CT in distinguishing benign and malignant lesions (28). Both modalities utilize size, morphology, and tissue contrast to differentiate benign from malignant lesions. Utilizing standard sequences to accentuate chemical shift differences, MRI may be more

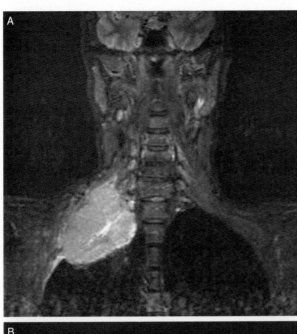

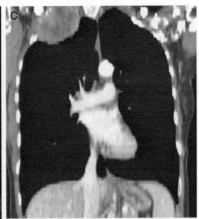

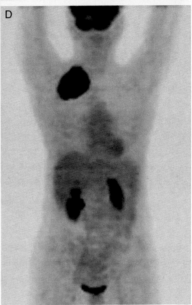

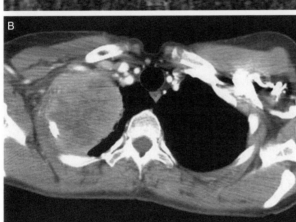

FIGURE 6.2 Incidentally discovered superior sulcus tumor in a woman presenting with brachial plexopathy (pathology proven adenocarcinoma; T4 N0 M0, stage IIIA). (A) Coronal STIR image from initial study, a cervical spine magnetic resonance, demonstrated 8 × 5 × 7 cm right superior sulcus mass. (B) and (C) Subsequent axial and coronal computed tomography images demonstrate superior sulcus tumor which is eroding through the 1st/2nd ribs. (D) Frontal maximum intensity projection positron emission tomography image demonstrates no distant metastatic disease.

specific than non–contrast-enhanced CT (29). However, contrast-enhanced CT utilizing washout characteristics increases specificity over non–contrast-enhanced examinations (30).

MRI is the most accurate modality for detecting suspected brain metastatic disease. Reasons for this include increased soft tissue contrast, significantly stronger enhancement with paramagnetic contrast agents, the lack of bone artifacts (particularly in the frontotemporal region), and fewer partial volume effects (Figure 6.3) (31).

Positron Emission Tomography

Positron emission tomography (PET) with fluorine-18-fluorodeoxyglucose (FDG) is a physiologic/metabolic imaging technique. After injection of FDG, which is a glucose analogue, the radiopharmaceutical is transported through the cell membrane and phosphorylated by glucose hexokinase through glycolytic pathways. However, the analogue remains unmetabolized by glucose-6-phosphatase in the cell and is imaged by coincidence detection of the emitted 511 KeV photons produced by positron annihilation (32).

Most cancer cells predominantly produce energy by glycolysis followed by lactic acid fermentation, even under aerobic conditions, termed the Warburg effect (33). Regions of high glucose metabolism, such as a cluster of malignant cells, demonstrate increased uptake compared with the background activity of cells. In addition, uptake of FDG is known to be proportional to tumor aggressiveness and growth rates (34). Uptake can be assessed qualitatively or quantitatively using standardized uptake values (SUV). However, visual assessment may lead to a tradeoff between sensitivity and specificity over quantitative SUV. As a guideline, uptake ratios of less than 2.5 are more likely benign (35, 36).

Overall, FDG-PET is excellent for characterization of solid pulmonary nodules. For solid pulmonary nodules 1 to 3 cm in diameter, meta-analyses have shown overall sensitivity at approximately 94% (37). However, this decreases significantly for smaller nodules in part due to lower spatial resolution compared with CT. Most current generation PET-cameras have a spatial resolution of 5 to 7 mm and the next generation cameras are expected to have improved resolution at 2 to 3 mm (38). False-negative results are also

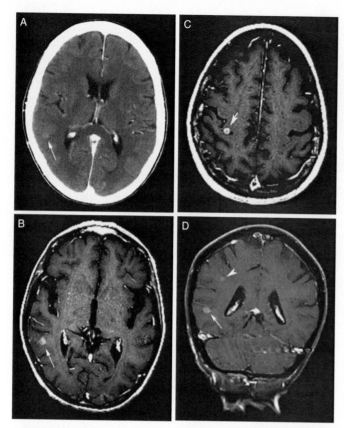

FIGURE 6.3 Lung cancer metastasis to the brain (pathology proven adenocarcinoma, M1b, stage IV). (A) Contrast-enhanced axial computed tomography (CT) image demonstrates subtle lesion in right posterior temporal gray-white matter junction (long arrow). (B) Contrast-enhanced axial T1-weighted magnetic resonance (MR) image shows lesion to better advantage (long arrow). (C) and (D) Axial and coronal contrast-enhanced T1-weighted MR images show additional lesions not seen on CT (short arrow, gray-white matter junction deep to central sulcus; arrowhead, right parietal lobe white matter).

seen with carcinoid tumors and bronchioloalveolar cell carcinoma (39,40). In addition, due to superior spatial resolution, CT is better for accurate anatomical assessment of primary tumor status (39). Overall specificity of FDG-PET for pulmonary nodule characterization has been reported at 83% (37). In certain instances, FDG-PET may be more specific than CT by distinguishing tumor from peritumoral atelectasis, thus preventing overestimation of tumor size (41). However, other diseases demonstrating increased metabolic activity may provide false positives, including focal active infection or granulomatous diseases (such as tuberculosis, histoplasmosis, and sarcoidosis) and rheumatoid lung disease (39,40).

Most studies and meta-analyses have found FDG-PET to be superior to CT in detecting pathologic mediastinal lymph nodes (Figures 6.4 and 6.7) (42–44). In a meta-analysis of 17 studies including 833 patients, the overall sensitivity of FDG-PET for detecting mediastinal lymph node metastasis was 83% and overall specificity was 92% (45). Smaller studies have shown the combination of PET and CT to be superior to either modality alone in detecting

mediastinal lymph node disease with combined sensitivity, specificity, and accuracy at 93%, 97%, and 96% (46). For this purpose, integrated PET-CT equipment has been developed and commercially manufactured. This combined equipment has been shown to further improve the detection and facilitate staging of bronchogenic carcinoma (47). In addition, integrated PET-CT has been shown to reduce both the total number of thoracotomies and the futile thoracotomies but did not affect overall mortality (48).

For extrathoracic disease, FDG-PET has been shown to be extremely helpful. With FDG-PET, occult extrathoracic metastases were found in up to 14% of patients selected for curative resection and altered management in up to 40% of cases (49–51). Currently, however, the cost-effectiveness of PET-based strategies in staging and workup of lung cancer are still being actively investigated (52–55).

■ IMAGING IN LUNG CANCER

The Solitary Pulmonary Nodule

A solitary pulmonary nodule (SPN) is defined as a round or oval opacity that is smaller than 3 cm in diameter and completely surrounded by pulmonary parenchyma without associated lymph node enlargement, atelectasis, or pneumonia (56). A number of clinical factors strongly affect the pretest probability of lung cancer, including whether or not the patient has a smoking history, the number of pack-years as a smoker (Brinkman Index), the duration of cessation in former smokers, age, sex, a history of pulmonary fibrosis of any etiology, immune status, and history of thoracic or extrathoracic cancer (57–64). Most SPNs are either inflammatory in etiology or primary lung cancers. Hamartomas (7%), solitary metastasis from an extrathoracic primary tumor (4%), and peripheral carcinoid tumors are other less frequent etiologies (65–68). The probability that an SPN represents a primary lung tumor rather than a metastasis varies depending on tumor type (e.g., 1:1.2 for colon cancer, 3.3:1 for breast and bladder cancer, and 8.3:1 for head and neck cancers).

There are several characteristics of SPNs that are helpful in determining the probability of malignancy, most of which are well evaluated by CT. These include size, morphology, border characteristics, location, tissue-specific, and metabolic features.

Size

Risk of malignancy is related to SPN size. The literature suggests that SPNs approaching 3 cm in diameter are more likely to be malignant, while more than 90% of nodules smaller than 2 cm are benign (3, 60, 70). In addition, lesions greater than 3 cm in size (which no longer fulfill the criteria for an SPN) have a likelihood of malignancy of greater than 93% (71).

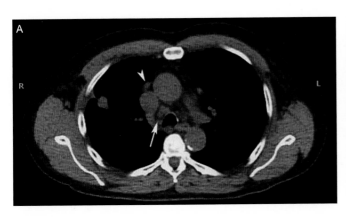
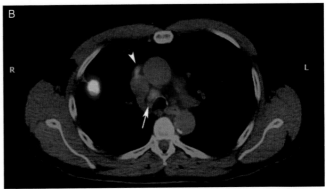

FIGURE 6.4 Right para-aortic fluorodeoxyglucose–positron emission tomography (FDG-PET) positive lymph node not enlarged by computed tomography (CT) size criteria (pathology proven adenocarcinoma; T1b N2 M0, stage IIIA). (A) and (B) Axial noncontrast CT and fused FDG-PET/CT images show 2.4 × 2.0 cm intensely hypermetabolic RUL nodule. Additionally hypermetabolic lymph nodes are noted at the right para-aortic (7 mm, arrowhead) and right paratracheal (11 mm, arrow) regions.

Comparison with any prior examinations is mandatory and essential in assessing the probability of malignancy. A solid SPN with absence of detectable growth over a 2-year period is more likely benign, although stability does not exclude the presence of malignancy (1,72,73). In addition, a very rapidly growing nodule is less likely to represent malignancy (74). These guidelines are based on data suggesting that the majority of lung cancers have doubling times between 20 and 400 days (73–75). In 1991, Lillington pointed out that "two year stability implies a doubling time of at least 730 days" (1). However, despite the widespread acceptance of the 2-year stability guideline, caution should be utilized because the biology of lung cancer varies considerably. Specifically, the relative lack of size change may not hold true for ground-glass opacities, which are typically slower growing malignancies (76,77) (refer to Tissue Specific and Metabolic Characteristics section) (78). Also, it may be difficult to reliably detect growth in very small nodules. For instance, if a 3-mm spherical nodule grows to 4 mm in size, it has more than doubled in volume (an increase in diameter by 26% implies doubling of volume). Recent data have shown that software volumetric evaluation has high reproducibility and negative predictive values of 98% (79,80).

Morphology

Morphologic characteristics worrisome for malignancy include spiculated margins, irregular margins, and lobulated margins (81). Spiculated margins have a positive predictive value for malignancy of approximately 90% (10,60). Irregular edges and spiculation seen radiographically are associated with histologic findings of radial extension of malignant cells along interlobular septa, lymphatics, small airways, or blood vessels (82). Lobulated margins are worrisome because they indicate uneven rates of growth (68, 81). Cavitation occurs in both benign and malignant nodules; however, cavity walls that are irregular and thicker

than 16 mm tend to be malignant, while cavities with thinner, smoother walls tend to be benign (Figure 6.5). In fact, approximately 95% of lesions with cavity walls thinner than 4 mm are benign (83,84).

Location

Location plays a factor in probability of malignancy as well since lung cancer is 1.5 times more likely to occur in the right lung compared with the left, 70% of lung cancers occur in the upper lobes, and 70% of lung cancers initially present as peripheral SPNs (85–87). In addition, patients with idiopathic pulmonary fibrosis have a 10% life-time risk of developing lung cancer and these tumors are more frequently seen in the regions where fibrosis occurs—the peripheral lower lobes (62). Different histopathologic tumor types tend to present in central or peripheral locations, although over the decades percentages have shifted due to several factors, including advances in diagnostic technology (ability to perform biopsies on smaller tumors in smaller, more distal airways), changes in cigarette designs (the adoption of filter tips), and changes in smoking practices (88,89). Regardless of cell type, central lung cancers can have very characteristic radiographic appearances, including a hilar mass or parenchymal collapse and consolidation of lung beyond the tumor with accompanying volume loss (Figure 6.6) (90).

Tissue-Specific and Metabolic Characteristics

Tissue-specific characteristics include presence and type of calcification, presence of fat, nodule attenuation on CT, and uptake of FDG-PET. The most important imaging feature that can be used to distinguish between benign and malignant SPNs is calcification. When nodules contain a central calcific nidus, or a laminated, popcorn, or diffuse pattern of calcification they are almost always benign (68,91). Popcorn calcifications are virtually pathognomonic for

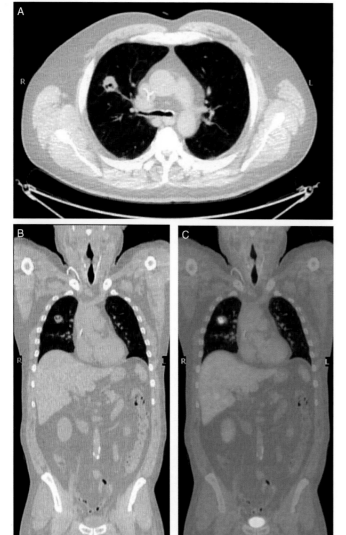

FIGURE 6.5 Right upper lobe (RUL) nodule with central cavitation. (A), (B), and (C) Axial noncontrast computed tomography (CT), coronal noncontrast CT, and fused fluorodeoxyglucose–positron emission tomography/CT images show 2.3 × 2.2 cm hypermetabolic RUL nodule with central cavitation.

pulmonary hamartomas, but are present only 5% to 10% of the time (92). The other patterns are often seen with granulomatous diseases such as tuberculosis or histoplasmosis (87). Calcification patterns worrisome for malignancy include amorphous, stippled, or eccentric (93,94). A stippled appearance or psammomatous calcification can be seen in SPNs that represent metastases from mucin-secreting tumors, such as colon or ovarian cancers (87). Presence of fat is also helpful in diagnosing pulmonary hamartoma. Focal fat attenuation is reliable in diagnosing pulmonary hamartomas; however, this is seen in only approximately 30% to 40% of hamartomas (10,95).

Nodules can be characterized by overall CT attenuation into nonsolid (ground-glass), part-solid (mixed), and solid.

After standardizing for size, nodules that were subsolid (nonsolid and part-solid) were much more likely to be malignant. The most worrisome type of nodule is the part-solid (mixed) type with frequency rates of malignancy as high as 63% (96). Malignant subsolid nodules tend to be bronchioloalveolar cell carcinomas or invasive mixed-subtype adenocarcinomas with bronchioloalveolar cell features. Solid nodules tend to represent other subtypes of adenocarcinoma (96).

Nodule avidity to FDG-PET has also been utilized to assess probability of malignancy (refer to Positron Emission Tomography section). Sensitivity and specificity for nodules 1 to 3 cm in diameter are 94% and 83%, respectively (37). In one study which evaluated the diagnostic accuracy of FDG-PET and CT in characterizing SPNs in 344 patients, FDG-PET proved to be more accurate and reliable than CT and resulted in far fewer indeterminate test results (97). In addition, PET was shown to have superior interobserver and intraobserver reliability compared with CT.

Imaging Guided Percutaneous Needle Biopsy

Once a pulmonary lesion has been discovered, the workup varies among institutions in regard to surgical resection, bronchoscopic biopsy, or the use of percutaneous needle biopsy (PCNB). In general, PCNB is useful for diagnosis of peripherally located lesions that are not accessible with bronchoscopy. These include nodules or masses in the peripheral lung, mediastinum, pleura, and chest wall (Figure 6.7). The most common indication for PCNB is the diagnosis of an SPN (98). PCNB can also be useful to determine the cytology (fine-needle aspiration) or histology (core biopsy) of suspected metastatic disease. Relative contraindications to percutaneous lung biopsy include severe obstructive pulmonary disease, moderate to severe pulmonary arterial hypertension, contralateral pneumonectomy, ventilator dependence, bleeding disorders, and inability to cooperate with breathing instructions (99).

Which imaging modality the interventional radiologist will use to perform the biopsy depends on a combination of availability and comfort level. A preprocedure CT is useful to plan all chest biopsies. Conventional fluoroscopy was previously commonly used to perform biopsies. However, CT guidance during biopsies is now the preferred technique of many interventionalists. Advances in CT fluoroscopy technology and technique have decreased both patient and radiologist radiation doses (100). Sonographic techniques can be utilized for chest wall, pleural, or subpleural lesions, and they utilize no ionizing radiation.

PCNB of the chest is very useful with overall high diagnostic yield and low clinically significant complication rate. Percutaneous biopsy is positive in patients with lung cancer approximately 90% of the time with a false-positive rate of less than 2% (101). However, caution must be used when interpreting a negative result because the false-negative rate is relatively high in up to one third of procedures. Patients

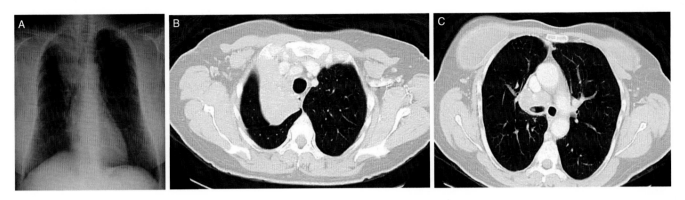

FIGURE 6.6 The "Golden S sign" (pathology proven adenocarcinoma, <5 cm and therefore T2a). (A) Frontal chest radiograph demonstrates right upper lobe (RUL) collapse secondary to a right hilar mass. (B) and (C) Two axial noncontrast chest computed tomography images confirm endobronchial mass causing complete atelectasis of the RUL.

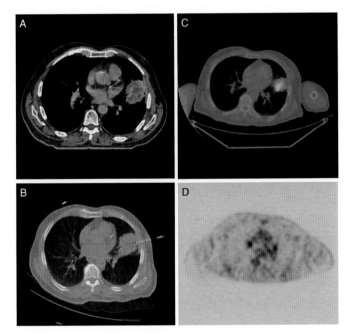

FIGURE 6.7 Percutaneous needle biopsy proven squamous cell carcinoma with fluorodeoxyglucose–positron emission tomography (FDG-PET) positive lymph nodes not initially seen on computed tomography (CT) (T2b N3 M0, stage IIIB). (A) Axial contrast-enhanced CT shows 5 cm heterogeneously enhancing mass in the left lower lobe. (B) Under CT guidance, coaxial 20-g needle was advanced to the peripheral margin of the lesion, and needle biopsies and cores were obtained for tissue analysis. (C) Axial FDG-PET/CT fusion image shows intense metabolic activity in mass with SUV measuring 8.4. (D) Axial FDG-PET image shows intense metabolic activity in bilateral hilar lymph nodes (SUV 3.1 on left and SUV 2.9 on right) which were subcentimeter on CT.

with a nonspecific biopsy result require close follow-up both clinically and radiologically, as well as consideration of repeat percutaneous biopsy.

The most common complication to occur is a pneumothorax, with a range reported in the literature from 5% to 57%, although most of these resolve without additional intervention (99). Many authors feel the true upper range of pneumothorax occurrence to be closer to 35% with 2%

to 15% requiring treatment and only a minority of which require a chest tube (98,99). Other less common complications include clinically significant pulmonary hemorrhage, hemothorax, and hemoptysis. Malignant needle tract seeding and systemic air embolism are extremely rare complications.

■ STAGING SMALL CELL LUNG CANCER

Small cell lung cancer (SCLC) is distinguished from NSCLC by its rapid tumor doubling time, early widespread metastasis (greater than 70% at the time of diagnosis), and almost exclusive occurrence in smokers (103). The Veteran's Administration Lung Cancer Study Group recommends two stages: limited disease and extensive disease (104). This distinction is clinically relevant as patients with limited stage disease are treated with combined radiation and chemotherapy while those with extensive disease stage receive chemotherapy alone.

Limited disease stage is defined as disease which can be confined to a single radiation portal. This includes tumor which has spread to the ipsilateral hilar or supraclavicular lymph nodes and cases with ipsilateral or contralateral mediastinal lymph node involvement (distinguishing this from the TNM staging of NSCLC; refer to Staging Non–Small Cell Lung Cancer section).

Extensive disease (ED) stage covers all other disease, including contralateral lung and distant extrathoracic metastasis. An area where this classification is problematic is with the presence of an ipsilateral malignant pleural effusion, a malignant pericardial effusion, or contralateral supraclavicular lymph node enlargement. Most authorities would categorize these as extensive disease stage, although the prognosis of patients with these findings remain controversial (Figure 6.8) (105–107). As previously mentioned, most patients with SCLC have extensive disease at presentation and common sites of metastasis

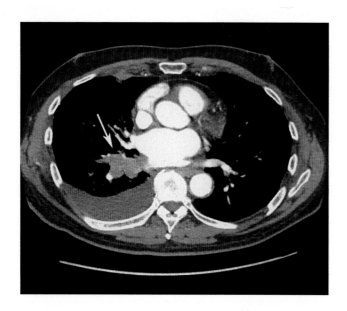

FIGURE 6.8 Small cell lung cancer, extensive disease stage. Axial contrast-enhanced computed tomography image demonstrates right lower lobe mass invading the pulmonary vein into the left atrium (arrow). Additionally, a moderate size right pleural effusion is seen compatible with metastatic pleural involvement.

include the liver, brain, retroperitoneal lymph nodes, and osseous structures (108).

There is no consensus regarding the imaging and invasive procedures that should be performed in the staging evaluation. To avoid performing an exhaustive staging workup, one alternative and cost-effective algorithm after detection and tissue diagnosis of SCLC includes a thorough history and physical examination, complete blood count, and blood chemistry (including liver function tests and bone enzymes) with positive findings directing the algorithm and terminated as soon as ED stage is documented (103,109).

However, there is literature supporting the use of noninvasive and invasive tests even in asymptomatic patients with SCLC. Head CT has been shown to be positive for metastatic disease in about 15% of patients at diagnosis including 5% to 8% of asymptomatic patients (2,103,100). MRI, with its increased sensitivity for intracranial metastatic disease, can be performed in all patients as an initial noninvasive test, and earlier identification and treatment of brain metastasis has been shown to lower the rate of chronic neurologic morbidity (111).

At presentation, 30% of patients have metastasis to the liver and 11% to the retroperitoneal lymph nodes. These patients can also be asymptomatic with normal routine liver function tests (104,112). Therefore, abdominal CT or MRI can be helpful to evaluate these structures as well as the adrenal glands (108). The osseous structures can also be well evaluated with Tc-99m-MDP scintigraphy, which is positive in up to 30% of patients, or with MRI (108,110,113).

FDG-PET in combination with CT has been shown in one study to be 100% sensitive in detecting intrathoracic disease and was also useful in staging patients as well as downstaging 18% of patients who were initially reported by CT alone to have extensive stage disease. FDG-PET has recently been shown to be useful in monitoring the treatment of SCLC, with visualization of a therapeutic response after one single cycle of chemotherapy (114).

■ STAGING NON–SMALL CELL LUNG CANCER

During the staging of NSCLC, a score is applied to each of three factors: the primary tumor, regional lymph node metastases, and distant metastases. The TNM staging system combines the tumor status score (T), lymph node score (N) and metastasis score (M) into a disease stage (see Table 6.1). Once a lung cancer has been staged the prognosis can be determined and appropriate therapy offered.

In 1996, the sixth edition of the TNM staging system was accepted as the standard for clinical use by the American Joint Committee on Cancer (AJCC) and Union Internationale Contre le Cancer (UICC). This system was based on survival analysis of 5,319 patients from University of Texas MD Anderson Cancer Center and the United States National Cancer Institute Cooperative Lung Cancer Study Group treated from 1975 through 1982 (116). In 2007, the IASLC proposed the seventh edition of the TNM staging system based on analysis of a database with 67,725 patients with NSCLC (117–119). We will base our figures and text on the seventh edition of the TNM staging system. As stated earlier, the rationale and data for this staging system is presented in Chapter 4 (*The New Lung Cancer Staging System*).

Tumor Status (T Stage)

To determine the T stage once malignancy has been diagnosed, a number of characteristics must be assessed including size, presence or absence of satellite nodules, extent of atelectasis if present, and invasion of adjacent structures. Most of these characteristics are best evaluated with CT, although as previously mentioned FDG-PET may offer increased specificity augmented by integrated FDG-PET/CT. The initial CT should be performed with intravenous contrast material to better assess potential vascular involvement of the superior vena cava, pulmonary veins, pulmonary arteries, systemic mediastinal arterial structures, and cardiopericardial structures.

Distinguishing between T3 and T4 stage is critical as this separates conventional surgical and nonsurgical

■ **Table 6.1** Proposed 7th edition TNM staging system for lung cancer

Primary tumor (T)

T1—Tumor ≤3 cm diameter, surrounded by lung or visceral pleura, without invasion more proximal than lobar bronchus

   T1a—Tumor ≤2 cm in diameter

   T1b—Tumor >2 cm but ≤3 cm in diameter

T2—Tumor >3 cm but ≤7 cm, or tumor with any of the following features:

      Involves main bronchus, ≥2 cm distal to carina

      Invades visceral pleura

      Associated with atelectasis or obstructive pneumonia that extends to the hilar region but does not involve the entire lung

   T2a—Tumor >3 cm but ≤ 5 cm

   T2b—Tumor >5 cm but ≤ 7 cm

T3—Tumor >7 cm or any of the following:

      Directly invades any of the following: chest wall, diaphragm, phrenic nerve, mediastinal pleura, parietal
         pericardium, main bronchus < 2 cm from carina (without involvement of carina)

      Atelectasis or obstructive pneumonia of the entire lung

      Separate tumor nodules in the same lobe

T4—Tumor of any size that invades the mediastinum, heart, great vessels, trachea, recurrent laryngeal nerve, esophagus, vertebral body, carina, or with separate tumor nodules in a different ipsilateral lobe

Regional lymph nodes (N)

N0—No regional lymph node metastases

N1—Metastasis in ipsilateral peribronchial and/or ipsilateral hilar lymph nodes and intrapulmonary nodes, including involvement by direct extension

N2—Metastasis in ipsilateral mediastinal and/or subcarinal lymph node(s)

N3—Metastasis in contralateral mediastinal, contralateral hilar, ipsilateral or contralateral scalene, or supraclavicular lymph node(s).

Distant metastasis (M)

M0—No distant metastasis

M1—Distant metastasis

   M1a—Separate tumor nodule(s) in a contralateral lobe; tumor with pleural nodules or malignant pleural or pericardial effusion

   M1b—Distant metastasis

Stage groupings

Stage IA	T1a–T1b	N0	M0
Stage IB	T2a	N0	M0
Stage IIA	T1a–T2a	N1	M0
	T2b	N0	M0
Stage IIB	T2b	N1	M0
	T3	N0	M0
Stage IIIA	T1a–T3	N2	M0
	T3	N1	M0
	T4	N0–N1	M0
Stage IIIB	T4	N2	M0
	T1a–T4	N3	M0
Stage IV	Any T	Any N	M1a or M1b

Source: Adapted from Ref. 115.

treatment. Some characteristics of tumors readily place them into the T4 stage, such as vertebral body invasion (Figure 6.9), invasion of the heart (Figure 6.10), or separate tumor nodules in a different ipsilateral lobe. T3 tumors can be more difficult to stage with noninvasive techniques such as defining the proximal extent of tumor within the airways, which can only be estimated by CT and requires bronchoscopy for confirmation. Distinguishing invasion of the mediastinal pleura can also be challenging as macroscopic contact is not sufficient to diagnose invasion (120). However, as previously described, MRI has been shown to be more sensitive than CT in determining mediastinal invasion, although subtle invasion can be missed (sensitivity 56–89%, specificity 50–93%). Occasionally

elevation of the hemidiaphragm may suggest phrenic nerve invasion (Figure 6.11). Also, satellite tumor nodules in the same lobe as the primary tumor were previously characterized as T4 lesions and now are T3 lesions in the seventh edition of the TNM classification (Figure 6.12).

MRI can be useful in evaluation of involvement of the brachial plexus or subclavian vessels, which are not defined by the standard AJCC staging system for lung cancer. However, it is generally regarded that limited involvement of the lower trunk or roots (C8, T1) of the brachial plexus constitutes T3 disease and more extensive invasion of the brachial plexus trunks or roots (C5–C7) or subclavian vessels constitutes T4 disease (Figure 6.2). A T4 classification for a superior sulcus tumor does not necessarily

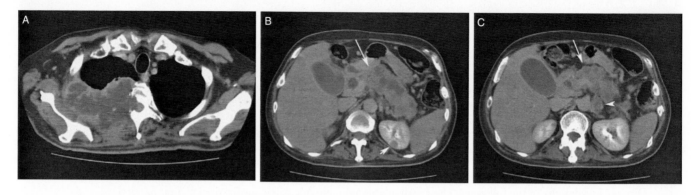

FIGURE 6.9 Superior sulcus tumor invading into spinal canal with intra-abdominal metastasis (T4 N3 M1b, stage IV). (A) Axial contrast-enhanced computed tomography (CT) image demonstrates heterogeneously enhancing right superior sulcus tumor which erodes the upper thoracic spine and right posterior rib cage, invading the spinal canal (T4). (B) and (C) Two axial contrast-enhanced CT images demonstrate metastatic disease to the pancreas (long arrow), left kidney (short arrow), and enlarged retroperitoneal lymph node (arrowhead).

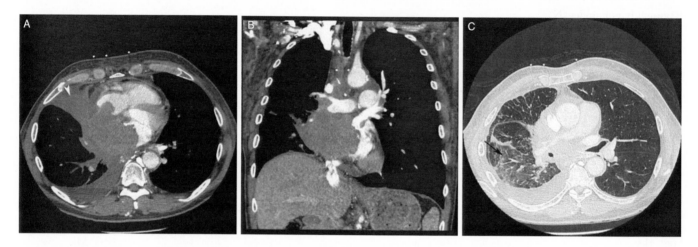

FIGURE 6.10 Non–small cell lung cancer invading into the heart with malignant pleural and pericardial effusions (T4 M1a, stage IV). (A), (B), and (C) Axial and coronal contrast-enhanced computed tomography images demonstrate gross invasion of tumor into the heart and presence of malignant pleural and pericardial effusions. Pulmonary venous obstruction causes right lower lobar pulmonary edema (black arrow). Partial collapse of the right middle lobe is also seen (arrowhead).

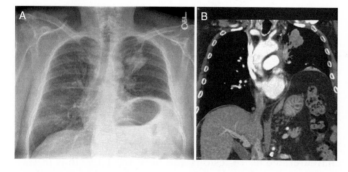

FIGURE 6.11 Elevation of the left hemidiaphragm due to phrenic nerve invasion by bronchogenic carcinoma (T3 N2 M0, stage IIIA). (A) and (B) Frontal chest radiograph and coronal contrast-enhanced computed tomography shows left upper lobe mass (>3 cm) extending toward the left hilum, elevation of the left hemidiaphragm due to phrenic nerve invasion by the tumor, and enlarged AP window and left hilar lymph nodes.

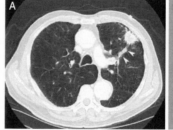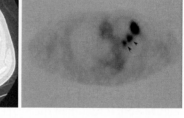

FIGURE 6.12 Satellite tumor nodules in the same lobe as the primary tumor (T3). (A) and (B) Axial computed tomography and fluorode-oxyglucose–positron emission tomography images demonstrate 2.5 cm metabolically active dominant left upper lobe nodule with adjacent satellite nodules (arrowheads).

imply nonsurgical management; however, invasion of the subclavian vessels does imply nonresectability (121).

Evaluation of Nodal Metastasis (N Stage)

Accurate staging of lymph node involvement is a critical aspect of the initial management of patients with non-metastatic NSCLC that influences decisions regarding the appropriateness and timing of treatment. Since the lung cancer staging system was first developed in 1973, lymph node involvement has been categorized as N0 (no nodes involved), N1 (peribronchial, interlobar, or perihilar lymph nodes involved), N2 (ipsilateral mediastinal nodes involved), or N3 (contralateral mediastinal or supraclavicular nodes involved) (122). Numerous studies have since validated the original N descriptors (119).

CT segregates normal from abnormal lymph nodes based upon their size in short axis (defined as the longest perpendicular diameter to the longest diameter of a lymph node or nodal mass) (11). The average mediastinal lymph node measures less than 10 mm in its short axis, although lymph nodes in the subcarinal region can reach a diameter of 13 mm. Nodes exceeding this size are presumed to be pathologic. Lymph nodes are rarely seen in the retrocrural region and in the pericardial fat and therefore lymph nodes exceeding 8 mm in these regions should be considered pathologic. Utilizing these guidelines, however, sensitivities are reported to be 79% and specificities to be 78% or lower (13,14).

Most studies and meta-analyses have found FDG-PET to be superior to CT for evaluation of nodal disease, with reported overall sensitivity for detecting mediastinal lymph node metastasis to be approximately 83% and overall specificity to be approximately 92% (Figures 6.4 and 6.7) (45). In addition, it has been reported that integrated FDG-PET and CT is superior to either modality interpreted separately for correct staging (123).

However, FDG-PET should be considered an adjunct rather than an alternative to invasive nodal staging (124,125). One meta-analysis found a post-test probability for N2 disease of 5% for lymph nodes measuring 10 to 15 mm on CT in patients with a negative FDG-PET result, suggesting that these patients should be planned for thoracotomy because the yield of mediastinoscopy will be extremely low. In patients with a negative FDG-PET and mediastinal lymph nodes measuring greater than 15 mm on CT, post-test probability for N2 disease was 21%, suggesting that these patients should undergo invasive mediastinal assessment by mediastinoscopy, endobronchial ultrasonography, and/or endoesophageal ultrasonography prior to possible thoracotomy to prevent too many unnecessary thoracotomies (126). In addition, due to the number of false-positive FDG-PET studies owing to infectious or inflammatory diseases, invasive nodal sampling should be performed for confirmation in patients where a change in result will impact management.

Evaluation of Metastasis (M Stage)

Metastases are graded as M0 (no distant metastases), M1a (malignant pleural effusion, pericardial effusion, pleural nodules, or metastatic nodules in the contralateral lung), and M1b (distant metastases).

Pleural effusions are present in up to one third of patients with NSCLC at the time of presentation (Figure 6.13) (13). Most of these are malignant; however, some will be of parapneumonic or sympathetic etiology. In cases where confirmation will influence disease stage, standard thoracentesis will detect approximately 65% of malignant effusions (13). If the initial thoracentesis is falsely negative, a repeat thoracentesis can be positive in up to 30% of cases (127). Thoracoscopy, with a reported sensitivity of 95%, should be performed if two thoracenteses are negative (13,128–130). FDG-PET has been reported to have a role in differentiating malignant from benign pleural effusions (sensitivity 55–95%, specificity 67–94%) (131–133). More recently, there has been some evidence that the combination of FDG-PET and CT may be superior to either modality alone (134).

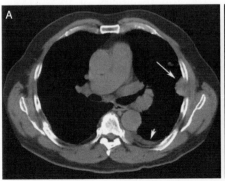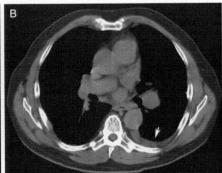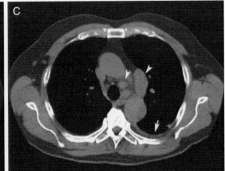

FIGURE 6.13 Malignant pleural effusion proven by thoracentesis, upgraded to stage IV disease (T3 N2 M1a, stage IV). (A), (B), and (C) Noncontrast axial computed tomography images demonstrate left upper lobe subpleural nodule (long arrow), small left effusion (short arrows), and enlarged AP window and left paratracheal lymph nodes (arrowheads).

Distant metastases are reported to occur in approximately 25% to 33% of all NSCLC patients at presentation (Figure 6.9) (135–140). Relative frequencies by site are reported to be brain:10%; bone: 7%; liver: 5%; and adrenal glands: 3%. Some authors have found that certain histology, such as adenocarcinoma, predisposes to increased risk of metastases (137, 140).

Most clinicians routinely assess the liver and adrenal glands for metastasis, even in asymptomatic patients, but do not look for metastasis to the brain, bones, or other organs unless the history, physical examination, or laboratory studies are suspicious for metastatic disease to these sites (13). This is supported by a meta-analysis of 25 studies with a total of 3,089 imaging examinations which found the risk of metastasis to be less than 3% if clinical examination was negative (71).

Brain Metastasis

The central nervous system (CNS) is the most frequent site of distant metastasis at presentation. However, most patients with brain metastasis are symptomatic and therefore CNS imaging in asymptomatic patients has been reported to be cost-ineffective and generally not recommended (71–141). However, with stage III patients who are being considered for aggressive local therapy (thoracic surgery or radiation), brain imaging is recommended (124). The rationale behind this recommendation is that the sample population of previous studies may have a selection bias toward those with early-stage disease and a lower prevalence of brain metastases, locally advanced disease being under-represented (121). This is supported by data which show that in patients with resected lung cancer, there is a substantial incidence of early postoperative recurrence of brain metastasis, especially in those with stage of disease higher than T1N0 or histology of large cell carcinoma or adenocarcinoma (121, 142–144). In one study of 27 patients, 22% with greater than T1N0M0 but surgically resectable disease had occult brain metastases (145).

Brain MRI is generally accepted to be more sensitive to brain metastases and is gaining popularity; however, there is insufficient evidence to recommend MRI over head CT in cases where cranial imaging is indicated (2). Reasons for the increased sensitivity were discussed in the Magnetic Resonance Imaging section. PET is not suited to the detection of brain metastases due to the physiologically high glucose uptake in the brain.

Bone Metastasis

Most patients with bony metastases are symptomatic or have laboratory abnormalities suggestive of osseous metastases (137). In patients where bone metastases are suspected, technetium 99m-methylene diphosphate (Tc-99m-MDP) scintigraphy has proven to be a fast and inexpensive initial test. Sensitivity is reported to be greater than 90%, although specificity can be somewhat limited (146).

In many centers, however, FDG-PET has become the preferred imaging modality for detection of skeletal metastases. FDG-PET has been reported to be of similar sensitivity to bone scan, but increased accuracy (accuracy of FDG-PET up to 96% vs. 73% for bone scan) (146,147).

Liver Metastasis

While the liver is a common place for metastasis, it is uncommon to have isolated liver metastases (135). Imaging of at least part, if not most, of the liver is included in the chest CT examination, and therefore routinely evaluated by the radiologist. However, in the absence of signs, symptoms, or laboratory abnormalities for lung cancer assessment, it is generally not recommended to perform dedicated CT or ultrasound of the abdomen and liver (93).

For detection of liver metastases, PET may be equal or slightly superior to CT. In some studies, PET has a reported sensitivity ranging from 97% to 100%. Most studies demonstrate increased accuracy for liver metastases of PET over CT (148,149). Further analysis of discovered lesions may be necessary, and contrast-enhanced ultrasound, CT, and MRI techniques have been helpful to delineate potentially metastatic lesions (150–152).

Adrenal Metastasis

The adrenal glands are generally included in the chest CT examination. However, most adrenal masses are benign adrenal adenomas, cysts, or myelolipomas. In fact, 6% to 10% of the general population have been reported to have benign adrenal adenomas (2,121). Both CT and MRI are useful in the evaluation of adrenal masses: features of malignancy include size greater than 3 cm, poorly defined margins, irregularly enhancing rim, invasion of adjacent structures, and high signal intensity on T2-weighted MR images (153). On noncontrast CT examinations, a threshold of less than 10 Hounsfield units can be utilized to differentiating a benign adenoma from a malignant lesion with sensitivity of 71% and specificity of 98% (154). Although this finding of low attenuation is helpful for diagnosing lipid-rich adenomas, up to 30% of adenomas do not contain enough lipid for the low attenuation to be a valid discriminator on routine noncontrast CT scanning (30). However, as previously mentioned, MRI is complementary to CT, and increased specificity can be achieved if chemical shift analysis and contrast kinetics analysis (washout characteristics) on contrast-enhanced CT scanning are used. FDG-PET has been reported to have a sensitivity of 100% and specificity of 80% to 90% in identifying adrenal masses (155, 156). In other words, in a patient with NSCLC and an isolated adrenal mass with increased FDG-PET uptake, the adrenal lesion should be biopsied before omitting curative resection.

■ SUMMARY

Imaging plays a vital role in the detection, diagnosis, staging, and follow-up of lung cancer. Chest CT should be obtained in all patients with suspected lung cancer. PET complements CT in the assessment of lung cancer, and its routine use can accurately characterize nodal and extrathoracic metastases.

■ REFERENCES

1. Lillington GA. Management of solitary pulmonary nodules. *Dis Mon*. 1991;37(5):271–318.

2. Hyer JD, Silvestri G. Diagnosis and staging of lung cancer. *Clin Chest Med*. 2000;21(1):95–106, viii.

3. Henschke CI, McCauley DI, Yankelevitz DF, et al. Early Lung Cancer Action Project: overall design and findings from baseline screening. *Lancet*. 1999;354(9173):99–105.

4. Henschke CI, Miettinen OS, Yankelevitz DF, Libby DM, Smith JP. Radiographic screening for cancer. Proposed paradigm for requisite research. *Clin Imaging*. 1994;18(1):16–20.

5. Kaneko M, Eguchi K, Ohmatsu H, et al. Peripheral lung cancer: screening and detection with low-dose spiral CT versus radiography. *Radiology*. 1996;201(3):798–802.

6. Malm HM. Medical screening and the value of early detection. When unwarranted faith leads to unethical recommendations. *Hastings Cent Rep*. 1999;29(1):26–37.

7. Sone S, Li F, Yang ZG, et al. Characteristics of small lung cancers invisible on conventional chest radiography and detected by population based screening using spiral CT. *Br J Radiol*. 2000;73(866):137–145.

8. Sone S, Takashima S, Li F, et al. Mass screening for lung cancer with mobile spiral computed tomography scanner. *Lancet*. 1998;351(9111):1242–1245.

9. Tillich M, Kammerhuber F, Reittner P, Riepl T, Stoeffler G, Szolar DH. Detection of pulmonary nodules with helical CT: comparison of cine and film-based viewing. *AJR Am J Roentgenol*. 1997;169(6):1611–1614.

10. Zwirewich CV, Vedal S, Miller RR, Müller NL. Solitary pulmonary nodule: high-resolution CT and radiologic-pathologic correlation. *Radiology*. 1991;179(2):469–476.

11. Glazer GM, Gross BH, Quint LE, Francis IR, Bookstein FL, Orringer MB. mediastinal lymph nodes: number and size according to American Thoracic Society mapping. *AJR Am J Roentgenol*. 1985;144(2):261–265.

12. Schwartz LH, Bogaerts J, Ford R, et al. Evaluation of lymph nodes with RECIST 1.1. *Eur J Cancer*. 2009;45(2):261–267.

13. Pretreatment evaluation of non-small-cell lung cancer. The American Thoracic Society and the European Respiratory Society. *Am J Respir Crit Care Med*. 1997;156(1):320–332.

14. McLoud TC, Bourgouin PM, Greenberg RW, et al. Bronchogenic carcinoma: analysis of staging in the mediastinum with CT by correlative lymph node mapping and sampling. *Radiology*. 1992;182(2):319–323.

15. Lewis JW, Jr, Pearlberg JL, Beute GH, et al. Can computed tomography of the chest stage lung cancer? Yes and no. *Ann Thorac Surg*.1990;49(4):591–595; discussion 5–6.

16. Gdeedo A, Van Schil P, Corthouts B, Van Mieghem F, Van Meerbeeck J, Van Marck E. Comparison of imaging TNM [(i) TNM] and pathological TNM [pTNM] in staging of bronchogenic carcinoma. *Eur J Cardiothorac Surg*. 1997;12(2): 224–227.

17. Cascade PN, Gross BH, Kazerooni EA, et al. Variability in the detection of enlarged mediastinal lymph nodes in staging lung cancer: a comparison of contrast-enhanced and unenhanced CT. *AJR Am J Roentgenol*. 1998;170(4):927–931.

18. Patz EF Jr, Erasmus JJ, McAdams HP, et al. Lung cancer staging and management: comparison of contrast-enhanced and nonenhanced helical CT of the thorax. *Radiology*. 1999;212(1): 56–60.

19. Bettmann MA, Heeren T, Greenfield A, Goudey C. Adverse events with radiographic contrast agents: results of the SCVIR Contrast Agent Registry. *Radiology*. 1997;203:611–620.

20. Kanal E, Barkovich AJ, Bell C, et al. ACR guidance document for safe MR practices: 2007. *AJR Am J Roentgenol*. 2007;188(6):1447–1474.

21. Batra P, Brown K, Steckel RJ, Collins JD, Ovenfors CO, Aberle D. MR imaging of the thorax: a comparison of axial, coronal, and sagittal imaging planes. *J Comput Assist Tomogr*. 1988;12(1):75–81.

22. Hatabu H, Stock KW, Sher S, et al. Magnetic resonance imaging of the thorax. Past, present, and future. *Clin Chest Med*. 1999;20(4):775–803, viii.

23. Dawn SK, Gotway MB, Webb WR. Multidetector-row spiral computed tomography in the diagnosis of thoracic diseases. *Respir care*. 2001;46(9):912–921.

24. Ueda T, Mori K, Minami M, Motoori K, Ito H. Trends in oncological CT imaging: clinical application of multidetector-row CT and 3D-CT imaging. *Int J Clin Oncol*. 2006;11(4):268–277.

25. Bae KT. Optimization of contrast enhancement in thoracic MDCT. *Radiol Clin North Am*. 2010;48(1):9–29.

26. Padovani B, Mouroux J, Seksik L, et al. Chest wall invasion by bronchogenic carcinoma: evaluation with MR imaging. *Radiology*. 1993;187(1):33–38.

27. Webb WR, Gatsonis C, Zerhouni EA, et al. CT and MR imaging in staging non-small cell bronchogenic carcinoma: report of the Radiologic Diagnostic Oncology Group. *Radiology*. 1991;178(3):705–713.

28. Toloza EM, Harpole L, McCrory DC. Noninvasive staging of non-small cell lung cancer: a review of the current evidence. *Chest*. 2003;123(1 suppl):137S–146S.

29. Israel GM, Korobkin M, Wang C, Hecht EN, Krinsky GA. Comparison of unenhanced CT and chemical shift MRI in evaluating lipid-rich adrenal adenomas. *AJR Am J Roentgenol*. 2004;183(1):215–219.

30. Peña CS, Boland GW, Hahn PF, Lee MJ, Mueller PR. Characterization of indeterminate (lipid-poor) adrenal masses: use of washout characteristics at contrast-enhanced CT. *Radiology*. 2000;217(3):798–802.

31. Schellinger PD, Meinck HM, Thron A. Diagnostic accuracy of MRI compared to CCT in patients with brain metastases. *J Neurooncol*. 1999;44(3):275–281.

32. Erasmus JJ, Patz EF Jr. Positron emission tomography imaging in the thorax. *Clin Chest Med*. 1999;20(4):715–724.

33. Kim JW, Dang CV. Cancer's molecular sweet tooth and the Warburg effect. *Cancer Res*. 2006;66(18):8927–8930.

34. Duhaylongsod FG, Lowe VJ, Patz EF Jr, Vaughn AL, Coleman RE, Wolfe WG. Lung tumor growth correlates with glucose metabolism measured by fluoride-18 fluorodeoxyglucose positron emission tomography. *Ann Thorac Surg*. 1995;60(5):1348–1352.

35. Lowe VJ, Duhaylongsod FG, Patz EF, et al. Pulmonary abities and PET data analysis: a retrospective study. *Radiology*. 1997;202(2):435–439.

36. Lowe VJ, Fletcher JW, Gobar L, et al. Prospective investigation of positron emission tomography in lung nodules. *J Clin Oncol*. 1998;16(3):1075–1084.

37. Gould MK, Maclean CC, Kuschner WG, Rydzak CE, Owens DK. Accuracy of positron emission tomography for diagnosis of pulmonary nodules and mass lesions: a meta-analysis. *JAMA*. 2001;285(7):914–924.

38. Vansteenkiste JF. FDG-PET for lymph node staging in NSCLC: a major step forward, but beware of the pitfalls. *Lung Cancer*. 2005;47(2):151–153.

39. Erasmus JJ, McAdams HP, Patz EF Jr. Non-small cell lung cancer: FDG-PET imaging. *J Thorac Imaging*. 1999;14(4):247–256.

40. Erasmus JJ, McAdams HP, Patz EF Jr, Coleman RE, Ahuja V, Goodman PC. Evaluation of primary pulmonary carcinoid tumors using FDG PET. *AJR Am J Roentgenol.* 1998;170(5):1369–1373.

41. Gámez C, Rosell R, Fernández A, et al. PET/CT fusion scan in lung cancer: current recommendations and innovations. *J Thorac Oncol.* 2006;1(1):74–77.

42. Dwamena BA, Sonnad SS, Angobaldo JO, Wahl RL. Metastases from non-small cell lung cancer: mediastinal staging in the 1990s–meta-analytic comparison of PET and CT. *Radiology.* 1999;213(2):530–536.

43. Farrell MA, McAdams HP, Herndon JE, Patz EF Jr. Non-small cell lung cancer: FDG PET for nodal staging in patients with stage I disease. *Radiology.* 2000;215(3):886–890.

44. Guhlmann A, Storck M, Kotzerke J, Moog F, Sunder-Plassmann L, Reske SN. Lymph node staging in non-small cell lung cancer: evaluation by [18F]FDG positron emission tomography (PET). *Thorax.* 1997;52(5):438–441.

45. Birim O, Kappetein AP, Stijnen T, Bogers AJ. Meta-analysis of positron emission tomographic and computed tomographic imaging in detecting mediastinal lymph node metastases in nonsmall cell lung cancer. *Ann Thorac Surg.* 2005;79(1):375–382.

46. Vansteenkiste JF, Stroobants SG, De Leyn PR, et al. Mediastinal lymph node staging with FDG-PET scan in patients with potentially operable non-small cell lung cancer: a prospective analysis of 50 cases. Leuven Lung Cancer Group. *Chest.* 1997;112(6):1480–1486.

47. Shim SS, Lee KS, Kim BT, et al. Non-small cell lung cancer: prospective comparison of integrated FDG PET/CT and CT alone for preoperative staging. *Radiology.* 2005;236(3):1011–1019.

48. Fischer B, Lassen U, Mortensen J, et al. Preoperative staging of lung cancer with combined PET-CT. *N Engl J Med.* 2009;361(1):32–39.

49. Lewis P, Griffin S, Marsden P, et al. Whole-body 18F-fluorodeoxyglucose positron emission tomography in preoperative evaluation of lung cancer. *Lancet.* 1994;344(8932):1265–1266.

50. Valk PE, Pounds TR, Hopkins DM, et al. Staging non-small cell lung cancer by whole-body positron emission tomographic imaging. *Ann Thorac Surg.* 1995;60(6):1573–81; discussion 1581.

51. Weder W, Schmid RA, Bruchhaus H, Hillinger S, von Schulthess GK, Steinert HC. Detection of extrathoracic metastases by positron emission tomography in lung cancer. *Ann Thorac Surg.* 1998;66(3):886–92; discussion 892.

52. Gambhir SS, Shepherd JE, Shah BD, et al. Analytical decision model for the cost-effective management of solitary pulmonary nodules. *J Clin Oncol.* 1998;16(6):2113–2125.

53. Herder GJ, Kramer H, Hoekstra OS, et al.; POORT Study Group. Traditional versus up-front [18F] fluorodeoxyglucose-positron emission tomography staging of non-small-cell lung cancer: a Dutch cooperative randomized study. *J Clin Oncol.* 2006;24(12):1800–1806.

54. van Tinteren H, Hoekstra OS, Smit EF, et al. Effectiveness of positron emission tomography in the preoperative assessment of patients with suspected non-small-cell lung cancer: the PLUS multicentre randomised trial. *Lancet.* 2002;359(9315):1388–1393.

55. Viney RC, Boyer MJ, King MT, et al. Randomized controlled trial of the role of positron emission tomography in the management of stage I and II non-small-cell lung cancer. *J Clin Oncol.* 2004;22(12):2357–2362.

56. Midthun DE, Swensen SJ, Jett JR. Approach to the solitary pulmonary nodule. *Mayo Clin Proc.* 1993;68(4):378–385.

57. Shopland DR, Burns DM; National Cancer Institute (U.S.). Smoking and Tobacco Control Program. *Changes in Cigarette-Related Disease Risks and Their Implication for Prevention and Control.* Bethesda, MD: National Institutes of Health, National Cancer Institute; 1997.

58. Tong L, Spitz MR, Fueger JJ, Amos CA. Lung carcinoma in former smokers. *Cancer.* 1996;78(5):1004–1010.

59. Wynder EL, Graham EA. Tobacco smoking as a possible etiologic factor in bronchiogenic carcinoma; a study of 684 proved cases. *J Am Med Assoc.* 1950;143(4):329–336.

60. Gurney JW, Lyddon DM, McKay JA. Determining the likelihood of malignancy in solitary pulmonary nodules with Bayesian analysis. Part II. Application. *Radiology.* 1993;186(2):415–422.

61. Jemal A, Chu KC, Tarone RE. Recent trends in lung cancer mortality in the United States. *J Natl Cancer Inst.* 2001;93(4):277–283.

62. Lee HJ, Im JG, Ahn JM, Yeon KM. Lung cancer in patients with idiopathic pulmonary fibrosis: CT findings. *J Comput Assist Tomogr.* 1996;20(6):979–982.

63. Parker MS, Leveno DM, Campbell TJ, Worrell JA, Carozza SE. AIDS-related bronchogenic carcinoma: fact or fiction? *Chest.* 1998;113(1):154–161.

64. Travis WD, Lubin J, Ries L, Devesa S. United States lung carcinoma incidence trends: declining for most histologic types among males, increasing among females. *Cancer.* 1996;77(12):2464–2470.

65. Bateson EM. AN Analysis of 155 solitary lung lesions illustrating the differential diagnosis of mixed tumours of the lung. *Clin Radiol.* 1965;16:51–65.

66. Murthy SC, Rice TW. The solitary pulmonary nodule: a primer on differential diagnosis. *Semin Thorac Cardiovasc Surg.* 2002;14(3):239–249.

67. Primack SL, Lee KS, Logan PM, Miller RR, Müller NL. Bronchogenic carcinoma: utility of CT in the evaluation of patients with suspected lesions. *Radiology.* 1994;193(3):795–800.

68. Siegelman SS, Khouri NF, Leo FP, Fishman EK, Braverman RM, Zerhouni EA. Solitary pulmonary nodules: CT assessment. *Radiology.* 1986;160(2):307–312.

69. Thanos L, Galani P, Mylona S, Pomoni M, Mpatakis N. Percutaneous CT-guided core needle biopsy versus fine needle aspiration in diagnosing pneumonia and mimics of pneumonia. *Cardiovasc Intervent Radiol.* 2004;27(4):329–334.

70. Swensen SJ, Jett JR, Hartman TE, et al. CT screening for lung cancer: five-year prospective experience. *Radiology.* 2005;235(1):259–265.

71. Silvestri GA, Littenberg B, Colice GL. The clinical evaluation for detecting metastatic lung cancer. A meta-analysis. *Am J Respir Crit Care Med.* 1995;152(1):225–230.

72. Nathan MH, Collins VP, Adams RA. Differentiation of benign and malignant pulmonary nodules by growth rate. *Radiology.* 1962;79:221–232.

73. Yankelevitz DF, Henschke CI. Does 2-year stability imply that pulmonary nodules are benign? *AJR Am J Roentgenol.* 1997;168(2):325–328.

74. Fishman AP, Elias JA. *Fishman's Pulmonary Diseases and Disorders.* 3rd ed. New York: McGraw-Hill, Health Professions Division; 1998.

75. Yankelevitz DF, Kostis WJ, Henschke CI, et al. Overdiagnosis in chest radiographic screening for lung carcinoma: frequency. *Cancer.* 2003;97(5):1271–1275.

76. Suzuki K, Kusumoto M, Watanabe S, Tsuchiya R, Asamura H. Radiologic classification of small adenocarcinoma of the lung: radiologic-pathologic correlation and its prognostic impact. *Ann Thorac Surg.* 2006;81(2):413–419.

77. Noguchi M, Morikawa A, Kawasaki M, et al. Small adenocarcinoma of the lung. Histologic characteristics and prognosis. *Cancer.* 1995;75(12):2844–2852.

78. Aoki T, Nakata H, Watanabe H, et al. Evolution of peripheral lung adenocarcinomas: CT findings correlated with histology and tumor doubling time. *AJR Am J Roentgenol.* 2000;174(3):763–768.

79. Revel MP, Merlin A, Peyrard S, et al. Software volumetric evaluation of doubling times for differentiating benign versus malignant pulmonary nodules. *AJR Am J Roentgenol.* 2006;187(1):135–142.

80. Revel MP, Lefort C, Bissery A, et al. Pulmonary nodules: preliminary experience with three-dimensional evaluation. *Radiology.* 2004;231(2):459–466.

81. Furuya K, Murayama S, Soeda H, et al. New classification of small pulmonary nodules by margin characteristics on high-resolution CT. *Acta Radiol.* 1999;40(5):496–504.

82. Heitzman ER, Markarian B, Raasch BN, Carsky EW, Lane EJ, Berlow ME. Pathways of tumor spread through the lung: radiologic correlations with anatomy and pathology. *Radiology.* 1982;144(1):3–14.

83. Woodring JH, Fried AM. Significance of wall thickness in solitary cavities of the lung: a follow-up study. *AJR Am J Roentgenol.* 1983;140(3):473–474.

84. Woodring JH, Fried AM, Chuang VP. Solitary cavities of the lung: diagnostic implications of cavity wall thickness. *AJR Am J Roentgenol.* 1980;135(6):1269–1271.

85. Proto AV, Thomas SR. Pulmonary nodules studied by computed tomography. *Radiology.* 1985;156(1):149–153.

86. Garland LH. Bronchial carcinoma. Lobar distribution of lesions in 250 cases. *Calif Med.* 1961;94:7–8.

87. Winer-Muram HT. The solitary pulmonary nodule. *Radiology.* 2006;239(1):34–49.

88. Thun MJ, Lally CA, Flannery JT, Calle EE, Flanders WD, Heath CW Jr. Cigarette smoking and changes in the histopathology of lung cancer. *J Natl Cancer Inst.* 1997;89(21):1580–1586.

89. Quinn D, Gianlupi A, Broste S. The changing radiographic presentation of bronchogenic carcinoma with reference to cell types. *Chest.* 1996;110(6):1474–1479.

90. Hollings N, Shaw P. Diagnostic imaging of lung cancer. *Eur Respir J.* 2002;19(4):722–742.

91. Zerhouni EA, Stitik FP, Siegelman SS, et al. CT of the pulmonary nodule: a cooperative study. *Radiology.* 1986;160(2):319–327.

92. Sinner WN. Fine-needle biopsy of hamartomas of the lung. *AJR Am J Roentgenol.* 1982;138(1):65–69.

93. McLoud TC, Swenson SJ. Lung carcinoma. *Clin Chest Med.* 1999;20(4):697–713, vii.

94. Mahoney MC, Shipley RT, Corcoran HL, Dickson BA. CT demonstration of calcification in carcinoma of the lung. *AJR Am J Roentgenol.* 1990;154(2):255–258.

95. Siegelman SS, Khouri NF, Scott WW Jr, et al. Pulmonary hamartoma: CT findings. *Radiology.* 1986;160(2):313–317.

96. Henschke CI, Yankelevitz DF, Mirtcheva R, McGuinness G, McCauley D, Miettinen OS; ELCAP Group. CT screening for lung cancer: frequency and significance of part-solid and non-solid nodules. *AJR Am J Roentgenol.* 2002;178(5):1053–1057.

97. Fletcher JW, Kymes SM, Gould M, et al.; VA SNAP Cooperative Studies Group. A comparison of the diagnostic accuracy of 18F-FDG PET and CT in the characterization of solitary pulmonary nodules. *J Nucl Med.* 2008;49(2):179–185.

98. Valji K. *Vascular and Interventional Radiology.* 2nd ed. Philadelphia, PA: Saunders Elsevier; 2006.

99. Perlmutt LM, Johnston WW, Dunnick NR. Percutaneous transthoracic needle aspiration: a review. *AJR Am J Roentgenol.* 1989;152(3):451–455.

100. Silit E, Kizilkaya E, Okutan O, et al. CT fluoroscopy-guided percutaneous needle biopsies in thoracic mass lesions. *Eur J Radiol.* 2003;48(2):193–197.

101. Charig MJ, Stutley JE, Padley SP, Hansell DM. The value of negative needle biopsy in suspected operable lung cancer. *Clin Radiol.* 1991;44(3):147–149.

102. Calhoun P, Feldman PS, Armstrong P, et al. The clinical outcome of needle aspirations of the lung when cancer is not diagnosed. *Ann Thorac Surg.* 1986;41(6):592–596.

103. Elias AD. Small cell lung cancer: state-of-the-art therapy in 1996. *Chest.* 1997;112(4 suppl):251S–258S.

104. Darling GE. Staging of the patient with small cell lung cancer. *Chest Surg Clin N Am.* 1997;7(1):81–94.

105. Argiris A, Murren JR. Staging and clinical prognostic factors for small-cell lung cancer. *Cancer J.* 2001;7(5):437–447.

106. Micke P, Faldum A, Metz T, et al. Staging small cell lung cancer: Veterans Administration Lung Study Group versus International Association for the Study of Lung Cancer–what limits limited disease? *Lung Cancer.* 2002;37(3):271–276.

107. Urban T, Chastang C, Vaylet F, et al. Prognostic significance of supraclavicular lymph nodes in small cell lung cancer: a study from four consecutive clinical trials, including 1,370 patients. "Petites Cellules" Group. *Chest.* 1998;114(6):1538–1541.

108. Jelinek JS, Redmond J 3rd, Perry JJ, et al. Small cell lung cancer: staging with MR imaging. *Radiology.* 1990;177(3):837–842.

109. Simon GR, Turrisi A. Management of small cell lung cancer: ACCP evidence-based clinical practice guidelines (2nd edition). *Chest.* 2007;132(3 suppl):324S–339S. http://www.nccn.org/professionals/physician_gls/f_guidelines.asp

110. Ihde DC, Makuch RW, Carney DN, et al. Prognostic implications of stage of disease and sites of metastases in patients with small cell carcinoma of the lung treated with intensive combination chemotherapy. *Am Rev Respir Dis.* 1981;123(5):500–507.

111. Lassman AB, DeAngelis LM. Brain metastases. *Neurol Clin.* 2003;21(1):1–23, vii.

112. Abrams J, Doyle LA, Aisner J. Staging, prognostic factors, and special considerations in small cell lung cancer. *Semin Oncol.* 1988;15(3):261–277.

113. Levitan N, Byrne RE, Bromer RH, et al. The value of the bone scan and bone marrow biopsy staging small cell lung cancer. *Cancer.* 1985;56(3):652–654.

114. Yamamoto Y, Kameyama R, Murota M, Bandoh S, Ishii T, Nishiyama Y. Early assessment of therapeutic response using FDG PET in small cell lung cancer. *Mol Imaging Biol.* 2009;11(6):467–472.

115. Goldstraw P, Crowley J, Chansky K, et al. The IASLC Lung Cancer Staging Project: proposals for the revision of the TNM stage groups in the forthcoming (seventh) edition of the TNM classification of malignant tumours. *J Thorac Oncol.* 2007;2:706.

116. Mountain CF. Revisions in the International System for Staging Lung Cancer. *Chest.* 1997;111(6):1710–1717.

117. Postmus PE, Brambilla E, Chansky K, et al.; International Association for the Study of Lung Cancer International Staging Committee; Cancer Research and Biostatistics; Observers to the Committee; Participating Institutions. The IASLC Lung Cancer Staging Project: proposals for revision of the M descriptors in the forthcoming (seventh) edition of the TNM classification of lung cancer. *J Thorac Oncol.* 2007;2(8):686–693.

118. Rami-Porta R, Ball D, Crowley J, et al.; International Staging Committee; Cancer Research and Biostatistics; Observers to the Committee; Participating Institutions. The IASLC Lung Cancer Staging Project: proposals for the revision of the T descriptors in the forthcoming (seventh) edition of the TNM classification for lung cancer. *J Thorac Oncol.* 2007;2(7):593–602.

119. Rusch VW, Crowley J, Giroux DJ, et al.; International Staging Committee; Cancer Research and Biostatistics; Observers to the Committee; Participating Institutions. The IASLC Lung Cancer Staging Project: proposals for the revision of the N descriptors in the forthcoming seventh edition of the TNM classification for lung cancer. *J Thorac Oncol.* 2007;2(7):603–612.

120. Glazer HS, Kaiser LR, Anderson DJ, et al. Indeterminate mediastinal invasion in bronchogenic carcinoma: CT evaluation. *Radiology.* 1989;173(1):37–42.

121. Erasmus JJ, Sabloff BS. CT, positron emission tomography, and MRI in staging lung cancer. *Clin Chest Med.* 2008;29(1):39–57, v.

122. Martini N. Mediastinal lymph node dissection for lung cancer. The Memorial experience. *Chest Surg Clin N Am.* 1995;5(2):189–203.

123. Antoch G, Stattaus J, Nemat AT, et al. Non-small cell lung cancer: dual-modality PET/CT in preoperative staging. *Radiology.* 2003;229(2):526–533.

124. Pfister DG, Johnson DH, Azzoli CG, et al.; American Society of Clinical Oncology. American Society of Clinical Oncology treatment of unresectable non-small-cell lung cancer guideline: update 2003. *J Clin Oncol.* 2004;22(2):330–353.

125. Reed CE, Harpole DH, Posther KE, et al.; American College of Surgeons Oncology Group Z0050 trial. Results of the American College of Surgeons Oncology Group Z0050 trial: the utility of positron emission tomography in staging potentially

operable non-small cell lung cancer. *J Thorac Cardiovasc Surg.* 2003;126(6):1943–1951.

126. de Langen AJ, Raijmakers P, Riphagen I, Paul MA, Hoekstra OS. The size of mediastinal lymph nodes and its relation with metastatic involvement: a meta-analysis. *Eur J Cardiothorac Surg.* 2006;29(1):26–29.

127. Roberts JR, Blum MG, Arildsen R, et al. Prospective comparison of radiologic, thoracoscopic, and pathologic staging in patients with early non-small cell lung cancer. *Ann Thorac Surg.* 1999;68(4):1154–1158.

128. Davenport RD. Rapid on-site evaluation of transbronchial aspirates. *Chest.* 1990;98(1):59–61.

129. Light RW, Erozan YS, Ball WC Jr. Cells in pleural fluid. Their value in differential diagnosis. *Arch Intern Med.* 1973;132(6):854–860.

130. Paone G, Nicastri E, Lucantoni G, et al. Endobronchial ultrasound-driven biopsy in the diagnosis of peripheral lung lesions. *Chest.* 2005;128(5):3551–3557.

131. Gupta NC, Rogers JS, Graeber GM, et al. Clinical role of F-18 fluorodeoxyglucose positron emission tomography imaging in patients with lung cancer and suspected malignant pleural effusion. *Chest.* 2002;122(6):1918–1924.

132. Prior J, Orcurto M, Nicod-Lalonde M, Allenbach G. Value of PET/CT for evaluating malignant exudative pleural effusions in patients with known cancer [Meeting Abstracts]. *J Nucl Med.* 2007;48.

133. Erasmus JJ, McAdams HP, Rossi SE, Goodman PC, Coleman RE, Patz EF. FDG PET of pleural effusions in patients with non-small cell lung cancer. *AJR Am J Roentgenol.* 2000;175(1):245–249.

134. Toaff JS, Metser U, Gottfried M, et al. Differentiation between malignant and benign pleural effusion in patients with extra-pleural primary malignancies: assessment with positron emission tomography-computed tomography. *Invest Radiol.* 2005;40(4):204–209.

135. Quint LE, Tummala S, Brisson LJ, et al. Distribution of distant metastases from newly diagnosed non-small cell lung cancer. *Ann Thorac Surg.* 1996;62(1):246–250.

136. Bell JW. Abdominal exploration in one-hundred lung carcinoma suspects prior to thoracotomy. *Ann Surg.* 1968;167(2):199–203.

137. Salvatierra A, Baamonde C, Llamas JM, Cruz F, Lopez-Pujol J. Extrathoracic staging of bronchogenic carcinoma. *Chest.* 1990;97(5):1052–1058.

138. Sider L, Horejs D. Frequency of extrathoracic metastases from bronchogenic carcinoma in patients with -sized hilar and mediastinal lymph nodes on CT. *AJR Am J Roentgenol.* 1988;151(5):893–895.

139. Smith RA. Evaluation of the long-term results of surgery for bronchial carcinoma. *J Thorac Cardiovasc Surg.* 1981;82(3):325–333.

140. Weiss W, Gillick JS. The metastatic spread of bronchogenic carcinoma in relation to the interval between resection and death. *Chest.* 1977;71(6):725–729.

141. Colice GL, Birkmeyer JD, Black WC, Littenberg B, Silvestri G. Cost-effectiveness of head CT in patients with lung cancer without clinical evidence of metastases. *Chest.* 1995;108(5):1264–1271.

142. Figlin RA, Piantadosi S, Feld R. Intracranial recurrence of carcinoma after complete surgical resection of stage I, II, and III non-small-cell lung cancer. *N Engl J Med.* 1988;318(20):1300–1305.

143. Robnett TJ, Machtay M, Stevenson JP, Algazy KM, Hahn SM. Factors affecting the risk of brain metastases after definitive chemoradiation for locally advanced non-small-cell lung carcinoma. *J Clin Oncol.* 2001;19(5):1344–1349.

144. Yokoi K, Kamiya N, Matsuguma H, et al. Detection of brain metastasis in potentially operable non-small cell lung cancer: a comparison of CT and MRI. *Chest.* 1999;115(3):714–719.

145. Earnest F 4th, Ryu JH, Miller GM, et al. Suspected non-small cell lung cancer: incidence of occult brain and skeletal metastases and effectiveness of imaging for detection–pilot study. *Radiology.* 1999;211(1):137–145.

146. Hsia TC, Shen YY, Yen RF, Kao CH, Changlai SP. Comparing whole body 18F-2-deoxyglucose positron emission tomography and technetium-99m methylene diophosphate bone scan to detect bone metastases in patients with non-small cell lung cancer. *Neoplasma.* 2002;49(4):267–271.

147. Bury T, Barreto A, Daenen F, Barthelemy N, Ghaye B, Rigo P. Fluorine-18 deoxyglucose positron emission tomography for the detection of bone metastases in patients with non-small cell lung cancer. *Eur J Nucl Med.* 1998;25(9):1244–1247.

148. Hustinx R, Paulus P, Jacquet N, Jerusalem G, Bury T, Rigo P. Clinical evaluation of whole-body 18F-fluorodeoxyglucose positron emission tomography in the detection of liver metastases. *Ann Oncol.* 1998;9(4):397–401.

149. Delbeke D, Martin WH, Sandler MP, Chapman WC, Wright JK Jr, Pinson CW. Evaluation of benign vs malignant hepatic lesions with positron emission tomography. *Arch Surg.* 1998;133(5):510–5; discussion 515.

150. Quaia E, Stacul F, Gaiani S, et al. Comparison of diagnostic performance of unenhanced vs SonoVue—enhanced ultrasonography in focal liver lesions characterization. The experience of three Italian centers. *La Radiologia Medica.* 2004;108(1–2): 71–81.

151. Tanimoto A, Wakabayashi G, Shinmoto H, Nakatsuka S, Okuda S, Kuribayashi S. Superparamagnetic iron oxide-enhanced MR imaging for focal hepatic lesions: a comparison with CT during arterioportography plus CT during hepatic arteriography. *J Gastroenterol.* 2005;40(4):371–380.

152. Seitz K, Strobel D, Bernatik T, et al. Contrast-enhanced ultrasound (CEUS) for the characterization of focal liver lesions—prospective comparison in clinical practice: CEUS vs. CT (DEGUM multicenter trial). Parts of this manuscript were presented at the Ultrasound Dreilandertreffen 2008, Davos. *Ultraschall Med.* 2009;30(4):383–389.

153. Mayo-Smith WW, Boland GW, Noto RB, Lee MJ. State-of-the-art adrenal imaging. *Radiographics.* 2001;21(4):995–1012.

154. Boland GW, Blake MA, Hahn PF, Mayo-Smith WW. Incidental adrenal lesions: principles, techniques, and algorithms for imaging characterization. *Radiology.* 2008;249(3):756–775.

155. Yun M, Kim W, Alnafisi N, Lacorte L, Jang S, Alavi A. 18F-FDG PET in characterizing adrenal lesions detected on CT or MRI. *J Nucl Med.* 2001;42(12):1795–1799.

156. Erasmus JJ, Patz EF Jr, McAdams HP, et al. Evaluation of adrenal masses in patients with bronchogenic carcinoma using 18F-fluorodeoxyglucose positron emission tomography. *AJR Am J Roentgenol.* 1997;168(5):1357–1360.

Treatment According to Stage

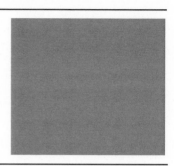

7 Early-Stage, Local Disease NSCLC, Surgical Therapy Options

PAUL C. Y. TANG

TODD L. DEMMY

SAI YENDAMURI

■ INTRODUCTION

A general thoracic surgeon, a subspecialist in cardiothoracic surgery, specializes in the treatment of benign and malignant diseases of the chest including those of the tracheobronchial tree, pulmonary parenchyma, pleura, pericardium, and mediastinum. Many of these professionals train either in thoracic-track training programs or perform additional fellowship training in the specialty at institutions with significant experience. However, several other acceptable training paradigms exist in different health systems. The general thoracic surgeon plays a role in the diagnosis, evaluation, staging, and treatment of lung cancer patients and should serve as a resource for the primary care physician in all facets of lung cancer care. It is optimal that such care is delivered in a multidisciplinary setting where the medical, radiation, and thoracic surgical oncologists provide impartial assessments and recommendations of care depending not only on the stage of disease but also on the comorbidities and personal goals of each patient. Thus, more than ever before, the general thoracic surgeon is a disease manager able to evaluate and advise patients with all stages of lung cancer. This chapter addresses issues relevant to the surgical management of lung cancer including preoperative assessment of adequacy of lung function, mediastinal staging and management, and techniques and extent of lung resection.

■ OVERVIEW OF THE SURGICAL TREATMENT OF NSCLC

Surgery is the major treatment modality for early-stage non–small cell lung cancer (NSCLC). It has the best survival for curative-intent treatment in this patient population. The 5-year survival rates after surgery are 70% for stage I,

50% for stage II, and 25% for selected patients with stage III disease (UICC 7 staging system) (1,2). The primary goal of surgical treatment is the complete resection of the tumor along with its regional lymphatic drainage (R0 is the goal, meaning that the gross and microscopic examination of the margin are free of tumor; R1 means that the margin has microscopic disease present, and R2 means that there is gross or visible tumor noted, usually at the time of resection). Depending on the extent of tumor, this may involve a sublobar resection (removing a segment of the lung or a wedge or extended wedge resection; definitions of an extended wedge resection vary, but usually means that the resection margin is 2–4 cm from the closest edge of tumor), lobectomy, or pneumonectomy. Any involved adjacent tissue should be resected en bloc. Tumor spillage must be avoided to prevent subsequent intrathoracic seeding. Margins are assessed with intraoperative frozen sections and any positive margins should be re-excised in an effort to achieve R0 resection (see R0, R1, and R2 classification described earlier) (3). The second goal of surgical therapy is tumor staging, which often determines the ultimate outcome of the patient. This can take the form of either a complete lymph node dissection or systematic lymph node sampling. The definitions of each are variable, but a complete lymph node dissection means that the surgical procedure resects all nodal tissue in the hilum and mediastinum, whereas lymph node sampling removes a few nodes in key nodal stations in the hilum and mediastinum. Commonly accepted definitions are described in the article by Allen et al. (4).

■ PREOPERATIVE PULMONARY LUNG FUNCTION ASSESSMENT FOR PLANNING SURGERY

One of the first issues facing the thoracic surgeon is the assessment of the patient eligibility for surgery based on pulmonary reserve. Identification of patients at risk for developing postoperative complications helps the practitioner pay special attention to prevention, early detection, and treatment of these complications. Spirometry represents an important aspect of this assessment. In general, a postoperative percentage predicted (ppo%) forced expiratory volume in the first second (FEV_1) and ppo% diffuse lung capacity of >40% are recommended (5,6). In patients with marginally acceptable pulmonary function tests, further testing can be performed to better assess the post–lung resection pulmonary reserve. A quantitative radionuclide perfusion scan can be performed to measure the relative function of each region of the lung and the subsidiary segments. Areas affected by cancer tend to have decreased perfusion. More advanced quantitation methods such as single-photon emission computed tomography (SPECT) may overcome the overlapping of lung areas in radionuclide imaging to provide a more accurate assessment. Thus, otherwise inoperable patients may tolerate resection of a nonfunctioning or poorly functioning area of the lung with acceptable risk of respiratory complications (6–8). Studies have shown that cardiopulmonary exercise tests (CPETs) can be used to predict oxygen uptake as well as cardiac and pulmonary reserve. Exercise testing has been shown to be a better predictor of postoperative complications than resting cardiac and pulmonary function. CPET allows the estimation of maximal oxygen consumption. The minimum recommended preoperative maximal oxygen consumption (VO_2 max) is 20 ml/kg/minute for pneumonectomy and a VO_2 max of 15 ml/kg/minute for a lobectomy. Other functional tests are the 6-minute walk distance test and stair-climbing test. However, these tests are less objective in their assessment and therefore uniform application is more difficult to assist in estimating postoperative morbidity and mortality (6,9,10). While the battery of tests mentioned earlier are useful guides, there is no single test that should be used to exclude patients from a potentially curative lung resection, and the expert general thoracic surgeon should review all of the data to determine the best course of action.

■ MEDIASTINAL ASSESSMENT

Another important preoperative consideration is mediastinal assessment for staging and treatment planning. Various options for mediastinal staging exist. Surgical methods include the cervical mediastinoscopy (Figure 7.1), the extended cervical mediastinoscopy, Chamberlain parasternal mediastinoscopy or mediastinotomy, the video-assisted mediastinal lymphadenectomy, the transcervical extended mediastinal lymphadenectomy (TEMLA), paramediastinoscopy, and thoracoscopic and open (via thoracotomy) mediastinal staging (11,12). Less invasive staging methods are computed tomography (CT), positron emission tomography (PET), PET-CT, magnetic resonance imaging (MRI), transbronchial needle aspiration (TBNA), endobronchial ultrasound with needle aspiration (EBUS-FNA—Figure 7.2), esophageal ultrasound with needle aspiration (EUS-FNA), and transthoracic needle

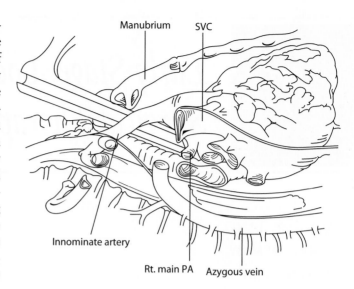

FIGURE 7.1 Cervical Mediastinoscopy.

aspiration (TTNA). A comparison of their relative effectiveness is summarized in Table 7.1. Of particular importance is the false negative rate which estimates the fraction of patients where the mediastinum is falsely declared free of tumor.

The choice of the ideal mediastinal staging techniques is disease, stage, and patient dependent. In patients with pathologically confirmed disease and who have gross evidence of extensive mediastinal involvement, CT and/or MRI may be sufficient to stage the mediastinum. PET or CT-PET can also be used to look for distant metastasis and can identify more extensive disease in 5% to 20% of patients (27). The finding of mediastinal lymph node enlargement ≥1 cm (e.g., N2,3) on CT has a cancer false positivity rate of approximately 56% (28). Furthermore, enlarged nodes by CT which are negative on PET have a false negative rate of 13% to 25% (29,30). PET-CT finding of mediastinal or hilar nodal enlargements demonstrated a false negative rate of 28% (31). In light of studies claiming superior results compared with this, one can infer that the effectiveness depends on the patient pool and that physician judgment and experience play a significant role in

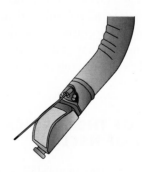

FIGURE 7.2 Endobronchial ultrasound. The ultrasound probe guides the insertion of the transbronchial needle into mediastinal lymph nodes, thereby minimizing vascular injury.

■ **Table 7.1** Summary of relative effectiveness for mediastinal staging modalities

Technique	Sensitivity (%)	Specificity (%)	False Negative Rate (%)	Invasiveness
Mediastinoscopy (13,14)	78 (85–92)	100	3–9	+++
TEMLA (15,16)	94	100	0	+++
CT (17,18)	51, 52	69, 86	16	+
PET (18,19)	72	85	8–20	+
PET-CT (19,20)	86	81	5	+
MRI (17)	48	64		+
TBNA (21,22)	58	100	10	++
EBUS-FNA (23,24)	92	100	5	++
EUS-FNA (14,25)	84, 89	100	19 (14–32)	++
TTNA (14,26)	88	100		++
VATS (14)	75	100	7	++++

CT, computed tomography; EBUS-FNA, endobronchial ultrasound–fine needle aspiration; EUS, endoscopic ultrasound; MRI, magnetic resonance imaging; PET, positron emission tomography—usually performed with fluorodeoxyglucose tracer and a PET scanning system rather than a SPECT (single-photon emission tomography) scanner; TBNA, transbronchial needle aspiration—performed without ultrasound guidance, instead using the bronchial airway anatomy and view on the CT to direct the needle; TEMLA, transcervical extended mediastinal lymphadenectomy—through a generous low transverse neck incision and with a specialized sternal retractor lymph nodes are completely resected from the major nodal stations; TTNA, transthoracic needle aspiration—usually performed by CT and/or fluoroscopic guidance; VATS, video-assisted thoracic surgery.

interpretation. In extrathoracic metastatic patients or in patients with grossly positive disease, invasive mediastinal staging is less likely to provide any additional prognostic or treatment-related information. For other patients, especially potential surgical candidates, most thoracic oncologists evaluate the mediastinum to either confirm or refute the noninvasive findings. A number of techniques like mediastinoscopy (with the numerous variations mentioned earlier), TBNA, endobronchial ultrasound with needle aspiration (EBUS-FNA), esophageal ultrasound with needle aspiration (EUS-FNA), TTNA, and video-assisted thoracic surgery (VATS) have been used to obtain a tissue diagnosis of lung cancer. The choice depends on local expertise as well as on the location of the suspicious nodes. It is important to note that the needle aspiration staging techniques are associated with a false negative rate of 20% to 28% and are operator dependent. In comparison, mediastinoscopy has a much lower false negative rate of 10% (14,32). Thus, negative findings on needle aspiration techniques are likely best evaluated by comparison with mediastinoscopy. In patients with a central lung tumor and/or N1 nodal involvement, both CT and PET are associated with high false negative rates of approximately 25% (33). In a prospective study of patients found to have N1 nodal involvement by integrated PET-CT, N2 disease was found by mediastinoscopy in 18% and EUS-FNA in 24% (31,34,35). Therefore, in this population, invasive staging is required even in the presence of a negative CT or PET scan.

Staging of peripheral tumors requires a different strategy. The false negative rate of PET (about 5%) (34–36) and CT (about 10%) (33) in detecting mediastinal disease in this population is relatively low. When using CT for staging, T1 tumors are associated with a lower false negative rate (9%) than T2 tumors (13%) (33). Thus, PET evaluation may be unnecessary following a negative CT assessment. This may be especially true for a T1 tumor. Follow-up studies after a negative integrated PET-CT scan shows that unsuspected N2 involvement can only be identified in 3% by mediastinoscopy and in 4% by EUS-FNA (37). Thus, invasive staging techniques are not routinely needed following a negative CT and/or PET assessment in small peripheral tumors. However, it is reasonable to do so if the lesion demonstrates unfavorable characteristics such as cavitation, peritumoral infiltration, or high standard uptake value (SUV) on PET scan.

Although patients diagnosed with stage IIIA lung cancer due to presence of N2 positive disease are generally considered to have a poor prognosis, recent studies have shown that these patients may be downstaged with neoadjuvant therapy. Subsequent surgical resection can still yield a significantly improved 5-year survival rate of 40% to 50%. Thus, restaging options constitute an important aspect of subsequent surgical treatment. A decrease of SUV by 80% or more predicts a complete response with 96% accuracy. For restaging, integrated PET-CT improves sensitivity without decreasing accuracy compared with PET alone (38). More invasive methods of staging such as TBNA, EBUS-FNA, and EUS-FNA have proved efficacious in restaging. For EBUS-FNA, the diagnostic statistics are sensitivity (76%), specificity (100%), positive predictive value (100%), and negative predictive value (20%) (39). For EUS-FNA, the diagnostic statistics are sensitivity (75%), specificity (100%), positive predictive value (100%), and negative predictive value (67%) (40). Restaging using redo-mediastinoscopy is technically challenging, particularly if radiation was used. Therefore, published results seem to be operator dependent. Low sensitivity of 29% with an accuracy of 60% has been reported by some (41) whereas others documented a sensitivity of 71%, specificity of 100%, and accuracy of 84% (42). It is disappointing that, in spite of all the available data and techniques available for accurate staging, inadequate mediastinal staging is common (43). Use of more mediastinal staging modalities is associated with improved outcomes, probably by avoiding mis-staging and the appropriate use of multi-modality treatment for the adequately staged advanced lung cancer patient (44).

■ SURGICAL TECHNIQUES—APPROACHES TO THE THORACIC CAVITY

Once a decision of surgical resection has been made in the appropriately selected and staged patient, lung resection can be performed through a thoracotomy or a median sterno-tomy, thoracotomy being the more common approach. The posterolateral thoracotomy (Figure 7.3) is a commonly used incision for lung resection. This incision is carried from the midpoint between the spine and the posterior border of the scapula to one fingerbreadth below the inferior tip of the scapula and then extended anteriorly the same dis-tance toward the inframammary fold. The serratus anterior muscle is usually preserved and retracted anteriorly. For the standard pulmonary resection, the chest cavity is reached by entering through an intercostal space that provides the best access for the procedure to be performed; ribs are usu-ally not resected (45). More recently, the posterior muscle sparing thoracotomy is preferred when possible as it spares all chest wall muscles by using the auscultatory triangle as the landmark. The initial skin incision is identical to the traditional thoracotomy. Subcutaneous skin flap are cre-ated superiorly and inferiorly. The latissimus dorsi muscle is identified and mobilized from the underlying serratus mus-cle for its entire length. The serratus muscle is then elevated. A rib can be partially excised to facilitate spreading and avoid fractures. The axillary thoracotomy (limited lateral thoracotomy) can be used for upper or middle lobe resec-tions or procedures confined to the anterior mediastinum or hilum. The incision is carried through the anterior aspect of the serratus muscle parallel to its fibers to the level of the fourth intercostal space. Care must be taken not to damage the long thoracic nerve posteriorly. With experience, this incision can be used for most situations. The anterior tho-racotomy is used to approach lesions in the anterior and middle thoracic cavity. An incision is made in the infra-mammary fold along the fifth rib. The pectoralis major muscle is divided at its insertion into the medial chest wall. The serratus anterior muscles are then incised to expose the fourth and fifth ribs with the chest cavity entered at the fourth intercostal space. Lateral serratus fibers are spared to avoid long thoracic nerve injury (45).

Increasingly, minimally invasive approaches to lung resection are being applied with benefits in postoperative

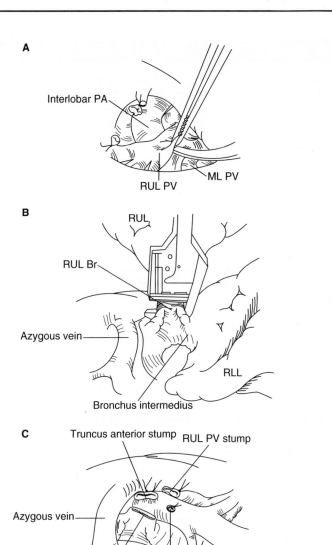

FIGURE 7.3 Open lobectomy.

morbidity without sacrificing oncologic outcomes. These approaches include thoracoscopic and robotic approaches. While several port placement strategies for VATS lobec-tomy exist, one is illustrated in Figure 7.4. A robotic approach sacrifices the tactile feel afforded by VATS in order to gain more control over dissection—this approach has been successfully utilized by several surgeons to obtain good outcomes (46).

■ SURGICAL TECHNIQUES—EXTENT OF RESECTION

Once a surgical approach has been selected, the extent of resection is determined by balancing the need for good surgical margins and the patient's pulmonary reserve.

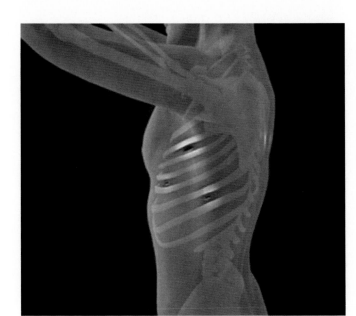

FIGURE 7.4 Incisions used for VATS lobectomy

Adequacy of Tumor Margins

Bronchial Margins

It is generally accepted that a microscopically negative margin is sufficient when performing an anatomic lung resection, such as a lobectomy (47). Estimation of adequate margin by gross examination is more difficult. Some have suggested more extensive margins of normal tissue between the tumor edge and the line of resection; one study recommended a margin as much as 1.9 cm (48). This recommendation is supported by studies showing that a bronchial resection margin of 1.5 cm maximum diameter from the macroscopic NSCLC tumor will provide negative margins in 93% of cases. NSCLC also differ in their infiltrative pattern. Adenocarcinomas demonstrate peribronchial extension whereas squamous cell carcinomas tend to extend proximally and may be microscopic in 24% (49). Positive margins with submucosal, peribronchial, and lymphatic space involvement is associated with worse outcomes than positive mucosal margins only (50–52). Because of differences in infiltrative patterns, some authors also recommend larger margins (2 cm) for adenocarcinoma and lesser margins (1.5 cm) for squamous cell carcinomas (50). For peripheral tumors, margins of 1.5 cm in a deflated lung or 2 cm in an inflated lung should be adequate (53).

Parenchymal Margins

The extent of resection appears to have a significant role in the likelihood of recurrence. For example, sublobar resection (wedge resections or segmentectomies) for all stage I NSCLC (combined IA and IB) has a local recurrence rate

three times that of lobectomy. Interestingly, there is no difference in postoperative disease-free survival between the two groups (54–57). Stratifying by substage, in the stage IB subgroup, survival is significantly lower with sublobar resections (56). However, sublobar resections have the advantage of preserving lung function with statistically superior postoperative spirometry data when compared with lobectomy (57) and improves quality of life of patients compared with patients who underwent a more extensive resection (58). Thus, sublobar resection is mostly reserved for small peripheral NSCLC in patients with high operative risk and/or poor cardiopulmonary reserve (59).

In 1995, a Lung Cancer Study Group (LCSG) report established lobectomy as the procedure of choice for stage 1A NSCLC (54). This study compared limited pulmonary resections (e.g., pulmonary segmentectomies and nonanatomic wedge resections) with lobectomies for stage 1 lung cancer and found increased mortality and locoregional recurrences in the limited resection group. However, LCSG included larger tumors (>3 cm) and nonanatomic wedge resections in approximately a third of the limited resection group (54). A number of subsequent studies have noted equivalent 5-year survival and freedom from local recurrence for early NSCLC less than or equal to 2 cm after segmentectomy compared with lobectomy (60–64). For subcentimeter tumors, limited wedge resections may be sufficient, but larger tumors may be better treated with segmentectomies (65) with greater tumor margins. Compared with lobectomy, limited sublobar resection of subcentimeter tumors appears to be associated with equivalent 5- and 10-year survival. In one retrospective review, an overall survival of 72% and a cancer-specific survival of 100% at 10 years were achieved (66). Okada and colleagues found that segmentectomy for tumors 2 to 3 cm in size achieved better 5-year survival than wedge resection (84.6 vs. 39.4%). Furthermore, for tumors >30 mm, segmentectomy confers an even greater survival benefit compared with wedge resection (62.9% vs. 0%) (67). Surgical judgment is critical in making the decision of wedge resection versus segmentectomy as wedge resections are more likely to be associated with a resection margin less than 1 cm (65).

Extent of Resection

Wedge Resection

Wedge resections are reserved for small peripheral lesions in patients with impaired cardiopulmonary reserve and are not candidates for lobectomy (54,68,69). VATS wedge resections that achieve shorter hospital stay and less patient morbidity than the open approach are standard of care (70). Criteria for wedge resection that have been suggested include (a) tumors less than 2 cm in diameter (T1a lesion); (b) tumors located in the outer third of lung and approachable by wedge resection by either staple, electrocautery, or laser; (c) no endobronchial extension; (d) frozen section evidence of negative pathologic resection margins; and (e) intraoperative mediastinal and hilar nodal staging (55). Recurrences vary with tumor size and nodal involvement. For node-negative patients with T1 and T2 tumors, the long-term local recurrence occurs in 5% to 12% whereas distant metastasis occurs in 7% to 30%. Failure rates increase with the presence of hilar or mediastinal nodal disease. In N1 and N2 disease, the local failure rate is 9% to 28% and 13% to 17%, respectively, and distant metastasis occurs in 22% to 61% (71–73). In patients with severe compromise of pulmonary function and harboring recurrent disease, the cause of clinical deterioration and death can be difficult to ascertain. Generally, death is more likely from cardiopulmonary deterioration rather than from tumor recurrence. A number of strategies decrease local recurrence after wedge resections. External beam radiation had promise(68), but in a prospective multi-institutional clinical trial of high-risk patients treated with post–wedge resection "postage stamp" radiotherapy, the results were disappointing (74). Alternatively, intraoperative radiotherapy reduces local recurrences from 19% to 1% in stage I NSCLC (75–79). Similarly, in patients unable to tolerate a lobectomy, brachytherapy appears to reduce local recurrence to levels seen in lobectomy patients (75–79). In general, brachytherapy can be applied to the lung by placing radioactive seeds embedded in mesh at the lung resection margin (76) or afterload catheters sewn to the resection margin. For the latter, the patient is isolated in a lead-lined room and radioactive seeds are instilled into the afterloading catheters for short periods over several days postoperatively. The catheters are then removed (80). Postoperative seed loading has the advantage of avoiding radiation exposure to operating room personnel and other individuals (80). Radioactive seed brachytherapy decreased local recurrence rate with sublobar resections to 6.1%, which is similar to that of lobectomies (6.4%) in the LCSG study (54,78). Using ^{125}I beaded sutures sewn into a polyglyconate mesh, Fernando et al. (77) reduced local recurrence in NSCLC to 3.3% in patients who underwent sublobar resections. For tumors less than 2 cm, no survival difference was demonstrated between lobectomy and sublobar resection with brachytherapy. Similar results have also been extended to stage IB tumors (79). At this point, this approach is reserved for those with compromised pulmonary function (80).

Segmentectomy

Segmentectomy is appropriate for select NSCLC patients. Examples are stage I and II NSCLC associated with impaired lung function, synchronous or metachronous lung cancer (as a lung preservation operation), and peripheral stage I lung cancer (81). Retrospective studies of selected patients have shown segmentectomies to confer equivalent survival rates to lobectomy. Major

complications include prolonged air leaks (5–16%) and a higher rate of recurrence (11–16% vs. 5% for lobectomy) (68,82–85). As expected, increased recurrence (22%) was seen in segmentectomies with margins less than 1 to 2 cm as well as proximity to the hilum (86,87). With underlying pulmonary compromise, segmentectomies were associated with a 30-day mortality benefit of 1.1% versus 3.3% for lobectomy (86). This is supported by findings that segmentectomy results in better residual pulmonary function than lobectomy (64). Thoracoscopic segmentectomy has been shown to result in shorter hospital stay as well as lower 30-day mortality compared with the open approach (88). Due to the improved tolerance of patients to adjuvant therapy, thoracoscopic segmentectomy may also yield better survival than the open technique (89). Commonly performed segmentectomies include lingula-sparing left upper lobectomy, lingulectomy, superior segmentectomy, and basilar segmentectomy. Anterior or posterior upper lobe segmentectomies are performed less commonly (90).

The adequacy of staging in sublobar resections has been examined by multiple investigators. One study found that no lymph nodes were sampled in 43% of patients who underwent sublobar resections. In comparison, only 2.7% did not have lymph node specimens after a lobectomy (56). However, when performing a sublobar resection, concerns have been raised about the inability to identify the nodal and parenchymal intransit disease (86). Segmentectomies address the biology of lung cancer and the segmental anatomical nature of the lymphatic drainage and blood supply, potentially allowing the intraoperative assessment of hilar, bronchial, and segmental lymph nodes (60,62,91). So, if requiring a less than lobectomy resection, segmentectomy with an adequate margin of parenchyma may meet the same goals as a lobectomy for many patients. There is an additional argument in support of performing a sublobar resection at the first presentation of a lung cancer. We know that NSCLC patients develop a new primary at a rate of 1% to 2% each year. Having performed a sublobar resection at the outset, a second surgical resection is less likely to compromise pulmonary reserve (92,93). Mortality rates are higher with repeat lung resections and correlate with the extent of resection. The mortality rates for repeat resections are 34% for pneumonectomy, 7% for lobectomy, 0% for segmentectomy, and 6% for a wedge resection (93). Limited resections were associated with less blood loss and air leaks in this setting (94).

Given the importance of the question whether sublobar resections are equivalent to anatomic lobectomy, there are several important trials that are underway or have just been completed. A multicenter phase III trial, CALGB 140503, is comparing sublobar resection to lobectomy in patients with peripheral primary NSCLC ≤ 2 cm. An additional multi-institutional phase III trial that has just completed accrual, ACOSOG Z4032, is comparing the local recurrence and survival of high-risk patients undergoing sublobar resection for stage I NSCLC with and without mesh brachytherapy. Finally, just approved by the National Cancer Institute is a multi-institutional phase III trial comparing feasibility, outcomes, and survival between wedge resection and brachytherapy to stereotactic body radiation therapy. These and many other forthcoming trials will help us to identify the role and type of surgery in early NSCLC.

Lobectomy

Open lobectomy has been the standard of care of early-stage NSCLC for many years. However, VATS lobectomy has recently emerged as an excellent alternative to open lobectomy. Complication (29,95,96) and survival (29,97,98) rates between VATS and open lobectomies are comparable. VATS lobectomies have several advantages over traditional open techniques: decreased postoperative pain (99,100), lower chest tube output and duration (29), less blood loss (101), superior pulmonary function (102), shorter hospital stay, and earlier return to normal activities (29,95). Equivalent survivals at 3 and 5 years were reported for VATS lobectomy (90% and 90%, respectively) and open lobectomy (93% and 85%) for stage I NSCLC (30,103,104). Others reported improved survival for VATS lobectomy at 4 years after resection (105). Importantly, VATS lobectomy patients were more tolerant of adjuvant therapy than their open lobectomy counterparts. Patients undergoing VATS lobectomy experienced fewer delayed doses (18% vs. 58%, $P < 0.001$) and tolerated more full-dose chemotherapy treatments (49% vs. 26%, $P = 0.02$). Furthermore, more VATS lobectomy patients received ≥75% of their planned regimen without delayed or reduced doses (60% vs. 40%, $P = 0.03$). Long-term outcome differences remain unproven (106). VATS lobectomy was also found to be feasible and safe after induction therapy (107). Robotic lobectomy has now been performed at several institutions with excellent outcomes and similar benefits as VATS lobectomy (46,108).

Tumors invading the chest wall should have the chest wall resected en bloc with their lobectomy. A special circumstance involving a chest wall resection is the resection of a Pancoast tumor. These tumors occur in the superior sulcus of the chest either in an anterior or posterior location. The most common approach to these tumors involves the administration of preoperative chemoradiation followed by surgical resection that includes a lobectomy along with resection of the ribs involved (109). The proximity of the tumor to the brachial plexus and the brachial vessels can make these resections technically challenging (Figure 7.5).

Pneumonectomy

Pneumonectomies involve removal of the entire left or right lung. Risk factors for mortality in pneumonectomies include right-sided pneumonectomies, older age (≥70 years), and low volume surgical centers. In addition, long-term sequelae of pneumonectomies include pulmonary hypertension, progression of emphysema, and increased right heart pressures during exercise (110,111). Pneumonectomies are considered when sleeve resections are considered technically not feasible (1). Impaired function and shortened long-term survival due to cardiorespiratory compromise have been cited as risks against pneumonectomies in favor of sleeve resection (111,112). Patients treated with pneumonectomy have poorer operative morbidity and mortality as well as poorer long-term survival compared with patients treated with lobectomy (113–115). Late death may also be increased by the long-term cardiopulmonary morbidity of pneumonectomies (115). Life-threatening complications following pneumonectomies are more likely when there is reduced preoperative diffusion capacity, preexisting compromising cardiopulmonary disease, excessive perioperative fluid administration, and a preoperative low hemoglobin (116). Others have found that after performing a multivariate analysis, pneumonectomy was not an independent determinate of long-term survival (117). Rather, it was the patient age, preoperative spirometry and T and N status that determined long-term survival. It has also been argued that pneumonectomies are associated with a lower rate of second primaries compared with lobectomies, presumably because there is less remaining lung tissue at risk for malignancy.

The safety of chemoradiation therapy with pneumonectomy is an important issue for patients with more advanced NSCLC. Single-institution experiences report that chemoradiation induction therapy can be performed with acceptable 30- and 100-day mortality rates of 6% and 10%, respectively with good oncologic outcomes (118). Long-term survival at 1 and 5 years for those receiving neoadjuvant therapy was 74% and 46% and similar to the surgery-only group with survival of 72% and 34% (119). Results from other similar reports were, however, less encouraging with 30- and 90-day mortality rates of 12% and 21%. Survival at 3 and 5 years were 35% and 25%, respectively (120). A consistent finding is that right pneumonectomies are associated with significantly greater morbidity and mortality and should be performed in carefully selected patients (121). Discrepant results are likely due to the retrospective nature of these studies that are subject to inherent biases. In addition, differences in perioperative management such as chest tube drainage options (balanced systems), pain control, steroid use, and fluid balance may lead to variations in outcomes.

Sleeve Resections

Bronchial sleeve lobectomy was introduced by Sir Clement Price-Thomas in 1947 to allow parenchyma sparing surgery. Allison subsequently performed the first sleeve lobectomy

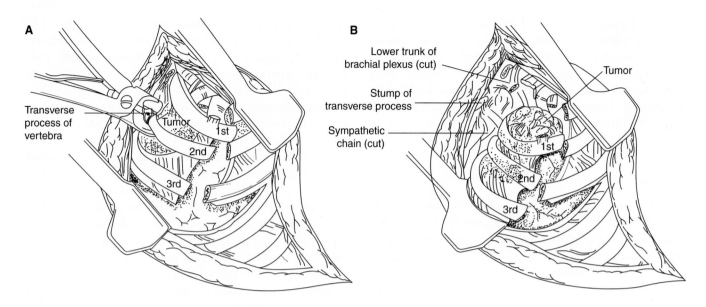

FIGURE 7.5 Superior sulcus tumor resection. (A) Division of ribs and (B) en-bloc resection of tumor.

for bronchogenic carcinoma (122). Bronchoplastic techniques are used in 3% to 13% of resectable pulmonary tumor accompanied by a corresponding decrease in pneumonectomies (122–124). The purpose is to provide adequate tumor resection margins while conserving as much healthy lung tissue as possible (125). Sleeve lobectomy (Figure 7.6) has become an alternative to pneumonectomy for patients with marked impairment in pulmonary function and for elderly patients, as well as for those with serious comorbidities, and should probably be considered in all patients where technically feasible. In particular, it is the procedure of choice for cancer extending to the left or right upper lobe bronchus orifice and adjacent main stem bronchus or for that extending to the proximal left lower lobe bronchus. Compared with pneumonectomy, it has provided an improved quality of life while achieving superior morbidity, mortality, and long-term survival (122,126) without sacrificing oncologic outcomes (127). Sleeve resections have a reported mortality of 5.5% with survival at 1 and 5 years of 84% and 42%, respectively. A sleeve lobectomy can reach the same functional result as a standard lobectomy. However, it takes 3 to 4 months for the reimplanted lobe to completely recover and contribute to residual postoperative pulmonary function (128). Given that the lifelong risk of developing a second lung cancer is about 2% per year after the resection, a subsequent lung resection can more safely be performed in patients who previously underwent a sleeve lobectomy versus those who had a prior pneumonectomy (126,129). The size of the tumor may limit the technical feasibility of sleeve lobectomy (130). However, chemotherapy and radiotherapy can downstage tumors in the presence of mediastinal disease to allow bronchoplastic therapy. Although chemotherapy has been associated with decreased mucosal blood flow and healing (131), clinical studies have shown that

sleeve lobectomy is safe after neoadjuvant chemotherapy (124,132). Operative mortality is high in patients with serious comorbidities (e.g., poor nutritional status, liver impairment, renal impairment, diabetes, cardiac compromise, peripheral vascular disease, stroke). Elderly patients must be very carefully selected as well (126).

Performance of sleeve resections involves a dissection of bronchus from its adjacent lung and pulmonary vessels at the lobar orifice level. A bronchotomy (sometimes performed under bronchoscopic guidance) may expose the tumor increasing the likelihood for recurrence. After determining the extent of the tumor, resection is performed en bloc with a portion of the airway and sometimes the associated pulmonary artery perfusing the remaining lung. The specimen is then sent for frozen section to confirm negative margins. An end-to-end anastomosis is then performed and covered with a vascularized pleural or pericardial flap for protection and prevention of pulmonary vessel erosion by suture knots and to provide extra blood supply to the anastomosis (125,133). The most common site of sleeve resection is the right upper lobe (134–140).

Bronchoplastic procedures have more postoperative complications than standard lobectomies thereby requiring intensive care monitoring in the immediate postoperative period. Early postoperative issues include partial atelectasis, lobar collapse, pneumonia, air leak, suture erosion of vessels, and transient vocal cord paralysis. Atelectasis commonly results from blood or mucus plugging. Routine postoperative flexible bronchoscopy and bronchial toilet is recommended for preemptive treatment prior to extubation. This also offers an opportunity for the surgeon to confirm the patency of the reconstructed bronchus. Pulmonary clearance mechanisms are compromised postoperatively, especially in elderly patients, so aggressive chest physiotherapy and steam inhalations

A

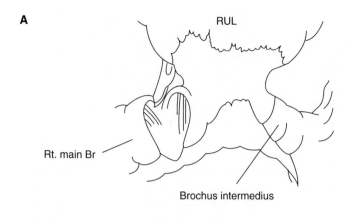

RUL

Rt. main Br

Brochus intermedius

B

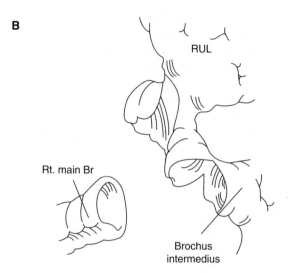

RUL

Rt. main Br

Brochus
intermedius

C

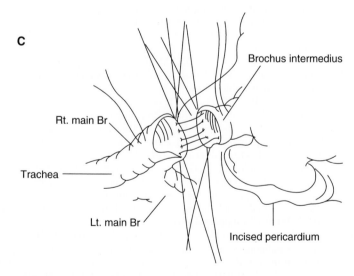

Brochus intermedius

Rt. main Br

Trachea

Lt. main Br

Incised pericardium

FIGURE 7.6 Sleeve right upper lobectomy.

may help prevent complications (125). Transection of bronchial lymphatics increases pulmonary fluid and likely contributes to increased infection risk (133). Other complications following sleeve resection are broncho-plasty site stenosis and dehiscence, bronchopleural fis-tulae, and bronchovascular fistulae (126,127). Late complications include bronchial stricture, bronchiectasis,

bronchopleural fistula, and empyema (122).The inci-dence of bronchial anastomotic complications is 6.4% with a bronchopleural fistula rate of 3% and a broncho-vascular fistula rate of 2.5%. There is also a 10% rate of pneumonia following sleeve resection (122). Predictive factors for postoperative complications include right-sided resections, smoking, and squamous cell carcino-mas (141). Technical points that can assist in minimizing complications include precise dissection and anasto-motic technique, avoidance of anastomotic stenosis dur-ing initial surgery, preservation of blood supply, using a buttress for the anastomosis, and interpositing healthy tissue between the bronchial and vascular structures (141). Anastomotic dehiscence or stenosis after sleeve lobectomy can require subsequent completion pneumo-nectomy (122). This occurs more frequently with com-promised patients (142), pathologic N2 status, and those with positive bronchial margins (142,143). Absorbable suture material such as Vicryl or polydioxanone has decreased the incidence of bronchial anastomotic com-plications which can more readily allow postoperative dilatation (144). Bronchoplastic procedures are techni-cally demanding and have better outcomes by surgeons specializing in general thoracic surgery.

Carinal Resection

Lung cancers in close proximity to, or involving the carina, are often not amenable to resection. However, complete resection may be possible for a select patient group that does not have dissemination or invasion of vital struc-tures (145,146) (Figure 7.7). Utilization of bronchoplastic techniques in these patients can greatly improve outcomes and survival (147). Recent studies have shown that bron-choplastic operations for carinal involvement can be done with an acceptable mortality rate of about 16% (147–153). Tracheobronchial junction tumors are particularly challeng-ing. While most of these tumors can be resected through the usual right posterolateral thoracotomy, Muscolino et al. used anterior thoracotomy through the fourth intercostal space to perform a right sleeve pneumonectomy. Good exposure for anastomosis as well as nodal clearance from the paratracheal and subcarinal areas can be achieved through this incision (129). Other exposures that have been described includes bilateral thoracotomies and combina-tions of thoracotomy with median sternotomy (151). Lethal complications of this operation are acute respiratory distress syndrome (ARDS) and noncardiogenic pulmonary edema. The etiology of post–lung resection ARDS is unknown but this complication has mortality rates approaching 90% (146,154). Nitric oxide can treat this devastating condition with modest success (155). Anastomotic complications are major complications of bronchoplastic resection of carinal tumors. Most commonly, these result from excessive tension on the anastomosis from long-segment airway resection or inadequate mobilization of the remaining lung and trachea.

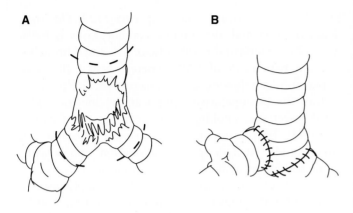

FIGURE 7.7 Carinal resection.

To avoid excessive airway resection, carinal resection should be limited to 4 cm (measured from proposed tracheotomy to left main stem bronchotomy). Other key factors include preservation of airway vascularity, meticulous anastomotic technique, and careful tissue handling (148). Prolonged postoperative mechanical ventilation increases mortality, so patients should be extubated immediately after surgery whenever possible (146).

■ MANAGEMENT OF THE MEDIASTINUM

Controversy exists regarding whether systematic nodal dissection during formal lung resection provides more benefit than mediastinal systematic lymph node sampling. Systematic lymph node dissection refers to the complete removal of mediastinal lymph node whereas mediastinal lymph node sampling describes the removal of limited number of representative lymph nodes. Lymph node sampling commonly refer to the removal of lymph node levels 3, 4, and 7 for right-sided tumors and levels 5, 6, and 7 for left-sided tumors (156). A recent prospective multi-institutional, randomized trial (ACOSOG Z0030) is examining if survival after lung resection is affected by systematic lymph node dissection versus sampling. Preliminary results found no difference in the operative mortality and morbidity of either procedure. Systematic dissection was associated with longer operative times and slightly greater, but clinically insignificant chest tube drainage. There was no difference in length of hospital stay. Long-term results from this trial are yet to be reported (4).

■ PULMONARY RESECTION IN THE ELDERLY

Pulmonary resections in elderly patients generally have increased morbidity and mortality. This was thought to be due to the increased incidence of comorbidities and age-related reduction in cardiopulmonary function (4). However, others suggest that ASA score, preoperative FEV_1, and tumor stage rather than chronological age are the main predictors of survival and outcome in elderly patients (157). Indeed, male gender, congestive heart failure, previous myocardial infarction, and those presenting with dyspnea are predictors of poor outcome in elderly populations (158,159). More limited resection may be indicated in this patient population even in patients who can tolerate a lobectomy (160). Indeed, it was shown that there is no survival difference between lobectomies and more limited resections in elderly patients (160). In the Japanese population, it was found that the 5-year survival after pulmonary resections in octogenarians (77.9% in c-stage IA and 66.9% for c-stage IB) was equivalent to the general Japanese population (161). However, these data have their limitations that temper the adoption of these recommendations. With the widespread adoption of VATS anatomic resections, a reappraisal of these recommendations is necessary to tailor surgical approaches to the elderly, frail patient.

■ REFERENCES

1. Baumann M, Stamatis G, Thomas M. Therapy of localized non-small cell lung cancer (take home messages). *Lung Cancer.* 2001;33(suppl 1):S47–S49.
2. Goldstraw P, Crowley J, Chansky K, et al.; International Association for the Study of Lung Cancer International Staging Committee; Participating Institutions. The IASLC Lung Cancer Staging Project: proposals for the revision of the TNM stage groupings in the forthcoming (seventh) edition of the TNM Classification of malignant tumours. *J Thorac Oncol.* 2007;2(8):706–714.
3. Saudi Thoracic Society. *Annals of Thoracic Medicine.* Mumbai, India: Medknow Publications.
4. Allen MS, Darling GE, Pechet TT, et al.; ACOSOG Z0030 Study Group. Morbidity and mortality of major pulmonary resections in patients with early-stage lung cancer: initial results of the randomized, prospective ACOSOG Z0030 trial. *Ann Thorac Surg.* 2006;81(3):1013–1019; discussion 1019.
5. Colice GL, Shafazand S, Griffin JP, Keenan R, Bolliger CT; American College of Chest Physicians. Physiologic evaluation of the patient with lung cancer being considered for resectional surgery: ACCP evidenced-based clinical practice guidelines (2nd edition). *Chest.* 2007;132(3 suppl):161S–177S.
6. van Tilburg PM, Stam H, Hoogsteden HC, van Klaveren RJ. Preoperative pulmonary evaluation of lung cancer patients: a review of the literature. *Eur Respir J.* 2009;33(5):1206–1215.
7. Markos J, Mullan BP, Hillman DR, et al. Preoperative assessment as a predictor of mortality and morbidity after lung resection. *Am Rev Respir Dis.* 1989;139(4):902–910.
8. Suga K, Tsukuda T, Awaya H, Matsunaga N, Sugi K, Esato K. Interactions of regional respiratory mechanics and pulmonary ventilatory impairment in pulmonary emphysema: assessment with dynamic MRI and xenon-133 single-photon emission CT. *Chest.* 2000;117(6):1646–1655.
9. Bobbio A, Chetta A, Carbognani P, et al. Changes in pulmonary function test and cardio-pulmonary exercise capacity in COPD patients after lobar pulmonary resection. *Eur J Cardiothorac Surg.* 2005;28(5):754–758.

10. Burke JR, Duarte IG, Thourani VH, Miller JI Jr. Preoperative risk assessment for marginal patients requiring pulmonary resection. *Ann Thorac Surg.* 2003;76(5):1767–1773.

11. Semik M, Netz B, Schmidt C, Scheld HH. Surgical exploration of the mediastinum: mediastinoscopy and intraoperative staging. *Lung Cancer.* 2004;45(suppl 2):S55–S61.

12. Whitson BA, Groth SS, Maddaus MA. Surgical assessment and intraoperative management of mediastinal lymph nodes in non-small cell lung cancer. *Ann Thorac Surg.* 2007;84(3):1059–1065.

13. Luke WP, Pearson FG, Todd TR, Patterson GA, Cooper JD. Prospective evaluation of mediastinoscopy for assessment of carcinoma of the lung. *J Thorac Cardiovasc Surg.* 1986;91(1):53–56.

14. Detterbeck FC, Jantz MA, Wallace M, Vansteenkiste J, Silvestri GA; American College of Chest Physicians. Invasive mediastinal staging of lung cancer: ACCP evidence-based clinical practice guidelines (2nd edition). *Chest.* 2007;132(3 suppl):202S–220S.

15. Zielinski M. Transcervical extended mediastinal lymphadenectomy: results of staging in two hundred fifty-six patients with non-small cell lung cancer. *J Thorac Oncol.* 2007;2(4):370–372.

16. Kuzdzal J, Zielinski M, Papla B, et al. The transcervical extended mediastinal lymphadenectomy versus cervical mediastinoscopy in non-small cell lung cancer staging. *Eur J Cardiothorac Surg.* 2007;31(1):88–94.

17. Webb WR, Gatsonis C, Zerhouni EA, et al. CT and MR imaging in staging non-small cell bronchogenic carcinoma: report of the Radiologic Diagnostic Oncology Group. *Radiology.* 1991;178(3):705–713.

18. Silvestri GA, Gould MK, Margolis ML, et al.; American College of Chest Physicians. Noninvasive staging of non-small cell lung cancer: ACCP evidenced-based clinical practice guidelines (2nd edition). *Chest.* 2007;132(3 suppl):178S–201S.

19. Allen-Auerbach M, Yeom K, Park J, Phelps M, Czernin J. Standard PET/CT of the chest during shallow breathing is inadequate for comprehensive staging of lung cancer. *J Nucl Med.* 2006;47(2):298–301.

20. Shim SS, Lee KS, Kim BT, et al. Non-small cell lung cancer: prospective comparison of integrated FDG PET/CT and CT alone for preoperative staging. *Radiology.* 2005;236(3):1011–1019.

21. Aono H, Okamoto H, Kunikane H, Nagatomo A, Watanabe K, Nagai A. Transbronchial needle aspiration cytology of subcarinal lymph nodes for the staging procedure in the diagnosis of lung cancer. *Respirology.* 2006;11(6):782–785.

22. Win T, Stewart S, Groves AM, Pepke-Zaba J, Laroche CM. The role of transbronchial needle aspiration in the diagnosis of bronchogenic carcinoma. *Respir Care.* 2003;48(6):602–605.

23. Annema JT, Versteegh MI, Veselič M, et al. Endoscopic ultrasound added to mediastinoscopy for preoperative staging of patients with lung cancer. *JAMA.* 2005;294(8):931–936.

24. Szlubowski A, Kuzdzal J, Kolodziej M, et al. Endobronchial ultrasound-guided needle aspiration in the non-small cell lung cancer staging. *Eur J Cardiothorac Surg.* 2009;35(2):332–335; discussion 335.

25. Silvestri GA, Hoffman BJ, Bhutani MS, et al. Endoscopic ultrasound with fine-needle aspiration in the diagnosis and staging of lung cancer. *Ann Thorac Surg.* 1996;61(5):1441–1445; discussion 1445.

26. Wilsher ML, Gurley AM. Transtracheal aspiration using rigid bronchoscopy and a rigid needle for investigating mediastinal masses. *Thorax.* 1996;51(2):197–199.

27. Detterbeck FC. Integration of mediastinal staging techniques for lung cancer. *Semin Thorac Cardiovasc Surg.* 2007;19(3):217–224.

28. Boyle EM, Vallieres E. Mediastinoscopy in the staging of lung cancer. *Curr Surg.* 2001;58(1):47–54.

29. McKenna RJ Jr, Houck W, Fuller CB. Video-assisted thoracic surgery lobectomy: experience with 1,100 cases. *Ann Thorac Surg.* 2006;81(2):421–425; discussion 425.

30. Onaitis MW, Petersen RP, Balderson SS, et al. Thoracoscopic lobectomy is a safe and versatile procedure: experience with 500 consecutive patients. *Ann Surg.* 2006;244(3):420–425.

31. Cerfolio RJ, Bryant AS, Ojha B, Eloubeidi M. Improving the inaccuracies of clinical staging of patients with NSCLC: a prospective trial. *Ann Thorac Surg.* 2005;80(4):1207–1213; discussion 1213.

32. Detterbeck FC, DeCamp MM, Jr, Kohman LJ, and Silvestri GA. Lung cancer. Invasive staging: the guidelines. *Chest.* 2003;123 (1 suppl):167S–175S.

33. Detterbeck FC. *Diagnosis and Treatment of Lung Cancer: An Evidence-Based Guide for the Practicing Clinician.* Philadelphia, PA: W.B. Saunders Co; 2001:14, 480 p.

34. Verhagen AF, Bootsma GP, Tjan-Heijnen VC, et al. FDG-PET in staging lung cancer: how does it change the algorithm? *Lung Cancer.* 2004;44(2):175–181.

35. Pozo-Rodríguez F, Martín de Nicolás JL, Sánchez-Nistal MA, et al. Accuracy of helical computed tomography and [18F] fluorodeoxyglucose positron emission tomography for identifying lymph node mediastinal metastases in potentially resectable non-small-cell lung cancer. *J Clin Oncol.* 2005;23(33): 8348–8356.

36. Meyers BF, Haddad F, Siegel BA, et al. Cost-effectiveness of routine mediastinoscopy in computed tomography- and positron emission tomography-screened patients with stage I lung cancer. *J Thorac Cardiovasc Surg.* 2006;131(4):822–829; discussion 822.

37. Cerfolio RJ, Bryant AS, Eloubeidi MA. Routine mediastinoscopy and esophageal ultrasound fine-needle aspiration in patients with non-small cell lung cancer who are clinically N2 negative: a prospective study. *Chest.* 2006;130(6):1791–1795.

38. Herth FJ, Ernst A, Eberhardt R. Restaging of the mediastinum. *Curr Opin Pulm Med.* 2009;15(4):308–312.

39. Herth FJ, Annema JT, Eberhardt R, et al. Endobronchial ultrasound with transbronchial needle aspiration for restaging the mediastinum in lung cancer. *J Clin Oncol.* 2008;26(20):3346–3350.

40. Annema JT, Veselič M, Versteegh MI, Willems LN, Rabe KF. Mediastinal restaging: EUS-FNA offers a new perspective. *Lung Cancer.* 2003;42(3):311–318.

41. Marra A, Hillejan L, Fechner S, Stamatis G. Remediastinoscopy in restaging of lung cancer after induction therapy. *J Thorac Cardiovasc Surg.* 2008;135(4):843–849.

42. Van Schil P, Stamatis G. Sensitivity of remediastinoscopy: influence of adhesions, multilevel N2 involvement, or surgical technique? *J Clin Oncol.* 2006;24(33):5338; author reply 5339–5338; author reply 5340.

43. Little AG, Rusch VW, Bonner JA, et al. Patterns of surgical care of lung cancer patients. *Ann Thorac Surg.* 2005;80(6):2051–2056; discussion 2056.

44. Farjah F, Flum DR, Ramsey SD, Heagerty PJ, Symons RG, Wood DE. Multi-modality mediastinal staging for lung cancer among medicare beneficiaries. *J Thorac Oncol.* 2009;4(3):355–363.

45. Nesbitt JC, Wind GG. *Thoracic Surgical Oncology: Exposures and Techniques.* Philadelphia, PA. London: Lippincott Williams & Wilkins; 2003.

46. Gharagozloo F, Margolis M, Tempesta B, Strother E, Najam F. Robot-assisted lobectomy for early-stage lung cancer: report of 100 consecutive cases. *Ann Thorac Surg.* 2009;88(2):380–384.

47. Rami-Porta R, Wittekind C, Goldstraw P; International Association for the Study of Lung Cancer (IASLC) Staging Committee. Complete resection in lung cancer surgery: proposed definition. *Lung Cancer.* 2005;49(1):25–33.

48. COTTON RE. The bronchial spread of lung cancer. *Br J Dis Chest.* 1959;53(2):142–150.

49. Kara M, Sak SD, Orhan D, Yavuzer S. Changing patterns of lung cancer; (3/4 in.) 1.9 cm; still a safe length for bronchial resection margin? *Lung Cancer.* 2000;30(3):161–168.

50. Law MR, Hodson ME, Lennox SC. Implications of histologically reported residual tumour on the bronchial margin after resection for bronchial carcinoma. *Thorax.* 1982;37(7):492–495.

51. Liewald F, Hatz RA, Dienemann H, Sunder-Plassmann L. Importance of microscopic residual disease at the bronchial margin after resection for non-small-cell carcinoma of the lung. *J Thorac Cardiovasc Surg.* 1992;104(2):408–412.

52. Passlick B, Sitar I, Sienel W, Thetter O, Morresi-Hauf A. Significance of lymphangiosis carcinomatosa at the bronchial resection margin in patients with non-small cell lung cancer. *Ann Thorac Surg.* 2001;72(4):1160–1164.

53. Pearson FG. *Thoracic Surgery.* 2nd ed. New York: Churchill Livingstone; 2002:25, 1942 p.

54. Ginsberg RJ, Rubinstein LV. Randomized trial of lobectomy versus limited resection for T1 N0 non-small cell lung cancer. Lung Cancer Study Group. *Ann Thorac Surg.* 1995;60(3):615–622; discussion 622.

55. Landreneau RJ, Sugarbaker DJ, Mack MJ, et al. Wedge resection versus lobectomy for stage I (T1 N0 M0) non-small-cell lung cancer. *J Thorac Cardiovasc Surg.* 1997;113(4):691–698; discussion 698.

56. El-Sherif A, Gooding WE, Santos R, et al. Outcomes of sublobar resection versus lobectomy for stage I non-small cell lung cancer: a 13-year analysis. *Ann Thorac Surg.* 2006;82(2):408–415; discussion 415.

57. Okada M, Koike T, Higashiyama M, Yamato Y, Kodama K, Tsubota N. Radical sublobar resection for small-sized non-small cell lung cancer: a multicenter study. *J Thorac Cardiovasc Surg.* 2006;132(4):769–775.

58. Schulte T, Schniewind B, Dohrmann P, Küchler T, Kurdow R. The extent of lung parenchyma resection significantly impacts long-term quality of life in patients with non-small cell lung cancer. *Chest.* 2009;135(2):322–329.

59. Lewis RJ. The role of video-assisted thoracic surgery for carcinoma of the lung: wedge resection to lobectomy by simultaneous individual stapling. *Ann Thorac Surg.* 1993;56(3):762–768.

60. Yoshikawa K, Tsubota N, Kodama K, Ayabe H, Taki T, Mori T. Prospective study of extended segmentectomy for small lung tumors: the final report. *Ann Thorac Surg.* 2002;73(4):1055–1058; discussion 1058.

61. Kodama K, Doi O, Higashiyama M, Yokouchi H. Intentional limited resection for selected patients with T1 N0 M0 non-small-cell lung cancer: a single-institution study. *J Thorac Cardiovasc Surg.* 1997;114(3):347–353.

62. Okada M, Yoshikawa K, Hatta T, Tsubota N. Is segmentectomy with lymph node assessment an alternative to lobectomy for non-small cell lung cancer of 2 cm or smaller? *Ann Thorac Surg.* 2001;71(3):956–960; discussion 961.

63. Koike T, Yamato Y, Yoshiya K, Shimoyama T, Suzuki R. Intentional limited pulmonary resection for peripheral T1 N0 M0 small-sized lung cancer. *J Thorac Cardiovasc Surg.* 2003;125(4):924–928.

64. Martin-Ucar AE, Nakas A, Pilling JE, West KJ, Waller DA. A case-matched study of anatomical segmentectomy versus lobectomy for stage I lung cancer in high-risk patients. *Eur J Cardiothorac Surg.* 2005;27(4):675–679.

65. El-Sherif A, Fernando HC, Santos R, et al. Margin and local recurrence after sublobar resection of non-small cell lung cancer. *Ann Surg Oncol.* 2007;14(8):2400–2405.

66. Lee PC, Korst RJ, Port JL, Kerem Y, Kansler AL, Altorki NK. Long-term survival and recurrence in patients with resected non-small cell lung cancer 1 cm or less in size. *J Thorac Cardiovasc Surg.* 2006;132(6):1382–1389.

67. Okada M, Nishio W, Sakamoto T, et al. Effect of tumor size on prognosis in patients with non-small cell lung cancer: the role of segmentectomy as a type of lesser resection. *J Thorac Cardiovasc Surg.* 2005;129(1):87–93.

68. Miller JI, Hatcher CR Jr. Limited resection of bronchogenic carcinoma in the patient with marked impairment of pulmonary function. *Ann Thorac Surg.* 1987;44(4):340–343.

69. Pastorino U, Valente M, Bedini V, Infante M, Tavecchio L, Ravasi G. Limited resection for Stage I lung cancer. *Eur J Surg Oncol.* 1991;17(1):42–46.

70. Landreneau RJ, Hazelrigg SR, Mack MJ, et al. Postoperative pain-related morbidity: video-assisted thoracic surgery versus thoracotomy. *Ann Thorac Surg.* 1993;56(6):1285–1289.

71. Feld R, Rubinstein LV, Weisenberger TH. Sites of recurrence in resected stage I non-small-cell lung cancer: a guide for future studies. *J Clin Oncol.* 1984;2(12):1352–1358.

72. Thomas P, Rubinstein L. Cancer recurrence after resection: T1 N0 non-small cell lung cancer. Lung Cancer Study Group. *Ann Thorac Surg.* 1990;49(2):242–246; discussion 246.

73. Pairolero PC, Williams DE, Bergstralh EJ, Piehler JM, Bernatz PE, Payne WS. Postsurgical stage I bronchogenic carcinoma: morbid implications of recurrent disease. *Ann Thorac Surg.* 1984;38(4):331–338.

74. Shennib H, Bogart J, Herndon JE, et al.; Cancer and Leukemia Group B; Eastern Cooperative Oncology Group. Video-assisted wedge resection and local radiotherapy for peripheral lung cancer in high-risk patients: the Cancer and Leukemia Group B (CALGB) 9335, a phase II, multi-institutional cooperative group study. *J Thorac Cardiovasc Surg.* 2005;129(4):813–818.

75. d'Amato TA, Galloway M, Szydlowski G, Chen A, Landreneau RJ. Intraoperative brachytherapy following thoracoscopic wedge resection of stage I lung cancer. *Chest.* 1998;114(4):1112–1115.

76. Santos R, Colonias A, Parda D, et al. Comparison between sublobar resection and 125Iodine brachytherapy after sublobar resection in high-risk patients with Stage I non-small-cell lung cancer. *Surgery.* 2003;134(4):691–697; discussion 697.

77. Fernando HC, Santos RS, Benfield JR, et al. Lobar and sublobar resection with and without brachytherapy for small stage IA non-small cell lung cancer. *J Thorac Cardiovasc Surg.* 2005;129(2):261–267.

78. Lee W, Daly BD, DiPetrillo TA, et al. Limited resection for non-small cell lung cancer: observed local control with implantation of I-125 brachytherapy seeds. *Ann Thorac Surg.* 2003;75(1):237–242; discussion 242.

79. Birdas TJ, Koehler RP, Colonias A, et al. Sublobar resection with brachytherapy versus lobectomy for stage Ib non-small cell lung cancer. *Ann Thorac Surg.* 2006;81(2):434–438; discussion 438.

80. McKenna RJ Jr, Mahtabifard A, Yap J, et al. Wedge resection and brachytherapy for lung cancer in patients with poor pulmonary function. *Ann Thorac Surg.* 2008;85(2):S733–S736.

81. Deslauriers J, Brisson J, Cartier R, et al. Carcinoma of the lung. Evaluation of satellite nodules as a factor influencing prognosis after resection. *J Thorac Cardiovasc Surg.* 1989;97(4):504–512.

82. Kutschera W. Segment resection for lung cancer. *Thorac Cardiovasc Surg.* 1984;32(2):102–104.

83. Bonfils-Roberts EA, Clagett OT. Contemporary indications for pulmonary segmental resections. *J Thorac Cardiovasc Surg.* 1972;63(3):433–438.

84. Jensik RJ, Faber LP, Kittle CF. Segmental resection for bronchogenic carcinoma. *Ann Thorac Surg.* 1979;28(5):475–483.

85. Bennett WF, Smith RA. Segmental resection for bronchogenic carcinoma: a surgical alternative for the compromised patient. *Ann Thorac Surg.* 1979;27(2):169–172.

86. Schuchert MJ, Pettiford BL, Keeley S, et al. Anatomic segmentectomy in the treatment of stage I non-small cell lung cancer. *Ann Thorac Surg.* 2007;84(3):926–932; discussion 932.

87. Sienel W, Stremmel C, Kirschbaum A, et al. Frequency of local recurrence following segmentectomy of stage IA non-small cell lung cancer is influenced by segment localisation and width of resection margins–implications for patient selection for segmentectomy. *Eur J Cardiothorac Surg.* 2007;31(3):522–527; discussion 527.

88. Houck WV, Fuller CB, McKenna RJ Jr. Video-assisted thoracic surgery upper lobe trisegmentectomy for early-stage left apical lung cancer. *Ann Thorac Surg.* 2004;78(5):1858–1860.

89. Atkins BZ, Harpole DH Jr, Mangum JH, Toloza EM, D'Amico TA, Burfeind WR Jr. Pulmonary segmentectomy by thoracotomy or thoracoscopy: reduced hospital length of stay with a minimally-invasive approach. *Ann Thorac Surg.* 2007;84(4):1107–1112; discussion 1112.

90. D'Amico TA. Thoracoscopic segmentectomy: technical considerations and outcomes. *Ann Thorac Surg.* 2008;85(2):S716–S718.

91. Keenan RJ, Landreneau RJ, Maley RH Jr, et al. Segmental resection spares pulmonary function in patients with stage I lung cancer. *Ann Thorac Surg.* 2004;78(1):228–233; discussion 228.

92. Johnson BE, Cortazar P, Chute JP. Second lung cancers in patients successfully treated for lung cancer. *Semin Oncol.* 1997;24(4):492–499.

93. Johnson BE. Second lung cancers in patients after treatment for an initial lung cancer. *J Natl Cancer Inst.* 1998;90(18):1335–1345.

94. Iwasaki A, Shirakusa T, Hamada T, et al. Less vigorous surgery for second primary lung cancer. *Thorac Cardiovasc Surg.* 2006;54(5):337–340.

95. Sugiura H, Morikawa T, Kaji M, Sasamura Y, Kondo S, Katoh H. Long-term benefits for the quality of life after video-assisted thoracoscopic lobectomy in patients with lung cancer. *Surg Laparosc Endosc Percutan Tech.* 1999;9(6):403–408.

96. Hoksch B, Ablassmaier B, Walter M, Müller JM. Complication rate after thoracoscopic and conventional lobectomy. *Zentralbl Chir.* 2003;128(2):106–110.

97. Sugi K, Sudoh M, Hirazawa K, Matsuda E, Kaneda Y. Intrathoracic bleeding during video-assisted thoracoscopic lobectomy and segmentectomy. *Kyobu Geka.* 2003;56(11):928–931.

98. Kaseda S, Aoki T. Video-assisted thoracic surgical lobectomy in conjunction with lymphadenectomy for lung cancer. *Nippon Geka Gakkai Zasshi.* 2002;103(10):717–721.

99. Walker WS. Video-assisted thoracic surgery (VATS) lobectomy: the Edinburgh experience. *Semin Thorac Cardiovasc Surg.* 1998;10(4):291–299.

100. Giudicelli R, Thomas P, Lonjon T, et al. Major pulmonary resection by video assisted mini-thoracotomy. Initial experience in 35 patients. *Eur J Cardiothorac Surg.* 1994;8(5):254–258.

101. Demmy TL, Curtis JJ. Minimally invasive lobectomy directed toward frail and high-risk patients: a case-control study. *Ann Thorac Surg.* 1999;68(1):194–200.

102. Nakata M, Saeki H, Yokoyama N, Kurita A, Takiyama W, Takashima S. Pulmonary function after lobectomy: video-assisted thoracic surgery versus thoracotomy. *Ann Thorac Surg.* 2000;70(3):938–941.

103. Sugi K, Kaneda Y, Esato K. Video-assisted thoracoscopic lobectomy achieves a satisfactory long-term prognosis in patients with clinical stage IA lung cancer. *World J Surg.* 2000;24(1):27–30; discussion 30.

104. Walker WS, Codispoti M, Soon SY, Stamenkovic S, Carnochan F, Pugh G. Long-term outcomes following VATS lobectomy for non-small cell bronchogenic carcinoma. *Eur J Cardiothorac Surg.* 2003;23(3):397–402.

105. Whitson BA, Groth SS, Duval SJ, Swanson SJ, Maddaus MA. Surgery for early-stage non-small cell lung cancer: a systematic review of the video-assisted thoracoscopic surgery versus thoracotomy approaches to lobectomy. *Ann Thorac Surg.* 2008;86(6):2008–2016; discussion 2016.

106. Bonadonna G, Valagussa P, Moliterni A, Zambetti M, Brambilla C. Adjuvant cyclophosphamide, methotrexate, and fluorouracil in node-positive breast cancer: the results of 20 years of follow-up. *N Engl J Med.* 1995;332(14):901–906.

107. Petersen RP, Pham D, Toloza EM, et al. Thoracoscopic lobectomy: a safe and effective strategy for patients receiving induction therapy for non-small cell lung cancer. *Ann Thorac Surg.* 2006;82(1):214–218; discussion 219.

108. Veronesi G, Galetta D, Maisonneuve P, et al. Four-arm robotic lobectomy for the treatment of early-stage lung cancer. *J Thorac Cardiovasc Surg.* 2010;140(1):19–25.

109. Rusch VW, Giroux DJ, Kraut MJ, et al. Induction chemoradiation and surgical resection for superior sulcus non-small-cell lung carcinomas: long-term results of Southwest Oncology Group Trial 9416 (Intergroup Trial 0160). *J Clin Oncol.* 2007;25(3):313–318.

110. van Meerbeeck JP, Damhuis RA, Vos de Wael ML. High postoperative risk after pneumonectomy in elderly patients with right-sided lung cancer. *Eur Respir J.* 2002;19(1):141–145.

111. Burrows B, Harrison RW, Adams WE, Humphreys EM, Long ET, Reimann AF. The postpneumonectomy state: clinical and physiologic observations in thirty-six cases. *Am J Med.* 1960;28:281–297.

112. Gaissert HA, Mathisen DJ, Moncure AC, Hilgenberg AD, Grillo HC, Wain JC. Survival and function after sleeve lobectomy for lung cancer. *J Thorac Cardiovasc Surg.* 1996;111(5):948–953.

113. Ginsberg RJ, Hill LD, Eagan RT, et al. Modern thirty-day operative mortality for surgical resections in lung cancer. *J Thorac Cardiovasc Surg.* 1983;86(5):654–658.

114. Rocco PM, Antkowiak JG, Takita H, Urschel JD. Long-term outcome after pneumonectomy for nonsmall cell lung cancer. *J Surg Oncol.* 1996;61(4):278–280.

115. Paulson DL, Reisch JS. Long-term survival after resection for bronchogenic carcinoma. *Ann Surg.* 1976;184(3):324–332.

116. Bernard A, Deschamps C, Allen MS, et al. Pneumonectomy for malignant disease: factors affecting early morbidity and mortality. *J Thorac Cardiovasc Surg.* 2001;121(6):1076–1082.

117. Kim DJ, Lee JG, Lee CY, Park IK, Chung KY. Long-term survival following pneumonectomy for non-small cell lung cancer: clinical implications for follow-up care. *Chest.* 2007;132(1):178–184.

118. Allen AM, Mentzer SJ, Yeap BY, et al. Pneumonectomy after chemoradiation: the Dana-Farber Cancer Institute/Brigham and Women's Hospital experience. *Cancer.* 2008;112(5):1106–1113.

119. Gudbjartsson T, Gyllstedt E, Pikwer A, Jönsson P. Early surgical results after pneumonectomy for non-small cell lung cancer are not affected by preoperative radiotherapy and chemotherapy. *Ann Thorac Surg.* 2008;86(2):376–382.

120. Doddoli C, Barlesi F, Trousse D, et al. One hundred consecutive pneumonectomies after induction therapy for non-small cell lung cancer: an uncertain balance between risks and benefits. *J Thorac Cardiovasc Surg.* 2005;130(2):416–425.

121. Martin J, Ginsberg RJ, Abolhoda A, et al. Morbidity and mortality after neoadjuvant therapy for lung cancer: the risks of right pneumonectomy. *Ann Thorac Surg.* 2001;72(4):1149–1154.

122. Tedder M, Anstadt MP, Tedder SD, Lowe JE. Current morbidity, mortality, and survival after bronchoplastic procedures for malignancy. *Ann Thorac Surg.* 1992;54(2):387–391.

123. Kim YT, Kang CH, Sung SW, Kim JH. Local control of disease related to lymph node involvement in non-small cell lung cancer after sleeve lobectomy compared with pneumonectomy. *Ann Thorac Surg.* 2005;79(4):1153–1161; discussion 1153.

124. Burfeind WR Jr, D'Amico TA, Toloza EM, Wolfe WG, Harpole DH. Low morbidity and mortality for bronchoplastic procedures with and without induction therapy. *Ann Thorac Surg.* 2005;80(2):418–421; discussion 422.

125. Jalal A, Jeyasingham K. Bronchoplasty for malignant and benign conditions: a retrospective study of 44 cases. *Eur J Cardiothorac Surg.* 2000;17(4):370–376.

126. Terzi A, Lonardoni A, Falezza G, et al. Sleeve lobectomy for non-small cell lung cancer and carcinoids: results in 160 cases. *Eur J Cardiothorac Surg.* 2002;21(5):888–893.

127. Ferguson MK, Karrison T. Does pneumonectomy for lung cancer adversely influence long-term survival? *J Thorac Cardiovasc Surg.* 2000;119(3):440–448.

128. Khargi K, Duurkens VA, Verzijlbergen FF, Huysmans HA, Knaepen PJ. Pulmonary function after sleeve lobectomy. *Ann Thorac Surg.* 1994;57(5):1302–1304.

129. Van Schil PE, Brutel de la Rivière A, Knaepen PJ, van Swieten HA, Defauw JJ, van den Bosch JM. Second primary lung cancer after bronchial sleeve resection. Treatment and results in eleven patients. *J Thorac Cardiovasc Surg.* 1992;104(5):1451–1455.

130. Bagan P, Berna P, Pereira JC, et al. Sleeve lobectomy versus pneumonectomy: tumor characteristics and comparative analysis of feasibility and results. *Ann Thorac Surg.* 2005;80(6):2046–2050.

131. Yamamoto R, Tada H, Kishi A, Tojo T. Effects of preoperative chemotherapy and radiation therapy on human bronchial blood flow. *J Thorac Cardiovasc Surg.* 2000;119(5):939–945.

132. Rendina EA, Venuta F, De Giacomo T, Flaishman I, Fazi P, Ricci C. Safety and efficacy of bronchovascular reconstruction after induction chemotherapy for lung cancer. *J Thorac Cardiovasc Surg.* 1997;114(5):830–835; discussion 835.

133. Mentzer SJ, Myers DW, Sugarbaker DJ. Sleeve lobectomy, segmentectomy, and thoracoscopy in the management of carcinoma of the lung. *Chest.* 1993;103(4 suppl):415S–417S.

134. Faber LP, Jensik RJ, Kittle CF. Results of sleeve lobectomy for bronchogenic carcinoma in 101 patients. *Ann Thorac Surg.* 1984;37(4):279–285.

135. Weisel RD, Cooper JD, Delarue NC, Theman TE, Todd TR, Pearson FG. Sleeve lobectomy for carcinoma of the lung. *J Thorac Cardiovasc Surg.* 1979;78(6):839–849.

136. Sartori F, Binda R, Spreafico G, et al. Sleeve lobectomy in the treatment of bronchogenic carcinoma. *Int Surg.* 1986;71(4):233–236.

137. Brusasco V, Ratto GB, Crimi P, Sacco A, Motta G. Lung function following upper sleeve lobectomy for bronchogenic carcinoma. *Scand J Thorac Cardiovasc Surg.* 1988;22(1):73–78.

138. Jensik RJ, Faber LP, Milloy FJ, Amato JJ. Sleeve lobectomy for carcinoma. A ten-year experience. *J Thorac Cardiovasc Surg.* 1972;64(3):400–412.

139. Van Schil PE, Brutel de la Rivière A, Knaepen PJ, van Swieten HA, Defauw JJ, van den Bosch JM. TNM staging and long-term follow-up after sleeve resection for bronchogenic tumors. *Ann Thorac Surg.* 1991;52(5):1096–1101.

140. Firmin RK, Azariades M, Lennox SC, Lincoln JC, Paneth M. Sleeve lobectomy (lobectomy and bronchoplasty) for bronchial carcinoma. *Ann Thorac Surg.* 1983;35(4):442–449.

141. Grillo HC. *Surgery of the Trachea and Bronchi.* Hamilton, ON: BC Decker; 2004:16, 872 p.

142. Hollaus PH, Wilfing G, Wurnig PN, Pridun NS. Risk factors for the development of postoperative complications after bronchial sleeve resection for malignancy: a univariate and multivariate analysis. *Ann Thorac Surg.* 2003;75(3):966–972.

143. Fadel E, Yildizeli B, Chapelier AR, Dicenta I, Mussot S, Dartevelle PG. Sleeve lobectomy for bronchogenic cancers: factors affecting survival. *Ann Thorac Surg.* 2002;74(3):851–858; discussion 858.

144. Tsang V, Goldstraw P. Endobronchial stenting for anastomotic stenosis after sleeve resection. *Ann Thorac Surg.* 1989;48(4):568–571.

145. Grillo HC. Carinal reconstruction. *Ann Thorac Surg.* 1982;34(4):356–373.

146. Mitchell JD, Mathisen DJ, Wright CD, et al. Clinical experience with carinal resection. *J Thorac Cardiovasc Surg.* 1999;117(1):39–52; discussion 52.

147. Wood DE, Vallières E. Tracheobronchial resection and reconstruction. *Arch Surg.* 1997;132(8):850–854; discussion 854.

148. Mitchell JD, Mathisen DJ, Wright CD, et al. Resection for bronchogenic carcinoma involving the carina: long-term results and effect of nodal status on outcome. *J Thorac Cardiovasc Surg.* 2001;121(3):465–471.

149. Jensik RJ, Faber LP, Kittle CF, Miley RW, Thatcher WC, El-Baz N. Survival in patients undergoing tracheal sleeve pneumonectomy for bronchogenic carcinoma. *J Thorac Cardiovasc Surg.* 1982;84(4):489–496.

150. Tsuchiya R, Goya T, Naruke T, Suemasu K. Resection of tracheal carina for lung cancer. Procedure, complications, and mortality. *J Thorac Cardiovasc Surg.* 1990;99(5):779–787.

151. Maeda M, Nakamoto K, Tsubota N, Okada T, Katsura H. Operative approaches for left-sided carinoplasty. *Ann Thorac Surg.* 1993;56(3):441–445; discussion 445.

152. Roviaro GC, Varoli F, Rebuffat C, et al. Tracheal sleeve pneumonectomy for bronchogenic carcinoma. *J Thorac Cardiovasc Surg.* 1994;107(1):13–18.

153. Dartevelle P, Macchiarini P. Carinal resection for bronchogenic cancer. *Semin Thorac Cardiovasc Surg.* 1996;8(4):414–425.

154. Kutlu CA, Williams EA, Evans TW, Pastorino U, Goldstraw P. Acute lung injury and acute respiratory distress syndrome after pulmonary resection. *Ann Thorac Surg.* 2000;69(2):376–380.

155. Mathisen DJ, Kuo EY, Hahn C, et al. Inhaled nitric oxide for adult respiratory distress syndrome after pulmonary resection. *Ann Thorac Surg.* 1998;66(6):1894–1902.

156. Takizawa H, Kondo K, Matsuoka H, et al. Effect of mediastinal lymph nodes sampling in patients with clinical stage I non-small cell lung cancer. *J Med Invest.* 2008;55(1–2):37–43.

157. Brock MV, Kim MP, Hooker CM, et al. Pulmonary resection in octogenarians with stage I nonsmall cell lung cancer: a 22-year experience. *Ann Thorac Surg.* 2004;77(1):271–277.

158. Dominguez-Ventura A, Cassivi SD, Allen MS, et al. Lung cancer in octogenarians: factors affecting long-term survival following resection. *Eur J Cardiothorac Surg.* 2007;32(2):370–374.

159. Dominguez-Ventura A, Allen MS, Cassivi SD, Nichols FC 3rd, Deschamps C, Pairolero PC. Lung cancer in octogenarians: factors affecting morbidity and mortality after pulmonary resection. *Ann Thorac Surg.* 2006;82(4):1175–1179.

160. Mery CM, Pappas AN, Bueno R, et al. Similar long-term survival of elderly patients with non-small cell lung cancer treated with lobectomy or wedge resection within the surveillance, epidemiology, and end results database. *Chest.* 2005;128(1):237–245.

161. Okami J, Higashiyama M, Asamura H, et al.; Japanese Joint Committee of Lung Cancer Registry. Pulmonary resection in patients aged 80 years or over with clinical stage I non-small cell lung cancer: prognostic factors for overall survival and risk factors for postoperative complications. *J Thorac Oncol.* 2009;4(10):1247–1253.

8 Surgical Treatment of Small Cell Lung Cancer

JAMES E. HARRIS, Jr.

MALCOLM V. BROCK

According to a recent analysis of the Surveillance, Epidemiology, and Results Database, small cell lung cancer (SCLC) consists of 13% of all newly diagnosed lung cancers each year in this country (1). But, because of the high case-fatality rate of SCLC, of roughly 26,000 new cases each year, 24,000 people succumb to the disease (2). SCLC has a very poor overall 5-year survival rate of less than 8% compared with approximately 15% for patients diagnosed with all stages of non–small cell lung cancer (NSCLC) (3). SCLC also has a stronger association with tobacco exposure than NSCLC and is very rarely seen among nonsmokers. With the downward trend in smoking in both men and women in the United States over the past several decades, there has also been a mirrored decline in the incidence of SCLC cases from 17% in 1986 to 13% in 2002 (1). Unlike NSCLC, SCLC has an early propensity to metastasize, and it is often found present outside the margins of surgical resection at the time of diagnosis. This lack of locally confined tumor effectively has historically rendered many patients with SCLC poor surgical candidates.

■ HISTORICAL PERSPECTIVE

Historically, the mainstay of therapy for SCLC has been chemotherapy, with the addition of either radiation therapy or occasionally surgery for local control. Two large prospective, randomized clinical trials conducted in the 1960s and 1970s by the British Medical Research Council, investigated the role of surgery versus radiation therapy in the treatment of limited disease SCLC (4,5). Both studies concluded that there was limited benefit of either surgery or radiation therapy in effectively controlling limited-stage disease (4,5). Advocates of surgical therapy in SCLC have questioned the validity and contemporary relevance of the studies' conclusions since they were performed in an era

where there were few preoperative tools to diagnose SCLC for regional nodal metastases. Hence, these trials suffered from the lack of inclusion of true limited disease (T1–T2, N0) SCLC patients due to an inability to predetermine the very group of patients who may benefit most from surgical intervention.

With advancements in diagnostic technology since the 1960s and 1970s, including high-resolution spiral computed tomography (CT), positron emission tomography (PET), improved methods of staging through diagnostic techniques via video-assisted mediastinoscopy, endoscopic ultrasound bronchoscopy, image-guided transthoracic biopsy, and video-assisted thoracoscopic surgery (VATS), we are now better able to identify those SCLC patients who are truly with limited, T1–T2, N0 disease. Despite these improvements, even today, fewer than 10% of SCLC cases are being diagnosed with very limited, stage I disease (T1–T2N0) (6).

The old nomenclature created by the Veterans' Affairs Lung Study Group for characterizing the extent of disease for SCLC codified the disease into two simple categories, either limited or extensive. Limited disease was defined as SCLC isolated to one hemithorax and within one radiation treatment field, whereas extensive disease referred to any lesions beyond the confines of regional radiation therapy. This broad categorization of limited disease includes the TNM stage I through III, wherein stage IV SCLC is defined as extensive disease. Although limited versus extensive disease was suitable for considering patients who were candidates for radiation therapy, the TNM nomenclature is adaptive and more broadly suited for clinical practice guidelines and the multidisciplinary nature of SCLC management today.

■ INDICATIONS FOR SURGERY AND PREOPERATIVE EVALUATION

For a long time, the National Comprehensive Cancer Network guidelines have recognized that surgery in very early T1–T2N0 disease is an effective means of maximizing local control in SCLC. However, it was only after more than a decade of experience with platinum-based chemotherapy that they revised their previous guidelines to include a salient recommendation that surgically resected early-stage SCLC patients should be treated with adjuvant chemotherapy (7). Furthermore, data from numerous retrospective and prospective studies seem to suggest a survival benefit when resected stage I SCLC (T1–T2N0) is followed with platinum-based adjuvant chemotherapy (8). In fact, 5-year survival rates as high as 86% have been achieved in some series when surgery and adjuvant platinum-based chemotherapy are employed for very early-stage T1N0 SCLC tumors (Figure 8.1) (8). The use of platinum in these patients also seems to be important as 5-year survival rates appear to be less when platinum is not administered to early-stage resected SCLC patients (8–10).

One hypothesis of the effectiveness of adjuvant chemotherapy in T1–T2N0 SCLC is that the disease is very chemosensitive to platinum agents and that any residual micrometastases in the circulation can be eradicated. Despite this, routine adjuvant administration of platinum-based chemotherapy in SCLC remains an area awaiting more definitive study. It should be remembered that with the much more prevalent NSCLC, it was not until 1995 that there was a meta-analysis which demonstrated that platinum-based chemotherapy resulted in a 27% reduction in the risk of death in advanced NSCLC. In this same study, platinum-based chemotherapy yielded only a 5% absolute survival advantage at 5 years in the adjuvant setting in NSCLC. In addition, it has only been in the last few years that three influential

clinical trials with adjuvant chemotherapy have been reported for resected patients with stage I–II NSCLC and in each, a definite survival benefit was observed for resected NSCLC patients with stage II disease, but no trial has shown benefit for the very earliest stage of NSCLC, T1N0 (9).

There are significant challenges to designing a large, multicenter trial to investigate the long-term survival benefits of surgically resected SCLC and adjuvant platinum-based chemotherapy. Only 5% to 6% of all SCLC cases have historically presented as solitary pulmonary nodules amenable to surgical intervention (11). This figure may be even further reduced when any patient who has nodal disease or any SCLC beyond the margins of surgical resection are excluded. In addition, it is rare that a patient presents with a solitary pulmonary nodule and a concomitant diagnosis of biopsy proven SCLC. Many of these patients with known SCLC on fine-needle aspiration are referred for surgical excision because of the chance that the mass may be of mixed histology (NSCLC/SCLC) on full pathologic review. However, most patients with early-stage SCLC who present with solitary pulmonary nodules of unknown etiology, undergo surgical resection on the assumption that the lesion is most likely of a pure NSCLC histology. The SCLC is subsequently discovered incidentally when a biopsy or frozen section histologic examination is performed during the operative intervention. Hence, any clinical trial investigating surgically resectable SCLC patients would have to be amenable to accepting patients who either had a preoperative diagnosis of very early-stage SCLC with no evidence of disseminated disease or patients with a single

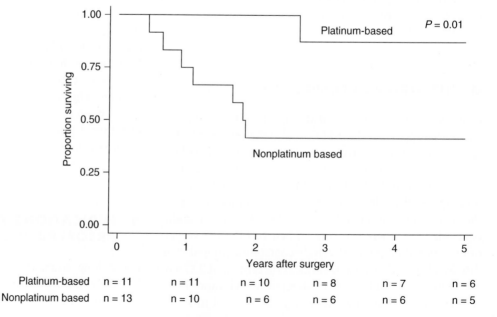

FIGURE 8.1 Kaplan-Meier survival curves of patients with stage 1 SCLC who received adjuvant chemotherapy (n = 24) according to whether platinum or nonplatinum chemotherapy was used. Five-year survival rates for patients who received platinum or nonplatinum therapy were 85.7% and 41.7%, respectively.

	0	1	2	3	4	5
Platinum-based	n = 11	n = 11	n = 10	n = 8	n = 7	n = 6
Nonplatinum based	n = 13	n = 10	n = 6	n = 6	n = 6	n = 5

nodule at surgery with no nodal disease who were found to have SCLC after pathology review. Despite these barriers to patient accrual, there is a considerable effort underway in a large, cooperative group setting to investigate the long-term survival of patients with T1–T2N0 who undergo surgery and then platinum-based adjuvant therapy.

If a preoperative biopsy does reveal SCLC in a patient with a solitary pulmonary nodule, at a minimum the patient work up should include a history and physical examination, complete blood count, comprehensive metabolic panel, LDH, chest x-ray, and high-resolution CT scan of the chest to evaluate the extent of the primary tumor along with the peribronchial, mediastinal, and supraclavicular lymph nodes. Special attention to the chest wall, spine, esophagus, and proximity of the tumor to the carina must also be taken into account in order to identify properly those patients who are surgical candidates. Every patient should also have a CT scan of the head or magnetic resonance imaging (preferred) to screen for subclinical brain metastasis and a CT of the abdomen and pelvis to look for intra-abdominal or pelvic metastases. In most large, academic centers in the United States, routine whole body screening for extrathoracic metastases is usually done with a PET-CT. PET-CT can also be included as part of the preoperative workup of SCLC to evaluate preliminarily the lymph nodes of the mediastinum and other regions which may be suspicious on CT alone for evidence of increased metabolic activity. It should be duly noted, however, that a high avidity PET-CT reading in a mediastinal or hilar lymph node is not necessarily consistent with metastatic disease, and most investigators recommend concomitant biopsy to rule out systemic inflammatory or infectious disease such as sarcoidosis or tuberculosis.

For appropriate staging of these mediastinal or hilar nodes, patients may undergo flexible bronchoscopy, endoscopic ultrasound bronchoscopy, and/or mediastinoscopy with biopsies of any suspicious lesions and/or mediastinal nodes either as a separate procedure or at the same time as the surgical resection of the primary tumor. If preoperative imaging, bronchoscopy, and mediastinoscopy/biopsy results are all consistent with stage I, T1–2, N0 SCLC, early elective surgery for curative resection should proceed. Postoperatively, all patients with histologically proven SCLC that are deemed medically suitable to receive chemotherapy should be offered four cycles of a standard 21-day regimen of etoposide/cisplatin (EP) chemotherapy. A reasonable dose to maximize postoperative tolerability that has been used in our institution is cisplatin 60 mg m^2 IV on day 1, and etoposide 120 mg/m^2 days 1, 2, and 3 every 21-day cycle. Spiral chest CT scan monitoring for recurrence every 3 months for 2 years, and then every 6 months thereafter is often done together by the surgeon and medical oncologist.

Adjuvant radiation therapy to the chest and mediastinum is indicated in surgically resected SCLC patients who have disease beyond stage 1. Such patients include those with proven microscopic or macroscopic tumor in the hilar or mediastinal nodes. Less clear is the role of prophylactic cranial irradiation (PCI) in patients with early-stage SCLC. There have been numerous recent studies that have shown a benefit of PCI in SCLC patients who are without clinical or radiographic evidence of brain metastasis; these patients have been shown to have both an overall lower incidence of symptomatic brain lesions as well as a significant survival benefit as compared with those who do not undergo PCI (12). Even among those with stage I disease who undergo surgery with adjuvant chemotherapy, PCI seems to give an additional survival benefit (12). Patients, however, can often be reluctant to undergo PCI because of the potential side-effects. It is the job of the surgeon as well as the radiation oncologist to have an informed, honest discussion with patients in this dilemma, and to allow the patient or their family to have a prominent role in deciding the best course of therapy for themselves.

■ LOBECTOMY VERSUS WEDGE RESECTION

In patients with SCLC who have T1–2, N0 disease, the most appropriate operation that would offer the highest survival rate, in most circumstances, would be a lobectomy. As observed with NSCLC, any resection that is less extensive can result in a lower survival benefit (13). For patients with chronic obstructive pulmonary disease or other underlying pulmonary disease, a less extensive resection may be warranted based on pulmonary function testing results. Although the oncologic benefit of a lobectomy will decrease the likelihood of recurrent disease, the risk of peri- and postoperative morbidity and mortality of doing a more extensive resection in a patient with baseline pulmonary disease may outweigh the benefits of performing a lobectomy.

■ ROLE FOR SURGICAL PALLIATIVE CARE IN SCLC

Given the aggressive nature of SCLC, there are few circumstances where there would be any benefit to curative surgical intervention in a patient with greater than stage I disease. However, surgery does have a role in palliative care especially in the patient with recurrent malignant pleural effusions. Pleurodesis or placement of a small-bore, indwelling intrapleural catheter is often indicated in the long-term management of chronic malignant pleural effusions in patients with extensive SCLC to avoid recurrent hospitalizations. Many of these patients have already had more than one thoracentesis and/or had chest tubes placed, requiring hospitalization for management of their effusions at the time of surgical consultation.

Pleurodesis is a procedure that is done to obliterate the pleural space so as to prevent the recurrence of effusions and/or pneumothorax. Pleurodesis can be achieved by chemical means with the introduction of a sclerosing chemical agent, usually talc, into the pleural space via a thoracostomy tube on the side of the effusion. The result is adherence of the overlying visceral pleura of the lung to the parietal pleura of the chest wall. Pleurodesis can also be achieved via VATS by applying talc under direct visualization or by mechanically causing pleurodesis with the use of an abrasive pad to irritate the parietal pleura lining of the chest wall.

An alternative for the management of malignant pleural effusions is through the placement of a small-bore, indwelling intrapleural catheter (14). These catheters are usually more comfortable than larger chest tubes which have been traditionally used in the hospital, and they allow the patient to be discharged home with the catheter in place. Pleural effusions can be managed by the patient through connecting the one-way catheter to a collection bag which can be easily hidden beneath the patients' clothing. This external drainage bag can be disconnected and capped off at times when output is low, or at the patients' convenience, and easily removed in the outpatient setting if it no longer becomes necessary. Most patients with malignant pleural effusions who receive these catheters are terminally ill, and often do not live long enough to ever have their catheters removed. Follow-up care can be easily managed for these patients in the outpatient clinic. Rarely is there the development of empyema, requiring removal of the catheter and VATS decortication.

Unlike patients with NSCLC, there is no indication for surgery in SCLC for those with tumors which involve the chest wall, superior sulcus tumors, or metastases to other distant sites. There are less invasive ways of managing these patients than surgery, but even with the utilization of all resources that are currently available, there is no survival benefit to any of these treatment modalities. The majority of patients can benefit from palliative radiation to regions of symptomatic metastatic or to locally invasive areas and most SCLCs are also very responsive to chemotherapy. For those who have tumor involving the airway, there has been some success in bronchoscopic placement of tracheal and bronchial stents in order to maintain airway patency; unfortunately all of these methods fail once disease has become extensive and almost all patients succumb to their disease within 6 months.

■ FUTURE DIRECTIONS

Despite numerous advances in diagnostic imaging, chemotherapeutic agents, and radiation therapy, the successful therapy that offers the best long-term survival benefit for early-stage SCLC still remains elusive. While it is our thesis that a pulmonary lobectomy combined with adjuvant platinum-based chemotherapy and PCI offers the greatest chance of survival to those patients with stage I (T1–T2N0) SCLC, this scenario only reflects 5% to 6% of all who are diagnosed with this cancer. To make some progress with this disease, we must not only improve our ability to diagnose patients at an early stage but also develop new methods to treat the majority of patients who are diagnosed beyond stage I disease. At the present time, etoposide and cisplatin combination chemotherapy is the standard of care for all who are afflicted, but invariably most who show an excellent initial response progress to recurrence and subsequently succumb to their disease.

We are now approaching an era of individualized cancer therapy where the genetic and epigenetic profile of specific cancers may be particularly informative not only about the prognosis of a specific cancer subtype, but also about the sensitivity or resistance of the cancers to certain chemotherapeutic agents. Much like the way we have the ability to culture bacteria from patient specimens and characterize which antibiotic agent offers the greatest therapeutic potential for that specific infection, research laboratories around the world are already working toward a similar model of personalizing treatment for cancer. Ultimately the goal of treating SCLC is to improve upon our ability to diagnose the disease in its earliest stages and establish a therapeutic strategy that offers the maximum survival to the patient.

■ REFERENCES

1. Govindan R, Page N, Morgensztern D, et al. Changing epidemiology of small-cell lung cancer in the United States over the last 30 years: analysis of the surveillance, epidemiologic, and end results database. *J Clin Oncol.* 2006;24(28):4539–4544.
2. Page NC, Read W, Tierney RM, et al. The epidemiology of small cell lung cancer. *Proc Am Soc Clin Oncol.* 2002;21:305a
3. Fry WA, Menck HR, Winchester DP. The National Cancer Data Base report on lung cancer. *Cancer.* 1996;77(9):1947–1955.
4. Miller AB, Fox W, Tall R. Five-year follow-up of the Medical Research Council comparative trial of surgery and radiotherapy for the primary treatment of small-celled or oat-celled carcinoma of the bronchus. *Lancet.* 1969;2:501–505.
5. Fox W, Scadding JG. Treatment of oat-celled carcinoma of the bronchus. *Lancet.* 1973;2:616–617.
6. Martini N, Wittes RE, Hilaris BS, Hajdu SI, Beattie EJ Jr, Golbey RB. Oat cell carcinoma of the lung. *Clin Bull.* 1975;5(4):144–148.
7. Ettinger D, Johnson B. Update: NCCN small cell and non-small cell lung cancer Clinical Practice Guidelines. *J Natl Compr Canc Netw.* 2005;3(suppl 1):S17–S21.

8. Brock MV, Hooker CM, Syphard JE, et al. Surgical resection of limited disease small cell lung cancer in the new era of platinum chemotherapy: Its time has come. *J Thorac Cardiovasc Surg.* 2005;129(1):64–72.

9. The International Adjuvant Lung Cancer Trial Collaborative Group. Cisplatin-based adjuvant chemotherapy in patients with completely resected non-small-cell lung cancer. *N Engl J Med.* 2004;350:351–360.

10. Agra Y, Pelayo M, Sacristan M, Sacristán A, Serra C, Bonfill X. Chemotherapy versus best supportive care for extensive small cell lung cancer. *Cochrane Database Syst Rev.* 2003;(4): CD001990.

11. Quoix E, Fraser R, Wolkove N, Finkelstein H, Kreisman H. Small cell lung cancer presenting as a solitary pulmonary nodule. *Cancer.* 1990;66(3):577–582.

12. Topkan E, Yildirim BA, Selek U, Yavuz MN. Cranial prophylactic irradiation in locally advanced non-small cell lung carcinoma: current status and future perspectives. *Oncology.* 2009;76(3):220–228.

13. Kraev A, Rassias D, Vetto J, et al. Wedge resection vs lobectomy: 10-year survival in stage I primary lung cancer. *Chest.* 2007;131(1):136–140.

14. Olden AM, Holloway R. Treatment of malignant pleural effusion: PleuRx catheter or talc pleurodesis? A cost-effectiveness analysis. *J Palliat Med.* 2010;13(1):59–65.

9

Evaluation, Management, and Medical Therapy of Small Cell Lung Cancer

RANDEEP SANGHA

PRIMO N. LARA, Jr.

■ INTRODUCTION

Lung cancer is a strikingly prevalent malignancy and is the leading cause of cancer-related deaths worldwide (1). Small cell lung cancer (SCLC) is a distinct clinicopathologic entity that represents 15% of all lung cancers. In 2009, an estimated 32,000 new cases were diagnosed within the United States (2). SCLC is highly smoking related and is characterized by aggressive growth kinetics and disseminated metastases, with 60% to 70% of patients presenting with advanced (or extensive-stage) disease. Despite high initial tumor response rates (RR) following platinum-based chemotherapy, rapid emergence of clinical drug resistance inevitably results in tumor progression and death of more than 90% of affected patients (3). Unfortunately, progress in the management of SCLC has been slow with no significant therapeutic advances within the past two decades. Given the high lethality of this malignancy, the need to improve outcomes is clearly apparent. Herein, the current strategies for evaluating and managing SCLC will be reviewed, and key research endeavors will be highlighted.

■ PATHOLOGY AND CLINICAL PRESENTATION

The World Health Organization has changed the classification for SCLC three times from 1967 to 2004 in an attempt to simplify the overall scheme and to better reflect pathology with clinical outcome. Currently, two histologic subtypes are recognized: small cell carcinoma and combined small cell carcinoma (Table 9.1). The former is defined as a malignant epithelial tumor consisting of small cells with scant cytoplasm, ill-defined cell borders, finely granular nuclear chromatin, and absent or inconspicuous nucleoli (4,5). In addition, the cells are round, oval, and spindle shaped with prominent nuclear molding and

necrosis is typically extensive. The mitotic count is characteristically high accounting for its rapid growth rate. In contrast, combined small cell carcinoma is not only distinguished by these characteristics but also consists of a ≥10% proportion of non–small cell lung cancer (NSCLC) tumor cells, commonly adenocarcinoma, squamous cell carcinoma, or large cell carcinoma. Although the diagnosis of SCLC rests primarily with morphologic assessment, immunocytochemistry plays a central role (6). Virtually, all SCLC tumors immunostain for keratin and epithelial membrane antigens, and alternative diagnoses are often sought if this pattern of immunoreactivity is not detected. SCLC is recognized as a neuroendocrine tumor, and ultrastructural and immunohistochemical analyses consistently display the presence of neurosecretory-type granules (7,8). Accordingly, 75% of SCLCs possess detectable markers of neuroendocrine differentiation, such as chromogranin, synaptophysin, neuron-specific enolase, and Leu-7.

The clinical presentation of SCLC is similar to other histologies of bronchogenic carcinoma, but typically develops in the central airways resulting in localized symptoms, such as cough and dyspnea. Other clinical manifestations arise from intrathoracic or extrathoracic spread, including neurologic symptoms related to central nervous system (CNS) metastases. Chest imaging commonly demonstrates hilar and mediastinal invasion with regional lymphadenopathy; the presence of a peripheral nodule or chest-wall involvement without central lymphadenopathy is rare. Given the neuroendocrine nature of SCLC, it is not surprising that it is associated with a spectrum of endocrine and neurologic paraneoplastic syndromes. For example, the inappropriate production of polypeptide hormones such as antidiuretic hormone or adrenocorticotropic hormone (ACTH) is linked notoriously to SCLC and ultimately result in the syndrome of inappropriate antidiuretic hormone or Cushing's syndrome, respectively. Laboratory features of ACTH oversecretion include hypokalemia and hyperglycemia. Neurologic paraneoplastic disorders can involve sensory, sensorimotor, and autoimmune neuropathies or encephalomyelitis (6). Mechanistically, antinuclear antibodies, such as anti-*Hu*, cross-react with SCLC antigens as well as to neuronal RNA-binding proteins, thereby triggering a diverse array of neurologic deficits (9).

■ **Table 9.1** Morphological features of SCLC histologic subtypes

	SCLC Histologic Subtype	Morphological Features
WHO Classification of SCLC	Small cell carcinoma	• Scant cytoplasm • Ill-defined cell borders • Finely granular chromatin • Absent or inconspicuous nucleoli • Prominent nuclear molding • High mitotic count
	Combined small cell carcinoma	• Scant cytoplasm • Ill-defined cell borders • Finely granular chromatin • Absent or inconspicuous nucleoli • Prominent nuclear molding • High mitotic count • 10% of tumor bulk comprised of NSCLC component

NSCLC, non–small cell lung cancer; SCLC, small cell lung cancer; WHO, World Health Organization.

Lambert-Eaton myasthenic syndrome, a disease of the neuromuscular junction, is associated with SCLC in 60% of all cases. Characterized by proximal muscle weakness and autonomic dysfunction, electrophysiologic studies pathognomonically display enhanced neurotransmission with repetitive stimulation. Lambert-Eaton syndrome manifests from impaired acetylcholine release due to autoantibodies targeting the presynaptic voltage-gated calcium channels of cholinergic nerve terminals, ultimately causing significant morbidity (10).

■ **STAGING AND EVALUATION**

Accurate staging provides prognostic information and stage aids the planning of treatment strategies in lung cancer (11). The tumor, node, metastases (TNM) staging system established by the American Joint Committee on Cancer Staging, is applicable to SCLC particularly with the forthcoming changes proposed by the IASLC (International Association for the Study of Lung Cancer) for the upcoming edition. The clinical utility of the TNM staging classification in identifying subgroups with differing prognoses was recently reported after a review of 349 cases of surgically resected SCLC within the IASLC database (11). However, patients seldom present where surgery is a therapeutic option and the TNM staging system has historically relied on surgical confirmation for accuracy. As a result, a long-standing two-stage system proposed by the Veterans' Administration Lung Study Group is still generally used (12). This system divides SCLC into two disease categories termed limited- or extensive-stage. Limited-stage SCLC (LS-SCLC) is characterized by disease confined to the ipsilateral hemithorax, which can be safely encompassed within a tolerable radiation field; all other presentations, including malignant pleural and

■ **Table 9.2** Initial evaluation of newly diagnosed SCLC

• History and physical examination
• Pathology review
• Complete blood count
• Complete biochemical panel including LDH and alkaline phosphatase
• Chest x-ray
• CT chest and abdomen (to include liver and adrenal glands)
• Bone scan
• MRI or CT brain[a]

[a] MRI is preferred over CT brain since it is more sensitive for identifying brain metastases.

CT, computed tomography; LDH, lactate dehydrogenase; MRI, magnetic resonance imaging; SCLC, small cell lung cancer.

pericardial effusions, are categorized as extensive-stage SCLC (ES-SCLC).

Considering SCLC has an aggressive clinical course and propensity for widespread metastases at diagnosis, 60% of patients present with hematogenous metastases which often involve the contralateral lung, liver, adrenal glands, brain, bone, and/or bone marrow. Complete evaluation of a patient with newly diagnosed SCLC consists of a history and physical examination, pathology confirmation, hematologic and biochemical profile, computed tomography (CT) of the chest and abdomen to include the liver and adrenal glands, bone scan, and a contrast-enhanced CT or magnetic resonance imaging (MRI) of the brain (Table 9.2) (13). These investigations are necessary to appropriately stage a patient and develop a suitable treatment plan. Bone marrow aspiration had been a routine practice, but has since been abandoned because of the infrequent incidence of bone marrow involvement in the absence of other sites of disseminated metastases. This is exemplified by a study of 403 patients with SCLC, where only seven patients (1.7%) had ES-SCLC based on bone marrow involvement alone (14).

The role for positron emission tomography (PET) is evolving, but no randomized or even large prospective studies have been conducted evaluating the role of PET as a staging tool for SCLC. Preliminary data supports avid uptake of [18F] fluorodeoxyglucose in SCLC tumors, suggesting that staging evaluation with PET could complement conventional staging (13).

■ ROLE OF SURGERY FOR EARLY-STAGE SCLC

In the rare circumstance where early-stage SCLC is suspected (<5%), curative-intent surgical resection may be offered based on several series showing long-term survival in patients treated with surgery (15). These favorable subsets of patients have stage I (T1–2, N0 tumors) identified at the time of surgery or at postoperative pathology examination (16–19). Because the number of patients presenting with this stage of disease is minimal, no randomized trials of adjuvant chemotherapy have been carried out. Despite a lack of a consensus for adjuvant therapy, common practice is to offer adjuvant platinum-based chemotherapy. Moreover, the current National Comprehensive Cancer Network guidelines recommend concurrent chemotherapy and postoperative mediastinal radiotherapy for patient with nodal metastases. Prophylactic cranial irradiation (PCI) after adjuvant therapy is also reasonable in this population in order to improve disease-free and overall survival (OS) (20).

Patients who present with node-positive SCLC do not benefit from surgery. The Lung Cancer Study Group completed a trial where the role of complete surgical resection was prospectively evaluated. Eligible LS-SCLC patients, excluding those with stage I disease, received five cycles of CAV (cyclophosphamide, doxorubicin, vincristine)

chemotherapy (21). Responding patients were randomized to undergo surgery or no surgery, and all patients received thoracic and cranial irradiation. Survival was equivalent between the two study arms with a reported median survival of 15 months, and a 2-year OS of 20% suggesting no benefit of surgery. Hence, patients being considered for surgical resection require mediastinal staging to rule out occult nodal disease (22). The presence of nodal metastases discards surgery as a modality of therapy since these patients would best be managed with concurrent chemotherapy and thoracic irradiation.

■ MANAGEMENT OF LS-SCLC

Current forms of treatment for LS-SCLC offer a median survival of 16 to 24 months, with 16% to 26% of patients surviving beyond 5 years (Table 9.3). The standard therapeutic approach, for patients who are not candidates for a clinical protocol, is four cycles of chemotherapy with concurrent thoracic irradiation. Based on its preclinical synergy and superiority in efficacy and tolerability with concomitant irradiation, cisplatin and etoposide chemotherapy has supplanted alkylator/anthracycline-based regimens as the chemotherapy backbone (23). Thoracic irradiation results in local control and a survival benefit; however, the timing of radiation appears critical (24,25). For example, early concurrent chemoradiation yields a small, but significant, survival advantage when compared to late concurrent or sequential thoracic irradiation (26,27). Moreover, the role of hyperfractionation remains controversial. For patients with excellent performance status and an adequate baseline pulmonary reserve, administration of twice-daily thoracic irradiation with cisplatin/etoposide has shown encouraging long-term survival results. In practice, this schedule is logistically difficult to administer and yet unknown to be

---

■ Table 9.3 Staging and prognosis of small cell lung cancer

Stage of Disease	% of Patients at Diagnosis	Survival		
		Untreated	Median with Treatment	2-year OS with Treatment
Limited stage Tumor confined to one hemithorax and regional lymph nodes within a radiation port[a]	30–35[c]	12 weeks	16–24 months	45%
Extensive stage Disease beyond the borders described for limited-stage disease[b]	65–70	6 weeks	7–12 months	<5%

[a] Contralateral hilar, mediastinal, and supraclavicular lymph nodes are commonly included in LS-SCLC.
[b] Malignant pericardial or pleural effusion is considered ES-SCLC.
[c] Less than 5% patients have surgically resectable stage I (T1N0 or T2N0) disease.

ES-SCLC, extensive-stage small cell lung cancer; LS-SCLC, limited-stage small cell lung cancer; OS, overall survival.

superior to a biologically equivalent dose of a once-daily thoracic irradiation regimen.

Chemotherapy

The ability to employ the optimal concurrent chemotherapy regimen with thoracic irradiation is determined by its efficacy and synergism with radiation. For LS-SCLC, the fundamental chemotherapy regimen is the combination of cisplatin and etoposide. A randomized phase III trial of 436 patients, initially designed to determine the superior regimen between cisplatin-etoposide (PE) with cyclophosphamide, epirubicin, vincristine (CEV), prospectively stratified patients according to extent of disease (LS-SCLC, n = 214; ES-SCLC, n = 222) (23). Patients received five cycles of PE or CEV, and for LS-SCLC cases, thoracic irradiation was given concurrent with cycle 3 of chemotherapy. Furthermore, PCI was administered to those achieving a complete response within the treatment period. In the LS-SCLC cohort, median survival reached 14.5 months versus 9.7 months in the PE and CEV arms, respectively (P = 0.001). The 2- and 5-year survival rates were 25% and 10% in the PE arm compared with 8% and 3% in the CEV arm (P = 0.0001). This trial illustrates the superiority of cisplatin/etoposide as the chemotherapy platform to be given concurrent with thoracic irradiation.

Radiation Therapy

In 1987, the Cancer and Leukemia Group B (CALGB) published a seminal report (CALGB 8083) describing the benefits of thoracic irradiation when given concurrently with chemotherapy for LS-SCLC patients (28). Local failure rates of 90% were seen in the chemotherapy alone arm and two subsequent meta-analyses showing improvements in local control and OS, thereby strengthening the case for shifting the standard of care to a chemoradiotherapy approach (24,25). Moreover, in the Pignon et al. meta-analysis, combined modality therapy resulted in a 14% reduction in death rate and an absolute 5.4% improvement in 3-year survival compared with the chemotherapy alone arm (24). Unfortunately, many questions still remain unanswered regarding the optimal delivery and dose of thoracic irradiation.

Randomized clinical trials have yielded conflicting data on whether concurrent irradiation is best administered early or late in the overall course of treatment. However, the existing evidence suggests that there may be a survival advantage for the early initiation of thoracic irradiation with cisplatin-based chemotherapy. For example, a National Cancer Institute of Canada Clinical Trials Group (NCIC-CTG) study randomized 308 patients to receive concurrent radiotherapy (40 Gray in 15 fractions) beginning at cycle 2 or cycle 6 of chemotherapy (26). The early administration of thoracic irradiation was associated with improved local

and systemic control as well as a statistically significant progression-free survival (PFS) and OS benefit. The phase III Japanese Clinical Oncology Group (JCOG) 9104 randomized 231 LS-SCLC patients to sequential or concurrent cycle 1 cisplatin/etoposide with thoracic irradiation given twice daily (45 Gray in 3 weeks) (29). Although the trial was underpowered, early concurrent therapy was found to be superior to sequential treatment. Median survival time was 27.2 months in the concurrent arm versus 19.7 months in the sequential arm. The trial also demonstrated that four cycles of cisplatin/etoposide with 45 Gray (Gy), given in accelerated fractionation, produced credible response, local control, and survival (6). Finally, a recent meta-analysis explored whether the timing of thoracic irradiation influenced patient survival in LS-SCLC. After reviewing data from seven eligible randomized clinical trials, early thoracic irradiation (defined as a start time within 30 days of chemotherapy) did not confer a clinically significant 2- or 5-year OS rate; however, for those trials using a platinum-backbone concurrent with thoracic irradiation, a significant 5-year OS was uncovered for early thoracic irradiation (P = 0.02). (30).

Although early thoracic irradiation appears to be favorable, the optimal dose and fractionation scheme for thoracic irradiation for LS-SCLC has not been clearly defined. Fractionation refers to the dose per treatment, number of treatments per day, and overall time of treatment (13). Hyperfractionation occurs when greater than one treatment is administered per day, whereas accelerated fractionation refers to the delivery of more than the common prescription of 10 Gy/week in standard daily fractions. CALGB has investigated a 70 Gy maximum-tolerated dose (MTD) of once-daily radiotherapy in the phase II setting (31,32). In addition, CALGB conducted the CALGB 39808 trial where 57 LS-SCLC patients were treated with 70 Gy in 35 once-daily fractions concurrently with carboplatin/etoposide following two cycles of induction paclitaxel and topotecan (33). The reported 2-year survival was 48%, while the incidence of grade 3 dysphagia was 16%. However, the experience with 70 Gy of concurrent thoracic chemoradiation remains limited and, as a consequence, the de facto practice still calls for once-daily radiotherapy to be delivered at a total dose of 50 to 60 Gy in 1.8 to 2.0 Gy fractions.

Hyperfractionating radiotherapy is believed to offer additional clinical benefits. An Intergroup 0096 phase II trial randomized 417 patients to receive four cycles of cisplatin/etoposide with either 45 Gy of concurrent thoracic irradiation given twice daily over three weeks or once daily for five weeks (34). Thoracic irradiation was scheduled to coincide with the start of chemotherapy. This pivotal trial found a significant 5-year OS benefit favoring twice-daily thoracic irradiation compared with once-daily fractionation (26% vs. 16%; P = 0.04), and a lower incidence of local failure (36% vs. 52%; P = 0.06). Grade 3 esophagitis was the most significant toxicity with twice-daily radiotherapy

(26% twice-daily vs. 11% once-daily) but the incidence of grade 4 esophagitis did not differ between regimens.

The Radiation Therapy Oncology Group (RTOG) has examined an alternative fractionation scheme using a concomitant-boost technique to escalate dose while keeping the total treatment duration at 5 weeks. Initially, thoracic irradiation is administered once daily for 3 weeks, followed by 2 weeks of twice-daily thoracic irradiation. This dose/fractionation regimen is hypothesized to counteract accelerated repopulation, the increased tumor cell growth rate that is known to often occur several weeks into treatment. The MTD for the concomitant-boost technique, when combined with cisplatin/etoposide chemotherapy, has been determined at 61.2 Gy (35). This schedule was found to be tolerable but associated with a high incidence of myelosuppression.(36) Thus, there are three plausible treatment regimens for delivering concurrent thoracic radiotherapy in LS-SCLC at relatively similar biologically effective doses: (a) CALGB's 70 Gy once-daily fractionation for 7 weeks; (b) Intergroup 0096 regimen of 45 Gy twice-daily fractionation for 3 weeks; and (c) RTOG's 61.2 Gy concomitant-boost technique for 5 weeks duration.

Prophylactic Cranial Irradiation in (PCI) LS-SCLC

At the time of initial presentation, only 18% of patients will have detectable brain metastases, but the cumulative incidence at 2 years is a profound 50%, which is consistent with autopsy series (37,38). Because brain metastases result in significant morbidity, a number of trials have evaluated the role of PCI in patients with SCLC. The pivotal report demonstrating the clinical utility of PCI stemmed from a meta-analysis assessing individual data of 987 patients with SCLC (composed primarily of LS-SCLC patients) in complete remission who took part in seven clinical trials comparing PCI with no PCI (20). A notable 5.4% improvement in 3-year OS (20.7% PCI-treated vs. 15.3% control) and a 25% reduction in the incidence of brain metastases (33.1% PCI-treated vs. 58.6 control) were observed. The reduced risk of CNS failure and improved survival at a reasonable toxicity expense justify PCI for LS-SCLC patients who attain a complete response.

The RTOG 0212 trial was designed to determine the optimal dose of PCI (39). Patients with LS-SCLC who were complete responders to primary treatment were randomized to receive standard (25 Gy/10 fractions/12 days) or higher PCI doses (36 Gy) administered using either conventional (18 fractions/24 days) or accelerated hyperfractionated radiotherapy (24 twice-daily fractions/16 days). A total of 720 patients were enrolled and although there was a nonsignificant trend for reduced 2-year brain metastases incidence with high-dose PCI compared with standard dose PCI (24% vs. 30%; $P = 0.13$), there was a significantly marked increase in chest relapse (48% vs. 40%; $P = 0.02$) and mortality (2-year OS 37% high-dose

PCI vs. 42% standard dose PCI; $P = 0.03$) (39). Based on this data, the prevailing PCI dose of 25 Gy remains the standard of care for LS-SCLC.

Key Clinical Trials in LS-SCLC

Many of the advances for LS-SCLC have come from trials evaluating the role of radiation therapy. Addressing the central question of optimal dose and fractionation scheme for thoracic irradiation has been a long-standing challenge. Fortunately, this is the basis of two key ongoing clinical trials.

CALGB 30610, a pivotal Intergroup phase III trial for treatment-naïve LS-SCLC patients, is the first of its kind in well over a decade (Figure 9.1). It consists of two parts. Part 1 has three treatment arms with patients randomized in a 1:2:2 fashion: arm A, 45 Gy (1.5 Gy twice daily × 3 weeks); arm B, 70 Gy (2.0 Gy once daily × 7 weeks); arm C, 61.2 Gy (1.8 Gy once daily × 16 days followed by 1.8 Gy twice daily × 9 days for a total duration of 5 weeks). Four cycles of cisplatin and etoposide are given concurrently, starting on day 1 of radiotherapy for all arms of this study. After interim analysis for toxicity assessment, only one experimental arm (arm B or arm C) will be selected for further accrual in part 2 of the study. The primary endpoint will be OS and the projected total accrual is approximately 712 patients.

Building upon the Intergroup 0096 study in LS-SCLC, the CONVERT (Concurrent ONce-daily VErsus Radiotherapy Twice-daily) trial, spearheaded by the European Organization for the Research and Treatment of Cancer cooperative group, hypothesizes that increasing the total dose of once-daily thoracic irradiation will improve efficacy and negate the benefit of twice-daily fractionation; thus making the once-daily regimen more practical and logistically easier to deliver. The CONVERT trial is a two-arm multicenter randomized phase III intergroup trial comparing a once-daily with twice-daily schedule, given concurrently with cisplatin and etoposide (Figure 9.2). The radiotherapy treatment regimen put forth by the Intergroup 0096 trial (45 Gy, twice-daily fractionation over 3 weeks) will be compared with 66 Gy, once-daily fractionation over 6.5 weeks. Unlike the CALGB 30610 trial, thoracic irradiation will commence with the second cycle of chemotherapy. The primary endpoint will be OS and the goal for accrual is 532 patients within a 4-year time span. The results of these trials are eagerly anticipated.

■ MANAGEMENT OF EXTENSIVE-STAGE SCLC

Progress in the treatment of ES-SCLC has disappointingly lagged behind LS-SCLC. For greater than 95% of patients,

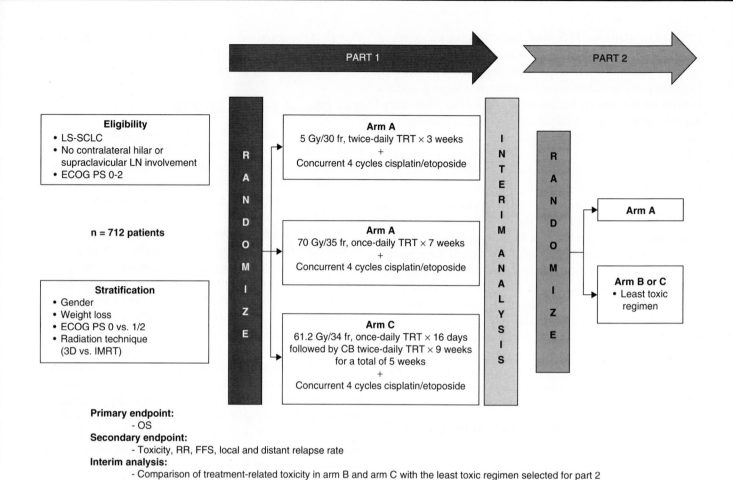

Primary endpoint:
- OS

Secondary endpoint:
- Toxicity, RR, FFS, local and distant relapse rate

Interim analysis:
- Comparison of treatment-related toxicity in arm B and arm C with the least toxic regimen selected for part 2

FIGURE 9.1 Phase III intergroup trial comparing thoracic radiotherapy regimens in LS-SCLC. 3D, 3D conformal radiation therapy; CB, concomitant boost; ECOG, Eastern Cooperative Oncology Group; FFS, failure-free survival; fr, fractions; Gy, Gray; IMRT, Intensity Modulated Radiation Therapy; LN, lymph node; LS-SCLC, limited-stage small cell lung cancer; OS, overall survival; PS, performance status; RR, response rate; TRT, thoracic radiation therapy.

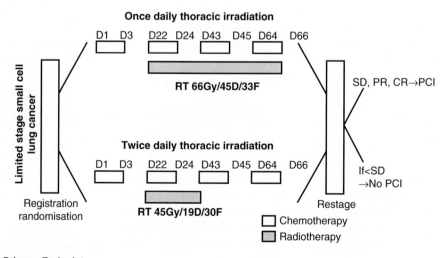

FIGURE 9.2 Phase III CONVERT Trial Schema. CR, complete response; D, day; F, fractions; Gy, gray; OS, overall survival; PCI, prophylactic cranial irradiation; PR, partial response; RT, radiotherapy; SD, stable disease.

Primary Endpoint:
-OS

Secondary Endpoint:
-Local progression-free survival, metastases-free survival, toxicity, chemotherapy and radiotherapy dose intensity

ES-SCLC is a fatal disease within 2 years of presentation. Despite overall RR of 60% to 80% to combination chemotherapy, the median survival only ranges from 7 to 12 months (40,41). The cornerstone of treatment in North America and Europe consists of platinum (cisplatin or carboplatin) and etoposide chemotherapy, which has been shown to be superior to older regimens such as CAV (cyclophosphamide, doxorubicin, vincristine). Unlike LS-SCLC, the primary role of radiotherapy is to palliate symptomatic sites of disease. PCI has also been incorporated into the treatment paradigm for ES-SCLC. Invariably, relapse occurs, and enrollment into a clinical trial is warranted in an attempt to improve upon the current outcomes.

Chemotherapy

During the 1970s, CAV was considered the standard combination chemotherapeutic regimen for SCLC, but in the mid-1980s platinum/etoposide chemotherapy was considered the optimal regimen for ES-SCLC and continues to be the current initial treatment recommendation. Maintenance or consolidation chemotherapy carries a greater risk of cumulative toxicity without increasing OS (42). The data available suggests that treatment with carboplatin/etoposide is as effective a treatment as cisplatin/etoposide chemotherapy, and is routinely used to reduce the incidence of emesis, neuropathy, and nephropathy, thereby, capitalizing on its favorable therapeutic ratio (43,44).

The addition of a third chemotherapeutic to the standard two-drug platinum/etoposide combination has largely failed to demonstrate survival advantages without significantly increasing toxicity. Phase II trials adding paclitaxel to cisplatin or carboplatin plus etoposide were initially promising, but a subsequent phase III study established unacceptable toxicity without an improvement in survival (45). Similarly, randomized trials using alternating or sequential combination therapies have been unsuccessful in improving upon the efficacy of the platinum/etoposide standard. Various randomized trials have evaluated the role of higher-dose therapy when compared with conventional dose treatment in SCLC. Although higher RR and modest improvements in survival are seen, there have not been consistent findings to endorse this philosophy.

Additional combinations have been evaluated against platinum/etoposide. A small, phase III study conducted solely in Japanese patients by JCOG (JCOG 9511) demonstrated the superiority of a cisplatin/irinotecan combination over cisplatin/etoposide in patients with chemotherapy-naïve ES-SCLC with respect to RR, PFS, and OS (46). The trial was closed early at interim analysis, after accruing only 154 patients, since prospectively defined efficacy parameters were reached. Because of its small sample size and possible effects from pharmacogenomic differences between Japanese and North American populations,

further confirmatory studies were prompted. In a North American and Australian phase III trial, coordinated by the Hoosier Oncology Group, 331 patients were randomized to receive a modified dose-schedule of cisplatin/irinotecan or cisplatin/etoposide (47). The modified treatment regimens were intended to improve delivery, reduce toxicity, and to be more consistent with the dosages and schedules administered in the United States (48). In this trial, there were no differences in outcome between cisplatin/irinotecan and cisplatin/etoposide. Because of the differing dose schedules, questions remained regarding the validity of cisplatin/irinotecan as an optimal regimen for ES-SCLC.

Subsequently, the Southwest Oncology Group completed a confirmatory, appropriately powered trial (S0124) that was identical in design to the JCOG 9511 trial. S0124 used the same cisplatin/irinotecan and cisplatin/etoposide treatment doses and schedules as was used in JCOG 9511 to determine whether the results were relevant and reproducible to a Western population (49). Correlative studies were incorporated to seek out the possible role of population-related pharmacogenomic variability in irinotecan metabolism due to genetic polymorphisms. Over a 4-year period, 671 patients were randomized to receive a maximum of four cycles of either cisplatin 60 mg/m^2 on day 1 plus irinotecan 60 mg/m^2 on days 1, 8, and 15 every 28 days or cisplatin 30 mg/m^2 on day 1 plus etoposide 100 mg/m^2 on days 1 to 3 every 21 days. Patients were stratified based on performance status, number of metastatic sites, weight loss, and lactate dehydrogenase levels. The primary endpoint was OS. S0124 failed to confirm the positive results of JCOG 9511. In S0124, cisplatin/irinotecan efficacy outcomes were similar to cisplatin/etoposide with an overall response rate (ORR) of 60% versus 57% (P = 0.56), median PFS of 5.8 months versus 5.2 months (P = 0.07), and a median OS of 9.9 months versus 9.1 month (P = 0.71), respectively.

Evaluation of the adverse events between the S0124 and JCOG 9511 trials demonstrated a significantly higher hematologic toxicity in Japanese patients when compared to North American patients with either treatment regimen ($P \leq 0.02$), but the incidence of nonhematologic toxicities did not differ significantly. Of those enrolled in the S0124 trial, 142 patient samples were analyzed for pharmacogenetic variability of select genes in irinotecan metabolism performed on genomic DNA from peripheral blood mononuclear cells. Intriguingly, significant correlations for genetic polymorphisms and hematologic and gastrointestinal toxicities were found (50).

Thus, S0124 was unable to replicate the results of JCOG 9511 in a Western population. The presumed mechanisms underlying the differences in efficacy and toxicity are hypothesized to be related to allelic variants of genes involved in irinotecan metabolism and transport. In North America, platinum/etoposide remains the standard of care for previously untreated ES-SCLC.

Relapsed Disease

Unfortunately, SCLC recurs in the majority of patients after initial treatment. Although second-line chemotherapy can result in tumor regression, responses are short-lived and median survival is often less than 6 months (51). A key factor guiding the selection of future therapy, and its possible efficacy, is the type of response gained after exposure to a first-line platinum-based regimen. Traditionally, patients are classified into one of three groups of relapsed disease: platinum-sensitive, platinum-resistant, or refractory. Platinum-sensitivity is arbitrarily defined as a chemotherapy-free interval greater than 90 days, whereas platinum-resistant patients have recurrent disease within 90 days of completing chemotherapy (51,52). Refractory SCLC refers to those who do not respond to, or progress during, first-line chemotherapy. Platinum-resistant and refractory patients are often grouped together and generally have poor responses to subsequent chemotherapy (10% or less) and shorter median survivals than platinum-sensitive patients. While there is no standard second-line treatment option, a number of agents have shown single-agent activity, such as the camptothecin analogs (topotecan, irinotecan), paclitaxel, vinorelbine, and gemcitabine (51). Multiple-agent regimens, such as retreatment with platinum/etoposide, are also a common treatment choice for platinum-sensitive tumors. In the late 1990s, a randomized phase III trial for patients with recurrent SCLC compared single-agent parenteral topotecan with CAV and found topotecan to be equally efficacious, but with greater palliative effects on common lung cancer symptoms (53). Two phase III trials have shown the benefit of oral topotecan when compared with best supportive care and with similar efficacy to parenteral topotecan (54,55). Neutropenia is a notable adverse event, and alternative doses are frequently used to limit toxicity in clinical practice, including weekly dosing or daily dosing for 3 days (56). Topotecan, as a result of its U.S. Food and Drug Administration approval for second-line therapy in platinum-sensitive relapse, has emerged as the standard of comparison in most phase III clinical trials (32).

Prophylactic Cranial Irradiation in ES-SCLC

Although PCI has become a standard therapy for patients with LS-SCLC, the data indicating a benefit in patients in ES-SCLC had been lacking. However, PCI has now been incorporated into the treatment algorithm on the basis of results from a phase III clinical trial randomizing 286 ES-SCLC patients with any response to initial chemotherapy to either PCI or observation (57). At 1 year, PCI significantly reduced the incidence of symptomatic brain metastases (14.4% PCI-treated vs. 40.4% control; hazard ratio [HR] = 0.27, $P < 0.001$) and increased OS (27.1% PCI-treated vs. 13.3% control; HR = 0.68, $P = 0.003$). Median disease-free survival was significantly longer in the PCI-treated arm than in the control group (14.7 weeks vs. 12.0 weeks; $P = 0.02$), as was median OS (6.7 months vs. 5.4 months; $P = 0.003$). Indeed, this study has created a role for PCI in ES-SCLC patients who respond to first-line chemotherapy.

Novel Therapeutics: The Future of SCLC Management

The high proliferative index and unique biology of SCLC lends itself to the development of novel treatment strategies incorporating innovative cytotoxic and biologic therapeutics. Several randomized clinical trials have attempted to build upon the foundation of platinum/etoposide chemotherapy for ES-SCLC; however, this has been met with less than desirable results. For example, the additions of topotecan consolidation, paclitaxel, Bec2 vaccination, or thalidomide to the platinum/etoposide backbone have not shown significant survival benefit (42,45,58–60). Fortunately, sound preclinical rationale is leading to the development of a new array of therapeutics that are under investigation, such as the cytotoxic agent amrubicin, anti-Bcl-2 family protein inhibitors, and Hedgehog pathway inhibitors (Table 9.4). These three select agents will be briefly highlighted to illustrate current research endeavors in SCLC.

Amrubicin

Amrubicin is a cytotoxic agent that has shown activity in relapsed SCLC including platinum-resistant or refractory disease (61,62). It is a fully synthetic 9-aminoanthracycline which is converted to amrubicinol by reduction of the 13-position ketone, which has a higher antitumor activity than its parent molecule (62). It exerts its effects as a DNA topoisomerase II inhibitor and not primarily as a DNA intercalator, although it is classified as an anthracycline agent. Moreover, amrubicin has been found to be less cardiotoxic than doxorubicin in animal models (63). As a single agent, amrubicin has demonstrated activity in refractory and sensitive relapsed SCLC patients. In this particular phase II Japanese trial, the ORR was approximately 50% in each group, and the median PFS, median OS, and 1-year survivals in the refractory and sensitive groups were 2.6 months and 4.4 months, 10.3 months and 11.6 months, and 40% and 46%, respectively (61). In addition, a phase II randomized trial comparing amrubicin with topotecan in previously treated SCLC reiterated the positive results observed previously. Sixty patients, stratified according to performance status and type of relapse (chemotherapy sensitive or refractory), were randomly assigned to receive amrubicin (40 mg/m² days 1–3) or topotecan (1 mg/m² days 1–5) for a minimum of three 21-day cycles. The primary endpoint of ORR was 38% for the amrubicin arm and 13% in the topotecan arm (62). In sensitive relapse,

■ **Table 9.4** Selected novel therapeutic agents investigated in SCLC

Target and Class of Agent	Therapy
Angiogenesis pathway	
VEGF mAb	Bevacizumab
Multitargeted VEGFR TKI	Sorafenib
	Cediranib
	Vandetanib
Antiangiogenic agent	Thalidomide
Apoptotic pathway	
Antisense Bcl-2 oligonucleotide	Oblimersen
Bcl-2 small-molecule inhibitors	AT-101
	ABT-263
	Obatoclax
CD56 (neural cell adhesion molecule)	
Conjugated anti-CD56 mAb with DM1 (cytotoxic maytansinoid)	BB-10901
c-Kit pathway	
c-kit TKI	Imatinib
Cytotoxic agents	
Anthracycline derivative	Amrubicin
	INNO-206
Microtubule inhibitor	Vinflunine
EGFR pathway	
EGFR TKI	Gefitinib
Farnesyltransferase	
Farnesyltransferase inhibitor of Ras	Tipifarnib
Hedgehog pathway	
Synthetic Hedgehog inhibitor	GDC-0449
Multidrug resistance inhibitor	
Pgp and MRP-1 inhibitor	Biricodar
PI3K/AKT/PTEN pathway	
mTOR inhibitor	Everolimus
	Temsirolimus
Protein degradation	
Proteosome inhibitor	Bortezomib
Src kinase	
Src TKI	Dasatinib
	AZD0530
Tumor cell invasion and metastases	
Matrix metalloproteinase inhibitor	Marimastat
	Tanomastat
Tumor vaccine	
Wild-type p53 tumor suppressor	Autologous dendritic cell-adenovirus p53 vaccine
GD3 ganglioside	Mitumomab

AKT, V-akt murine thymoma viral oncogene homolog; EGFR, epidermal growth factor receptor; mAb, monoclonal antibody; MRP-1, multidrug resistance-associated protein; mTOR, mammalian target of rapamycin; Pgp, P-glycoprotein; PI3K, phosphatidylinositol 3 kinase; PTEN, phosphatase and tensin homolog; SCLC, small cell lung cancer; TKI, tyrosine kinase inhibitor; VEGF, vascular endothelial growth factor; VEGFR, vascular endothelial growth factor receptor.

the ORR for amrubicin compared with topotecan was 53% and 21%, and in refractory relapse, 17% and 0%, respectively. There were no significant advantages of either therapy in median PFS and OS. Neutropenia was severe for those treated with amrubicin with 93% of patients experiencing grade 3 or 4 neutropenia and 14% of patients with febrile neutropenia. Moreover, one treatment-related death was observed resulting from sepsis. Amrubicin is approved in Japan and is currently being investigated in the United States in chemotherapy-naive ES-SCLC patients and for those who do not respond to first-line therapy. Considerable hope exists for this agent, particularly in the chemotherapy-refractory setting, which has notoriously been difficult to treat.

Anti-Bcl-2 Family Protein Inhibitors

Apoptotic dysregulation is a common occurrence in many malignancies. The Bcl-2 family of proteins is a central regulator of apoptosis and is implicated in cell survival, tumorigenesis, and chemotherapy resistance, which is of particular importance in SCLC (64,65). To date, the Bcl-2 family is comprised of a total of 25 known gene products that are either proapoptotic or antiapoptotic (41). Overexpression of Bcl-2 has been reported in approximately 80% of SCLC tumors and, thus, forms the rationale of Bcl-2 as a prime therapeutic target (66,67). Strategies to inhibit Bcl-2 have included antisense oligonucleotides and small-molecule inhibitors.

Oblimersen, an antisense oligonucleotide to Bcl-2, has shown a lack of efficacy in a phase II randomized trial when combined with carboplatin/etoposide in untreated patients with ES-SCLC (68). In fact, median survival was worse for patients receiving oblimersen. It is hypothesized that the lack of efficacy may be related to insufficient suppression of Bcl-2 in vivo (41). Despite the negative results with this particular antisense oligonucleotide strategy, oral small-molecule inhibitors of Bcl-2 have shown initial promise (56). ABT-263, AT-101, and obatoclax are examples of such agents that are in phase I and/or phase II of clinical development.

Hedgehog Pathway Inhibitors

The Hedgehog (Hh) pathway is an essential embryonic signaling cascade implicated as an oncogenic catalyst in a variety of malignancies. This developmental pathway is known to regulate the proliferation of stem cell, and dysregulation has been associated with tumorigenesis (69). The transmembrane protein smoothened (Smo) is required for downstream activation of the Hh pathway transcriptional effectors Gli1, Gli2, and Gli3 (64). Patched, an inhibitory cell surface receptor, constitutively suppresses the activation of the Hh pathway by inhibiting Smo. The Patched ligands (Sonic, Indian, and Desert Hh) can individually bind to and inactivate Patched, suppressing Smo and causing pathway activation. In SCLC, persistent ligand-dependent activation of the Hg pathway occurs with elevated levels of expression of Sonic Hh ligand (64). Potent Hh inhibitors, such as cyclopamine, cause significant growth inhibition in vitro (70). The development of synthetic Hg inhibitors is an active area of research. GDC-0449 is an example of an orally bioavailable synthetic inhibitor of Hh signal transduction which has shown safety and clinical benefit in a phase I trial for patients with advanced solid tumors (71). Phase II studies with this compound are currently underway.

■ CONCLUSION

This chapter summarizes the evaluation and management of SCLC, while underscoring the importance of ongoing research efforts. Although the treatment for SCLC has not significantly changed over the last 2 decades, a sobering fact given the poor clinical outcomes, the future appears encouraging. The current SCLC research portfolio is focusing on answering relevant questions regarding the optimal delivery of known effective treatments, such as thoracic irradiation, while developing novel treatment strategies and therapeutics. As the biology and molecular mechanisms underlying SCLC tumorigenesis, proliferation, and chemotherapy resistance become unraveled, new targets are being discovered offering hope that a significant breakthrough will soon result.

■ REFERENCES

1. Jemal A, Siegel R, Ward E, Hao Y, Xu J, Thun MJ. Cancer statistics, 2009. *CA Cancer J Clin.* 2009;59(4):225–249.
2. Govindan R, Page N, Morgensztern D, et al. Changing epidemiology of small-cell lung cancer in the United States over the last 30 years: analysis of the surveillance, epidemiologic, and end results database. *J Clin Oncol.* 2006;24(28): 4539–4544.
3. Stupp R, Monnerat C, Turrisi AT 3rd, Perry MC, Leyvraz S. Small cell lung cancer: state of the art and future perspectives. *Lung Cancer.* 2004;45(1):105–117.
4. Hann CL, Ettinger DS. The change in pattern and pathology of small cell lung cancer. *American Society of Clinical Oncology 2009 Educational Book* 2009:451–454.
5. Brambilla E, Travis WD, Colby TV, Corrin B, Shimosato Y. The new World Health Organization classification of lung tumours. *Eur Respir J.* 2001;18(6):1059–1068.
6. DeVita Jr VT, Hellman S, Rosenberg SA, eds. *Cancer: Principles and Practice of Oncology, Lung Cancer.* Baltimore: Lippincott Williams & Wilkins; 2005;246–279.
7. Bensch KG, Corrin B, Pariente R, Spencer H. Oat-cell carcinoma of the lung. Its origin and relationship to bronchial carcinoid. *Cancer.* 1968;22(6):1163–1172.
8. Travis WD, Linnoila RI, Tsokos MG, et al. Neuroendocrine tumors of the lung with proposed criteria for large-cell neuroendocrine carcinoma. An ultrastructural, immunohistochemical, and flow cytometric study of 35 cases. *Am J Surg Pathol.* 1991;15(6):529–553.
9. Dalmau J, Furneaux HM, Gralla RJ, Kris MG, Posner JB. Detection of the anti-Hu antibody in the serum of patients with small cell lung cancer–a quantitative western blot analysis. *Ann Neurol.* 1990;27(5):544–552.
10. Meriney SD, Hulsizer SC, Lennon VA, Grinnell AD. Lambert-Eaton myasthenic syndrome immunoglobulins react with multiple types of calcium channels in small-cell lung carcinoma. *Ann Neurol.* 1996;40(5):739–749.
11. Vallières E, Shepherd FA, Crowley J, et al.; International Association for the Study of Lung Cancer International Staging Committee and Participating Institutions. The IASLC Lung Cancer Staging Project: proposals regarding the relevance of TNM in the pathologic staging of small cell lung cancer in the forthcoming (seventh) edition of the TNM classification for lung cancer. *J Thorac Oncol.* 2009;4(9):1049–1059.
12. Micke P, Faldum A, Metz T, et al. Staging small cell lung cancer: Veterans Administration Lung Study Group versus International Association for the Study of Lung Cancer–what limits limited disease? *Lung Cancer.* 2002;37(3):271–276.
13. Simon GR, Turrisi A; American College of Chest Physicians. Management of small cell lung cancer: ACCP evidence-based

clinical practice guidelines (2nd edition). *Chest.* 2007;132 (3 suppl):324S–339S.

14. Campling B, Quirt I, DeBoer G, Feld R, Shepherd FA, Evans WK. Is bone marrow examination in small-cell lung cancer really necessary? *Ann Intern Med.* 1986;105(4):508–512.

15. Simon G, Ginsberg RJ, Ruckdeschel JC. Small-cell lung cancer. *Chest Surg Clin N Am.* 2001;11(1):165–88, ix.

16. Higgins GA, Shields TW, Keehn RJ. The solitary pulmonary nodule. Ten-year follow-up of veterans administration-armed forces cooperative study. *Arch Surg.* 1975;110(5):570–575.

17. Lennox SC, Flavell G, Pollock DJ, Thompson VC, Wilkins JL. Results of resection for oat-cell carcinoma of the lung. *Lancet.* 1968;2(7575):925–927.

18. Shields TW, Higgins GA Jr, Matthews MJ, Keehn RJ. Surgical resection in the management of small cell carcinoma of the lung. *J Thorac Cardiovasc Surg.* 1982;84(4):481–488.

19. Miyazawa N, Tsuchiya R, Naruke T, et al. A clinico-pathological study of surgical treatment for small cell carcinoma of the lung. *Jpn J Clin Oncol.* 1986;16(3):297–307.

20. Aupérin A, Arriagada R, Pignon JP, et al. Prophylactic cranial irradiation for patients with small-cell lung cancer in complete remission. Prophylactic Cranial Irradiation Overview Collaborative Group. *N Engl J Med.* 1999;341(7):476–484.

21. Lad T, Piantadosi S, Thomas P, Payne D, Ruckdeschel J, Giaccone G. A prospective randomized trial to determine the benefit of surgical resection of residual disease following response of small cell lung cancer to combination chemotherapy. *Chest.* 1994;106(6 suppl):320S–323S.

22. Inoue M, Nakagawa K, Fujiwara K, Fukuhara K, Yasumitsu T. Results of preoperative mediastinoscopy for small cell lung cancer. *Ann Thorac Surg.* 2000;70(5):1620–1623.

23. Sundstrøm S, Bremnes RM, Kaasa S, et al.; Norwegian Lung Cancer Study Group. Cisplatin and etoposide regimen is superior to cyclophosphamide, epirubicin, and vincristine regimen in small-cell lung cancer: results from a randomized phase III trial with 5 years' follow-up. *J Clin Oncol.* 2002;20(24): 4665–4672.

24. Pignon JP, Arriagada R, Ihde DC, et al. A meta-analysis of thoracic radiotherapy for small-cell lung cancer. *N Engl J Med.* 1992;327(23):1618–1624.

25. Warde P, Payne D. Does thoracic irradiation improve survival and local control in limited-stage small-cell carcinoma of the lung? A meta-analysis. *J Clin Oncol.* 1992;10(6):890–895.

26. Murray N, Coy P, Pater JL, et al. Importance of timing for thoracic irradiation in the combined modality treatment of limited-stage small-cell lung cancer. The National Cancer Institute of Canada Clinical Trials Group. *J Clin Oncol.* 1993;11(2):336–344.

27. Fried DB, Morris DE, Poole C, et al. Systematic review evaluating the timing of thoracic radiation therapy in combined modality therapy for limited-stage small-cell lung cancer. *J Clin Oncol.* 2004;22(23):4837–4845.

28. Perry MC, Eaton WL, Propert KJ, et al. Chemotherapy with or without radiation therapy in limited small-cell carcinoma of the lung. *N Engl J Med.* 1987;316(15):912–918.

29. Takada M, Fukuoka M, Kawahara M, et al. Phase III study of concurrent versus sequential thoracic radiotherapy in combination with cisplatin and etoposide for limited-stage small-cell lung cancer: results of the Japan Clinical Oncology Group Study 9104. *J Clin Oncol.* 2002;20(14):3054–3060.

30. De Ruysscher D, Pijls-Johannesma M, Vansteenkiste J, Kester A, Rutten I, Lambin P. Systematic review and meta-analysis of randomised, controlled trials of the timing of chest radiotherapy in patients with limited-stage, small-cell lung cancer. *Ann Oncol.* 2006;17(4):543–552.

31. Choi NC, Herndon JE 2nd, Rosenman J, et al. Phase I study to determine the maximum-tolerated dose of radiation in standard daily and hyperfractionated-accelerated twice-daily radiation schedules with concurrent chemotherapy for limited-stage small-cell lung cancer. *J Clin Oncol.* 1998;16(11):3528–3536.

32. Lally BE, Urbanic JJ, Blackstock AW, Miller AA, Perry MC. Small cell lung cancer: have we made any progress over the last 25 years? *Oncologist.* 2007;12(9):1096–1104.

33. Bogart JA, Herndon JE 2nd, Lyss AP, et al.; Cancer and Leukemia Group B study 39808. 70 Gy thoracic radiotherapy is feasible concurrent with chemotherapy for limited-stage small-cell lung cancer: analysis of Cancer and Leukemia Group B study 39808. *Int J Radiat Oncol Biol Phys.* 2004;59(2):460–468.

34. Turrisi AT 3rd, Kim K, Blum R, et al. Twice-daily compared with once-daily thoracic radiotherapy in limited small-cell lung cancer treated concurrently with cisplatin and etoposide. *N Engl J Med.* 1999;340(4):265–271.

35. Komaki R, Swann RS, Ettinger DS, et al. Phase I study of thoracic radiation dose escalation with concurrent chemotherapy for patients with limited small-cell lung cancer: Report of Radiation Therapy Oncology Group (RTOG) protocol 97–12. *Int J Radiat Oncol Biol Phys.* 2005;62(2):342–350.

36. Komaki R, Moughan J, Ettinger D, et al. Toxicities in a phase II study of accelerated high dose thoracic radiation therapy (TRT) with concurrent chemotherapy for limited small cell lung cancer (LSCLC) (RTOG 0239) [abstract 7717]. *J Clin Oncol.* 2007;25.

37. Seute T, Leffers P, Wilmink JT, ten Velde GP, Twijnstra A. Response of asymptomatic brain metastases from small-cell lung cancer to systemic first-line chemotherapy. *J Clin Oncol.* 2006;24(13):2079–2083.

38. Hirsch FR, Paulson OB, Hansen HH, Vraa-Jensen J. Intracranial metastases in small cell carcinoma of the lung: correlation of clinical and autopsy findings. *Cancer.* 1982;50(11):2433–2437.

39. Le Pechoux C, Hatton M, Kobierska A, et al. Randomized trial of standard dose to a higher dose prophylactic cranial irradiation (PCI) in limited-stage small cell cancer (SCLC) complete responders (CR): primary endpoint analysis (PCI99–01, IFCT 99–01, EORTC 22003–08004, RTOG 0212) [abstr LBA7514]. *J Clin Oncol.* 2008;26.

40. Jackman DM, Johnson BE. Small-cell lung cancer. *Lancet.* 2005;366(9494):1385–1396.

41. Rossi A, Maione P, Palazzolo G, et al. New targeted therapies and small-cell lung cancer. *Clin Lung Cancer.* 2008;9(5):271–279.

42. Schiller JH, Adak S, Cella D, DeVore RF 3rd, Johnson DH. Topotecan versus observation after cisplatin plus etoposide in extensive-stage small-cell lung cancer: E7593–a phase III trial of the Eastern Cooperative Oncology Group. *J Clin Oncol.* 2001;19(8):2114–2122.

43. Skarlos DV, Samantas E, Kosmidis P, et al. Randomized comparison of etoposide-cisplatin vs. etoposide-carboplatin and irradiation in small-cell lung cancer. A Hellenic Co-operative Oncology Group study. *Ann Oncol.* 1994;5(7):601–607.

44. Lassen U, Kristjansen PE, Osterlind K, et al. Superiority of cisplatin or carboplatin in combination with teniposide and vincristine in the induction chemotherapy of small-cell lung cancer. A randomized trial with 5 years follow up. *Ann Oncol.* 1996;7(4):365–371.

45. Niell HB, Herndon JE 2nd, Miller AA, et al.; Cancer and Leukemia Group. Randomized phase III intergroup trial of etoposide and cisplatin with or without paclitaxel and granulocyte colony-stimulating factor in patients with extensive-stage small-cell lung cancer: Cancer and Leukemia Group B Trial 9732. *J Clin Oncol.* 2005;23(16):3752–3759.

46. Noda K, Nishiwaki Y, Kawahara M, et al.; Japan Clinical Oncology Group. Irinotecan plus cisplatin compared with etoposide plus cisplatin for extensive small-cell lung cancer. *N Engl J Med.* 2002;346(2):85–91.

47. Hanna N, Bunn PA Jr, Langer C, et al. Randomized phase III trial comparing irinotecan/cisplatin with etoposide/cisplatin in patients with previously untreated extensive-stage disease small-cell lung cancer. *J Clin Oncol.* 2006;24(13):2038–2043.

48. Sher T, Dy GK, Adjei AA. Small cell lung cancer. *Mayo Clin Proc.* 2008;83(3):355–367.

49. Lara PN Jr, Natale R, Crowley J, et al. Phase III trial of irinotecan/cisplatin compared with etoposide/cisplatin in extensive-stage

small-cell lung cancer: clinical and pharmacogenomic results from SWOG S0124. *J Clin Oncol*. 2009;27(15):2530–2535.

50. Lara PN, Redman M, Lenz HJ, et al. Cisplatin (Cis)/etoposide (VP16) compared to cis/irinotecan (CPT11) in extensive-stage small cell lung cancer (E-SCLC): pharmacogenomic (PG) and comparative toxicity analysis of JCOG 9511 and SWOG 0124 [abstract 7524]. *J Clin Oncol*. 2007;25.

51. Davies AM, Evans WK, Mackay JA, Shepherd FA. Treatment of recurrent small cell lung cancer. *Hematol Oncol Clin North Am*. 2004;18(2):387–416.

52. Sangha R, Lara PN Jr, Adjei AA, et al. Cooperative group research endeavors in small-cell lung cancer: current and future directions. *Clin Lung Cancer*. 2009;10(5):322–330.

53. von Pawel J, Schiller JH, Shepherd FA, et al. Topotecan versus cyclophosphamide, doxorubicin, and vincristine for the treatment of recurrent small-cell lung cancer. *J Clin Oncol*. 1999;17(2):658–667.

54. Eckardt JR, von Pawel J, Pujol JL, et al. Phase III study of oral compared with intravenous topotecan as second-line therapy in small-cell lung cancer. *J Clin Oncol*. 2007;25(15):2086–2092.

55. O'Brien ME, Ciuleanu TE, Tsekov H, et al. Phase III trial comparing supportive care alone with supportive care with oral topotecan in patients with relapsed small-cell lung cancer. *J Clin Oncol*. 2006;24(34):5441–5447.

56. Allen J, Jahanzeb M. Extensive-stage small-cell lung cancer: evolution of systemic therapy and future directions. *Clin Lung Cancer*. 2008;9(5):262–270.

57. Slotman B, Faivre-Finn C, Kramer G, et al.; EORTC Radiation Oncology Group and Lung Cancer Group. Prophylactic cranial irradiation in extensive small-cell lung cancer. *N Engl J Med*. 2007;357(7):664–672.

58. Gandara DR, Lara PN Jr, Natale R, Belani C. Progress in small-cell lung cancer: the lowest common denominator. *J Clin Oncol*. 2008;26(26):4236–4238.

59. Giaccone G, Debruyne C, Felip E, et al. Phase III study of adjuvant vaccination with Bec2/bacille Calmette-Guerin in responding patients with limited-disease small-cell lung cancer (European Organisation for Research and Treatment of Cancer 08971–08971B; Silva Study). *J Clin Oncol*. 2005;23(28):6854–6864.

60. Pujol JL, Breton JL, Gervais R, et al. Phase III double-blind, placebo-controlled study of thalidomide in extensive-disease small-cell lung cancer after response to chemotherapy: an intergroup study FNCLCC cleo04 IFCT 00–01. *J Clin Oncol*. 2007;25(25):3945–3951.

61. Onoda S, Masuda N, Seto T, et al.; Thoracic Oncology Research Group Study 0301. Phase II trial of amrubicin for treatment of refractory or relapsed small-cell lung cancer: Thoracic Oncology Research Group Study 0301. *J Clin Oncol*. 2006;24(34):5448–5453.

62. Inoue A, Sugawara S, Yamazaki K, et al. Randomized phase II trial comparing amrubicin with topotecan in patients with previously treated small-cell lung cancer: North Japan Lung Cancer Study Group Trial 0402. *J Clin Oncol*. 2008;26(33):5401–5406.

63. Suzuki T, Minamide S, Iwasaki T, Yamamoto H, Kanda H. Cardiotoxicity of a new anthracycline derivative (SM-5887) following intravenous administration to rabbits: comparative study with doxorubicin. *Invest New Drugs*. 1997;15(3):219–225.

64. Johnson BE, Rudin CM, Salgia R. Novel and targeted agents for small cell lung cancer. *American Society of Clinical Oncology 2008 Educational Book*. 2008:363–367.

65. Adams JM, Cory S. The Bcl-2 apoptotic switch in cancer development and therapy. *Oncogene*. 2007;26(9):1324–1337.

66. Jiang SX, Sato Y, Kuwao S, Kameya T. Expression of bcl-2 oncogene protein is prevalent in small cell lung carcinomas. *J Pathol*. 1995;177(2):135–138.

67. Ikegaki N, Katsumata M, Minna J, Tsujimoto Y. Expression of bcl-2 in small cell lung carcinoma cells. *Cancer Res*. 1994;54(1):6–8.

68. Rudin CM, Salgia R, Wang X, et al. Randomized phase II Study of carboplatin and etoposide with or without the bcl-2 antisense oligonucleotide oblimersen for extensive-stage small-cell lung cancer: CALGB 30103. *J Clin Oncol*. 2008;26(6):870–876.

69. Subramanian J, Govindan R. Small cell, big problem! Stem cells, root cause? *Clin Lung Cancer*. 2008;9(5):252–253.

70. Watkins DN, Berman DM, Burkholder SG, Wang B, Beachy PA, Baylin SB. Hedgehog signalling within airway epithelial progenitors and in small-cell lung cancer. *Nature*. 2003;422(6929):313–317.

71. LoRusso PM, Rudin CM, Borad MJ, et al. A first-in-human, first-in-class, phase (ph) I study of systemic Hedgehog (Hh) pathway antagonist, GDC-0449, in patients (pts) with advanced solid tumors [abstract 3516]. *J Clin Oncol*. 2008;26.

10

Stages IB to IIIA NSCLC: The Case for Induction versus Adjuvant Chemotherapy

STEPHANIE L. GRAFF

KAREN KELLY

Patients with resectable non–small cell lung cancer (NSCLC) have an opportunity to be cured with 5-year survival rates ranging from 73% for patients with pathologic stage IA disease to 24% for patients with pathologic stage IIIA disease (1). The inability to cure more patients is the result of distant failure rather than local recurrence. This failure pattern suggests that micrometastatic disease is present at the time of diagnosis. Thus, the use of systemic chemotherapy to eradicate micrometastases with the hope of increasing the cure rate deserves investigation. This chapter will critically review the results from randomized trials evaluating chemotherapy given after surgery (adjuvant chemotherapy), before surgery (induction chemotherapy), or, in rare instances, both (perioperative chemotherapy), followed by a discussion on optimizing systemic treatment.

■ ADJUVANT CHEMOTHERAPY

The evaluation of adjuvant chemotherapy after surgical resection for early-stage lung cancer began its arduous journey in the 1960s. After 30 years and numerous randomized trials, no survival benefit for adjuvant treatment was observed. To better understand the issues surrounding the role of adjuvant chemotherapy, the Non-Small Cell Lung Cancer Collaborative Group conducted a meta-analysis based on individual patient data (2). It revealed that the early randomized trials using alkylating agents were detrimental producing a hazard ratio (HR) for death of 1.15. After the introduction of cisplatin-based regimens, the meta-analysis noted a favorable effect with an HR of 0.87 ($P = 0.08$). Although not statistically significant, this data spurred investigators to continue to pursue adjuvant therapy. Subsequently, several large randomized clinical trials have been conducted and their data published.

The first trial reported in this century was the North American Intergroup Trial INT01159 (3). This trial was designed to evaluate the role of adjuvant cisplatin and etoposide, when added to postoperative radiation versus radiation alone, in patients with stage II and III NSCLC. A total of 488 patients were enrolled in the study. There was no difference in overall survival (OS) between the two arms. The median survival for the chemotherapy plus radiation arm was 38 months compared with 39 months for patients assigned to radiation alone ($P = 0.56$). The risk of recurrence was also not diminished for the bimodality arm at 0.98. In retrospect, the routine use of postoperative radiotherapy (PORT), as mandated in this study, was abandoned in 1998 when the PORT meta-analysis showed it produced a harmful effect (4).

In the United Kingdom, the Big Lung Trial (BLT) set out to corroborate the results of the meta-analysis by exploring three cycles of a variety of cisplatin-based adjuvant regimens versus observation in 381 patients with resected stage I–III NSCLC (5). This study was underpowered and unable to show a survival benefit for chemotherapy with an HR of 1.02; 95% confidence interval (CI) 0.77 to 1.35; $P = 0.90$.

In 2003, the first report from a series of large, mature adjuvant trials was released (Table 10.1). Adjuvant Lung Project Italy (ALPI) unfortunately failed to demonstrate a survival benefit for chemotherapy (6). In this study, 1,209 patients with stage I, II, and IIIA NSCLC were randomized to receive chemotherapy with mitomycin C, vindesine, and cisplatin every 21 days for three cycles versus no therapy after complete surgical resection. Optional chest radiation was allowed. There was no statistically significant benefit in OS or progression-free survival (PFS) between the two groups (HR 0.96; 95% CI, 0.81–1.13; $P = 0.589$ and HR 0.89; 95% CI 0.76–1.03; $P = 0.128$, respectively). Poor compliance with chemotherapy was thought to contribute to the negative result with 69% of patients completing the planned treatment, but half required dose modifications, and 48 patients (9%) did not receive any chemotherapy (7). Furthermore, a significant number of patients (43%) received postoperative radiation that may have masked a potential benefit from the systemic therapy. One intriguing observation was seen in a subgroup analysis by stage whereby patients with stage II disease receiving chemotherapy had a PFS and OS survival benefit of 10% at

■ **Table 10.1** Phase III trials of adjuvant chemotherapy in resectable NSCLC

Study	Stage	No. of Patients	Treatment	Median OS	5-Year OS	HR (95% CI)	*P* Value
ALPI	I–IIIA	603	Observation	48.0 months	NR	0.96	*P* = 0.589
2003		606	MVP	55.2 months	NR	(0.81–1.13)	
IALT	I–III	935	Observation	NR	40%	0.91	*P* = 0.10
2004		932	Cisplatin-doublets	NR	45%	(0.81–1.02)	
JBR 10	IB–II	240	Observation	73.0 months	56%	0.78	*P* = 0.04
2005		242	VNR/P	94.0 months	67%	(0.62–0.99)	
ANITA	IB–IIIA	433	Observation	43.7 months	43%	0.80	*P* = 0.017
2006		407	VNR/P	65.7 months	51%	(0.66–0.96)	
CALGB 9633	IB	171	Observation	78.0 months	43%	0.83	*P* = 0.12
2008		173	PC	95.0 months	47%	(0.64–1.08)	

Cisplatin-doublets: Cisplatin, Etoposide; Vinorelbine, Cisplatin; Vinblastine, Cisplatin; Vindesine, Cisplatin; MVP: Mitomycin C, Vindesine, Cisplatin; VNR/P: Vinorelbine, Cisplatin; PC: Paclitaxel, Carboplatin.

ALPI, Adjuvant Lung Project Italy; ANITA, Adjuvant Navelbine International Trialist Association; CALGB, Cancer and Leukemia Group B; HR, hazard ratio; IALT, International Adjuvant Lung Cancer Trial; NR, not reported; OS, overall survival.

5 years (HR 0.78; 95% CI 0.60–1.03 and 0.80; 95% CI 0.60–1.06, respectively) although this was not statistically significant (7).

The first trial to demonstrate a survival advantage for adjuvant chemotherapy was the International Adjuvant Lung Cancer Trial Cooperative Group (IALT) study (8). This trial enrolled 1,867 patients; 932 patients were randomized to receive chemotherapy (cisplatin plus etoposide, vinorelbine, vinblastine, or vindesine every 21 days for 3–4 cycles), and 935 patients were randomized to observation. Postoperative radiation therapy was allowed. The 5-year OS rate significantly favored the chemotherapy arm (HR 0.86; 95% CI 0.76–0.98; *P* < 0.03). Disease-free survival (DFS) was also superior in the treated arm (HR 0.83; 95% CI 0.74–0.94; *P* = 0.003). With longer follow-up of 8 years the HR for OS was not significant (NS) (HR 91; 95% CI 0.81–1.02; *P* = 0.10) while the HR for DFS retained significance (HR 0.88; 95% CI 0.78–0.98; *P* = 0.02) (9). The loss of the OS benefit was thought to be due to a higher rate of noncancer-related deaths in the chemotherapy arm (HR 1.34; *P* = 0.06), raising the possibility of a latent harmful effect from treatment.

In 2005, the National Cancer Institute of Canada Cancer Treatment Group reported the results of JBR10 (10). Patients with completely resected stage IB or stage II NSCLC were randomized to receive cisplatin plus vinorelbine for 16 weeks (242 patients) or observation (240 patients). An impressive OS benefit was observed for the treated group (HR 0.69; 95% CI 0.52–0.91; *P* = 0.04) corresponding to an absolute survival improvement of 15%. In a subgroup analysis, the survival benefit was restricted to patients with stage II disease. An update of this study, with >9 years of follow up, was recently

presented and continued to show a survival benefit for the treated group with an absolute improvement in the 5-year OS rate of 11% (67% vs. 56%, respectively) with a HR of 0.78; 95% CI 0.62 to 0.99; *P* = 0.04 (11). In contrast to the updated IALT data, there was no difference in the incidence of death from other causes between the two arms (*P* = 0.62). Patients with stage II disease continued to derive the maximal benefit with a 5-year OS rate of 59% for the chemotherapy group compared with 44% for the observation group (HR 0.68; 95% CI 0.50–0.92; *P* = 0.01). An additional analysis of patients with stage IB disease with tumors <4 cm or ≥4 cm revealed that those patients with smaller tumors did not benefit from adjuvant therapy (HR 1.73; 95% CI 0.98–3.04; *P* = 0.07). Median 5-year OS rates were 73% for chemotherapy and 79% for observation. Treated patients with tumors ≥4 cm had a favorable 5-year OS rate of 79% compared with 59% for untreated patients (HR 0.66; 95% CI 0.39–1.14; *P* = 0.13). The positive data from these two studies led to the widespread adoption of adjuvant chemotherapy, especially in patients with stage II and IIIA disease.

Subsequently, the results from the Adjuvant Navelbine International Trialist Association (ANITA) trial solidified the role of adjuvant systemic treatment (12). A total of 840 patients with stage IB, II, and IIIA were randomized to cisplatin plus vinorelbine for 16 weeks versus observation. The HR for death was significantly lower for the chemotherapy group (HR = 0.80, 95% CI 0.66–0.96; *P* = 0.017). The 5- and 7-year OS was improved by 8.6% and 8.4% in the chemotherapy group, respectively. No benefit was seen in the subset of patients with stage IB disease (HR 1.10; 95% CI 0.76–1.57; *P* = NS). In an unplanned retrospective analysis evaluating the value of postoperative chest radiation, there was a determintal effect in the overall population with HR of 1.34 (95% CI 1.10 - 1.63; p - 0.003) (13). However patients with N2 disease benefited from the addition of radiation. Patients receiving PORT after chemotherapy had a 5-year OS rate of 47.4% compared with a 5-year OS rate of 34% for patients treated with chemotherapy alone. N2 patients receiving PORT on the observation arm also had an improved 5-year OS rate of 21.3% compared with 16.6%. Patients with N1 disease were harmed if they received PORT after chemotherapy. The 5-year OS rate was 40% with PORT versus 56.3% if no PORT was given. In contrast, N1 patients on the observation arm benefited from PORT with a 5-year OS rate of 42.6% versus 31.4% without PORT. This limited data suggest that PORT should be prospectively evaluated in resected N2 disease.

The only U.S. study addressing the role of adjuvant treatment was the Cancer and Leukemia Group B (CALGB) trial 9633, conducted in stage IB patients (14). The goal was to randomize 384 patients to four cycles of carboplatin and paclitaxel after surgery versus surgery alone. The trial closed early due to poor accrual with 344 patients enrolled. The preliminary data presented in 2004 reported a survival benefit at 4 years for patients receiving chemotherapy but with a more mature follow up of 74 months, OS was not significantly different between the two groups (HR 0.83; 95% CI 0.64–1.08; P = 0.12). Nor was there a significant improvement in DFS. However, there was an encouraging finding in an unplanned subgroup analysis based on tumor size, whereby a survival advantage for paclitaxel and carboplatin was seen in patients who had tumors ≥4 cm (HR 0.69; 95% CI 0.48–0.99; P = 0.043).

To identify which patients might have the greatest benefit from adjuvant chemotherapy, the Lung Adjuvant Cisplatin Evaluation (LACE) meta-analysis was conducted (15). Individual patient data were collected and pooled from 4,584 patients in five trials (BLT, ALPI, IALT, JBR10, and ANITA). The HR of death was 0.89; 95% CI 0.82 to 0.96; P = 0.005, which corresponded to a 5-year absolute survival benefit of 5.4% with chemotherapy. This benefit varied with stage of disease and was not seen for stage IA patients. The HR for stage IA disease was 1.40 (95% CI 0.95–2.06), for IB 0.93 (95% CI 0.78–1.10), for stage II 0.83 (95% CI 0.73–0.95), and for stage III 0.83 (95% CI 0.72–0.94). A positive chemotherapy effect was seen in patients with performance status (PS) 0 to 1, whereas chemotherapy was potentially harmful for patients with a PS of 2. Other subgroups analyzed including age, sex, histology, type of surgical resection, planned radiation, dose of cisplatin, or the second agent used did not affect OS or DFS. As a note of caution, a 1.4% excess in noncancer-related deaths occurred in the pooled chemotherapy group after 5 years.

Since the majority of patients diagnosed with lung cancer are 70 years or older, an additional analysis of the LACE data set by age was conducted (16). Elderly

patients, defined as 70 years or older, accounted for 9% of the patients. Their HR of death was better with treatment at 0.90 (95% CI 0.74–1.16) and was similar to the HR of death for treated patients younger than 65 years at 0.86 (95% CI 0.78–0.94). Patients between 65 and 69 years did not show a treatment effect with an HR of 1.10 (95% CI 0.85–1.21), but this subgroup was noted to have multiple unfavorable patient characteristics compared with the other two groups that may have contributed to the lack of benefit. Elderly patients achieved a survival benefit despite having received lower cisplatin doses and fewer number of chemotherapy cycles than their younger counterparts. Older patients died more frequently from noncancer causes at 22% compared with 19% for patients older than 65 to 69 years and 12% for patients younger than 65 years.

In Japan, the oral agent UFT (uracil/tegafur) has been extensively studied as an adjuvant treatment. The most notable trial was the randomized phase III study of UFT daily for 2 years or observation for patients with pathologic stage I adenocarcinoma (17). Nine hundred and ninety-nine patients were enrolled in the study. Patients receiving UFT had a superior survival time and an HR of death of 0.71 (95% CI 0.53 to 0.98; P = 0.04). This benefit was limited to the patients with stage IB disease (HR 0.48; 95% CI 0.29–0.81; P = 0.005). Overall six randomized trials have been conducted with UFT versus observation in predominantly pathologic stage I NSCLC patients. A meta-analysis of these trials with 2,003 patients revealed the 5- and 7-year survival rate was higher for the treated groups (18). The pooled HR was 0.74 (95% CI 0.61 to 0.88; P = 0.001). UFT is approved in Japan for adjuvant treatment but is not available in the United States.

■ INDUCTION CHEMOTHERAPY

Enthusiasm for induction chemotherapy has multiple potential advantages over adjuvant chemotherapy. It provides the earliest possible attack on micrometastases, could increase treatment compliance, and could lead to higher resectability rates. Initial studies were conducted in patients with stage III NSCLC. Roth et al. (19) randomized 60 stage IIIA patients to perioperative chemotherapy (n = 28) versus surgery alone (n = 32). The trial was terminated early following an unplanned interim analysis that revealed a substantial treatment effect with chemotherapy. Patients randomized to perioperative chemotherapy received three cycles of cyclophosphamide, etoposide, and cisplatin followed by surgery. Patients with ≥35% radiographic tumor regression were eligible to receive three additional cycles of chemotherapy after surgery. Patients treated with perioperative chemotherapy had an estimated median survival of 64 months compared with 11 months for patients who had surgery alone ($P < 0.008$). Reanalysis of the study with a follow-up time of 82 months revealed the median survival for the chemotherapy group was still prolonged at 21 months with a 5-year OS rate of 36% compared with a median survival of 14 months and a 5-year OS rate of 15% for the surgery-alone arm (20).

A similar study conducted in Spain randomized 60 stage IIIA patients to induction chemotherapy with mitomycin, ifosfamide, and cisplatin (MIP) for three cycles followed by surgery and mediastinal radiation or surgery followed by radiation therapy (21). The median survival increased from 8 months (95% CI 7–10) in the control arm to 26 months (95% CI 16–34) in the chemotherapy arm ($P < 0.001$). The HR of death was 5; (95% CI 2 to 17) for the surgery-alone arm. Median DFS was 5 months (95% CI 4–7) and 20 months (95% CI 12–30) in the control and chemotherapy arms respectively ($P < 0.001$). At 7 years the median survival was 22 months (95% CI 13.4–30.6) in the chemotherapy arm as compared with 10 months (95% CI 7.4–12.6) in the control arm ($P = 0.005$) (22). Interestingly, at 5 years 17% of the chemotherapy-treated patients were alive versus no patients in the surgery-alone group.

The exceptional results from these two small randomized trials led to larger randomized phase III trials (Table 10.2). Our French colleagues evaluated preoperative MIP in patients with stage IB–IIIA NSCLC (23). Three hundred and fifty-five patients were randomized to two cycles of MIP followed by surgery or surgery alone. Two additional cycles of MIP were given postoperatively to responsive patients. Radiation therapy was administered to patients with pT3 or pN2 disease in both arms. The median survival was 37 months (95% CI 26.7–48.3)

in the MIP arm and 26 months (95% CI 19.8–33.6) in the control arm ($P = 0.15$). At 4 years the survival rate was 44% (95% CI 36–51) versus 35% (95% CI 28–42) respectively. The HR of death for the induction arm was 0.78 (95% CI 0.60–1.02). DFS strongly favored chemotherapy with a median DFS time of 27.6 months (95% CI 17.3–39.8) compared with 12.9 months (95% CI 10–12.6). The relative risk (RR) of recurrence or death for patients receiving MIP was 0.76 (95% CI 0.59–0.98; $P = 0.033$). A treatment interaction by nodal status was observed with N0–1 patients having a survival benefit with chemotherapy (RR 0.68; 95% CI 0.49–0.96; $P = 0.027$) whereas no survival advantage was seen in patients with N2 disease treated with induction MIP. A concern that chemotherapy would increase surgical complication rates was not substantiated. The postoperative mortality rates were 6.7% in the MIP group and 4.5% in the surgery group ($P = 0.38$).

In the United States the multi-institutional Bimodality Lung Oncology Team evaluated the feasability of administering paclitaxel and carboplatin in the perioperative period (two cycles before surgery and three cycles after surgery) for patients with stage IB–IIIA NSCLC (24). Ninety-four patients entered into this pilot study. The objective response rate to induction chemotherapy was 56%. Overall, the chemotherapy was well tolerated and only two postoperative deaths were reported. Compliance with the induction chemotherapy was high at 96%, but only 45% of patients received adjuvant therapy. The 5-year OS rate was 42% (25).

Based on these results, the Southwest Oncology Group (SWOG) launched S9900 comparing surgery alone with three cycles of induction paclitaxel and carboplatin

■ **Table 10.2**　Phase III studies of induction chemotherapy in resectable NSCLC

Study	Stage	No. of Patients	Treatment	Median OS	5-Year OS	HR (95% CI)	P Value
Depierre 2002	I–IIIA	186	Surgery	26.0 months	35% (4 years)	0.78 (0.60–1.02)	0.15
		187	MIC→Surgery	37.0 months	44% (4 years)		
SWOG 9900 2007	IB–IIIA	167	Surgery	75.0 months	50%	0.81 (0.6–1.1)	0.19
		169	PC→Surgery	46.0 months	43%		
LU 22 2007	I–III	261	Surgery	55.0 months	45%	1.02 (0.80–1.3)	0.86
		258	MIC, MVP, NP→Surgery	54.0 months	44%		
ChEST 2008	IB–IIIA (T3N1)	141	Surgery	4.8 years	60% (3 years)	0.63 (0.42–0.93)	0.005
		129	GC→Surgery	NR	67% (3 years)		
NATCH 2009	IA (>2 cm), IB II IIIA (T3N1)	210	Surgery	48.8 months	44%		
		199	PC→Surgery	55.2 months	47%	0.96 (0.84–1.1)	0.56
		210	Surgery→PC	50.2 months	46%	0.99 (0.75–1.3)	0.93

GC: gemcitabine, cisplatin; MIC: mitomycin, ifosfamide, cisplatin; MVP: mitomycin C, vindesine, cisplatin; NP: vinorelbine, cisplatin; PC: paclitaxel, carboplatin.

HR, hazard ratio; NR: not reported; OS, overall survival.

followed by surgery in patients with clinical stage T2N0, T1–2N1, and T3N0–1 NSCLC (26,27). This trial closed prematurely with 354 patients due to slow accrual, after adjuvant chemotherapy was shown to be beneficial. Seventy-nine percent of patients completed the drug regimen, and 41% of patients had a major radiographic response. Updated survival with a median follow-up time of 53 months revealed that OS and PFS continued to favor the chemotherapy arm (27). The median OS was 75 months for the chemotherapy arm and 46 months for the surgical-alone arm with a 5-year OS rate of 50% and 43% respectively (HR 0.81; 95% CI 0.60–1.10; $P = 0.19$). The median and 5-year PFS was 33 months and 42% for patients receiving paclitaxel and carboplatin compared with 21 months and 32% for patients who did not receive chemotherapy (HR 0.77; 95% CI 0.59–1.02; $P = 0.07$).

A similarly designed phase III trial conducted by our Scandinavian colleagues (28) was closed prematurely because of slow accrual. A total of 90 patients were enrolled; 44 patients were randomized to induction paclitaxel and carboplatin followed by surgery, and 46 patients were randomized to surgery alone. A nonsignificant increase in the median survival time and 5-year survival rate was seen for induction therapy at 34.4 months and 36% compared with 22.5 months and 24% respectively, for resection alone.

A large European trial (LU 22) randomized patients to three cycles of a platinum-based chemotherapy regimen followed by surgery versus surgery alone in patients with resectable stage I–III NSCLC (29). Due to the standard use of adjuvant chemotherapy, the study closed with 519 of 600 planned patients randomized. Seventy-five percent of patients received three cycles of chemotherapy and 49% achieved an objective response. OS was not different between the arms (HR 1.02; 95% CI 0.80–1.31; $P = 0.86$). The estimated median survival time and 5-year OS rate was 54 months and 44% for the chemotherapy arm and 55 months and 45% for the surgery-alone arm. No difference in PFS survival was seen (HR 0.96; 95% CI 0.77–1.21; $P = 0.74$).

The Italian ChEST trial evaluated the role of three cycles of induction gemcitabine and cisplatin in patients with stage I–IIIA disease (30). The primary endpoint of this trial was the 3-year PFS rate. Here again, the trial was closed prematurely due to the routine use of adjuvant chemotherapy. A total of 270 patients were randomized; 129 patients to the induction chemotherapy arm and 141 patients to the surgery arm. A radiographic response was seen in 35% of all patients and 86% of patients who completed the cycles of therapy. There was no statistical difference in the 3-year PFS rate but it favored the induction arm with an HR of 0.71; (95% CI 0.50 to 0.99; $P = 0.109$). The median PFS time was 4 years for the chemotherapy group and 2.9 years for the surgical group. The 3-year

OS rate was 67% and 60% (HR 0.63; 95% CI 0.42–0.93; $P = 0.053$). The 5-year OS rate has not been reported. In the subgroup of patients with stage IIB–IIIA, disease PFS and OS were significantly increased for patients receiving induction chemotherapy with a 3-year PFS rate of 55% versus 36% ($P = 0.002$) and a 3-year OS rate of 70% versus 47% ($P = 0.001$) respectively.

■ INDUCTION VERSUS ADJUVANT CHEMOTHERAPY

One phase III trial has evaluated induction or adjuvant chemotherapy compared with surgical resection in patients with stage I (>2 cm), II, and III (T3N1) (31). The NATCH trial completed its enrollment with 624 patients and has a short median follow-up time of 51 months. Its primary endpoint was 5-year DFS. The preliminary data showed all three arms were similar in outcomes (Table 10.2). Induction treatment compared with surgery alone revealed a 5-year DFS rate of 38% versus 34% (HR 0.92; 95% CI 0.81–1.04; $P = 0.176$) with a median DFS time of 31.5 months and 25.1 months, respectively. For the adjuvant treatment arm the 5-year DFS rate was 36.6% versus 34.1% (HR 0.96; 95% CI 0.75–1.22; $P = 0.73$) with a median DFS time of 26 months and 25.1 months, respectively. The median and 5-year OS data were 48.8 months and 44% for the surgery-alone arm, 50.3 months and 45.5% (HR 0.99; 95% CI 0.75–1.31; $P = 0.95$) for the adjuvant arm, and 55.2 months and 46.6% (HR 0.96; 95% CI 0.84–1.1; $P = 0.56$) for the induction arm. We look forward to the reanalysis of the data with longer follow-up time. Compliance with chemotherapy was higher in the induction arm at 97%, while only 66% of patients received adjuvant chemotherapy.

A meta-analysis of induction versus adjuvant chemotherapy was recently reported by Lim et al. (32) from the United Kingdom. A total of 32 randomized trials with over 10,000 patients from 1992 to 2007 were included in the analysis. Twenty-two trials evaluated adjuvant therapy versus surgery and 10 trials evaluated induction therapy with three trials exploring perioperative therapy versus surgical resection. There was no difference in survival based on chemotherapy timing. The OS and DFS HR of adjuvant chemotherapy compared with induction chemotherapy was 0.99 (95% CI 0.81–1.21) and 0.96 (95% CI 0.74–1.26), respectively.

In summary, the data overwhelmingly supports the routine use of systemic chemotherapy in good PS patients with resectable NSCLC II–IIIA and suggests a beneficial role for patients with stage IB ≥4-cm tumors. The most compelling data favor the administration of adjuvant chemotherapy, but there is a role for induction chemotherapy in selected patients. However, evidence for the role of chemotherapy in patients with comorbidities, the very elderly patients, and patients with stage IA disease with aggressive tumors is lacking, leading us to face significant dilemmas. We strongly recommend discussion of all patients at a multidisciplinary tumor board to determine the appropriate patient and timing of systemic chemotherapy in this setting. Finally, the decision to receive chemotherapy is ultimately that of the patient and must include a discussion of the side effects of treatment; while the regimens were well tolerated in the studies outlined above, it is imperative that a detailed discussion of the risks and benefits of treatment be conveyed to the patient.

■ FUTURE DIRECTIONS

Now that a proven benefit for systemic chemotherapy has been achieved in resectable NSCLC, our research efforts must focus on optimizing this therapy and further increasing the cure rate. Two broad approaches are being investigated: (a) the evaluation of new agents particularly molecularly targeted agents and (b) molecular tumor profiling for predictive markers of response and survival and prognostic markers for recurrence.

Novel Therapeutic Agents

In this era of molecular biology, drug discovery and development has turned toward molecularly targeted anticancer agents. In advanced lung cancer, epidermal growth factor receptor (EGFR) and vascular endothelial growth factor (VEGF) inhibitors have been successful and justify their evaluation in earlier stages of disease (Table 10.3) (33,34). The Randomized Double-blind Trial in Adjuvant NSCLC with Tarceva (RADIANT) study is an ongoing international study to determine if 2 years of maintenance therapy with erlotinib improves DFS over placebo in patients with resected, pathologic stage IB–IIIA (N2-) NSCLC who have EGFR-positive tumors by immunohistochemistry (IHC) or fluorescent in situ hybridization. Patients may or may not have received adjuvant chemotherapy. The trial is nearing its target accrual of 945 patients. Bevacizumab, a VEGF inhibitor, is being examined by the Eastern Oncology Cooperative Group (ECOG) in ECOG 1505, a randomized phase III trial of a cisplatin-based doublet with or without bevacizumab for four cycles. Patients on the bevacizumab arm will continue with bevacizumab maintenance for 1 year. Patients with stage IB (tumors ≥4 cm)–IIIA (N2-) are eligible. OS is the primary endpoint and will require 1,500 patients.

No randomized phase III trials of induction chemotherapy are planned and an immunologic strategy is also

under investigation. A randomized phase II study with the MAGE-A3 vaccine or placebo in 182 resected stage IB-II NSCLC patients whose tumors expressed MAGE-A3 showed prolonged DFS for the vaccine (35). The MAGRIT (MAGE-A3 Adjuvant Non–Small Cell LunG cancer ImmunoTherapy) study is a double-blind, randomized phase III trial enrolling 2,270 resected patients with stage IB–IIIA (Table 10.3). Patients receive the MAGE-A3 vaccine or placebo weekly for 5 weeks and then every 3 months for eight treatments. The coprimary endpoints are DFS in patients receiving or not receiving adjuvant chemotherapy.

Patient Selection

Selecting patients most likely to benefit from systemic chemotherapy and avoiding it in patients who are cured with resection alone is the hallmark of personalized medicine. Efforts to accomplish this goal require the identification of predictive and prognostic markers in tumor and/or blood samples. A predictive marker determines a tumor's sensitivity to treatment and a prognostic marker determines outcome regardless of treatment. Several of the randomized adjuvant trials previously discussed examined subsets of patients with tumor samples amenable for marker testing. The first promising predictive/prognostic marker to emerge was excision repair cross-complementation group 1 (ERCC1). ERCC1 is involved in DNA repair. Low levels of ERCC1 expression suggests a tumor may not be able to repair cisplatin-induced DNA damage while tumors with high ERCC1 expression could repair such an insult. A retrospective analysis of ERCC1 protein expression by IHC in tumor specimens from 761 patients on the IALT trial revealed that ERCC1-negative tumors had a survival advantage from adjuvant cisplatin-containing regimens with an HR of 0.76 (95% CI 0.59–0.98) as compared with observation (36). Patients with ERCC1-positive tumors did not benefit from chemotherapy with an HR of 1.20 (95% CI 0.91–1.59). Moreover, patients in the control group with ERCC1-positive tumors had a superior survival compared with patients with ERCC1-negative tumors (HR 0.66; 95% CI 0.49–0.90; $P = 0.009$), suggesting ERCC1 is also a prognostic marker. A related gene, RRM1 (the regulatory subunit of ribonucleotide reductase), has been shown to correlate with ERCC1 expression and to be associated with gemcitabine sensitivity (37,38).

Additional analysis of IALT specimens by IHC for cell cycle regulators p27Kip1, p16NK4A, cyclin D1, cyclin D3, cyclin E, and Ki-67 were not prognostic or predictive, but a subset of patients with p27Kip1-negative tumors enjoyed a longer survival (HR 0.66; 95% CI 0.50–0.88; $P = 0.006$) with adjuvant treatment compared with no treatment controls (39).

JBR 10 prospectively studied KRAS and p53 in 253/482 patients with viable samples (40). Mutations in

■ Table 10.3 Current phase III studies in resectable NSCLC

Study	Stage	No. of Patients	Design
Novel therapy			
RADIANT	IB–IIIA	945	Surgery → ± Adjuvant → EGFR + Tumors by / Placebo chemotherapy IHC/FISH \ Erlotinib
ECOG 1505	IB–IIIA	1500	Surgery / Chemotherapy \ Chemotherapy + bevacizumab
MaGRIT	IB–IIIA	2270	Surgery → ± Adjuvant / MAGE-A3 vaccine chemotherapy \ Placebo
Prognostic			
Pharmacogenomics			
ITACA	II–IIIA	700	Surgery → High → TS / High → Taxane vs. control* / \ Low → Pem vs. control* ERCC1 \ Low → TS / High → Cis/Gem vs. control* \ Low → Cis/Pem vs. control*
TASTE	II–IIIA	910	Surgery / Control CDDP-Pem \ / EGFR → Erlotinib Experimental \ mutated customized EGFR / ERCC1+ → Observation wt \ ERCC1- → CDDP-Pem
SCAT	II–IIIA	432	Surgery / Control → Docetaxel/Cis → T1 RAP80 → Gem/Cis (T1–T3 BRCA1) \ Experimental → T2–T3 RAP80 → DocetaxelCis (T1–T2 BRCA1) → T2–T3 RAP80 → Docetaxel (T3 BRCA1)
CALGB 30506	I	1300	Surgery → High risk → / Chemotherapy \ Observation Low risk → / Chemotherapy \ Observation

CALGB, Cancer and Leukemia Group B; ECOG, Eastern Cooperative Oncology Group; EGFR, epidermal growth factor receptor; ERCC1, excision repair cross-complementation group 1; FISH, fluorescent in situ hybridization; ITACA, The International Tailored Chemotherapy Adjuvant Trial; RADIANT, Randomized Double-blind Trial in Adjuvant NSCLC with Tarceva; SCAT, Spanish Customized Adjuvant Trial; TASTE, Tailored Post-Surgical Therapy in Early Stage Lung Cancer; TS, thymidylate synthetase.

KRAS or p53 were not prognostic for survival or predictive of a benefit to adjuvant chemotherapy. However, P53 protein overexpression by IHC was associated with a shorter survival (HR 1.89; 95% CI 1.07–3.34, $P = 0.03$) and a positive treatment effect (HR 0.54; $P = 0.02$; interaction $P = 0.02$).

Efforts continue to identify and validate promising prognostic and/or predictive markers. Three large randomized trials are ongoing in Europe (Table 10.3). The International Tailored Chemotherapy Adjuvant Trial (ITACA) will select patients first by ERCC1 expression (high or low) and then by thymidylate synthetase (TS) levels (high or low). TS mRNA expression has been shown to play a role in pemetrexed activity (41). Based on the ERCC1 and TS expression patterns patients will be randomized to

the experimental pharmacogenomic-selected treatment or standard treatment. OS is the primary endpoint of the study. TASTE (Tailored Post-Surgical Therapy in Early Stage Lung Cancer) takes a slightly different approach. Patients will be randomized upfront to chemotherapy or to the experimental pharmacogenomics tailored arm whereby all tumors will be tested for EGFR mutations. If positive, these patients will receive erlotinib based upon the results of the Iressa-Pan Asian Study (IPASS) that showed an impressive DFS benefit for stage IV patients with EGFR mutations (42). EGFR wild-type tumor patients will then undergo ERCC1 testing to determine if they will receive chemotherapy. The trial is looking for an 8% improvement in the 3-year DFS rate. The Spanish Customized Adjuvant Trial (SCAT) builds on phase II data which demonstrate that BRCA1 (a DNA repair gene) and receptor-associated protein 80 (RAP80), which is required for BRCA1 accumulation at DNA break sites, are both prognostic and predictive markers in advanced lung cancer (43). High levels of both are associated with shorter survival. Low BRCA1 levels confer cisplatin sensitivity while high levels confer taxane sensitivity. High levels of RAP80 confers cisplatin resistance. In the United States, SWOG is conducting a feasibility study to determine the prognostic and predictive value of ERCC1 and RRM1 protein expression in patients with stage I (>2 cm) NSCLC. Patients will be assigned treatment with gemcitabine and cisplatin or observation based on the pattern of protein expression in their resected tumor specimen.

Concern that a single prognostic/predictive biomarker may not be ideal has led investigators to perform DNA arrays. Several gene signatures have shown prognostic value in resected NSCLC tumors (44–46). The lung metagene model developed by the Duke group was shown to predict recurrence in 109 patients with resected stage IB–IIIA disease better than clinical factors (44). This model is being further investigated validated in a randomized phase III trial CALGB 30506 (Table 10.3). Patients with resected stage I (1.7–6 cm) will be stratified into a high-risk or low-risk group and then randomized to receive adjuvant chemotherapy versus observation. The primary objective is to determine if adjuvant chemotherapy impacts survival.

Additional support for a gene signature approach comes from JBR 10. A 15-gene signature was determined to have both prognostic and predictive value. Patients with IB disease with a high-risk profile (n = 14) had a dramatically worse survival (HR 13.32; 95% CI 2.86–62.11; P < 0.001), than the 20 patients with the low-risk profile (47). Interestingly the 15-gene signature was also predictive. High-risk patients who received chemotherapy had prolonged survival compared with high-risk patients on the observation arm (HR 0.33; 95% CI 0.17–0.63; P = 0.005). Low-risk patients who received chemotherapy had inferior survival (HR 3.67; 95% CI 1.22–11.06; P = 0.013) (47).

CONCLUSION

The ability of systemic chemotherapy to cure more patients with resectable lung cancer represents the most significant treatment advance of this century. However, its benefit is modest, and lung cancer remains a deadly disease. We must continue to focus our efforts on enhancing cure rates through novel treatment approaches that include not only novel agents but also innovative surgical and radiation techniques. In addition, we must aggressively identify and validate molecular markers that can be used to appropriately select therapy.

KEY POINTS

- Three randomized phase III trials (IALT, JBR 10, ANITA) have demonstrated a survival benefit for adjuvant cisplatin-based chemotherapy in patients with stage I–IIIA non–small cell lung cancer (NSCLC).
- LACE meta-analysis of data from 4,584 individual patients from five trials (ALPI, IALT, JBR 10, ANITA, BLT) reported a hazard ratio (HR) of death of 0.89 (95% confidence interval [CI] 0.82–0.96; P = 0.005), which corresponded to a 5-year absolute survival benefit of 5.4% with adjuvant chemotherapy.
- Stage-specific analysis showed harm for stage IA patients receiving chemotherapy (HR 1.40; 95% CI 0.95–2.06).
- Eight-year follow-up of IALT showed the HR for overall survival (OS) was not significant (HR 0.91; 95% CI 0.81–1.02; P = 0.10) while the HR for disease-free survival retained significance (HR 0.88; 95% CI 0.78–0.98; P = 0.02). Loss of OS benefit may be secondary to an excess in noncancer-related deaths.
- Nine-year follow-up of JBR 10 continued to show a survival benefit for the treated group with an absolute improvement in the 5-year OS rate of 11% (67% vs. 56%, respectively) with an HR of 0.78 (95% CI 0.62–0.99; P = 0.04).
- CALGB 9633 conducted in stage IB patients and administered carboplatin with paclitaxel did not yield a statistically significant survival advantage for chemotherapy.
  - An unplanned subgroup analysis showed a survival benefit for adjuvant therapy for patients with tumors ≥4 cm.
  - JBR 10 has also shown a survival advantage with chemotherapy for stage IB patients with ≥4-cm tumors.
- In Japan, a randomized phase III trial showed benefit for oral UFT (Tegafur Uracil) as an adjuvant treatment for patients with stage IB adenocarcinoma.
- Several randomized phase III trials evaluating induction chemotherapy (SWOG 9900, the European LU22, and Italian ChEST trial) closed prematurely due to the routine use of adjuvant chemotherapy.
- NATCH compared induction chemotherapy versus adjuvant chemotherapy versus surgery alone. Preliminary 5-year survival data showed similar outcomes for all arms.
- A meta-analysis comparing induction versus adjuvant chemotherapy showed no difference in survival based on timing of chemotherapy.
- The data overwhelmingly supports the routine use of systemic chemotherapy in good performance status patients with resectable NSCLC II–IIIA and suggests a beneficial role for patients with stage IB >4-cm tumors.

- Research is focused on identifying and validating patient selection markers for systemic treatment and evaluating novel therapeutics.

■ REFERENCES

1. Goldstraw P, Crowley J, Chansky K, et al.; International Association for the Study of Lung Cancer International Staging Committee; Participating Institutions. The IASLC Lung Cancer Staging Project: proposals for the revision of the TNM stage groupings in the forthcoming (seventh) edition of the TNM Classification of malignant tumours. *J Thorac Oncol.* 2007;2(8):706–714.

2. Non-small Cell Lung Cancer Collaborative Group. Chemotherapy in non-small cell lung cancer: a meta-analysis using updated data on individual patients from 52 randomised clinical trials. *BMJ.* 1995;311(7010):899–909.

3. Keller SM, Adak S, Wagner H, et al. A randomized trial of postoperative adjuvant therapy in patients with completely resected stage II or IIIA non-small-cell lung cancer. Eastern Cooperative Oncology Group. *N Engl J Med.* 2000;343(17):1217–1222.

4. PORT Meta-analysis Trialists Group. Postoperative radiotherapy in non-small cell lung cancer: systematic review and meta-analysis of individual patient data from nine randomised controlled trials. *Lancet.* 1998;52(9124):257–263.

5. Waller D, Peake MD, Stephens RJ, et al. Chemotherapy for patients with non-small cell lung cancer: the surgical setting of the Big Lung Trial. *Eur J Cardiothorac Surg.* 2004;26(1):173–182.

6. Scagliotti GV, Fossati R, Torri V, et al.; Adjuvant Lung Project Italy/European Organisation for Research Treatment of Cancer-Lung Cancer Cooperative Group Investigators. Randomized study of adjuvant chemotherapy for completely resected stage I, II, or IIIA non-small-cell Lung cancer. *J Natl Cancer Inst.* 2003;95(19):1453–1461.

7. Scagliotti GV. The ALPI Trial: the Italian/European experience with adjuvant chemotherapy in resectable non-small cell lung cancer. *Clin Cancer Res.* 2005;11(13 Pt 2l):5011s–5016s.

8. Arriagada R, Bergman B, Dunant A, Le Chevalier T, Pignon JP, Vansteenkiste J; International Adjuvant Lung Cancer Trial Collaborative Group. Cisplatin-based adjuvant chemotherapy in patients with completely resected non-small-cell lung cancer. *N Engl J Med.* 2004;350(4):351–360.

9. Arriagada R, Dunant A, Pignon JP, et al. Long-term results of the international adjuvant lung cancer trial evaluating adjuvant Cisplatin-based chemotherapy in resected lung cancer. *J Clin Oncol.* 2010;28(1):35–42.

10. Winton T, Livingston R, Johnson D, et al.; National Cancer Institute of Canada Clinical Trials Group; National Cancer Institute of the United States Intergroup JBR.10 Trial Investigators. Vinorelbine plus cisplatin vs. observation in resected non-small-cell lung cancer. *N Engl J Med.* 2005;352(25):2589–2597.

11. Butts CA, Ding K, Seymour L, et al. Randomized phase III trial of vinorelbine plus cisplatin compared with observation in completely resected stage IB and II non-small-cell lung cancer: updated survival analysis of JBR-10. *J Clin Oncol.* 2010;28(1):29–34.

12. Douillard JY, Rosell R, De Lena M, et al. Adjuvant vinorelbine plus cisplatin versus observation in patients with completely resected stage IB-IIIA non-small-cell lung cancer (Adjuvant Navelbine International Trialist Association [ANITA]): a randomised controlled trial. *Lancet Oncol.* 2006;7(9):719–727.

13. Douillard JY, Rosell R, De Lena M, Riggi M, Hurteloup P, Mahe MA; Adjuvant Navelbine International Trialist Association. Impact of postoperative radiation therapy on survival in patients with complete resection and stage I, II, or IIIA non-small-cell lung cancer treated with adjuvant chemotherapy: the adjuvant Navelbine International Trialist Association (ANITA) Randomized Trial. *Int J Radiat Oncol Biol Phys.* 2008;72(3):695–701.

14. Strauss GM, Herndon JE 2nd, Maddaus MA, et al. Adjuvant paclitaxel plus carboplatin compared with observation in stage IB non-small-cell lung cancer: CALGB 9633 with the Cancer and Leukemia Group B, Radiation Therapy Oncology Group, and North Central Cancer Treatment Group Study Groups. *J Clin Oncol.* 2008;26(31):5043–5051.

15. Pignon JP, Tribodet H, Scagliotti GV, et al.; LACE Collaborative Group. Lung adjuvant cisplatin evaluation: a pooled analysis by the LACE Collaborative Group. *J Clin Oncol.* 2008;26(21):3552–3559.

16. Früh M, Rolland E, Pignon JP, et al. Pooled analysis of the effect of age on adjuvant cisplatin-based chemotherapy for completely resected non-small-cell lung cancer. *J Clin Oncol.* 2008;26(21):3573–3581.

17. Kato H, Ichinose Y, Ohta M, et al.; Japan Lung Cancer Research Group on Postsurgical Adjuvant Chemotherapy. A randomized trial of adjuvant chemotherapy with uracil-tegafur for adenocarcinoma of the lung. *N Engl J Med.* 2004;350(17):1713–1721.

18. Hamada C, Tanaka F, Ohta M, et al. Meta-analysis of postoperative adjuvant chemotherapy with tegafur-uracil in non-small-cell lung cancer. *J Clin Oncol.* 2005;23(22):4999–5006.

19. Roth JA, Fossella F, Komaki R, et al. A randomized trial comparing perioperative chemotherapy and surgery with surgery alone in resectable stage IIIA non-small-cell lung cancer. *J Natl Cancer Inst.* 1994;86(9):673–680.

20. Roth JA, Atkinson EN, Fossella F, et al. Long-term follow-up of patients enrolled in a randomized trial comparing perioperative chemotherapy and surgery with surgery alone in resectable stage IIIa non-small-cell lung cancer. *Lung Cancer.* 2000;28(3):247–251.

21. Rosell R, Gómez-Codina J, Camps C, et al. A randomized trial comparing preoperative chemotherapy plus surgery with surgery alone in patients with non-small-cell lung cancer. *N Engl J Med.* 1994;330(3):153–158.

22. Rosell R, Gómez-Codina J, Camps C, et al. Preresectional chemotherapy in stage IIIA non-small-cell lung cancer: a 7-year assessment of a randomized controlled trial. *Lung Cancer.* 1999;26(1):7–14.

23. Depierre A, Milleron B, Moro-Sibilot D, et al.; French Thoracic Cooperative Group. Preoperative chemotherapy followed by surgery compared with primary surgery in resectable stage I (except T1N0), II, and IIIa non-small-cell lung cancer. *J Clin Oncol.* 2002;20(1):247–253.

24. Pisters KM, Ginsberg RJ, Giroux DJ, et al. Induction chemotherapy before surgery for early-stage lung cancer: A novel approach. Bimodality Lung Oncology Team. *J Thorac Cardiovasc Surg.* 2000;119(3):429–439.

25. Pisters K, Ginsberg R, Giroux D, et al. Bimodality Lung Oncology Team (BLOT) trial in induction paclitaxel/carboplatin in early stage non-small cell lung cancer (NSCLC): long term follow up of a phase II trial. *Proc Am Soc Clin Oncol.* 2003;22(a2544):633.

26. Pisters K, Vallieres E, Bunn PA, et al. S9900: a phase III trial of surgery alone or surgery plus preoperative (preop) paclitaxel/carboplatin (PC) chemotherapy in early stage non-small cell lung cancer (NSCLC): preliminary results. *Proc Am Soc Clin Oncol.* 2005;23(16s):624s.

27. Pisters K, Vallieres E, Bunn PA, et al. S9900: surgery alone or surgery plus induction (ind) paclitaxel/carboplatin (PC) chemotherapy in early stage non-small cell lung cancer (NSCLC): follow-up on a phase III trial. *J Clin Oncol.* 2007;25(18s):7520.

28. Sorensen J, Riska H, Ravn J, et al. Scandinavian phase III trial of neoadjuvant chemotherapy in NSCLC stages IB-IIA/T3. *J Clin Oncol.* 2005;23(16s):7146.

29. Gilligan D, Nicolson M, Smith I, et al. Preoperative chemotherapy in patients with resectable non-small cell lung cancer: results of the MRC LU22/NVALT 2/EORTC 08012 multicentre randomised trial and update of systematic review. *Lancet.* 2007;369(9577):1929–1937.

30. Scagliotti GV, Pastorino U, Vansteenkiste JF, et al. A phase III randomized study of surgery alone or surgery plus

preoperative gemcitabine-cisplatin in early-stage non-small cell lung cancer (NSCLC): follow-up data of Ch.E.S.T. *J Clin Oncol.* 2008;26(a7508):399s.

31. Felip E, Massuti B, Alonso G, et al. Surgery (S) alone, preoperative (preop) paclitaxel/carboplatin (PC) chemotherapy followed by S, or S followed by adjuvant (adj) PC chemotherapy in early-stage non-small cell lung cancer (NSCLC): results of the NATCH multicenter, randomized phase III trial. *J Clin Oncol.* 2009;27(a7500):15s.

32. Lim E, Harris G, Patel A, et al. Preoperative versus postoperative chemotherapy in patients with resectable non-small cell lung cancer: systematic review and indirect comparison meta-analysis of randomized trials. *J Clin Oncol.* 2008;26(a7546):408s.

33. Shepherd FA, Rodrigues Pereira J, Ciuleanu T, et al.; National Cancer Institute of Canada Clinical Trials Group. Erlotinib in previously treated non-small-cell lung cancer. *N Engl J Med.* 2005;353(2):123–132.

34. Sandler A, Gray R, Perry MC, et al. Paclitaxel-carboplatin alone or with bevacizumab for non-small-cell lung cancer. *N Engl J Med.* 2006;355(24):2542–2550.

35. Vansteenkiste J, Zielinski M, Linder A, et al. Final results of a multi-center, double-blind, randomized, placebo-controlled phase II study to assess the efficacy of MAGE-A3 immunotherapeutic as adjuvant therapy in stage IB/II non-small cell lung cancer (NSCLC). *J Clin Oncol.* 2007;25(18S):7554.

36. Olaussen KA, Dunant A, Fouret P, et al.; IALT Bio Investigators. DNA repair by ERCC1 in non-small-cell lung cancer and cisplatin-based adjuvant chemotherapy. *N Engl J Med.* 2006;355(10):983–991.

37. Zheng Z, Chen T, Li X, Haura E, Sharma A, Bepler G. DNA synthesis and repair genes RRM1 and ERCC1 in lung cancer. *N Engl J Med.* 2007;356(8):800–808.

38. Rosell R, Danenberg KD, Alberola V, et al.; Spanish Lung Cancer Group. Ribonucleotide reductase messenger RNA expression and survival in gemcitabine/cisplatin-treated advanced non-small cell lung cancer patients. *Clin Cancer Res.* 2004;10(4): 1318–1325.

39. Filipits M, Pirker R, Dunant A, et al. Cell cycle regulators and outcome of adjuvant cisplatin-based chemotherapy in completely resected non-small-cell lung cancer: the International Adjuvant Lung Cancer Trial Biologic Program. *J Clin Oncol.* 2007;25(19):2735–2740.

40. Tsao MS, Aviel-Ronen S, Ding K, et al. Prognostic and predictive importance of p53 and RAS for adjuvant chemotherapy in non small-cell lung cancer. *J Clin Oncol.* 2007;25(33): 5240–5247.

41. Hanauske AR, Eismann U, Oberschmidt O, et al. *In vitro* chemosensitivity of freshly explanted tumor cells to pemetrexed is correlated with target gene expression. *Invest New Drugs.* 2007;25(5):417–423.

42. Mok TS, Wu YL, Thongprasert S, et al. Gefitinib or carboplatin-paclitaxel in pulmonary adenocarcinoma. *N Engl J Med.* 2009;361(10):947–957.

43. Rosell R, Perez-Roca L, Sanchez JJ, et al. Customized treatment in non-small-cell lung cancer based on EGFR mutations and BRCA1 mRNA expression. *PLoS ONE.* 2009;4(5):e5133.

44. Potti A, Mukherjee S, Petersen R, et al. A genomic strategy to refine prognosis in early-stage non-small-cell lung cancer. *N Engl J Med.* 2006;355(6):570–580.

45. Chen HY, Yu SL, Chen CH, et al. A five-gene signature and clinical outcome in non-small-cell lung cancer. *N Engl J Med.* 2007;356(1):11–20.

46. Lau SK, Boutros PC, Pintilie M, et al. Three-gene prognostic classifier for early-stage non small-cell lung cancer. *J Clin Oncol.* 2007;25(35):5562–5569.

47. Tsao MS, Zhu C, Ding K. A 15-gene expression signature prognostic for survival and predictive for adjuvant chemotherapy benefit in JBR.10 patients [abstract 7510]. *J Clin Oncol.* 2008;26:399s.

Stage IIIA–N2 NSCLC: The Case Against Surgical Involvement

I.K. DEMEDTS

JAN P. VAN MEERBEECK

■ INTRODUCTION

Lung cancer is the leading cause of death among cancers worldwide. Non–small cell lung cancer (NSCLC) accounts for approximately 85% of all cases and has a poor overall 5-year survival of about 15%. At the time of presentation, about one third have locally advanced (stage III) disease, which is a heterogeneous stage. According to the 6th edition of the tumor, node, metastases (TNM) classification, stage IIIA includes patients with either T3N1 tumors or malignant involvement of one or several ipsilateral mediastinal lymph node(s) (1). In the new proposed classification, T4 tumors without mediastinal lymph node invasion (N0–1) will be added to this substage (2). Importantly, an ipsilateral nodule in a different lobe is now classified as T4 (previously classified as M1) and thus also stage IIIA. On the other hand, tumors larger than 7 cm will be classified as T3 (previously T2) and considered stage IIIA whenever there is hilar lymph node involvement (N1) (Table 11.1).

In this chapter, we will only review the treatment options in stage IIIA–N2 NSCLC. As the role of surgery after induction chemotherapy in patients with stage IIIA–N2 NSCLC remains debated, we will argue against surgery for stage IIIA–N2 disease, by unveiling the biases for the unwary in surgical series (3).

■ TREATMENT OF STAGE IIIA–N2 NSCLC

Survival of patients with N2 disease treated with surgery alone is worse than in those with stages I–II NSCLC (4). The cause of treatment failure is local and/or distant relapse, the latter originating from occult micrometastatic disease missed at clinical staging. This pattern of failure has led several investigators to study the benefit of adding systemic and local therapy to surgery, in order to improve long-term survival by reducing both the distant and locoregional relapses, respectively. Different approaches have been evaluated (pre- or postoperative chemo- and/or radiotherapy), which we will only briefly summarize here (5).

Several meta-analyses have shown an improved survival with cisplatin-based *postoperative chemotherapy* (5–7), also in patients with pIIIA. *Postoperative radiotherapy* (PORT) was shown to have a significant detrimental effect on overall survival in stage pI–II, and pooled data in pN2 patients show a small nonsignificant reduction in local recurrence (8). Results from a subgroup analysis of a randomized trial addressing adjuvant chemotherapy (9) and from a retrospective epidemiologic study (10) suggest a benefit of PORT on overall outcome in stage IIIA. This issue is currently further studied in the ongoing LUNG-ART trial (11).

Parallel to the aforementioned adjuvant therapies, the same nonsurgical approaches were added *preoperatively* in order not only to reduce the distant relapse rate but also to aim at a possible parenchyma-sparing resection and better compliance to chemotherapy. Twelve randomized trials have compared *neoadjuvant chemotherapy* followed by surgery versus surgery alone in patients with stage IIIA NSCLC with variable numbers of N2 involvement (12). It can be concluded that a significant survival benefit in favor of neoadjuvant chemotherapy is present, ranging at 5 years from 6% to 14%, albeit weakened by confounding factors as the inhomogeneity of the patients included, the inadequate sample size, the variable addition of postoperative treatments, and the premature closure of some trials (12).

Three randomized trials have compared chemotherapy and chemoradiotherapy as an induction regimen in stage III NSCLC (13–15); one more is ongoing and one has been prematurely closed due to a lack of accrual (16–18). Taken together, these trials suggest that *induction chemoradiotherapy* results in better rates of resectability, pathologic downstaging, and pathologic complete remissions than chemotherapy alone, without significantly affecting overall or progression-free survival (PFS).

Based on the observed improvement with neoadjuvant chemotherapy followed by surgery, this treatment strategy quickly became the new standard of care for clinical stage IIIA NSCLC. Prospective series and studies in homogenous

■ **Table 11.1** Stage IIIA according to successive editions of the UICC TNM-staging classification of lung cancer

UICC Edition	5	6	7 (Proposed)
T and N categories included in IIIA	**T3N0–1** **T1–3N2**	T3N1 T1–3N2	T3N1 T1–3N2 T4N0–1

M, Metastasis; N, Node; UICC, Union Internationale Contre Le Cancer; T, Tumor.

Subgroups discussed in this review are set in bold.

N2 subgroups confirmed the earlier results with even better outcomes, albeit selection and stage migration biases cannot be excluded, and the results look less favorable when analyzed on an intention-to-treat basis than on per-protocol basis (19–21).

■ INDUCTION CHEMOTHERAPY FOLLOWED BY SURGERY OR BY RADIOTHERAPY?

For many years, surgery was regarded as the best local treatment. However, as dose localization techniques in radiotherapy continue to improve, the role of surgery for locoregional control was increasingly questioned and investigators embarked on strategies comparing which local treatment modality was the more effective. In a systematic review from 2006, two randomized trials were mentioned (22). In one study, the inclusion criteria required the presence of biopsy-proven N2 disease (23) but the TNM status of participants was not well described in the other study (24). In one study there were two treatment-related deaths in the chemotherapy/surgery group and one in the chemotherapy/radiotherapy group (23). Treatment-related deaths were not described in the other trial (24). These trials were statistically heterogeneous and therefore not suitable for a pooled analysis. In none of the studies was the surgical treatment arm found to be significantly superior to the nonsurgical approach in terms of overall survival.

Taylor et al. (25) observed an equivalent outcome in patients randomized to either concurrent chemoradiation or induction chemotherapy followed by resection. However, patients undergoing induction chemotherapy followed by resection often needed postoperative radiotherapy to achieve local control equivalent to that achieved with concurrent chemoradiation.

The European Organization for Research and Treatment of Cancer (EORTC) performed a large multicenter randomized trial to compare surgery with radiotherapy in patients with stage IIIA–N2 NSCLC who showed response to induction chemotherapy (26) (Table 11.2). There was no significant difference in median survival or PFS. Patients randomized to radiotherapy tended to relapse more frequently in the chest, whereas those randomized to surgery had more distant metastases. However, a substantial fraction of operated patients had PORT, which could explain the observed difference in recurrence and PFS. In a post hoc unplanned univariate subgroup analysis of the surgical arm, 5-year survival was longer if a radical resection was performed, if nodal downstaging was present, or if a lobectomy was performed. The authors concluded that, after a radiologic response to induction chemotherapy, surgery is not superior to radiotherapy, which remained the preferred treatment in view of its lower morbidity and mortality.

U.S. investigators conducted the Intergroup trial 0139, wherein patients with T1–3 tissue-proven N2M0 NSCLC and performance status of 0 to 1 were randomized between induction chemoradiotherapy followed by either surgery or consolidation radiotherapy to 61 Gy and the same chemotherapy for two adjuvant cycles (27). Here too, PORT was optional in case of incomplete resection. Both arms received consolidation chemotherapy with two cycles of cisplatin/etoposide. PFS was significantly improved in the surgery group but overall survival did not differ, most probably because of the operative mortality. Factors associated with better outcome were female gender, absence of weight loss, and single N2 involvement at diagnosis. Pathologic downstaging was associated with improved outcome after surgery. An unplanned exploratory "matched pair" analysis showed a significantly better survival for patients who underwent lobectomy compared with irradiated patients. The authors conclude that chemotherapy with radiotherapy both with and without resection, preferably lobectomy, are options.

An ongoing Danish trial compares consolidation radiotherapy versus surgery with postoperative radiotherapy, both following induction chemotherapy in stage IIIA–N2 NSCLC (28). This trial started its accrual in 1998 and was expected to have its last patient enrolled in January 2008. Mature results are not to be expected before 2010 at the earliest.

Successful interventions to increase local control with radiotherapy include dose escalation, altered fractionation, and the integration with concurrent chemotherapy. These interventions increase the tumor cell kill by a variety of mechanisms, inflicting more initial radiation damage, decreasing repair, or counteracting the effects of cancer-cell proliferation (29). Despite the fact that randomized controlled trials failed to show a formal superiority of surgery over radiotherapy as optimal treatment for locoregional control in stage IIIA NSCLC, postinduction surgery is still advocated as the gold standard by some. This absence of solid evidence is strengthened by the following critical appraisals of the biases of those proponents of surgery (3).

■ **Table 11.2** Randomised trials in stage IIIA-N2 NSCLC comparing surgery and radiotherapy as locoregional modalities after induction chemo(radio)-therapy

Study (reference)	EORTC 08941 (26)		Intergroup 0139 (27)	
Treatment arm	Induction chemotherapy + surgery	Induction chemotherapy + radiotherapy	Induction chemoradiotherapy + surgery	Chemoradiotherapy
Number of patients with IIIA–N2	167	166	202	194
Chemotherapy regimen	Platinum based		Cisplatin-etoposide	
Radiotherapy total dose (Gray)	–	60	45	61
Rate of pneumonectomy/ (bi-)lobectomy/exploratory thoracotomy (%)	47/38/14	–	27/49/4	–
R0 resection rate (%)	50	–	88	–
PORT (% of patients)	40	–	?	–
Treatment related mortality rate (%)	4	<1	8	2
Pathological nodal downstaging rate (%)	41 (pN0–1)	–	38 (pN0)	–
Pathological complete respons rate (%)	5	–	15	–
Median PFS (months)	9.0	11.3	12.8	10.5
Locoregional failure rate (%)	32	55	10	22
Site of recurrence				
Local only[a] (%)	32	55	10	22
Brain (%)	NA	NA	11	15
Other distant sites (%)	NA	NA	37	42
Median OS (months) with 95% CI	16.4 (13.3–19.0)	17.5 (15.8–23.2)	23.6	22.2
5-year SR (%) with 95% CI	15.7 (10–22)	14 (9–20)	27.2	20.3

[a] Local relapse = relapse in primary tumor site; hilar, mediastinal or supraclavicular nodes.

PFS, progression-free survival.

■ HISTORICAL BIAS

Surgery has historically been the cornerstone for the loco(regional) treatment of most cancers. Radical surgery for stage III NSCLC started in the 1980s. The authors of the many surgical series that were published since tend to conclude that surgery still confers the survival advantage. This belief would seem to be widespread. In the methods section of many chemoradiation study reports, there is a statement that "candidates have to have irresectable stage III." The clear implication is that surgical cure can be achieved. The distinction, between the surgically operable and inoperable cancers, has been negotiated since the early reports of radical surgery for stage III NSCLC. Whether stage III is as such resectable is as much a matter of debate as the limits of that resectability. In the early days of thoracic surgery, pneumonectomy was considered the standard procedure, no matter what the tumor extent. Nowadays, surgeons consider sublobar resections for selected cases of ground glass opacities with malignant features. Similarly, the limits of resectability of stage

III have often been left to the discretion and the expertise of the surgeon, as clear definitions were only recently drafted.

■ CAUSATION BIAS

Multivariate analyses of registries and retrospective series tend to confine a survival benefit to operated patients. Does this prove that surgery favorably influenced the outcome for these patients? The problem is that many factors are used by experienced and knowledgeable teams when they decide to operate on one patient but not another. These factors include all available clinical information but cannot account for all: some are not consciously recognized, some are not made explicit, and some are unknown unknowns. It would be indeed surprising if these choices did not produce a cohort of patients who did better than those not selected, that is, unless the authors are suggesting that the decision to operate is some sort of haphazard event. Hence association is the correct word for the relation found at multivariate analysis.

■ PRESUMPTION OF EFFICACY BIAS

When surgeons perform very extensive surgery on many patients, there is a deep-felt belief, held by doctors and the public alike, that the operation must be doing some good. This very human tenet, called here the presumption of efficacy, holds despite increasing evidence that other modalities might result in equivalent results without the surgical morbidity, for example, radiotherapy in early-stage prostatic, cervical, and laryngeal cancer. In limited stage small cell lung cancer, radiotherapy was shown already in the 1970s to be superior to surgery (30). Promising results have been obtained with stereotactic body radiotherapy in selected medically inoperable patients with early-stage NSCLC, with cancer specific overall and recurrence-free survival rates similar to operated patients (31). A randomized trial comparing stereotactic radiotherapy to surgery in early-stage NSCLC is currently ongoing (32).

■ COMPARISON BIAS

Survival times after surgery are given in isolation as if there is some gold standard of the natural history against which these can be compared, which is certainly not the case. Survival data vary between observational series and are amenable to lead-time bias. Reference to an expected average survival has no validity. Comparison groups have a different case mix. Many surgical reports are retrospective, with differently staged patients and variations in treatment schedules. In the earliest series using chemotherapy and surgery, patients were included according to the 5th edition of the TNM classification, and some of these would be reclassified now as having stage II. Similarly, by the introduction of positron emission tomography scan and minimally invasive endoscopic ultrasound techniques, stage migration has improved the outcome of both stage IIIA and IIIB patients, as compared with the pool of patients treated before their introduction (33).

■ ANALYTICAL BIAS

It is common for authors of case series to report an analysis of those patients who completed the full treatment schedule under review. They are reporting on the

outcomes for a particular management strategy. This is the contrary of "intention-to-treat" analysis, which is the generally accepted standard of reporting for prospective studies and randomized clinical trials. The lapse into "per-protocol" analysis is perhaps natural inasmuch as these are the data retrieved by the author's team—the patients who were treated in a particular way. The most obvious breach of intention-to-treat analysis is to exclude from the survival curves the patients who died in the immediate postoperative period. In an extreme scenario, the patient pool under consideration is reduced at each of the multiple stages through both clinical selection and survival and the denominator on which survival is estimated shrinks at each step. The patients had to be worked up; they had to undergo, survive, and recover from each of the components. All take time, each step may eliminate some patients, and each intervention takes its toll on patients. Those who arrive at the end are clinically and self-selected survivors. The question arises whether these survivors survive because of the treatment or because they are the fittest.

■ REPORTING BIAS

Promising phase 2 trials must be confirmed by an appropriate randomized study. The history of medicine and of lung cancer is replete of treatments that did not stand up under the scrutiny of the randomized comparison, despite "very promising" uncontrolled results. This argument has been further developed in an aforementioned section of this chapter, discussing the randomized trials in IIIA–N2 NSCLC.

■ PROGNOSTIC FACTOR BIAS

There are no surgical outcome studies with an internal control group. Instead, the investigators analyze the predictors of survival within their study group. The arguments that surgery should be offered to patients who are likely to be downstaged, and/or in whom a complete resection can be obtained with a lobectomy, are of a circular kind. However, inasmuch as these factors are derived from a multivariable analysis and then used to categorize the same data, this is not surprising. The validity of these factors as predictors should be proven by applying them to a new series, independent of the one from which they were derived. Even if they have been validated as predictive factors associated with survival after surgery, such analysis cannot be used to select those likely to "benefit most" from surgery because the notion of differential benefit is based entirely on the presumption of efficacy.

SELECTION BIAS

Criteria for case selection must be applicable before surgery. There is a separate flaw in the promulgation of the aforementioned factors to select patients who are most likely to benefit from radical surgery, in that they were all defined a posteriori. Completeness of resection can only be defined post hoc, lymph node status is revised as part of pathologic staging, and surgeons are not likely to claim before the operation that a pneumonectomy will definitely not be necessary for an individual patient with stage III, even in one showing radiologic evidence of response. This fact is illustrated by the high rates of pneumonectomy in the surgical series mentioned (19–21). If we are to have a set of criteria upon which to select or counsel patients, these criteria must be available before surgery and be validated, before they can be used. The search for these factors is still ongoing. At present, the preoperative estimation of mediastinal downstaging or completeness of resection by noninvasive or (minimally) invasive techniques is controversial and uncertain.

EXPLORATORY SUBGROUP ANALYSIS BIAS

In the Intergroup trial, an exploratory analysis was performed wherein a group of patients operated by lobectomy were compared with a matched group treated with radiotherapy (27). According to this analysis, patients undergoing a lobectomy fared better and those undergoing a pneumonectomy fared worse than their irradiated counterparts, and this analysis was used as further proof that resection was preferable. This kind of matched analysis is however prone to severe bias in favor of surgery in downstaged patients and in favor of radiotherapy in non-downstaged patients. Furthermore, pneumonectomy is a known negative prognostic factor (34). A similar matched analysis was conducted in the EORTC 08941 trial and did not observe a differential survival for lobectomized patients as compared with irradiated ones (35).

CONCLUSION

Whereas surgical resection after induction treatment can certainly be radical and result in impressive survival, it remains unproven that this approach is superior to radical adequate modern thoracic radiotherapy. The optimal treatment in locally advanced NSCLC is by itself a moving target. There is a strong conviction that modern radiotherapy, as part of a multimodality approach of stage III patients, will further improve the outcome. The last decade has seen the advent of several novel radiation techniques, which are likely to improve the local control by the delivery of higher radiation doses to smaller volumes, allowing for lesser toxicity. Pending further randomized evidence, patients should be given a balanced view of both treatments, taking into account the availability of the expertise and the complications of treatment. The use of surgery in stage IIIA–N2 should not be uncritically recommended in guidelines and be restrictive, preferably treatment should be done as part of clinical trials, in large centers with sufficient expertise (12). A defeatism against the use of a nonsurgical consolidation treatment—even after downstaging—is not justified.

REFERENCES

1. Mountain CF. Revisions in the International System for Staging Lung Cancer. *Chest.* 1997;111(6):1710–1717.
2. Goldstraw P, Crowley J, Chansky K, et al.; International Association for the Study of Lung Cancer International Staging Committee; Participating Institutions. The IASLC Lung Cancer Staging Project: proposals for the revision of the TNM stage groupings in the forthcoming (seventh) edition of the TNM Classification of malignant tumours. *J Thorac Oncol.* 2007;2(8):706–714.
3. Treasure T, Utley M. Ten traps for the unwary in surgical series: a case study in mesothelioma reports. *J Thorac Cardiovasc Surg.* 2007;133(6):1414–1418.
4. Detterbeck F, Socinski M. Induction therapy and surgery for I-IIIA, B non-small cell lung cancer. In: Detterbeck F, Socinski M, Rivera M, Rosenman J, eds. *Diagnosis and Treatment of Lung Cancer. An Evidence-Based Guide for the Practicing Clinician.* Philadelphia, PA: WB Saunders; 2001.
5. van Meerbeeck JP, Surmont VF. Stage IIIA-N2 NSCLC: a review of its treatment approaches and future developments. *Lung Cancer.* 2009;65(3):257–267.
6. Pignon JP, Tribodet H, Scagliotti GV, et al.; LACE Collaborative Group. Lung adjuvant cisplatin evaluation: a pooled analysis by the LACE Collaborative Group. *J Clin Oncol.* 2008;26(21):3552–3559.
7. Stewart LA, Burdett S, Tierney JF, Pignon J, on behalf of the NSCLC Collaborative Group. Surgery and adjuvant chemotherapy (CT) compared to surgery alone in non-small cell lung cancer (NSCLC): a meta-analysis using individual patient data (IPD) from randomized clinical trials (RCT) [Meeting Abstracts]. *J Clin Oncol.* 2007;25:7552.
8. Group PM-aT. Postoperative radiotherapy for non-small cell lung cancer. Cochrane Database of Systematic Reviews. 2005 Issue 2; John Wiley & Sons, Ltd Chichester, UK DOI: 101002/14651858CD002142pub2 2005.
9. Douillard JY, Rosell R, De Lena M, et al. Adjuvant vinorelbine plus cisplatin versus observation in patients with completely resected stage IB-IIIA non-small-cell lung cancer (Adjuvant Navelbine International Trialist Association [ANITA]): a randomised controlled trial. *Lancet Oncol.* 2006;7(9):719–727.
10. Lally BE, Zelterman D, Colasanto JM, Haffty BG, Detterbeck FC, Wilson LD. Postoperative radiotherapy for stage II or III non-small-cell lung cancer using the surveillance, epidemiology, and end results database. *J Clin Oncol.* 2006;24(19):2998–3006.
11. National Library of Medicine. Radiation therapy in treating patients with non-small cell lung cancer that has been completely removed by surgery. (Clinical Trials.gov no NCT 00410683.) http://www.clinicaltrials.gov/NCT 00410683. Accessed July 15, 2009.
12. Robinson LA, Ruckdeschel JC, Wagner H Jr, Stevens CW; American College of Chest Physicians. Treatment of non-small

cell lung cancer-stage IIIA: ACCP evidence-based clinical practice guidelines (2nd edition). *Chest*. 2007;132(3 suppl):243S–265S.

13. Sauvaget J, Rebischung J, Vannetzel J, et al. Phase III study of neo-adjuvant MVP versus MVP plus chemo-radiation in stage III NSCLC. *Proc ASCO*. 2000;19:495a.

14. Fleck J, Carmargo J, Godoy D, al. e. Chemoradiation therapy (CRT) versus chemotherapy (CT) alone as a neoadjuvant treatment for stage III non-small cell lung cancer (NSCLC). Preliminary report of a phase III prospective randomized trial. Proc ASCO 1993; 12: abstract 1108.

15. Thomas M, Rübe C, Hoffknecht P, et al.; German Lung Cancer Cooperative Group. Effect of preoperative chemoradiation in addition to preoperative chemotherapy: a randomised trial in stage III non-small-cell lung cancer. *Lancet Oncol*. 2008;9(7):636–648.

16. Phase III randomized trial of preoperative chemotherapy versus preoperative concurrent chemotherapy and thoracic radiotherapy followed by surgical resection and consolidation chemotherapy in favorable prognosis patients with stage IIIA (N2) non-small cell lung cancer: RTOG 0412/SWOG S0332. http://www.rtog.org/members/protocols/0412/0412.pdf. Accessed January 2, 2009.

17. Preoperative chemotherapy versus concurrent chemoradiotherapy in N2 positive IIIA non small cell lung cancer (NSCLC). (Clinical Trials.gov no NCT 00452803.) National Library of Medicine, 2009. http://www.clinicaltrials.gov/NCT 00452803). Accessed July 15, 2009.

18. Chemotherapy with or without radiation therapy before surgery in treating patients with stage iiia non-small cell lung cancer. (Clinical Trials.gov no NCT00030771.) National Library of Medicine, 2009. http://www.clinicaltrials.gov/NCT00030771. Accessed July 15, 2009.

19. Lorent N, De Leyn P, Lievens Y, et al.; Leuven Lung Cancer Group. Long-term survival of surgically staged IIIA-N2 non-small-cell lung cancer treated with surgical combined modality approach: analysis of a 7-year prospective experience. *Ann Oncol*. 2004;15(11):1645–1653.

20. Garrido P, González-Larriba JL, Insa A, et al. Long-term survival associated with complete resection after induction chemotherapy in stage IIIA (N2) and IIIB (T4N0–1) non small-cell lung cancer patients: the Spanish Lung Cancer Group Trial 9901. *J Clin Oncol*. 2007;25(30):4736–4742.

21. Betticher DC, Hsu Schmitz SF, Tötsch M, et al. Mediastinal lymph node clearance after docetaxel-cisplatin neoadjuvant chemotherapy is prognostic of survival in patients with stage IIIA pN2 non-small-cell lung cancer: a multicenter phase II trial. *J Clin Oncol*. 2003;21(9):1752–1759.

22. Wright G, Manser RL, Byrnes G, Hart D, Campbell DA. Surgery for non-small cell lung cancer: systematic review and meta-analysis of randomised controlled trials. *Thorax*. 2006;61(7):597–603.

23. Johnstone DW, Byhardt RW, Ettinger D, Scott CB. Phase III study comparing chemotherapy and radiotherapy with preoperative chemotherapy and surgical resection in patients with non-small-cell lung cancer with spread to mediastinal lymph nodes (N2); final report of RTOG 89–01. Radiation Therapy Oncology Group. *Int J Radiat Oncol Biol Phys*. 2002;54(2):365–369.

24. Stathopoulos G, Papakostas P, Malamos N, et al. Chemoradiotherapy versus chemo-surgery in stage IIIA non-small cell lung cancer. *Oncol Rep*. 1996;3:673–6.

25. Taylor NA, Liao ZX, Cox JD, et al. Equivalent outcome of patients with clinical Stage IIIA non-small-cell lung cancer treated with concurrent chemoradiation compared with induction chemotherapy followed by surgical resection. *Int J Radiat Oncol Biol Phys*. 2004;58(1):204–212.

26. van Meerbeeck JP, Kramer GW, Van Schil PE, et al.; European Organisation for Research and Treatment of Cancer-Lung Cancer Group. Randomized controlled trial of resection versus radiotherapy after induction chemotherapy in stage IIIA–N2 non-small-cell lung cancer. *J Natl Cancer Inst*. 2007;99(6):442–450.

27. Albain KS, Swann RS, Rusch VW, et al. Radiotherapy plus chemotherapy with or without surgical resection for stage III non-small-cell lung cancer: a phase III randomised controlled trial. *Lancet*. 2009;374(9687):379–386.

28. Neoadjuvant chemotherapy plus/minus surgery in non-small-cell lung cancer (NSCLC) stage IIIA/N2. (Clinical Trials.gov no NCT00273494.) National Library of Medicine, 2009. http://www.clinicaltrials.gov/NCT00273494. Accessed July 15, 2009.

29. van Meerbeeck JP, Meersschout S, De Pauw R, Madani I, De Neve W. Modern radiotherapy as part of combined modality treatment in locally advanced non-small cell lung cancer: present status and future prospects. *Oncologist*. 2008;13(6):700–708.

30. Fox W, Scadding JG. Medical Research Council comparative trial of surgery and radiotherapy for primary treatment of small-celled or oat-celled carcinoma of bronchus. Ten-year follow-up. *Lancet*. 1973;2(7820):63–65.

31. Baumann P, Nyman J, Hoyer M, et al. Outcome in a prospective phase II trial of medically inoperable stage I non-small-cell lung cancer patients treated with stereotactic body radiotherapy. *J Clin Oncol*. 2009;27(20):3290–3296.

32. Trial of either surgery or stereotactic radiotherapy for early stage (IA) lung cancer (ROSEL). (Clinical Trials.gov no NCT 00687986.). National Library of Medicine, 2008. http://www.clinicaltrials.gov/NCT 00687986. Accessed July 15, 2009.

33. Chee KG, Nguyen DV, Brown M, Gandara DR, Wun T, Lara PN Jr. Positron emission tomography and improved survival in patients with lung cancer: the Will Rogers phenomenon revisited. *Arch Intern Med*. 2008;168(14):1541–1549.

34. van Meerbeeck JP, Damhuis RA, Vos de Wael ML. High postoperative risk after pneumonectomy in elderly patients with right-sided lung cancer. *Eur Respir J*. 2002;19(1):141–145.

35. Van Meerbeeck JP, Kramer GW, Legrand C, et al. Does downstaging in patients (pts) with IIIA-N2 non-small cell lung cancer (NSCLC) and a response to induction chemotherapy (ICT) influence outcome with surgery (S) or radiotherapy (RT)? An exploratory analysis of EORTC 08941 [Meeting Abstracts] . *J Clin Oncol*. 2006;24: 7047.Current Multidisciplinary Oncology: Lung Cancer

JUSTIN D. BLASBERG

HARVEY I. PASS

JESSICA S. DONINGTON

12 Stage IIIA NSCLC: The Case for Surgical Involvement

■ OVERVIEW

Stage IIIA non–small cell lung cancer (NSCLC) treatment has an evolving therapeutic foundation based on innovations and advancements in surgery, chemotherapy, and tailored radiation therapy, as well as improvements in the identification of metastatic basins. This stage of disease encompasses a heterogeneous group of patients, and optimal therapy including the role of surgical resection has not been clearly defined. Over the past 3 decades several randomized trials have helped guide decision-making algorithms. In patients with T3N1 tumors, surgical resection with adjuvant chemotherapy is the mainstay of treatment, and little controversy exists about this management scheme. However, in the larger proportion of stage IIIA disease patients with mediastinal lymph node involvement (N2), a multimodality treatment approach is required. The exact role and timing of chemotherapy, radiation, and surgical resection is unclear. Overall, patients with micrometastatic N2 disease and single station nodal involvement have the greatest chance for cure. For these patients, surgical resection has the potential to play a significant role in treatment. In addition to surgery, sterilization of mediastinal lymph nodes with the use of induction chemotherapy alone or chemotherapy with radiation has been shown to correlate strongly with survival. Conversely, bulky multistation disease is frequently not amendable to complete resection by surgery and is best approached with definitive chemotherapy and radiation. The biological and therapeutic variability of stage IIIA NSCLC will be the primary focus of this chapter; to better define the role of surgical management in NSCLC patients with mediastinal lymph node involvement.

■ INTRODUCTION

Advances in the use of modern imaging technology, chemotherapy, and radiation, as well as research which is focused on improving surgical outcomes in lung cancer, have created new decision-making algorithms for locally advanced NSCLC. Unlike stage I and II NSCLC, which are treated primarily by surgical resection, multimodality treatment in stage IIIA disease is the foundation of therapy. Despite recent controversy, the role of surgical resection for stage IIIA NSCLC, in combination with pre- or postoperative chemotherapy and radiation, continues to be the most important discussion point at tumor boards which present such patients. Debate continues to exist regarding the role and the timing of all three arms of treatment.

Many features contribute to the heterogeneity of stage IIIA disease, including the number, size, and location of involved mediastinal lymph nodes. The identification of mediastinal disease either pre- or postresection is also relevant in regard to expected outcome. Finally, the completeness of mediastinal evaluation with intraoperative sampling versus complete lymph node dissection is a heavily debated topic (1). Surgeons are learning that the degree of mediastinal lymph node involvement is an important parameter to consider when approaching stage IIIA disease surgically, and that bulky mediastinal disease can be prohibitive.

Conventional wisdom dictates that the definition of bulky disease includes presentation with matted, involved lymph node masses which approach 3 cm in size, and which are contiguous with the primary tumor. A subset of these patients are those with so-called "extracapsular disease." Moreover, multistation lymph node involvement certainly implies extensive disease even if the "size" of involvement is not bulky. Even more confounding is the fact that in such bulky presentations, protocols of chemotherapy and radiation alone are not considered sufficient by many practicing thoracic oncologists (2,3). There is uniform agreement, however, that the most important components, as well as the timing and dose of those components, include those which can achieve sterilization of mediastinal lymph nodes, decrease rates of loco-regional recurrence, and ultimately improved outcome. Currently there is no consensus regarding how these characteristics affect outcome. This chapter serves to explore the surgical management of stage IIIA NSCLC and its appropriateness in patients with varying degrees of mediastinal lymph node involvement.

■ DEFINITION

Stage IIIA NSCLC is a heterogeneous classification that encompasses locally advanced ipsilateral disease. The American Joint Committee on Cancer staging defines IIIA disease as tumor stage T1, T2, or T3, with either metastatic disease in the ipsilateral mediastinal lymph nodes, subcarinal nodes, or both (N2), as well as T3 tumors with metastatic disease to the ipsilateral peribronchial, ipsilateral hilar lymph nodes, or both (N1) (4). The presence of N2 disease confers an overall worse prognosis, with optimal 5-year survival data ranging from 16% to 30% with concurrent chemotherapy and radiation followed by surgery (5–8). Recently the International Association for the Study of Lung Cancer (IASLC) has proposed changes to the stage classifications for patients with NSCLC (9). The intricacies of the 2009 staging system will be discussed further as they specifically relate to stage IIIA disease (9) (Table 4.1, Chapter 4).

Surgical management of stage IIIA NSCLC is based on the extent of local and regional disease, the degree of medical comorbidities which may limit a patient's ability to tolerate resection, and tumor response to induction chemotherapy and radiation. *Surgical intervention confers a survival advantage only when an R0 resection can be performed and all tumor containing tissue completely excised.* Therefore, adequately defining the presence of mediastinal lymph node metastasis (N2) is clinically important due to the necessary shift in primary management from surgical resection to neoadjuvant therapy.

■ STAGING GUIDELINES: NEW VERSUS OLD

The reclassification by the IASLC has resulted in some stage migration to improve the prognostic utility of the system. Changes that effect stage IIIA specifically include the inclusion of tumors greater than 7 cm, which are now classified as stage IIIA regardless of nodal status. T4 tumors without mediastinal lymph node involvement, previously classified as IIIB, have more appropriately been placed with other potentially resectable locally advanced disease in stage IIIA.

In a recent evaluation presented at the American Association of Thoracic Surgery in 2008, a comparison of the IASLC and Union Internationale Contre le Cancer (UICC)-6 staging systems was performed by retrospectively evaluating 1,154 surgical patients from MD Anderson Cancer Center to determine how stage migration directed by the 2009 IASLC system compared with outcome data. Based on IASLC staging, 17.5% of all NSCLC patients were reassigned, with an increase in the number of stage IIIA patients from 153 (13.3%) to 216 (18.7%); the majority of which were prior stage IIIB. Ten patients were upstaged to IIIA from IIB. Five-year survival was 37% and median survival 35 months for the reclassified IIIA patients. Implementation of IASLC IIIA in place of UICC-6 IIIB did not reduce survival for the newly characterized IIIA cohort (10). Overall, enhanced stratification of survival and limited heterogeneity among patients within any given stage will have important implications for adjuvant treatment algorithms. In the case of stage IIIA disease, it will likely produce a larger cohort of surgical patients, some previously treated with definitive chemotherapy and radiation.

■ T3N1 TUMORS

Patients who present with hilar or intralobar lymph node involvement (N1) and primary tumors invading resectable structures including the chest wall, diaphragm, and pericardium, or tumors within 2 cm of the carina (T3), represent a small subgroup of stage IIIA disease. In the absence of gross mediastinal lymph node involvement, T3N1 patients are usually candidates for surgical resection with mediastinal lymph node sampling or dissection. By definition, T3N1 tumors may require complex surgical intervention to achieve an R0 resection. This usually consists of either bronchoplastic procedures for centrally located tumors or necessitates en bloc resection of the chest wall, diaphragm, or pericardium with lobectomy for peripheral lesions. Complete tumor resection without mediastinal lymph node involvement is associated with a cure rate of 39%, which is significantly higher than for stage IIIA patients with N2 disease (11).

Data from the IALT (International Adjuvant Lung Cancer Trial) (12), ANITA (Adjuvant Navelbine International Trialist Association) (13), and the LACE (Lung Adjuvant Cisplatin Evaluation) (14) meta-analysis now provide strong evidence supporting the use of adjuvant platinum-based chemotherapy in T3N1 patients, as they represent a completely resected IIIA population. To date, there is no phase III evidence to support the use of induction over adjuvant chemotherapy in this group. However, theoretical advantages of neoadjuvant therapy include early treatment of micrometastatic tumor deposits and increased patient compliance.

Adjuvant radiotherapy also has a limited role in the management of T3N1 tumors because, by definition, disease of this stage should be completely resectable. However, there is a role for postoperative radiotherapy (PORT) in select patients with close or compromised surgical margins, which is currently the only indication for radiotherapy in T3N1 patients (15).

■ MANAGEMENT OF N2 DISEASE/ MEDIASTINAL LYMPH NODE INVOLVEMENT

Patients with NSCLC tumor metastasis to ipsilateral mediastinal lymph nodes (N2) represent the majority of stage IIIA disease. N2 lymph node involvement independently confers a poor prognosis, and surgery as the initial and definitive therapy has been a point of contention for decades (16). In the 1970s and 1980s, the presence of N2 disease was considered prohibitive to surgical resection, and patient management was limited to radiotherapy. One- and 2-year survival rates ranged from 4% to 11% (17), the risk of distant failure was greater than 50% at 2 years, and local control rates were less than 20% (18). The addition of chemotherapy, either sequentially or concurrently with radiation, improved outcome; however, cure rates remained less than 20% with poor local control (2,3). The addition of chemotherapy and radiation to surgical resection has created a multimodality treatment protocol aimed at improving loco-regional control and decreasing the risk of distant relapse. Currently, for patients in whom complete resection is feasible by lung resection and mediastinal lymph node dissection, surgery is an important component of treatment. The addition of chemotherapy and radiation protocols either pre- or postresection has been the focus of much research surrounding stage IIIA N2 disease, and continues to be an area of significant controversy in part due to the heterogeneous nature of the N2 patient population.

To appropriately apply the principles of multimodality therapy, pretreatment identification of mediastinal nodal involvement is mandatory. Current recommendations for noninvasive staging of the mediastinum in NSCLC include both computed tomography (CT) and positron emission tomography (PET), either individually or as an integrated study. Combination PET and CT has rates of sensitivity and specificity of greater than 93%, with positive and negative predictive values also greater than 93% (19). However, the presence of suspicious nodes by PET and CT usually mandates tissue sampling prior to treatment. Currently, the gold standard for pathologic assessment of N2 lymph node involvement is cervical mediastinoscopy or Chamberlain procedure with biopsy. In a recent meta-analysis of 5,678 patients, mediastinoscopy was associated with low rates of morbidity and mortality, as well as 81% sensitivity and 100% specificity for detection of N2 involvement in NSCLC (20,21).

Ultrasound guided minimally invasive mediastinal lymph node assessment for preoperative staging has gained considerable interest over the past decade and in some institutions has become an integral component of the stage IIIA diagnostic algorithm. Theoretical advantages of this technique include potential avoidance of general anesthesia, less pain, minimal recovery, and the lack of surgical manipulation of regional lymph node basins, facilitating easier access if postinduction sampling is required. Although the popularity of minimally invasive lymph node sampling continues to grow, limitations precluding its recommendation over surgical mediastinoscopy include the inability to access all lymph node stations. In addition, an experienced operator is necessary to properly identify and sample mediastinal lymph nodes and reduce the risk of false-negative results. Endobronchial ultrasound with transbronchial fine-needle aspiration (EBUS-TBNA) is associated with a false-negative rate of 13% to 24%, necessitating cervical mediastinoscopy in the event of negative cytology for radiographically suspicious lymph nodes (22).

Esophageal endoscopic ultrasound with TBNA (EUS-TBNA) for mediastinal lymph node assessment may be performed concurrently with EBUS-TBNA, but is a more challenging technique with fewer anatomic clues for the operator. In experienced hands EUS has a sensitivity of 71% to 96% (23–28), a false-negative rate of 15% to 22%, and a false positive rate of 4% to 7% for mediastinal lymph node evaluation in NSCLC (22,23,26–31). Like EBUS, negative pathology in a lymph node basin that is radiographically suspicious requires confirmation by surgical biopsy. The combination of EBUS–fine-needle aspiration (FNA) and EUS-FNA can provide near-complete mediastinal access with a combined sensitivity of 93%, a false-negative rate as low as 3%, and low associated morbidity (30). A helpful diagnostic algorithm, described by Detterbeck, utilizes both traditional and minimally invasive lymph node sampling in the work up of a potential stage IIIA NSCLC patient. This algorithm can be broken down into four classifications based on findings from preoperative imaging (22,29) (Table 12.1).

Minimally invasive lymph node sampling techniques play an important role in the staging and treatment of stage IIIA NSCLC. For patients with obvious evidence of malignant mediastinal disease by CT or chest radiograph, pathologic confirmation by EUS-TBNA, EBUS-TBNA, or conventional transbronchial biopsy eliminates the need for surgical biopsy. This may facilitate expeditious initiation of systemic therapy and the possibility for future evaluation by cervical mediastinoscopy postinduction therapy. Repeat mediastinoscopy, which is associated with increased morbidity due to fibrosis and scarring from prior surgery (32), also has reduced diagnostic yield compared with initial mediastinoscopy, with a sensitivity of only 29% and an accuracy of

■ Table 12.1 Recommendations for evaluation of mediastinum based upon radiographic assessment of NSCLC

Description of Mediastinal Disease by Radiographic Assessment	Inaccuracy of Radiologic Assessment	Mediastinal Nodal Tissue Sampling	Initial Biopsy Techniques
Bulky, unresectable multistation		Not required if another location is easier to biopsy	Least invasive method to access any tumor
Discrete enlargement	False positive rate 20% with PET/CT	Required	EBUS/EUS with surgical biopsy if negative
None, with central tumor or hilar disease	False negative up to 20% with PET/CT	Recommended	EBUS/EUS with surgical biopsy if negative
None, with peripheral tumor	False negative <5% with PET/CT	Not required	Intraoperative lymph node sampling or dissection

CT, computed tomography; EBUS, endobronchial ultrasound; EUS, endoscopic ultra sound; PET, positron emission tomography.
From Ref. 29.

60% (33). For these reasons, the use of EBUS and EUS as a primary staging tool in NSCLC will likely continue to increase.

improved survival with mediastinal dissection; likely due to increased use of adjuvant therapy in patients upstaged following mediastinal lymph node dissection (14,35–37).

■ MEDIASTINAL LYMPH NODE EVALUATION DURING SURGICAL RESECTION

Pathologically defining the extent of N2 disease during definitive surgical resection is necessary for complete and adequate mediastinal staging, and guides the use of adjuvant therapy. Controversy exists as to the equivalence of mediastinal nodal sampling versus complete ispsilateral mediastinal dissection to appropriately identify N2 disease. The American College of Surgeons Oncology Group recently completed a large phase III trial (ACOSOG Z0030), which randomized 1,000 patients to compare mediastinal lymph node dissection versus lymph node sampling to address this question. Initial results from Allen et al. suggest that nodal dissection is associated with clinically insignificant increases in intraoperative blood loss, operative time, and chest tube drainage but does not prolong length of stay or rates of postoperative complications. Survival data for this series is not yet available, but will likely influence operative practice in the future (34). Several small studies have indicated that complete dissection may be superior to nodal sampling. Massard evaluated 208 patients with clinically negative N2 nodes, for which patients underwent nodal sampling followed by mediastinal lymph node dissection. Sixty patients were identified with N2 disease following dissection, while sampling unsuccessfully staged 29 (48%) of those patients. In patients with multilevel disease, nodal sampling identified 10 (40%) of 25 patients (35). These results were replicated by investigations from Wu and Keller (35–37), and suggests that complete mediastinal lymph node dissection more accurately stages N2 disease than selective nodal sampling. In these trials, only Wu was able to demonstrate

■ SINGLE VERSUS MULTISTATION DISEASE

N2 disease is a heterogeneous classification with varying degrees of mediastinal lymph node involvement at the time a patient presents for consultation, and vast differences in survival when patients are stratified by the extent and bulkiness of disease. Several studies have shown that 5-year survival for mediastinoscopy negative postresection positive N2 disease is significantly higher than for bulky N2 disease recognized clinically prior to resection (38–41). Multilevel and clinically evident N2 nodes are negative prognostic factors for IIIA NSCLC (41), and suggest that bulky mediastinal involvement be considered clinically distinct from microscopic N2 disease. The prognosis of bulky N2 lymph node involvement is so poor that some consider it to be more accurately categorized as stage IIIB disease (39).

The presence of multistation N2 disease is another commonly cited factor influencing survival in stage IIIA NSCLC (1). A recent assessment by Riquet (42) of 586 patients with N2 disease undergoing curative resection found a significant survival advantage for single-level mediastinal lymph node involvement compared with multilevel disease (28.5% vs. 17.2% respectively). Differences in survival were independent of histology, location of the primary tumor, capsular rupture, number, or size of involved lymph nodes (43–47).

Multilevel disease was also shown to confer worse prognostic significance by Lee, who demonstrated improved 5-year survival for resected single-level N2 NSCLC (33.8%) compared with multistation N2 involvement (20.4%). Survival associated with multilevel N2 disease was similar to patients with stage IIIB disease (15.5%), and further demonstrated the heterogeneous survival profile of mediastinal lymph node involvement (48). Casali (16), who retrospectively reviewed 183 patients with pathologically diagnosed N2 disease following complete surgical resection, also described a survival advantage of single-level (23.8%) compared with multilevel N2 disease at 5 years (14.7%). Data from Andre in 686 surgically resected patients with histologic evidence of N2 involvement also demonstrated multilevel disease to be associated with poorer prognosis and reduced 5-year survival of 11% compared with 34% for single-level disease. Clinical evidence of N2 disease at multiple stations was associated with a bleak 3% 5-year survival (39). This trend was also appreciated by Ichinose, who reported similar results in 209 patients, and found single-level N2 disease to be a favorable prognostic factor in patients with completely resected stage IIIA NSCLC (43% 5-year survival vs. 17% 5-year survival for multilevel N2 involvement) (49) (Table 12.2).

The influence of extensive N2 involvement on survival following surgical resection was also evaluated by Andre, who investigated over 700 patients with varying degrees of N2 disease on preoperative imaging. The absence of radiographic N2 involvement or microscopic evidence (mN2) was associated with a 5-year survival rate of 29% compared with 7% for patients with radiologic evidence of bulky N2 disease. There was also a significant survival advantage for patients with single station versus multistation N2 involvement (39,41,50). Patients with microscopic disease at one station had a 5-year survival of 34% and a prognosis similar to stage IIB, while multistation disease was associated with a 3% to 11% survival rate, similar to that observed in stage IIIB(39). The site of nodal spread was also shown to have prognostic relevance; right upper lobe tumors that spread to right paratracheal lymph nodes, and left upper lobe tumors with aorta-pulmonary window node involvement, had significantly better survival than patients with lower lobe tumors that spread to lower mediastinal nodes (39).

In summary, the presence of multistation N2 disease confers an overall worse prognosis, and the extent of lymph node involvement is an important predictive variable with significant relevance to survival profiles.

SINGLE MODALITY SURGICAL MANAGEMENT OF N2 DISEASE

Primary surgical management of stage IIIA NSCLC with involvement of mediastinal lymph nodes has been evaluated by multiple investigators. An early trial from Memorial Sloan-Kettering Cancer Center of 400 patients with N2 disease demonstrated limited 5-year survival (9%) and low rates of resectability (18%) for those patients with clinically overt N2 involvement. Patients with unsuspected N2 disease had 5-year survival of 34%, and increased rates of resection in up to 53% of investigation participants (50). This investigation provided early evidence that NSCLC with clinical evidence of metastatic mediastinal disease is associated with poor prognosis, and survival of N2 disease can vary based upon the bulk and degree of lymph node involvement. These factors, in addition to tumor size and location, determine resectability and ultimately affect outcome (50).

Currently, the benefit of primary surgical management for N2 disease is limited to patients in whom complete resection can be obtained and all involved mediastinal disease resected. However, the overall survivability associated with surgical resection alone for N2 disease is poor due to the high risk for both loco-regional and distant recurrence. These results have led to a variety of investigations into induction therapy in lieu of primary surgical intervention.

INDUCTION CHEMOTHERAPY FOR N2

Induction chemotherapy affords an opportunity for improved outcome in patients with N2 disease, with the possibility of reducing, or even eliminating, gross mediastinal and undetected micrometastatic disease, as well as the theoretical advantage of primary tumor reduction for easier resectability (51). The addition of induction chemotherapy in the N2 patient population has been shown to improve survival in a variety of studies (52–54). An early evaluation from MD Anderson Cancer Center of stage IIIA NSCLC patients treated with perioperative

■ **Table 12.2** Review of trials which evaluate survival based upon extent and volume of mediastinal lymph node involvement

			5-Year Overall Survival		
Author	Stage	No. of Patients	Single Station N2 Disease (%)	Multistation N2 Disease (%)	Clinically Evident N2 Disease
Riquet et al. (42)	IIIA	586	28.5	17.2	NR
Lee et al. (48)	IIIA–IIIB	262	33.8	20.4	NR
Casali et al. (16)	IIIA	183	23.8	14.7	NR
Andre et al. (39)	IIIA	686	34	11	3%
Ichinose et al. (49)	IIIA	209	43	17	NR

NR, not reported.

cyclophosphamide, etoposide, and cisplatin followed by surgical resection demonstrated improved median survival from 11 months to 64 months compared with primary surgical management (54). Additional small studies in the 1990s confirmed these results, although many were criticized for small sample size, inconsistent application of PORT, and inclusion of patients who are not considered stage IIIA by current staging (55–57). However, based on these data, induction chemotherapy for stage IIIA disease has become widely accepted. Subsequent randomized trials from the Japanese Cooperative Oncology Group and the French Thoracic Cooperative Group have raised questions about the overall efficacy of neoadjuvant therapy for stage IIIA NSCLC (58,59), demonstrating low chemotherapy response rates and insignificant survival differences between induction therapy and surgery alone. Poor results from these two large trials may be due to older platinum-based chemotherapy regiments and a significant number of patients with bulky N2 disease. More recent phase II trials with third generation platinum-based chemotherapy have validated the utility of induction therapy compared with surgery alone. Third generation platinum-based chemotherapy is now a mainstay of treatment for most stage IIIA NSCLC disease (60–63), with objective response rates of 60% to 74%, and rates of complete surgical resection following induction chemotherapy between 48% and 80%. Three- and 5-year survival rates are also improved over historical controls.

■ INDUCTION CHEMOTHERAPY/ RADIOTHERAPY FOR N2

Concurrent chemotherapy and radiation was initially evaluated in patients with unresectable NSCLC and later applied as neoadjuvant therapy for potentially resectable locally advanced disease. Friess (64), who evaluated definitive chemotherapy and radiation in unresectable stage III patients, found that combination therapy with cisplatin, etoposide, and 60Gy radiation resulted in a median survival of 16 months and a 2-year survival of 30%. This protocol was later applied to the Southwest Oncology Group trial (SWOG) 8805 evaluating 126 patients with stage IIIA or IIIB disease. Patients received two cycles of cisplatin and etoposide with concurrent radiotherapy to 45Gy. Surgical resection was employed in cases without evidence of disease progression (54,65). Three-year survival for stage IIIA patients was 27%, with an 85% complete resection rate following favorable response to neoadjuvant therapy. This was a significant improvement compared with historical controls of patients treated with chemotherapy alone. The SWOG 8805 trial also demonstrated the significant predictive value in sterilization of mediastinal lymph nodes. In patients with

eradication of mediastinal disease by preoperative chemoradiation, 3-year survival was 44%, compared with 18% in patients with an incomplete pathologic response to therapy (54,65).

The importance of mediastinal node sterilization by induction therapy has been the focus of several single institution studies. Bueno evaluated 103 patients with stage IIIA N2 NSCLC; 29 were down staged to pathologic N0 disease by neoadjuvant platinum-based chemotherapy with vival compared to 74 patients with residual mediastinal disease at the time of surgery. Median survival was 21.3 months for N0 disease versus 15.9 months in patients with an incomplete pathologic response, with 5-year survival of 35.8% versus 9% respectively (66). Similar response rates and improved survival was noted by Barlesi (67) in patients treated with platinum-based chemotherapy and radiation of 20 to 45Gy. Based on this data, many feel that stage IIIA patients with a complete N2 pathologic response following induction chemoradiotherapy are ideal candidates for surgical resection; however, others question the utility of resection in this population due to the belief that induction therapy has likely cured the patient. The recent North American Intergroup trial 0139 (INT 0139) was designed to answer that question, but its results have increased the controversy surrounding this topic. Due to the significant difference in survival between patients with and without persistent mediastinal disease, there is considerable interest in detecting residual tumor burden following induction therapy. Patients with evidence of residual disease achieve no survival benefit with surgical resection, and require additional chemotherapy and radiation. To adequately define the presence of residual disease, restaging is accomplished by traditional radiographic methods, including combination PET and CT scans, and more recently EUS/EBUS. While mediastinoscopy with biopsy is the most accurate method of establishing a pretreatment pathologic diagnosis of N2 disease, lymph node sampling following induction therapy or surgery is plagued with inaccuracies due to post-treatment adhesions and fibrosis (68,69). As a result, integrated before PET/CT is the preferred modality for noninvasive reassessment of the mediastinum following induction therapy. After induction therapy reoperative mediastinoscopy has a poorer sensitivity and specificity than integrated PET-CT (68). Interest in EUS-TBNA and EBUS-TBNA for lymph node sampling in this capacity is increasing, but has not been validated in a large prospective trial.

Recent investigations to assess optimization of induction chemotherapy and radiation include the Radiation Oncology Group trial (RTOG) 0412/SWOG 0332; a trial designed for patients with limited N2 disease who were randomized to cisplatin and docetaxel alone or with concurrent radiotherapy (50.4Gy). This protocol was limited to patients with resectable, low volume mediastinal lymph node involvement, and was first trial evaluating induction chemoradiotherapy in stage IIIA NSCLC disease with these specific features. Unfortunately, accrual was poor and the trial closed early without answering the question of optimal treatment in this highly selective group of patients.

■ SURGICAL MANAGEMENT FOLLOWING NEOADJUVANT CHEMOTHERAPY AND RADIATION

Following neoadjuvant therapy, the appropriate selection of patients for surgical resection continues to represent a significant clinical challenge. Operative management following induction therapy in patients with residual disease has been associated with increased risk of morbidity and mortality, especially when larger, more complicated resections are required. Fowler reported a mortality rate of 43% in patients undergoing pneumonectomy after chemotherapy and radiation (60Gy), compared with 0% mortality in patients undergoing lobectomy following neoadjuvant therapy. Similarly the SWOG 8805 trial reported a 29% mortality rate associated with pneumonectomy following neoadjuvant radiation therapy to 45Gy (65,70).

Comparison of 5-year survival for stage IIIA N2 patients undergoing induction chemotherapy followed by surgical resection was assessed in the European Organisation for Research and Treatment of Cancer (EORTC) 08941 trial. One hundred and fifty-four randomized patients underwent surgical resection after demonstrating tumor response to induction chemotherapy, while an additional 154 patients were treated with radiotherapy after tumor cytoreduction. Median and 5-year survival for resection was 16.4 months and 15.7% versus 17.5 months and 14% for patients treated by radiotherapy alone. Progression-free survival was also similar between groups. In this investigation, surgical resection did not improve overall or progression-free survival compared with radiotherapy after a response to induction chemotherapy was achieved (71).

Critics of the EORTC 08941 trial cite a lack of survival associated with surgical intervention to an inappropriate study population which was deemed "resectable" but in fact represented "unresectable" disease. In this study 50% of patients in the surgical arm underwent incomplete resection. In addition, heterogeneous induction-chemotherapy protocols which varied among treatment centers and a high proportion of patients undergoing pneumonectomy have also cast doubt on these conclusions (72,73).

The role of surgical resection following induction chemoradiotherapy was also assessed by a phase III trial (National Cancer Institute R9309, INT 0139) of 396 patients with pathologic N2 disease who were randomized to induction therapy with cisplatin, etoposide, and 45Gy

radiation followed by surgery, or definitive treatment with chemoradiotherapy to 60Gy. Both groups received consolidation chemotherapy with two cycles of cisplatin and etoposide. Progression-free survival favored the trimodality treatment group (12.8 months vs. 10.5 months respectively), as did 5-year survival with rates of 27.2% versus 20.3% in the nonsurgical arm (although this difference did not reach statistical significance). Pathologic evidence of disease remission at N2 stations was associated with a 5-year survival of 41% compared with 24% in the presence of residual nodal disease. Increased postoperative deaths associated with trimodality therapy were predominately in patients undergoing complex resections or pneumonectomy, with only one postoperative death in a patient undergoing lobectomy. An unplanned post-hoc analysis demonstrated favorable median and 5-year survival for patients undergoing nonsurgical management if pneumonectomy was necessary to complete the resection (24% vs. 22% with trimodality treatment). For patients undergoing lobectomy with matched controls treated nonsurgically, trimodality treatment was associated with a significant survival advantage (median survival 24 months vs. 22 months, and 5-year survival 36% vs. 18%) (6,74). Pneumonectomy was associated with inferior operative mortality of 17.6% versus 1.1% for lobectomy (6,74), an observation which has been validated in similar investigations (70,75,76). This assessment also highlighted the importance of loco-regional control in select stage IIIA patients (73). For stage IIIA N2 disease with a favorable response to induction therapy, the INT 0139 trial does support the selective use of surgical resection in patients who require less complex operative procedures (i.e., lobectomy) (73).

Morbidity commonly associated with preoperative radiotherapy followed by pneumonectomy includes the development of pulmonary edema and/or bronchopleural fistula (which occurs due to the nonspecific damage incurred by healthy lung tissue), reduced vascularity of the resection stump, and sclerosis of the mediastinal lymphatics. Complications are more common following right pneumonectomy than left, and are thought to be due to the increased volume of lung tissue resected, limited vascular supply, and less available soft tissue coverage for the bronchial stump compared with the left. These are important considerations when evaluating a patient who might require pneumonectomy after induction therapy.

Several additional European and U.S. investigations have demonstrated improved outcome for surgical resection following neoadjuvant chemoradiotherapy (even with increased dosing up to 60Gy) compared with the INT 0139 and EORTC 08941. Five-year survival data following a response to induction chemotherapy and surgical resection, particularly for cases in which pneumonectomy is avoided, can exceed 30% (6–8,77). Continued improvement in the detection of residual N2 disease following

induction therapy by PET/CT, EBUS, and EUS to identify patients with resectable IIIA disease will likely further
improve the survival rate associated with multimodality
therapy (78,79). Improved morbidity and mortality in
these trials is attributed to enhanced three-dimensional
radiation planning systems that maximize tumor exposure
and minimize unwanted damage to adjacent structures.
Likewise, improved quality control associated with surgery, meticulous surgical technique, appropriate fluid
management, and the use of vascularized muscle flaps on
bronchial stumps have all been associated with improved
outcome after complex resection (including pneumonectomy) following induction therapy (78,79).

ADJUVANT CHEMOTHERAPY FOR N2

The use of adjuvant chemotherapy following surgical resection for pathologically defined N2 disease is an extension
of the work in early-stage NSCLC (stage I and II), where a
13% reduction in 5-year mortality was observed following
treatment (12–14). Adjuvant chemotherapy specifically for
stage III NSCLC was first assessed in a subgroup analysis
of the IALT and the ANITA. In each of these trials patients
were randomized to three or four cycles of cisplatin-based
adjuvant chemotherapy versus observation. Overall results
supported the use of adjuvant therapy for completely
resected patients and planned subset analysis confirmed
a significant survival benefit in resected stage III patients
(12,13). More recently, Pignon's LACE meta-analysis of
4,585 resected NSCLC patients treated with adjuvant cisplatin demonstrated a lower hazard ratio (HR) for death
with the use of adjuvant chemotherapy in resected stage
III patients (HR = 0.83 vs. 0.92). This translated into a
5.5% absolute survival benefit at 5 years and suggested
a survival advantage for adjuvant chemotherapy following resection in patients with incidentally discovered N2
disease (14).

RADIATION THERAPY

In 1998, the PORT meta-analysis for NSCLC assessed over
2,100 patients in nine randomized trials, demonstrating
an overall detrimental effect with the use of PORT on survival for completely resected NSCLC. Two-year survival
for all stages was 48% compared with 55% with surgery
alone. A higher rate of mortality associated with PORT
was thought to be due to increased intercurrent deaths,
and inferior results were greater for patients with N0 or
N1 disease, while a nonsignificant survival advantage was
noted for N2 disease compared with surgery alone (80).
Following this analysis, PORT was reserved for use only

in instances of close surgical margins, evidence of extran-
odal extension, or in the presence of residual disease following surgery. Improvements in technology associated
with imaging and radiation planning have increased interest in the utility of PORT following surgical resection for
stage IIIA patients.

In a recent retrospective review from the Surveillance,
Epidemiology, and End Results database of 7,000 NSCLC
patients, overall survival for patients who received PORT
was inferior to matched controls (81). Subgroup analysis by stage demonstrated that patients with stage I and
II disease fared worse following PORT, but a significant
survival advantage was noted with the use of PORT for
stage IIIA patients (HR = 0.855; 95% confidence interval,
0.762–0.959) (81). These findings suggest that in patients
with N2 disease, the high risk of local/regional recurrence
outweighs the toxicity associated with radiotherapy.

Radiation oncologists now utilize three-dimensional
targeting systems to more accurately isolate tumor radiation delivery, enhancing the overall therapeutic ratio
and increasing the ability to improve local control with
decreased toxicity to surrounding normal structures.
The advent of enhanced-resolution CT scan, magnetic
resonance imaging, and combination PET/CT have further helped to delineate a biologically relevant tumor
target. This technology has allowed focused research
on dose escalation to 60Gy and beyond for enhanced
tumor destruction. Historically, radiation dosing in the
range of 80 to 100Gy was required for tumor sterilization (82). However, without accurate targeting technology, patients receiving greater than 70Gy are at risk for
significant adverse events due to inadvertent radiation of
normal tissues (82).

New outcome data from large volume centers treating stage IIIA patients with resectable N2 disease support
the use of PORT. A phase II trial from RTOG #9705,
studied adjuvant paclitaxel and carboplatin with PORT
for resected stage II and IIIA NSCLC, and demonstrated
1-, 2-, and 3-year survival of 86%, 70%, and 61% (83).
These survival rates were markedly improved from historical controls.

Dose escalation trials in concert with chemotherapy
regimens have recently been underway to determine
the safety and efficacy of combination therapy. The
University of North Carolina–based consortium studied
62 unresectable stage III NSCLC patients receiving 60 to
74Gy of radiation with concurrent chemotherapy (carboplatin and paclitaxel) and demonstrated survival rates
at 1, 2, 3, and 4 years of 71%, 52%, 40%, and 36%
respectively, with a median survival of 26 months (84).
This was followed by an RTOG #9311, a study of 177
unresectable NSCLC patients treated with similar chemotherapy and escalating radiation dosing to 75Gy, with
a median survival for patients receiving full dose therapy
of 22 months (85). The North Central Cancer Treatment

Group also reported on dose escalation in 20 locally advanced NSCLC patients receiving between 70 and 74Gy of radiation, with a median survival of 37 months (86). An upcoming RTOG trial will compare survival of 60Gy against 70Gy in an adjuvant chemoradiotherapy protocol, and further characterize the efficacy of radiation dose escalation.

Future trials will delineate the role of radiotherapy and dose escalation both in the pre- and postoperative periods. Improved localization technology may also allow radiation dose escalation for improved efficacy in patients with N2 disease.

■ CONCLUSION

Stage IIIA NSCLC represents a heterogeneous group of patients with a spectrum of mediastinal lymph node involvement and resultant variety of treatment protocols. For the small group of patients with T3N1 disease, surgical resection remains the mainstay of current management. Adjuvant chemotherapy in this setting is clinically indicated and has been associated with a survival benefit in multiple randomized trials. Patients with N2 disease represent the majority of stage IIIA disease. PET/CT, cervical mediastinoscopy, or EBUS/EUS with FNA are the main tools used in pretreatment assessment of mediastinal lymph node involvement. The current recommended management of N2 disease is multimodality therapy; however, the optimal role and timing of chemotherapy, radiation, and surgery continues to be an issue of great debate. Overall, lower volume lymph node involvement and the ability to sterilize the mediastinum are associated with a favorable prognosis and correlates strongly with survival. Future investigations are aimed at improving stratification of patients based upon the volume of mediastinal involvement, increasing preoperative identification of mediastinal disease, optimizing adjuvant and neoadjuvant treatments, and improving the safety of resection.

■ REFERENCES

1. Kassis ES, Vaporciyan AA. Defining N2 disease in non-small cell lung cancer. *Thorac Surg Clin.* 2008;18(4):333–337.
2. Sause W, Kolesar P, Taylor S IV, et al. Final results of phase III trial in regionally advanced unresectable non-small cell lung cancer: Radiation Therapy Oncology Group, Eastern Cooperative Oncology Group, and Southwest Oncology Group. *Chest.* 2000;117(2):358–364.
3. Curran WJ, Scott C, Langer C, et al. Long-term benefit is observed in phase III comparison for sequential versus concurrent chemoradiation for patients with unresected stage III NSCLC. *Proc ASCO.* 2003;22:621.
4. Mountain CF. Revisions in the International System for Staging Lung Cancer. *Chest.* 1997;111(6):1710–1717.
5. DeCamp MM Jr, Ashiku S, Thurer R. The role of surgery in N2 non-small cell lung cancer. *Clin Cancer Res.* 2005;11(13 Pt 2):5033s–5037s.
6. Albain KS, Swann RS, Rusch VW. Phase III study of concurrent chemotherapy and radiotherapy (CT/RT) vs. CT/RT followed by surgical resection for stage IIIA (pN2) non-small cell lung cancer (NSCLC): outcomes update of North American Intergroup 0139 (RTOG 9309). *J Clin Oncol.* 2005;23:16S.
7. Lorent N, De Leyn P, Lievens Y, et al.; Leuven Lung Cancer Group. Long-term survival of surgically staged IIIA-N2 non-small-cell lung cancer treated with surgical combined modality approach: analysis of a 7-year prospective experience. *Ann Oncol.* 2004;15(11):1645–1653.
8. Eberhardt W, Wilke H, Stamatis G, et al. Preoperative chemotherapy followed by concurrent chemoradiation therapy based on hyperfractionated accelerated radiotherapy and definitive surgery in locally advanced non-small-cell lung cancer: mature results of a phase II trial. *J Clin Oncol.* 1998;16(2):622–634.
9. Goldstraw P, Crowley J, Chansky K, et al.; International Association for the Study of Lung Cancer International Staging Committee; Participating Institutions. The IASLC Lung Cancer Staging Project: proposals for the revision of the TNM stage groupings in the forthcoming (seventh) edition of the TNM Classification of malignant tumours. *J Thorac Oncol.* 2007;2(8): 706–714.
10. Kassis ES, Vaporciyan AA, Swisher SG, et al. Application of the revised lung cancer staging system (IASLC Staging Project) to a cancer center population. *J Thorac Cardiovasc Surg.* 2009;138(2):412–418.e1.
11. Oda M, Watanabe S, Tsukayama S, et al. [Results of resection of T3N0–2M0 non-small cell lung cancer according to involved organ and nodal status]. *Kyobu Geka.* 1998;51(11):902–906.
12. Arriagada R, Bergman B, Dunant A, Le Chevalier T, Pignon JP, Vansteenkiste J; International Adjuvant Lung Cancer Trial Collaborative Group. Cisplatin-based adjuvant chemotherapy in patients with completely resected non-small-cell lung cancer. *N Engl J Med.* 2004;350(4):351–360.
13. Douillard JY, Rosell R, Delena M. ANITA: phase III adjuvant vinorelbine (N) and cisplatin (P) versus observation in completely resected (stage I-III) non-small cell lung cancer (NSCLC) patients: final results after 70 month median follow-up. On behalf of the Adjuvant Navelbine International Trialist Association. *J Clin Oncol.* 2005;23:624.
14. Pignon JP, Tribodet H, Scagliotti GV, et al.; LACE Collaborative Group. Lung adjuvant cisplatin evaluation: a pooled analysis by the LACE Collaborative Group. *J Clin Oncol.* 2008;26(21):3552–3559.
15. Roy MS, Donington JS. Management of locally advanced non small cell lung cancer from a surgical perspective. *Curr Treat Options Oncol.* 2007;8(1):1–14.
16. Casali C, Stefani A, Natali P, Rossi G, Morandi U. Prognostic factors in surgically resected N2 non-small cell lung cancer: the importance of patterns of mediastinal lymph nodes metastases. *Eur J Cardiothorac Surg.* 2005;28(1):33–38.
17. Le Chevalier T, Arriagada R, Quoix E, et al. Radiotherapy alone versus combined chemotherapy and radiotherapy in unresectable non-small cell lung carcinoma. *Lung Cancer.* 1994;10(suppl 1):S239–S244.
18. Le Chevalier T, Arriagada R, Tarayre M, et al. Significant effect of adjuvant chemotherapy on survival in locally advanced non-small-cell lung carcinoma. *J Natl Cancer Inst.* 1992;84(1):58.
19. Vansteenkiste JF, Stroobants SG, Dupont PJ, et al. FDG-PET scan in potentially operable non-small cell lung cancer: do anatometabolic PET-CT fusion images improve the localisation of regional lymph node metastases? The Leuven Lung Cancer Group. *Eur J Nucl Med.* 1998;25(11):1495–1501.
20. Toloza EM, Harpole L, Detterbeck F, McCrory DC. Invasive staging of non-small cell lung cancer: a review of the current evidence. *Chest.* 2003;123(1 suppl):157S–166S.

21   Toloza EM, Harpole L, McCrory DC. Noninvasive staging of non-small cell lung cancer: a review of the current evidence. *Chest.* 2003;123(1 suppl):137S–146S.

22. Detterbeck FC, Jantz MA, Wallace M, Vansteenkiste J, Silvestri GA; American College of Chest Physicians. Invasive mediastinal staging of lung cancer: ACCP evidence-based clinical practice guidelines (2nd edition). *Chest.* 2007;132(3 suppl): 202S–220S.

23. Fritscher-Ravens A, Soehendra N, Schirrow L, et al. Role of transesophageal endosonography-guided fine-needle aspiration in the diagnosis of lung cancer. *Chest.* 2000;117(2):339–345.

24. Gress FG, Savides TJ, Sandler A, et al. Endoscopic ultrasonography, fine-needle aspiration biopsy guided by endoscopic ultrasonography, and computed tomography in the preoperative staging of non-small-cell lung cancer: a comparison study. *Ann Intern Med.* 1997;127(8 Pt 1):604–612.

25. Mortensen MB, Fristrup C, Holm FS, et al. Prospective evaluation of patient tolerability, satisfaction with patient information, and complications in endoscopic ultrasonography. *Endoscopy.* 2005;37(2):146–153.

26. Silvestri GA, Hoffman BJ, Bhutani MS, et al. Endoscopic ultrasound with fine-needle aspiration in the diagnosis and staging of lung cancer. *Ann Thorac Surg.* 1996;61(5):1441–5; discussion 1445.

27. Wallace MB, Silvestri GA, Sahai AV, et al. Endoscopic ultrasound-guided fine needle aspiration for staging patients with carcinoma of the lung. *Ann Thorac Surg.* 2001;72(6):1861–1867.

28. Wiersema MJ, Vazquez-Sequeiros E, Wiersema LM. Evaluation of mediastinal lymphadenopathy with endoscopic US-guided fine-needle aspiration biopsy. *Radiology.* 2001;219(1):252–257.

29. Detterbeck FC. Integration of mediastinal staging techniques for lung cancer. *Semin Thorac Cardiovasc Surg.* 2007;19(3):217–224.

30. Wallace MB, Pascual JM, Raimondo M, et al. Minimally invasive endoscopic staging of suspected lung cancer. *JAMA.* 2008;299(5):540–546.

31. Annema JT, Versteegh MI, Veseliç M, et al. Endoscopic ultrasound added to mediastinoscopy for preoperative staging of patients with lung cancer. *JAMA.* 2005;294(8):931–936.

32. Goldstraw P. Selection of patients for surgery after induction chemotherapy for N2 non-small-cell lung cancer. *J Clin Oncol.* 2006;24(21):3317–3318.

33. Van Schil P, Stamatis G. Sensitivity of remediastinoscopy: influence of adhesions, multilevel N2 involvement, or surgical technique? *J Clin Oncol.* 2006;24(33):5338; author reply 5339–5338; author reply 5340.

34. Allen MS, Darling GE, Pechet TT, et al.; ACOSOG Z0030 Study Group. Morbidity and mortality of major pulmonary resections in patients with early-stage lung cancer: initial results of the randomized, prospective ACOSOG Z0030 trial. *Ann Thorac Surg.* 2006;81(3):1013–9; discussion 1019.

35. Massard G, Ducrocq X, Kochetkova EA, Porhanov VA, Riquet M. Sampling or node dissection for intraoperative staging of lung cancer: a multicentric cross-sectional study. *Eur J Cardiothorac Surg.* 2006;30(1):164–167.

36. Keller SM, Adak S, Wagner H, Johnson DH. Mediastinal lymph node dissection improves survival in patients with stages II and IIIa non-small-cell lung cancer. Eastern Cooperative Oncology Group. *Ann Thorac Surg.* 2000;70(2):358–65; discussion 365.

37. Wu Y, Huang ZF, Wang SY, Yang XN, Ou W. A randomized trial of systematic nodal dissection in resectable non-small cell lung cancer. *Lung Cancer.* 2002;36(1):1–6.

38. Pearson FG, DeLarue NC, Ilves R, Todd TR, Cooper JD. Significance of positive superior mediastinal nodes identified at mediastinoscopy in patients with resectable cancer of the lung. *J Thorac Cardiovasc Surg.* 1982;83(1):1–11.

39. Andre F, Grunenwald D, Pignon JP, et al. Survival of patients with resected N2 non-small-cell lung cancer: evidence for a subclassification and implications. *J Clin Oncol.* 2000;18(16):2981–2989.

40. Martini N, Flehinger BJ, Zaman MB, Beattie EJ Jr. Results of resection in non-oat cell carcinoma of the lung with mediastinal lymph node metastases. *Ann Surg.* 1983;198(3):386–397.

41. Vansteenkiste JF, De Leyn PR, Deneffe GJ, Lerut TE, Demedts MG. Clinical prognostic factors in surgically treated stage IIIA-N2 non-small cell lung cancer: analysis of the literature. *Lung Cancer.* 1998;19(1):3–13.

42. Riquet M, Bagan P, Le Pimpec Barthes F, et al. Completely resected non-small-cell lung cancer: reconsidering prognostic value and significance of N2 metastases. *Ann Thorac Surg.* 2007;84(6):1818–1824.

43. Cybulsky IJ, Lanza LA, Ryan MB, Putnam JB Jr, McMurtrey MM, Roth JA. Prognostic significance of computed tomography in resected N2 lung cancer. *Ann Thorac Surg.* 1992;54(3):533–537.

44. Hata E, Miyamoto H, Sakao Y. [Investigation into mediastinal lymph node metastasis of lung cancer and rationale for decision of the extent of mediastinal dissection]. *Nippon Geka Gakkai Zasshi.* 1997;98(1):8–15.

45. Maggi G, Casadio C, Cianci R, et al. Results of surgical resection of stage IIIa (N2) non small cell lung cancer, according to the site of the mediastinal metastases. *Int Surg.* 1993;78(3):213–217.

46. Miller DL, McManus KG, Allen MS, et al. Results of surgical resection in patients with N2 non-small cell lung cancer. *Ann Thorac Surg.* 1994;57(5):1095–100; discussion 1100.

47. Nakanishi R, Osaki T, Nakanishi K, et al. Treatment strategy for patients with surgically discovered N2 stage IIIA non-small cell lung cancer. *Ann Thorac Surg.* 1997;64(2):342–348.

48. Lee JG, Lee CY, Park IK, et al. The prognostic significance of multiple station N2 in patients with surgically resected stage IIIA N2 non-small cell lung cancer. *J Korean Med Sci.* 2008;23(4):604–608.

49. Ichinose Y, Kato H, Koike T, et al.; Japanese Clinical Oncology Group. Completely resected stage IIIA non-small cell lung cancer: the significance of primary tumor location and N2 station. *J Thorac Cardiovasc Surg.* 2001;122(4):803–808.

50. Martini N, Flehinger BJ. The role of surgery in N2 lung cancer. *Surg Clin North Am.* 1987;67(5):1037–1049.

51. Choi NC, Carey RW, Daly W, et al. Potential impact on survival of improved tumor downstaging and resection rate by preoperative twice-daily radiation and concurrent chemotherapy in stage IIIA non-small-cell lung cancer. *J Clin Oncol.* 1997;15(2): 712–722.

52. Pass HI, Pogrebniak HW, Steinberg SM, Mulshine J, Minna J. Randomized trial of neoadjuvant therapy for lung cancer: interim analysis. *Ann Thorac Surg.* 1992;53(6):992–998.

53. Rosell R, Maestre J, Font A, et al. A randomized trial of mitomycin/ifosfamide/cisplatin preoperative chemotherapy plus surgery versus surgery alone in stage IIIA non-small cell lung cancer. *Semin Oncol.* 1994;21(3 suppl 4):28–33.

54. Roth JA, Fossella F, Komaki R, et al. A randomized trial comparing perioperative chemotherapy and surgery with surgery alone in resectable stage IIIA non-small-cell lung cancer. *J Natl Cancer Inst.* 1994;86(9):673–680.

55. Meko J, Rusch VW. Neoadjuvant therapy and surgical resection for locally advanced non-small cell lung cancer. *Semin Radiat Oncol.* 2000;10(4):324–332.

56. Martini N, Kris MG, Flehinger BJ, et al. Preoperative chemotherapy for stage IIIa (N2) lung cancer: the Sloan-Kettering experience with 136 patients. *Ann Thorac Surg.* 1993;55(6):1365–73; discussion 1373.

57. Rosell R, Gómez-Codina J, Camps C, et al. A randomized trial comparing preoperative chemotherapy plus surgery with surgery alone in patients with non-small-cell lung cancer. *N Engl J Med.* 1994;330(3):153–158.

58. Depierre A, Milleron B, Moro-Sibilot D, et al.; French Thoracic Cooperative Group. Preoperative chemotherapy followed by surgery compared with primary surgery in resectable stage I (except T1N0), II, and IIIa non-small-cell lung cancer. *J Clin Oncol.* 2002;20(1):247–253.

59. Tada H, Tsuchiya R, Ichinose Y, et al. A randomized trial comparing adjuvant chemotherapy versus surgery alone for completely resected pN2 non-small cell lung cancer (JCOG9304). *Lung Cancer.* 2004;43(2):167–173.

60. Betticher DC, Hsu Schmitz SF, Tötsch M, et al. Mediastinal lymph node clearance after docetaxel-cisplatin neoadjuvant chemotherapy is prognostic of survival in patients with stage IIIA pN2 non-small-cell lung cancer: a multicenter phase II trial. *J Clin Oncol.* 2003;21(9):1752–1759.

61. Cappuzzo F, Selvaggi G, Gregorc V, et al. Gemcitabine and cisplatin as induction chemotherapy for patients with unresectable Stage IIIA-bulky N2 and Stage IIIB nonsmall cell lung carcinoma: an Italian Lung Cancer Project Observational Study. *Cancer.* 2003;98(1):128–134.

62. O'Brien ME, Splinter T, Smit EF, et al.; EORTC Lung Cancer Group. Carboplatin and paclitaxol (Taxol) as an induction regimen for patients with biopsy-proven stage IIIA N2 non-small cell lung cancer. an EORTC phase II study (EORTC 08958). *Eur J Cancer.* 2003;39(10):1416–1422.

63. Splinter TA, van Schil PE, Kramer GW, et al. Randomized trial of surgery versus radiotherapy in patients with stage IIIA (N2) non small-cell lung cancer after a response to induction chemotherapy. EORTC 08941. *Clin Lung Cancer.* 2000;2(1):69–72; discussion 73.

64. Friess GG, Baikadi M, Harvey WH. Concurrent cisplatin and etoposide with radiotherapy in locally advanced non-small cell lung cancer. *Cancer Treat Rep.* 1987;71(7–8):681–684.

65. Albain KS, Rusch VW, Crowley JJ, et al. Concurrent cisplatin/etoposide plus chest radiotherapy followed by surgery for stages IIIA (N2) and IIIB non-small-cell lung cancer: mature results of Southwest Oncology Group phase II study 8805. *J Clin Oncol.* 1995;13(8):1880–1892.

66. Bueno R, Richards WG, Swanson SJ, et al. Nodal stage after induction therapy for stage IIIA lung cancer determines patient survival. *Ann Thorac Surg.* 2000;70(6):1826–1831.

67. Barlési F, Doddoli C, Chetaille B, et al. Survival and postoperative complication in daily practice after neoadjuvant therapy in resectable stage IIIA-N2 non-small cell lung cancer. *Interact Cardiovasc Thorac Surg.* 2003;2(4):558–562.

68. De Leyn P, Stroobants S, De Wever W, et al. Prospective comparative study of integrated positron emission tomography-computed tomography scan compared with remediastinoscopy in the assessment of residual mediastinal lymph node disease after induction chemotherapy for mediastinoscopy-proven stage IIIA-N2 Non-small-cell lung cancer: a Leuven Lung Cancer Group Study. *J Clin Oncol.* 2006;24(21):3333–3339.

69. Mateu-Navarro M, Rami-Porta R, Bastus-Piulats R, Cirera-Nogueras L, González-Pont G. Remediastinoscopy after induction chemotherapy in non-small cell lung cancer. *Ann Thorac Surg.* 2000;70(2):391–395.

70. Fowler WC, Langer CJ, Curran WJ Jr, Keller SM. Postoperative complications after combined neoadjuvant treatment of lung cancer. *Ann Thorac Surg.* 1993;55(4):986–989.

71. van Meerbeeck JP, Kramer GW, Van Schil PE, et al.; European Organisation for Research and Treatment of Cancer-Lung Cancer Group. Randomized controlled trial of resection versus radiotherapy after induction chemotherapy in stage IIIA-N2 non-small-cell lung cancer. *J Natl Cancer Inst.* 2007;99(6):442–450.

72. Vansteenkiste J, Betticher D, Eberhardt W, De Leyn P. Randomized controlled trial of resection versus radiotherapy after induction chemotherapy in stage IIIA-N2 non-small cell lung cancer. *J Thorac Oncol.* 2007;2(8):684–685.

73. Eberhardt WE, Stamatis G, Stuschke M. Surgery in stage III non-small-cell lung cancer. *Lancet.* 2009;374(9687):359–360.

74. Albain KS, Swann RS, Rusch VW, et al. Radiotherapy plus chemotherapy with or without surgical resection for stage III non-small-cell lung cancer: a phase III randomised controlled trial. *Lancet.* 2009;374(9687):379–386.

75. Deutsch M, Crawford J, Leopold K, et al. Phase II study of neoadjuvant chemotherapy and radiation therapy with thoracotomy in the treatment of clinically staged IIIA non-small cell lung cancer. *Cancer.* 1994;74(4):1243–1252.

76. Pisters KM, Ginsberg RJ, Giroux DJ, et al. Induction chemotherapy before surgery for early-stage lung cancer: A novel approach. Bimodality Lung Oncology Team. *J Thorac Cardiovasc Surg.* 2000;119(3):429–439.

77. Betticher DC, Hsu Schmitz SF, Tötsch M, et al.; Swiss Group for Clinical Cancer Research (SAKK). Prognostic factors affecting long-term outcomes in patients with resected stage IIIA pN2 non-small-cell lung cancer: 5-year follow-up of a phase II study. *Br J Cancer.* 2006;94(8):1099–1106.

78. Sonett JR, Suntharalingam M, Edelman MJ, et al. Pulmonary resection after curative intent radiotherapy (>59 Gy) and concurrent chemotherapy in non-small-cell lung cancer. *Ann Thorac Surg.* 2004;78(4):1200–5; discussion 1206.

79. Daly BD, Fernando HC, Ketchedjian A, et al. Pneumonectomy after high-dose radiation and concurrent chemotherapy for nonsmall cell lung cancer. *Ann Thorac Surg.* 2006;82(1):227–231.

80. Postoperative radiotherapy in non-small-cell lung cancer: systematic review and meta-analysis of individual patient data from nine randomised controlled trials. PORT Meta-analysis Trialists Group. *Lancet.* 1998;352(9124):257–263.

81. Lally BE, Zelterman D, Colasanto JM, Haffty BG, Detterbeck FC, Wilson LD. Postoperative radiotherapy for stage II or III non-small-cell lung cancer using the surveillance, epidemiology, and end results database. *J Clin Oncol.* 2006;24(19):2998–3006.

82. Fletcher GH. Clinical dose response curves of human malignant epithelial tumours. *Br J Radiol.* 1973;46(542):151.

83. Bradley JD, Paulus R, Graham MV, et al.; Radiation Therapy Oncology Group. Phase II trial of postoperative adjuvant paclitaxel/carboplatin and thoracic radiotherapy in resected stage II and IIIA non-small-cell lung cancer: promising long-term results of the Radiation Therapy Oncology Group–RTOG 9705. *J Clin Oncol.* 2005;23(15):3480–3487.

84. Socinski MA, Rosenman JG, Halle J, et al. Dose-escalating conformal thoracic radiation therapy with induction and concurrent carboplatin/paclitaxel in unresectable stage IIIA/B nonsmall cell lung carcinoma: a modified phase I/II trial. *Cancer.* 2001;92(5):1213–1223.

85. Bradley J, Graham MV, Winter K, et al. Toxicity and outcome results of RTOG 9311: a phase I-II dose-escalation study using three-dimensional conformal radiotherapy in patients with inoperable non-small-cell lung carcinoma. *Int J Radiat Oncol Biol Phys.* 2005;61(2):318–328.

86. Schild SE, Wong WW, Vora SA, et al. The long-term results of a pilot study of three times a day radiotherapy and escalating doses of daily cisplatin for locally advanced non-small-cell lung cancer. *Int J Radiat Oncol Biol Phys.* 2005;62(5):1432–1437.

13 Management of Unresectable Stage III NSCLC

ANJALI BHARNE

LYUDMILA BAZHENOVA

BARBARA GITLITZ

After a patient is confirmed to have stage III non–small cell lung cancer (NSCLC), a variety of therapeutic options exist to treat this heterogeneous group of tumors. Unlike the earlier stages of NSCLC, which can be treated definitively with surgical resection with or without adjuvant chemotherapy, or radiation therapy, or other modalities such as radiofrequency ablation, stage III disease often requires the incorporation of multiple modalities of treatment. These tumors are, by definition, locoregionally advanced due to primary tumor extension into extrapulmonary structures or mediastinal lymph node involvement without evidence of distant metastases. In this chapter, we will focus on the key issues in formulating a treatment plan after a patient has been assessed to have unresectable stage III NSCLC disease.

■ CLASSIFICATION

NSCLC is staged according to the TNM (Tumor, Node, Metastasis) system, and according to AJCC 6.0 stage III NSCLC can be subdivided into IIIA disease, and IIIB (dry) and IIIB (wet) disease. Since stage IIIB (wet) disease is defined by the presence of a malignant pleural or pericardial effusion, which is generally incurable and treated as metastatic disease, our discussion will be centered on IIIA and IIIB—dry disease. In the new seventh edition of the TNM staging guidelines for lung cancer, these IIIB (wet) patients are reclassified as stage IV (M1a), reflecting the natural history of the pleural or pericardial involvement (1).

Stage IIIA patients can be clinically separated into those with bulky or nonbulky mediastinal lymph node involvement. Bulky disease is defined generally by lymph nodes >2 cm measured by computed tomography, groupings of multiple smaller lymph nodes, or involvement of more than 2 lymph node stations (2). This delineation now helps select patients appropriate for surgical resection after neoadjuvant therapy. Prior to the use of combined modality treatment, patients with bulky stage III disease were considered inoperable, while patients with nonbulky stage IIIA cancer were considered for curative resection. Now in light of data showing that surgery alone rarely cures even nonbulky stage IIIA patients, the presence or absence of mediastinal lymph node involvement can guide treatment toward a combined modality approach although this is a noted area of controversy.

Patients with stage IIIA disease are distinguished from IIIB patients by ipsilateral hilar (N1) or mediastinal lymph node involvement (N2); invasion of the chest wall (including superior sulcus), diaphragm, mediastinal pleura, parietal pericardium; or proximity to the carina (all T3). Stage IIIB (dry) patients, in contrast, have either involvement of the contralateral mediastinal lymph nodes (N3) or extrapulmonary mediastinal structures such as the great vessels, heart, trachea, esophagus, or vertebral body (all T4).

As described earlier, the heterogeneity of stage III NSCLC necessitates creating tumor and node-specific treatment plans, with cure as the overall intent of treatment. From the medical oncology, radiation oncology, and surgical standpoints, performance status and pulmonary function are key components of formulating this plan. If a patient has a compromised performance status, then potentially curative combined modality treatments may be contraindicated due to their increased morbidity and mortality. The American Society of Clinical Oncology (ASCO) guidelines indicate those patients best suited for combined modality therapy have an Eastern Cooperative Oncology Group (ECOG) performance status score of 0 or 1; adequate pulmonary function generally defined as a forced expiratory ventilation in 1 second (FEV_1) >800 to 1,000 cm^3; and adequate hematologic, renal, and hepatic function (3).

■ DEFINITION OF UNRESECTABLE DISEASE

Medical Unresectability

The median age of diagnosis of lung cancer is approximately 71 years, an age at which many patients have developed serious comorbid medical conditions. These underlying physiologic medical problems can include chronic obstructive pulmonary disease, coronary artery disease, certain connective tissue diseases, or diabetes, some of which are directly related to the patient's smoking history. Patients with these baseline conditions have a low probability of tolerating general anesthesia, the operation, the postoperative recovery period, or the removal of adjacent functioning lung and their lung cancer is generally considered medically unresectable.

Surgical Unresectability

When determining the suitability of a patient with locally advanced NSCLC for surgical resection, the absence of lung cancer in the mediastinal lymph nodes is an important factor in determining treatment. If mediastinal lymph nodes are pathologically proven to contain cancer, then the patient has stage III disease, and a multimodality approach should be utilized with input from a medical oncologist, radiation oncologist, and thoracic surgeon.

From a purely surgical standpoint, N2 lymph nodes (at least on the right side) are considered resectable since they are within the field of resection of a right thoracotomy or right thoracoscopic procedure (4). N3 lymph nodes, in contrast, are considered unresectable because they are contralateral to the tumor or in the supraclavicular region, which are both outside the field of the procedure. Some authors also deem disease anatomically unresectable if there is invasion of vertebral bodies, heart, or great vessels (5).

■ OVERVIEW OF MANAGEMENT

Owing to the varied nature of stage III NSCLC, the natural history of this stage of the disease is dependent upon tumor size and lymph node involvement. Roswit et al. (6) early on showed that best supportive care alone for stage III NSCLC patients resulted in survival of 14% at 1 year. Treatment with standard radiation therapy alone to 60 Gy has shown 5-year survival rates ranging from 4% to 6%, and median survival from 9 to 11 months (7–12). When utilizing chemotherapy and radiation therapy as part of the treatment plan, 5-year survival rates can improve to 15% to 17%, and median survival 13 to 17 months (7,10,13).

■ TREATMENT

Radiation Alone

Throughout the 1980s, radiation therapy remained the definitive treatment for unresectable stage III NSCLC. In an oft-quoted early clinical trial, Roswit et al. (6) showed that standard external beam radiation to 40–50 Gy resulted in improved survival compared to best supportive care. Building on this study, the Radiation Therapy Oncology Group (RTOG) attempted to determine the influence of radiation dose on outcome. In RTOG 73–01 which included patients with stages I–IIIA NSCLC and RTOG 73–02 which included those with stage IIIB disease (14,15), a total of 551 patients with medically or surgically inoperable NSCLC were treated with radiation according to two different protocols depending on the stage of the tumor. Patients with T1–3, N0–2 tumors were randomized to four different regimens: 40 Gy given split course or 40, 50, or 60 Gy given continuously (five fractions per week). Patients with T4 or N3 tumors were randomized to three different regimens: 30 Gy given continuously (five fractions per week), 40 Gy given split course, or 40 Gy given continuous course. There was no difference in survival among the four different regimens, but local control was improved with higher radiation doses. RTOG 73–01 demonstrated the lowest intrathoracic failure rate with 60 Gy relative to lower doses, and that became the standard dose for unresectable stage III NSCLC (Table 13.1).

Yet based on their data, the authors believed that higher doses of radiation therapy would be necessary in order to achieve better local control, especially with large masses. In fact, in a trial of patients with locally advanced NSCLC, Arriagada et al. (10,12,16) randomized patients to either standard radiation therapy to 65 Gy or the same radiation regimen preceded and followed by three cycles of systemic dose chemotherapy to control distant metastases. Although the radiation therapy + chemotherapy arm did have a lower rate of distant metastasis of 45% compared to 67% in the radiation therapy–alone arm (P < 0.001), the 2-year survival rates were not very different at 21% versus 14%, respectively (P = 0.08). In fact, they found that local control at 1 year was low in both groups, 15% and 17%, respectively. This led to the conclusion that local thoracic tumor control is a key element of improving survival in these unresectable patients.

Therefore, certain approaches have been investigated to improve local control of the lung tumor. These include altered fractionation schemes, dose escalation, radiation sensitization, and better tumor targeting.

Altered Fractionation

Although studies have shown that higher doses of radiation can result in higher rates of local control, the main limitation of increasing the radiation dose is resulting toxicity

Table 13.1 Results of Radiation Therapy Oncology Group 73–01				
	Radiation Regimen			
	4,000 Gy—Split Course	**4,000 Gy—Continuous**	**5,000 Gy—Continuous**	**6,000 Gy—Continuous**
Intrathoracic failure rate (within irradiated lung)	38%	48%	38%	27%

Source: Adapted from Ref. 14.

to normal tissues. To address this toxicity problem and improve the therapeutic index, altered fractionation has been explored to shorten the schedule of radiation therapy and change the dose delivered per fraction.

- Hyperfractionation—One strategy of altered fractionation is pure hyperfractionation where two or more daily fractions are administered to the same total dose with the purpose of reducing the late effects of radiation. It is hypothesized that shortening the radiation therapy schedule will produce more tumor cell kill but also more severe acute side effects, so that the total dose of radiation must be partly reduced (17). However, when smaller doses are used per fraction, more fractions can be delivered which enables a higher total dose of radiation to be given. This also results in less late toxicity to normal tissues.

- Using this theory, the RTOG 83–11 trial was a prospective, dose-seeking randomized phase I/II study of hyperfractionation in patients with stage III NSCLC conducted from 1983 to 1987 (18). During this time, 848 patients were randomized to total doses of 62 Gy, 64.8 Gy, 69.6 Gy, 74.4 Gy, or 79.2 Gy, delivered in 1.2 Gy fractions twice daily. There were no significant differences in the risks of acute or late effects in normal tissues among all the patients analyzed in the five arms. Among the 350 stage III patients with favorable prognostic factors, including Karnofsky performance status of 70 or higher and weight loss of less than 5%, there was a survival benefit for the tumor dose of 69.6 Gy compared with lower doses (median, 13.0 months; 2 years, 29%, *P* = 0.02).

- Building on the results of RTOG 83–11, the 69.6 Gy arm of that trial was examined further in a phase III, 3-arm trial in patients with locally advanced NSCLC (8). In this trial, RTOG 88–08/ECOG 4588, 490 patients were randomized to standard radiation therapy to 60 Gy (2 Gy fractions daily for 6 weeks) or hyperfractionated treatment to 69.6 Gy (1.2 Gy fractions twice daily for 6 weeks) or induction chemotherapy of cisplatin and vinblastine followed by standard radiation therapy. Preliminary data showed 1-year survival (%) and median survival as follows: standard radiation therapy—46%, 11.4 months; chemotherapy

plus radiotherapy—60%, 13.8 months; and hyperfractionated radiation therapy—51%, 12.3 months. The chemotherapy plus radiotherapy arm was statistically superior to the other two treatment arms (*P* = 0.03). With longer follow-up, the curves for the chemotherapy plus radiotherapy and hyperfractionation arms began to overlap, with 3-year survivals of 13% versus 14% and 5-year survivals of 8% and 6%, respectively (9). Considering RTOG 83–11 and RTOG 88–08/ECOG 4588 together, hyperfractionation alone does not show clear benefit and is not widely practiced.

- Accelerated fractionation is another type of altered fractionation. With this approach, the same total dose of radiation therapy is condensed in an attempt to decrease the likelihood of tumor regeneration during treatment. This results in a decrease in overall treatment time and more tumor kill since there is less time for rapidly growing cells to repopulate.

- Combining the concepts of hyperfractionation and accelerated fractionation, continuous hyperfractionated accelerated radiation therapy, or CHART, was developed. Small fractions are given up to three times daily, allowing the overall treatment time to be reduced. In a trial comparing CHART (given in 1.5 Gy fractions three times daily for 12 consecutive days to a total 54 Gy) to standard radiation therapy of 60 Gy (given in 2 Gy daily fractions), 563 patients with locally advanced NSCLC and good performance status were randomized to the above arms (19,20). The CHART arm showed a statistically significantly better 2-year survival of 29% versus 20% in the standard radiation therapy arm (*P* = 0.004), as well as improved local control of 23% versus 15%, respectively. The patients in the CHART arm did experience a significantly higher incidence of severe dysphagia during the first 3 months (19% vs. 3%), but this mainly occurred after completion of the radiation therapy, and there were no significant differences in late toxicities.

- Yet other large randomized trials have failed to show a clear benefit with combined modality treatment and hyperfractionated accelerated radiation therapy (HART). The ECOG 2597 trial treated 141 patients with induction chemotherapy of carboplatin and paclitaxel and then randomized them to either HART

(57.6 Gy in 1.5 Gy fractions three times/day, with 2 weekend breaks) or conventional radiation therapy (64 Gy in 2 Gy daily fractions) (21). The trial closed early secondary to slow accrual, but the trend in improvement in median survival did not reach statistical significance (20.3 months vs. 14.9 months, $P = 0.28$).

Although the theoretical benefit of altered fractionation schemes seems appealing, the evidence to support these approaches is unconvincing. Moreover, the practical challenges of delivering treatment more than once daily and continuous treatment over weekend days can be major obstacles in pursuing further altered fractionation strategies.

Sequential Chemotherapy Followed by Radiation

Given the importance of establishing local tumor control and decreasing the risk of developing distant metastasis, systemic chemotherapy was then added to radiation therapy in the treatment of locally advanced unresectable NSCLC. A landmark clinical trial which evaluated the role of induction chemotherapy prior to radiation was the Cancer and Leukemia Group B (CALGB) 8433 trial which randomized 155 patients with stage III disease to conventional radiation therapy alone (60 Gy over 6 weeks) or two cycles of cisplatin and vinblastine followed by the same radiation treatment (7). The addition of chemotherapy resulted in an improved median survival of 13.7 months compared to 9.6 months in the radiation treatment–alone group ($P = 0.012$) and improved 5-year survival of 17% compared to 6%. It should be noted that the patients included in this study had high performance status (ECOG/CALGB 0–1) and less than 5% weight loss in the 3 months prior to diagnosis. Although systemic chemotherapy did improve survival, the authors acknowledged that still 80% to 85% of stage III patients still died within 5 years due to both local and distant failure. Based on the original publication (22), when both treatment groups were considered together, 41% to 45% had relapse in the lung alone, 39% to 45% had lung and distant metastases, and 4% to 6% had metastatic disease alone.

Additionally, the results of CALGB 8433 were confirmed by the US Intergroup trial, an effort of the RTOG, ECOG, and Southwest Oncology Group (SWOG) cooperative groups (9). They randomized 458 patients with surgically unresectable stage II, IIIA, and IIIB disease to standard radiation therapy alone (60 Gy in 2 Gy daily fractions) or hyperfractionated radiation therapy (69.6 Gy in 1.2 Gy fractions twice daily) or induction chemotherapy with cisplatin and vinblastine followed by standard radiation therapy. Overall survival (OS) was superior in the arm receiving chemotherapy and irradiation compared with those arms receiving standard radiation or hyperfractionated radiation alone ($P = 0.04$), with median survival of 13.2 months compared to 11.4 months versus 12 months,

respectively. At 5 years, survival was 8% in the sequential chemoradiotherapy group, 5% in the standard radiation group, and 6% in the hyperfractionated radiation group.

Meta-analyses of patients with locally advanced NSCLC have also shown the survival advantage of combined treatment with cisplatin-based chemotherapy followed by radiation compared to radiation alone (23,24). A review of CALGB trial patients with stage III NSCLC evaluating combined modality therapy showed that treatment with thoracic radiation alone predicted for poorer survival (hazard ratio 1.58; 95% confidence interval [CI] 1.22–2.05; $P = 0.001$) (24).

Concurrent Chemotherapy with Radiation

Building on the evidence that systemic chemotherapy improves survival likely by decreasing the rate of distant metastasis (12), exploration of concurrent delivery of chemotherapy with radiation therapy seemed the most intuitive next step in both eradicating micrometastatic disease and sensitizing radiation to improve local control.

Concurrent modality treatment was initially shown to be beneficial relative to radiation treatment alone. The European Organization for Research and Treatment of Cancer conducted a 3-arm phase III trial of 331 patients comparing split-course radiotherapy over 7 weeks (2 weeks of 3 Gy given 10 times followed by a 3-week rest period and then radiotherapy for 2 more weeks of 2.5 Gy given 10 times); radiotherapy on the same schedule, combined with weekly cisplatin 30 mg/m^2; or radiotherapy on the same schedule, combined with daily cisplatin 6 mg/m^2) (25). Survival was significantly improved in the radiotherapy-daily-cisplatin group as compared to the radiotherapy group: 54% versus 46% at 1 year, 26% versus 13% at 2 years, and 16% versus 2% at 3 years ($P = 0.009$). Survival in the radiotherapy-weekly-cisplatin group was intermediate and not significantly different from survival in either of the other two groups. The survival benefit of daily combined treatment was due to improved control of local disease ($P = 0.003$). Time to local recurrence was prolonged in the groups that received cisplatin chemotherapy, but there was no difference in time to distant metastases among all the groups. Because of the improvement in local control for patients receiving systemic chemotherapy with radiation, it has been hypothesized that this may have been primarily responsible for the improvement observed in OS.

Multiple large randomized trials by Jeremic et al. (26,27) also explored concurrent modality therapy but used hyperfractionated radiation as the control arm. One of these trials randomized 131 patients to hyperfractionated radiation alone or carboplatin and etoposide given daily with hyperfractionated radiation (27). The group treated with concurrent chemoradiation had a longer median survival of 22 months compared to 14 months in the hyperfractionated radiation group, with 4-year survival rates of 23% and 9%, respectively ($P = 0.021$). The local recurrence-free survival rates also favored the concurrently treated group but there was no difference in the rate of distant metastasis, emphasizing the importance of local tumor control in improving OS.

Concurrent modality therapy has now been examined in several trials head-to-head with sequential chemotherapy followed by radiation. The West Japan Lung Cancer Group conducted a phase III trial which randomized 320 patients to chemotherapy consisting of cisplatin 80 mg/m², vindesine 3 mg/m², and mitomycin 8 mg/m² given concurrent with split-course radiation of 56 Gy or given prior to the same radiotherapy regimen (13). Survival favored the group receiving concurrent treatment, with a median survival of 16.5 months compared to 13.3 months in the sequential treatment group ($P = 0.04$). Moreover, the concurrent therapy group had a 5-year survival of 15.8% compared to 8.9% in the sequentially treated group. In regard to toxicity, myelosuppression occurred more frequently in the concurrently treated arm, but there was no difference in the incidence of esophageal toxicity, which may have been due to split-course treatment.

In the largest phase III trial reaffirming the benefit of concurrent chemoradiation, the RTOG 94–10 trial randomized 610 patients with stage II or III NSCLC to three different treatment regimens, one of which included hyperfractionated radiation (28). The treatment groups were once-daily radiation (60 Gy) after induction chemotherapy with cisplatin (100 mg/m²) and vinblastine (5 mg/m²); once-daily radiation (60 Gy) concurrent with the same chemotherapy; or hyperfractionated radiation (69.6 Gy) with concurrent chemotherapy with cisplatin (50 mg/m²) and oral etoposide (50 mg twice daily). Survival was improved in the group treated with concurrent chemotherapy and daily radiation, with a median survival of 17.1 months and 4-year survival of 21% compared to 14.6 months and 12%, respectively, in the sequential group ($P = 0.046$). The rates of acute grade 3 to 4 nonhematologic toxicity were higher with concurrent than sequential therapy, but late toxicity rates were similar. Zatloukal et al. (29) also examined concurrent chemoradiotherapy compared to sequential

treatment using cisplatin and vinorelbine in a randomized phase II trial of 102 patients, and found a similar survival benefit (median survival 16.6 vs. 12.9 months ($P = 0.023$). The study also detailed the increased toxicity profile of using concurrent therapy: increased grade 3 to 4 leukopenia (53% compared to 19% in the sequential group, $P = 0.009$) and nausea/vomiting (39% compared to 15%, $P = 0.044$). There was no significant difference in grade 3 to 4 neutropenia, febrile neutropenia, and esophagitis (Table 13.2).

The most effective chemotherapy regimen to be delivered concurrently with radiation therapy is not clearly established, but a majority of the trials have used cisplatin-based chemotherapy. In fact, cisplatin and etoposide have been rigorously studied, showing efficacy in a population of patient with bulky stage IIIB NSCLC (30). In that multicenter phase II trial, SWOG 9019, 50 patients were treated with cisplatin 50 mg/m² on days 1, 8, 29, and 36; etoposide 50 mg/m² on days 1 to 5 and 29 to 33 and concurrent radiotherapy (to 61 Gy). Of note, patients were re-evaluated at the 45-Gy mark with imaging and pulmonary function testing to ensure there was no evidence of disease progression. This regimen resulted in a median survival of 15 months and a 5-year survival of 15%.

Having established that concurrent therapy results in improved survival compared to sequential therapy, the role of induction therapy in the concurrent setting has been explored (31). The CALGB 39801 trial randomized 366 patients to weekly carboplatin (area under the curve [AUC] 2) and paclitaxel (50 mg/m²) concurrent with radiation (66 Gy) [=Arm A] or two cycles of carboplatin (AUC 6) and paclitaxel (200 mg/m²) followed by identical chemoradiation [=Arm B]. There was no significant difference in survival; in fact, the median survival on arm A was 12 months versus 14 months on arm B, with 2-year survivals of 29% and 31%, respectively. However, neutropenia and overall toxicity were higher in the induction chemotherapy arm. There was no difference in radiotherapy-related toxicities of esophagitis or pneumonitis. Based on these results, induction chemotherapy prior to definitive chemoradiation should be reserved only to downstage those tumors which cannot fit into a safe radiation field. Additionally,

■ **Table 13.2** Results of Radiation Therapy Oncology Group 94–10

	Radiation Regimen		
	Sequential—CT→RT	Concurrent—CT + Daily RT	Concurrent—CT + Hyperfractionated RT
Median survival	14.6 months	17.0 months	15.2 months
4-year survival	12%	21%	17%
P value vs SEQ		0.046	0.296

CT, computed tomography, RT, radiation therapy.

Source: Adapted from Ref. 28.

weekly carboplatin and paclitaxel should not be utilized unless the patient cannot tolerate full-dose platinum and etoposide.

Thus, the current evidence-based approach to patients with locally advanced, unresectable NSCLC who have a good performance status without significant weight loss is the administration of cisplatin-based chemotherapy concurrent with conventional daily radiation to at least 60 Gy. Many institutions, however, have extrapolated the use of carboplatin-based regimens from the data, which is a reasonable alternative.

■ CONSOLIDATION CHEMOTHERAPY

Based on the disappointing survival rates of patients with stage III unresectable disease, SWOG decided to examine the role of non–cross-reactive chemotherapy after completion of concurrent chemoradiation in their SWOG 9504 phase 2 trial (32). This was a single-arm trial of 81 patients accrued from 1996 to 1998. It used identical staging, eligibility criteria, and concurrent chemotherapy arm as SWOG 9019, which accrued from 1992 to 1995 (30). This was done intentionally to allow historical comparison between those 2 trials. Consolidation docetaxel was given to patients with nonprogressive disease after two cycles of concurrent chemoradiation. Doses of docetaxel were set to be 75 mg/m^2 for cycle number 1 and 100 mg/m^2 for cycles 2 and 3 in the absence of protocol-defined toxicities. Stage distribution of patients enrolled in this trial was T4N0/1: 31 patients; T4N2: 22 patients; and N3: 30 patients. Positron emission tomography scanning was not mandated as it was not a standard of care at that time, although a very strict histologic criteria for confirmation of N3 involvement was mandated. Upon completion of concurrent chemoradiotherapy 65 patients (78%) proceeded to consolidation arm. Forty-nine patients (75% of those starting consolidation) completed all three cycles, 28 of them on the intended dose schedule. With a median follow-up of 32 months, median progression-free survival was 16 months and median survival was 26 months. OS rates at 1, 2, and 3 years were 76%, 54%, and 37%, respectively. When S9019 and S9504 were compared, toxicities were similar, but survival was better: 26 versus 15 months for median survival and 34% versus 54% and 17% versus 37 % for 2- and 3-year survival, respectively. The reported survival was the highest seen for stage III NSCLC which generated a lot of enthusiasm and was accepted as a new standard without properly conducted randomized trial. Gandara updated S9504 results in 2006. At a median follow-up of 71 months, median progression-free survival was still robust at 16 months; median survival 26 months; and 3-, 4-, and 5-year survival rates were 40%, 29%, and 29%, respectively. In the

predecessor trial S9019, 3-, 4-, and 5-year survival rates were 17%, 17%, and 17% (33).

Hoosier Oncology group (HOG) embarked upon proving improved survival with consolidation docetaxel with a randomized phase III study (34). This trial enrolled 203 patients and was terminated early based on an interim analysis for futility. It utilized a typical SWOG regimen of cisplatin 50 mg/m^2 days 1 and 8 and etoposide 50 mg/m^2 days 1 to 5 repeated every 4 weeks for two cycles. Patients were then randomized to either docetaxel at 75 mg/m^2 or observation. Docetaxel arm resulted in more toxicity, specifically a 5.5% death rate attributed to docetaxel and increase in hospitalization rate 28.8% versus 8.1%. With a median follow-up of 41.6 months there was no difference in survival between 2 arms, with the median OS time of 23.2 months in the observation arm and 21.2 months in the docetaxel arm (log rank P = 0.883) and 3-year OS rates of 26.1% and 27.1%. Based on the HOG randomized clinical trial, consolidation therapy with at least docetaxel cannot be recommended.

S9504 and HOG trials had several important differences; inclusion of patients with stage IIIA disease into the HOG trial (40% of the trial participants) and less strict cutoff for FEV1. For the HOG, FEV had to exceed 1 L versus ≥ 2 L for S9504 trial. We know from the past trials that baseline FEV1 levels predict for outcomes. In HOG there was a very slight imbalance between arms for the patients who have an FEV1 ≥2 L favoring the control arm (P = not significant). Despite those minor differences it is difficult to argue with its results.

HOG trial also raised an important question regarding the optimal duration of chemotherapy in unresectable stage III lung cancer. There was no difference in survival in patients receiving four cycles of chemotherapy or two, thus showcasing the need for further investigation into an optimal duration of chemotherapy (Table 13.3).

Other phase III trials have examined the role of consolidation therapy in unresectable stage III disease. S0023 looked at a role of an epidermal growth factor receptor (EGFR) tyrosine kinase inhibitor gefitinib after concurrent chemoradiation therapy. Patients who have completed SWOG 9540 regime with cisplatin and etoposide, followed by consolidation docetaxel were then registered and randomly assigned to gefitinib at 250 mg/day or placebo (35). Study was closed early for futility based on unplanned interim analysis, which was triggered by a negative Iressa Survival Evaluation in Lung Cancer trial (phase III randomized trial comparing gefitinib and best supportive care in second-line metastatic disease setting) (36). With 243 randomly assigned patients, median survival time was 23 months for gefitinib and 35 months for placebo (n = 125); two-sided P = 0.013). One- and 2-year survival rates were 73% and 46% for the gefitinib arm and 81% and 59% for the placebo arm, respectively. It is difficult to explain

■ Table 13.3 Comparison of S9019, S9504 and Hoosier Oncology group

Trial	Median Survival (months)	1-Year Survival	2-Year Survival	3-Year Survival
S9019 4 cycles of cisplatin/etoposide concurrently with radiation (30)	15	58%	35%	17%
S9504 2 cycles of cisplatin/etoposide concurrent with radiation followed by docetaxel (32)	26	76%	54%	37%
HOG 2 cycles of cisplatin/etoposide concurrent with radiation, followed by observation or docetaxel (34)	23.2 obs 21.2 docetaxel	NR	NR	26.1% 27.1%

NR, non reported.

an inferior survival for gefitinib in this study. Majority of deaths were cancer related and there were no toxic deaths. There was no statistically significant imbalance in the arms. Although smoking status was not collected, it is unlikely to have made a difference. Based on the results of BR21 trial (randomized trial of erlotinib vs. best supportive care in second-line metastatic setting), erlotinib was not detrimental in either former or current smokers. In fact the benefit of erlotinib remained in this subgroup of patients, albeit not as dramatic as in nonsmokers (37). Imbalance in EGFR or KRAS mutations and absence of data on subsequent therapies may explain inferior results of this trial.

This detrimental effect is also surprising based on the recently reported SATURN trial showing small but statistically significant improvement in survival for maintenance erlotinib after completion of a first-line therapy for stage IV disease (38). Ongoing investigations looking at a role of adjuvant erlotinib for early-stage lung cancer might give us some clues to explain S0023 results.

Other phase II single-arm clinical trials have examined the role of consolidation therapy added to different combination of concurrent backbone. Different agents were used including carboplatin and taxanes, topotecan, and oral vinorelbine (39–42)

■ PROPHYLACTIC CRANIAL IRRADIATION

Although the combination of chemotherapy and radiation has resulted in improved survival for patients with unresectable stage III NSCLC by improving locoregional control and decreasing the risk of visceral metastasis, isolated brain metastasis remains a problem for these patients. Studies have shown that 30% to 43% of patients with stage III (N2) disease treated with preoperative chemotherapy and irradiation subsequently developed a brain metastasis (43,44). In fact, the brain is the first site of failure for approximately 25% of patients (45).

A retrospective review of 422 patients with stage III NSCLC treated with cisplatin-based chemotherapy and concurrent radiation showed that brain metastases developed early during treatment, with almost half of the relapses occurring in the first 16 weeks after treatment (46). Nonsquamous histology and young patient age predicted for increased risk of early relapse with brain metastases.

In light of this discouraging data, prophylactic cranial irradiation (PCI) presents a worthwhile method of decreasing the risk of disease recurrence in the brain, a very problematic sanctuary site. Multiple prospective randomized trials in the 1970s and 1980s suggested PCI decreased brain metastasis in patients with advanced NSCLC (47–49), but a meta-analysis of these trials concluded that PCI did not improve survival in these patients (50). It should be noted that these were earlier studies which used less efficacious chemotherapy and radiation regimens.

More recent randomized trials have attempted to identify a role for PCI. Pöttgen et al. randomized 112 patients with operable stage III NSCLC to either primary resection followed by adjuvant radiation therapy (50–60 Gy); or preoperative chemotherapy followed by concurrent chemoradiotherapy (45 Gy; 1.5 Gy twice per day) and definitive surgery (51). Patients in the preoperative combined modality arm received PCI (30 Gy; 2 Gy daily fractions). The results showed that PCI reduced the probability of brain metastases as the first site of failure at 5 years (7.8% compared to 34.7%; $P = 0.02$) as well as the overall brain relapse rate (9.1% at 5 years vs. 27.2%; $P = 0.04$).

The previous study, however, was not powered to detect the effect of PCI on survival. To investigate this question, the RTOG 0214 trial attempted to randomize patients with stage III NSCLC who had stable disease following definitive therapy to either whole brain radiation therapy (30 Gy in 15 fractions) or observation. Unfortunately, the trial closed prematurely due to slow accrual. At this time, the evidence is not convincing to offer PCI to all patients who have been definitively treated for stage III NSCLC.

■ FUTURE DIRECTIONS

Radiation

Dose Escalation + "Radiation-Sensitizing" Doses of Chemotherapy

In an effort to improve on the locoregional failures seen with radiation therapy alone and to minimize toxicity relative to concurrent full-dose chemotherapy, the concept of radiation dose escalation with concurrent "radiation-sensitizing" doses of chemotherapy has been explored through multiple trials. Phase I/II data from the RTOG 0117 trial where patients received weekly carboplatin (AUC 2) and paclitaxel (50 mg/m²) and concurrent dose-escalated radiation showed a maximum-tolerated dose of 74 Gy (52). For the 24 patients who have been treated to this dose, the median survival is 21.6 months.

The CALGB 30105 trial built on this earlier data and their own phase I trial that escalated radiation doses to 74 Gy from a starting dose of 60 Gy (53). In the phase I trial, all patients received induction chemotherapy of carboplatin (AUC 6) and paclitaxel (225 mg/m²) for two cycles followed by concurrent chemoradiotherapy. During radiation treatment, weekly carboplatin (AUC 2) and paclitaxel (45 mg/m²) were given. Radiation was delivered as three-dimensional conformal radiation therapy in 2 Gy fractions to totals of 60, 66, 70, and 74 Gy, with a median survival of 24 months. For the phase II trial, patients were randomized to either the same induction chemotherapy and concurrent chemoradiotherapy regimen as mentioned earlier or induction carboplatin (AUC 5) and gemcitabine (1,000 mg/m²) followed by concurrent gemcitabine twice weekly (35 mg/m²) during radiation to 74 Gy (54). At a median follow-up of 44 months, the median survival was 24.3 months for the carboplatin/paclitaxel group and 12.5 months for the carboplatin/gemcitabine group. In fact, the gemcitabine arm was closed early due to a high rate of pulmonary toxicity (37% with grade 3–5). Based on these results, the carboplatin/paclitaxel regimen will be compared to standard radiation therapy in further randomized trials in the United States.

Chemotherapy

Previous trials have shown that treatment of locally advanced head and neck cancer with concomitant high-dose radiotherapy plus cetuximab improves locoregional control and median OS (54,55). CALGB 30407 was a phase II randomized clinical trial which tested an addition of cetuximab to carboplatin (AUC5) and pemetrexed 500 mg/m² given concurrently with radiation. All patients received total of eight cycles of chemotherapy. Cetuximab was given for 6 weeks during the radiation phase. Preliminary results of this trial were reported at ASCO 2009 (56) and showed similar rates of partial response in chemotherapy versus cetuximab arm, respectively 73%

(95% CI 59–83)/71% (95% CI 57–81%). Median failure-free survival (months) 12.9 (95% CI 8.6–18.0)/10.3 (95% CI 8.7–18.9); 18-month survival 57% (95% CI 41–79)/47% (95% CI 33–67); and median survival (months) 22.3/18.7 was also similar in chemotherapy versus cetuximab arm. The trial was later updated at world lung conference (57), still showing no dramatic differences. Further evaluation of this regimen is ongoing.

Further studies of consolidation approach is still underway with a PROCLAIM study (58). This is a trial comparing two cycles SWOG 9019 chemoradiation regimen followed by a two additional cycles—"dealers choice" of consolidation schemas using one of the following regimens: etoposide and cisplatin; vinorelbine and cisplatin; or paclitaxel and carboplatin. The investigational arm will include three cycles of cisplatin and pemetrexed concurrently with radiation followed by two more cycles of single-agent pemetrexed.

In summary managing of unresectable stage III disease continues to evolve and a lot of questions remain unanswered. It is important, however, to enlist a multi-disciplinary team which should, at a minimum, include a thoracic surgeon, a radiation oncologist, and a medical oncologist.

■ REFERENCES

1. Goldstraw P, Crowley J, Chansky K, et al.; International Association for the Study of Lung Cancer International Staging Committee; Participating Institutions. The IASLC Lung Cancer Staging Project: proposals for the revision of the TNM stage groupings in the forthcoming (seventh) edition of the TNM Classification of malignant tumours. *J Thorac Oncol.* 2007;2(8):706–714.
2. Robinson LA, Ruckdeschel JC, Wagner H Jr, Stevens CW; American College of Chest Physicians. Treatment of non-small cell lung cancer-stage IIIA: ACCP evidence-based clinical practice guidelines (2nd edition). *Chest.* 2007;132(3 suppl):243S–265S.
3. Pfister DG, Johnson DH, Azzoli CG, et al.; American Society of Clinical Oncology. American Society of Clinical Oncology treatment of unresectable non-small-cell lung cancer guideline: update 2003. *J Clin Oncol.* 2004;22(2):330–353.
4. Patel V, Shrager JB. Which patients with stage III non-small cell lung cancer should undergo surgical resection? *Oncologist.* 2005;10(5):335–344.
5. Caglar HB, Baldini EH, Othus M, et al. Outcomes of patients with stage III nonsmall cell lung cancer treated with chemotherapy and radiation with and without surgery. *Cancer.* 2009;115(18):4156–4166.
6. Roswit B, Patno ME, Rapp R, et al. The survival of patients with inoperable lung cancer: a large-scale randomized study of radiation therapy versus placebo. *Radiology.* 1968;90(4):688–697.
7. Dillman RO, Herndon J, Seagren SL, Eaton WL Jr, Green MR. Improved survival in stage III non-small-cell lung cancer: seven-year follow-up of cancer and leukemia group B (CALGB) 8433 trial. *J Natl Cancer Inst.* 1996;88(17):1210–1215.
8. Sause WT, Scott C, Taylor S, et al. Radiation Therapy Oncology Group (RTOG) 88–08 and Eastern Cooperative Oncology Group (ECOG) 4588: preliminary results of a phase III trial in regionally advanced, unresectable non-small-cell lung cancer. *J Natl Cancer Inst.* 1995;87(3):198–205.

9. Sause W, Kolesar P, Taylor S IV, et al. Final results of phase III trial in regionally advanced unresectable non-small cell lung cancer: Radiation Therapy Oncology Group, Eastern Cooperative Oncology Group, and Southwest Oncology Group. *Chest.* 2000;117(2):358–364.

10. Le Chevalier T, Arriagada R, Quoix E, et al. Radiotherapy alone versus combined chemotherapy and radiotherapy in nonresectable non-small-cell lung cancer: first analysis of a randomized trial in 353 patients. *J Natl Cancer Inst.* 1991;83(6):417–423.

11. Johnson DH, Einhorn LH, Bartolucci A, et al. Thoracic radiotherapy does not prolong survival in patients with locally advanced, unresectable non-small cell lung cancer. *Ann Intern Med.* 1990;113(1):33–38.

12. Le Chevalier T, Arriagada R, Tarayre M, et al. Significant effect of adjuvant chemotherapy on survival in locally advanced non-small-cell lung carcinoma. *J Natl Cancer Inst.* 1992;84(1):58.

13. Furuse K, Fukuoka M, Kawahara M, et al. Phase III study of concurrent versus sequential thoracic radiotherapy in combination with mitomycin, vindesine, and cisplatin in unresectable stage III non-small-cell lung cancer. *J Clin Oncol.* 1999;17(9):2692–2699.

14. Perez CA, Pajak TF, Rubin P, et al. Long-term observations of the patterns of failure in patients with unresectable non-oat cell carcinoma of the lung treated with definitive radiotherapy. Report by the Radiation Therapy Oncology Group. *Cancer.* 1987;59(11):1874–1881.

15. Perez CA, Bauer M, Edelstein S, Gillespie BW, Birch R. Impact of tumor control on survival in carcinoma of the lung treated with irradiation. *Int J Radiat Oncol Biol Phys.* 1986;12(4):539–547.

16. Arriagada R, Le Chevalier T, Quoix E, et al. ASTRO (American Society for Therapeutic Radiology and Oncology) plenary: Effect of chemotherapy on locally advanced non-small cell lung carcinoma: a randomized study of 353 patients. GETCB (Groupe d'Etude et Traitement des Cancers Bronchiques), FNCLCC (Féderation Nationale des Centres de Lutte contre le Cancer) and the CEBI trialists. *Int J Radiat Oncol Biol Phys.* 1991;20(6):1183–1190.

17. Thames HD, Jr, Peters LJ, Withers HR, et al. Accelerated fractionation vs hyperfractionation: rationales for several treatments per day. *Int J Radiat Oncol Biol Phys.* 1983;9:127–138.

18. Cox JD, Azarnia N, Byhardt RW, Shin KH, Emami B, Pajak TF. A randomized phase I/II trial of hyperfractionated radiation therapy with total doses of 60.0 Gy to 79.2 Gy: possible survival benefit with greater than or equal to 69.6 Gy in favorable patients with Radiation Therapy Oncology Group stage III non-small-cell lung carcinoma: report of Radiation Therapy Oncology Group 83–11. *J Clin Oncol.* 1990;8(9):1543–1555.

19. Saunders M, Dische S, Barrett A, Harvey A, Gibson D, Parmar M. Continuous hyperfractionated accelerated radiotherapy (CHART) versus conventional radiotherapy in non-small-cell lung cancer: a randomised multicentre trial. CHART Steering Committee. *Lancet.* 1997;350(9072):161–165.

20. Saunders M, Dische S, Barrett A, Harvey A, Griffiths G, Palmar M. Continuous, hyperfractionated, accelerated radiotherapy (CHART) versus conventional radiotherapy in non-small cell lung cancer: mature data from the randomised multicentre trial. CHART Steering committee. *Radiother Oncol.* 1999;52(2):137–148.

21. Belani CP, Wang W, Johnson DH, et al. Phase III study of the Eastern Cooperative Oncology Group (ECOG 2597): induction chemotherapy followed by either standard thoracic radiotherapy or hyperfractionated accelerated radiotherapy for patients with unresectable stage IIIA and B non-small-cell lung cancer. *J Clin Oncol.* 2005;23:3760–3767.

22. Dillman RO, Seagren SL, Propert KJ, et al. A randomized trial of induction chemotherapy plus high-dose radiation versus radiation alone in stage III non-small-cell lung cancer. *N Engl J Med.* 1990;323(14):940–945.

23. Marino P, Preatoni A, Cantoni A. Randomized trials of radiotherapy alone versus combined chemotherapy and radiotherapy in stages IIIa and IIIb nonsmall cell lung cancer. A meta-analysis. *Cancer.* 1995;76(4):593–601.

24. Socinski MA, Zhang C, Herndon JE 2nd, et al. Combined modality trials of the Cancer and Leukemia Group B in stage III non-small-cell lung cancer: analysis of factors influencing survival and toxicity. *Ann Oncol.* 2004;15(7):1033–1041.

25. Schaake-Koning C, van den Bogaert W, Dalesio O, et al. Effects of concomitant cisplatin and radiotherapy on inoperable non-small-cell lung cancer. *N Engl J Med.* 1992;326(8):524–530.

26. Jeremic B, Shibamoto Y, Acimovic L, Djuric L. Randomized trial of hyperfractionated radiation therapy with or without concurrent chemotherapy for stage III non-small-cell lung cancer. *J Clin Oncol.* 1995;13(2):452–458.

27. Jeremic B, Shibamoto Y, Acimovic L, Milisavljevic S. Hyperfractionated radiation therapy with or without concurrent low-dose daily carboplatin/etoposide for stage III non-small-cell lung cancer: a randomized study. *J Clin Oncol.* 1996;14(4):1065–1070.

28. Curran WJ, Scott C, Langer C, et al. Long-term benefit is observed in a phase III comparison of sequential vs concurrent chemo-radiation for patients with unresected stage III NSCLC: RTOG 9410 [abstract 2499]. *Proc Am Soc Clin Oncol.* 2003;22.

29. Zatloukal P, Petruzelka L, Zemanova M, et al. Concurrent versus sequential chemoradiotherapy with cisplatin and vinorelbine in locally advanced non-small cell lung cancer: a randomized study. *Lung Cancer.* 2004;46(1):87–98.

30. Albain KS, Crowley JJ, Turrisi AT 3rd, et al. Concurrent cisplatin, etoposide, and chest radiotherapy in pathologic stage IIIB non-small-cell lung cancer: a Southwest Oncology Group phase II study, SWOG 9019. *J Clin Oncol.* 2002;20(16):3454–3460.

31. Vokes EE, Herndon JE 2nd, Kelley MJ, et al.; Cancer and Leukemia Group B. Induction chemotherapy followed by chemoradiotherapy compared with chemoradiotherapy alone for regionally advanced unresectable stage III Non-small-cell lung cancer: Cancer and Leukemia Group B. *J Clin Oncol.* 2007;25(13):1698–1704.

32. Gandara DR, Chansky K, Albain KS, et al.; Southwest Oncology Group. Consolidation docetaxel after concurrent chemoradiotherapy in stage IIIB non-small-cell lung cancer: phase II Southwest Oncology Group Study S9504. *J Clin Oncol.* 2003;21(10):2004–2010.

33. Gandara DR, Chansky K, Albain KS, et al. Long-term survival with concurrent chemoradiation therapy followed by consolidation docetaxel in stage IIIB non-small-cell lung cancer: a phase II Southwest Oncology Group Study (S9504). *Clin Lung Cancer.* 2006;8(2):116–121.

34. Hanna N, Neubauer M, Yiannoutsos C, et al.; Hoosier Oncology Group; US Oncology. Phase III study of cisplatin, etoposide, and concurrent chest radiation with or without consolidation docetaxel in patients with inoperable stage III non-small-cell lung cancer: the Hoosier Oncology Group and U.S. Oncology. *J Clin Oncol.* 2008;26(35):5755–5760.

35. Kelly K, Chansky K, Gaspar LE, et al. Phase III trial of maintenance gefitinib or placebo after concurrent chemoradiotherapy and docetaxel consolidation in inoperable stage III non-small-cell lung cancer: SWOG S0023. *J Clin Oncol.* 2008;26(15):2450–2456.

36. Thatcher N, Chang A, Parikh P, et al. Gefitinib plus best supportive care in previously treated patients with refractory advanced non-small-cell lung cancer: results from a randomised, placebo-controlled, multicentre study (Iressa Survival Evaluation in Lung Cancer). *Lancet.* 2005;366(9496):1527–1537.

37. Shepherd FA, Rodrigues Pereira J, Ciuleanu T, et al.; National Cancer Institute of Canada Clinical Trials Group. Erlotinib in previously treated non-small-cell lung cancer. *N Engl J Med.* 2005;353(2):123–132.

38. Cappuzzo F, Coudert B, Wierzbicki R, et al. Efficacy and safety of erlotinib as first-line maintenance in NSCLC following non-progression with chemotherapy: results from the phase III SATURN study. In: 13th World Conference on Lung Cancer; 2009; San Francisco, CA. Abstract A 2.1.

39. Davies AM, Chansky K, Lau DH, et al.; SWOG S9712. Phase II study of consolidation paclitaxel after concurrent chemoradiation

in poor-risk stage III non-small-cell lung cancer: SWOG S9712. *J Clin Oncol.* 2006;24(33):5242–5246.

40. Jain AK, Hughes RS, Sandler AB, et al. A phase II study of concurrent chemoradiation with weekly docetaxel, carboplatin, and radiation therapy followed by consolidation chemotherapy with docetaxel and carboplatin for locally advanced inoperable non-small cell lung cancer (NSCLC). *J Thorac Oncol.* 2009;4(6):722–727.

41. Reck M, Macha HN, Del Barco S, et al. Phase II study of oral vinorelbine in combination with carboplatin followed by consolidation therapy with oral vinorelbine as single-agent in unresectable localized or metastatic non-small cell lung carcinoma. *Lung Cancer.* 2009;64(3):319–325.

42. Sekine I, Nokihara H, Sumi M, et al. Docetaxel consolidation therapy following cisplatin, vinorelbine, and concurrent thoracic radiotherapy in patients with unresectable stage III non-small cell lung cancer. *J Thorac Oncol.* 2006;1(8):810–815.

43. Eberhardt W, Wilke H, Stamatis G, et al. Preoperative chemotherapy followed by concurrent chemoradiation therapy based on hyperfractionated accelerated radiotherapy and definitive surgery in locally advanced non-small-cell lung cancer: mature results of a phase II trial. *J Clin Oncol.* 1998;16(2):622–634.

44. Kumar P, Herndon J 2nd, Langer M, et al. Patterns of disease failure after trimodality therapy of nonsmall cell lung carcinoma pathologic stage IIIA (N2). Analysis of Cancer and Leukemia Group B Protocol 8935. *Cancer.* 1996;77(11):2393–2399.

45. Carolan H, Sun AY, Bezjak A, et al. Does the incidence and outcome of brain metastases in locally advanced non-small cell lung cancer justify prophylactic cranial irradiation or early detection? *Lung Cancer.* 2005;49(1):109–115.

46. Gaspar LE, Chansky K, Albain KS, et al. Time from treatment to subsequent diagnosis of brain metastases in stage III non-small-cell lung cancer: a retrospective review by the Southwest Oncology Group. *J Clin Oncol.* 2005;23(13):2955–2961.

47. Russell AH, Pajak TE, Selim HM, et al. Prophylactic cranial irradiation for lung cancer patients at high risk for development of cerebral metastasis: results of a prospective randomized trial conducted by the Radiation Therapy Oncology Group. *Int J Radiat Oncol Biol Phys.* 1991;21(3):637–643.

48. Cox JD, Stanley K, Petrovich Z, Paig C, Yesner R. Cranial irradiation in cancer of the lung of all cell types. *JAMA.* 1981;245(5):469–472.

49. Umsawasdi T, Valdivieso M, Chen TT, et al. Role of elective brain irradiation during combined chemoradiotherapy for limited disease non-small cell lung cancer. *J Neurooncol.* 1984;2(3):253–259.

50. Lester JF, MacBeth FR, Coles B. Prophylactic cranial irradiation for preventing brain metastases in patients undergoing radical treatment for non-small-cell lung cancer: a Cochrane Review. *Int J Radiat Oncol Biol Phys.* 2005;63(3):690–694.

51. Pöttgen C, Eberhardt W, Grannass A, et al. Prophylactic cranial irradiation in operable stage IIIA non small-cell lung cancer treated with neoadjuvant chemoradiotherapy: results from a German multicenter randomized trial. *J Clin Oncol.* 2007;25(31):4987–4992.

52. Bradley JD, Graham M, Suzanne S, et al. Phase I Results of RTOG L-0117; a phase I/II dose intensification study using 3DCRT and concurrent chemotherapy for patients with inoperable NSCLC. ASCO Annual Meeting Proceedings [abstract 7063]. *J Clin Oncol.* 2005;23:16S(Part I of II, June 1 suppl).

53. Socinski MA, Rosenman JG, Halle J, et al. Dose-escalating conformal thoracic radiation therapy with induction and concurrent carboplatin/paclitaxel in unresectable stage IIIA/B nonsmall cell lung carcinoma: a modified phase I/II trial. *Cancer.* 2001;92(5):1213–1223.

54. Bonner JA, Harari PM, Giralt J, et al. Radiotherapy plus cetuximab for squamous-cell carcinoma of the head and neck. *N Engl J Med.* 2006;354(6):567–578.

55. Bonner JA, Harari PM, Giralt J, et al. Radiotherapy plus cetuximab for locoregionally advanced head and neck cancer: 5-year survival data from a phase 3 randomised trial, and relation between cetuximab-induced rash and survival. *Lancet Oncol.* 2010;11(1):21–28.

56. Govindan R, Bogart J, Wang X, et al. Phase II study of pemetrexed, carboplatin, and thoracic radiation with or without cetuximab in patients with locally advanced unresectable non small cell lung cancer: CALGB 30407 [abstract 7505]. *J Clin Oncol.* 2009;2:15s.

57. Govindan R, Bogart J, Wang X, et al. A phase II study of pemetrexed, carboplatin and thoracic radiation with or without cetuximab in patients with locally advanced unresectable non-small cell lung cancer: CALGB 30407. In: 13th World Conference on Lung Cancer; 2009; San Friancisco, CA. Abstract C6.2.

58. Vokes EE, Senan S, Treat JA, Iscoe NA. PROCLAIM: A phase III study of pemetrexed, cisplatin, and radiation therapy followed by consolidation pemetrexed versus etoposide, cisplatin, and radiation therapy followed by consolidation cytotoxic chemotherapy of choice in locally advanced stage III non-small-cell lung cancer of other than predominantly squamous cell histology. *Clin Lung Cancer.* 2009;10(3):193–198.

14 Surgery for T4 and N3 NSCLC, Additional Pulmonary Nodules, and Isolated Distant Metastases

ANTHONY W. KIM

FRANK C. DETTERBECK

■ INTRODUCTION

Non–small cell lung cancer (NSCLC) that has extended to major mediastinal structures, N3 nodes, or distant sites is typically considered to be a nonsurgical disease. Nevertheless, there are exceptions, and these situations are the focus of this chapter. Specifically, this chapter includes patients with T4 tumors that invade major mediastinal structures and patients with N3 node involvement. The role of multimodality treatment pertains to both of these situations. This chapter also includes patients with additional pulmonary nodules of cancer, with ipsilateral pleural involvement as well as those with limited distant metastases. Pancoast tumors are addressed elsewhere (chapter __).

We have approached this chapter by focusing on particular T, N, and M categories, and in fact subsets within these categories, rather than overall stage groups (e.g., IIIb and IV). This is because the 7th edition of the AJCC/UICC stage classification system is somewhat different than the 5th and 6th editions (1). Simply describing the patients in question by T, N, and M characteristics avoids the awkwardness of discussing the existing literature that uses the old grouping in the context of the current grouping schema.

This chapter focuses on peer-reviewed literature published over the 20-year period ending December 1, 2009. Every effort was made to include all studies providing relevant information. We have also drawn from earlier comprehensive reviews of literature published between 1980 and 2000 (2–4). In some categories the limited amount of data available necessitated including a longer time period (so noted in tables and text).

■ T4 TUMORS BY LOCAL INVASION

Tumors invading major mediastinal structures (i.e., trachea, carina, superior vena cava [SVC], aorta, atrium,

esophagus, or vertebral bodies) are designated as T4$_{Inv}$. Under the appropriate circumstances curative-intent resection of these structures in concert with the primary NSCLC can be considered. Both the appropriate patient selection and safe conduct of the resection and reconstruction are challenging.

Unfortunately, the prospective studies of T4 involvement have generally not provided much detail regarding the specific mediastinal structures actually involved (5–9). Neoadjuvant therapy and downstaging may account for the marked discrepancy between the pretreatment T4 designation and what was actually resected in many studies (5,7,10). Much more data regarding outcomes of involvement of specific mediastinal structures is available from retrospective studies..

T4—Carinal Resection

A carinal resection, usually combined with pneumonectomy, is a formidable procedure, but the perioperative mortality is approximately 7% in current series (Table 14.1) (11–27). Older series or those spanning into the pre-1980 era generally report a mortality of 15% to 30%. This is corroborated by Mitchell et al. (21), who found that mortality decreased from 20% to 10% between the first and second half of the 26-year study. The definition of perioperative mortality varied from 1 to 2 months (11,16,18), vaguely defined in-hospital mortality (15,17), but most commonly included any death even beyond 90 days if due to a complication (15,17,19–21,23,24). Adult respiratory distress syndrome is the most common cause of death. Intraoperative deaths were extremely rare.

The 5-year-survival results are difficult to interpret; being 40% to 45% in almost half of the studies and approximately 25% in the rest (Table 14.1). It is not clear why this is the case. It does not appear to be related to the time period of the series, the extent of preoperative mediastinal staging, the size of the study, or the use of neoadjuvant or adjuvant treatment. Although the data justify surgical resection of tumors invading the trachea or carina, the procedure is complex and should not be done sporadically, but rather be undertaken in centers with experience.

Approximately 20% to 25% of the patients undergoing carinal resection were found to have pN2 node status.

■ **Table 14.1** Surgery for carinal involvement

Study	Years Included	Total N	Preop Med	% p/ypN2	% Preop CH	% Preop RT	% Postop CH	% Postop RT	Periop Mort.	% 5-Year Survival All	% 5-Year Survival R0	% 5-Year Survival p/ypN2
Yamamoto (11)	1987–2004	29	Some	34[a]	21	—	—	—	8	27	—	0
Roviaro (12–14)	1983–2004	49	Some	24	45	45	6	51	7	24	—	—
Rea (15)	1982–2005	49	Some	18	16	26	16	31	6	27	—	0
Yildizeli (16)	1981–2006	92	Some	21	21[b]	21[b]	29[b]	29[b]	6	42	43	17[c]
Regnard (17)	1982–2002	65	Some	35	17[d]	0	12[d]	45[d]	8	26	—	5
De Perrot (18)	1981–2004	100	Majority	26	23[d]	5[d]	38[b,e]	38[b,e]	8	44	—	15[c]
Dartevelle (19)	1981–1996	60	Unknown	22	20	—	2	—	7	42	42	7
Porhanov (20)	1979–2001	147	Some	7	1	18	2	16[e]	16	25	—	7
Mitchell (21)	1973–1998	60	Majority	18[c]	—	7	—	7	15	42	—	12[c]
Maeda (22)	before 1993	31	Unknown	—	—	—	—	—	19	41	—	—
Mathisen (23)	1973–1990	37	Majority	—	8	11	—	51	18	19	—	—
Tsuchiya (24)	1977–1989	20	Minority	60	—	—	—	—	30	59[f]	—	—
Average[g]				22					10	33		8

Inclusion criteria: Retrospective series of T4 resections for NSCLC with ≥20 carinal resections published in peer-reviewed journals from December, 1989, to December, 2009. Excluded are three studies (25–27) that did not provide specific outcome data for tracheal/carinal resections.

5-Year survival includes perioperative mortality.

[a] Includes 50% with T3N2 disease; [b] distribution between chemotherapy or radiation therapy not provided; [c] includes N2 and N3 lymph node disease; [d] some concurrently as chemoradiation therapy; [e] distribution of bronchogenic carcinomas receiving postoperative radiation therapy not provided; [f] 2-year survival; [g] excluding values in parentheses.

All, all patients undergoing resection; CH, chemotherapy; Periop mort, perioperative mortality; Preop med, preoperative mediastinoscopy; preop, preoperative (neoadjuvant); postop, postoperative (adjuvant); p/ypN2, pN2 or ypN2 (after neoadjuvant treatment); R0, complete resection; RT, radiotherapy.

This number is fairly consistent among the different series, and does not correlate with the method of preoperative mediastinal staging or the use of neoadjuvant therapy. One study (18) specifically tried to exclude any N2 patients and another (21) consistently gave neoadjuvant therapy if N2 involvement was found, but pN2 patients were still found at the time of resection. In all series, the presence of pN2 disease has uniformly poor outcome (11,15,16,18,20). Such patients should be excluded from surgery, but the ability to reliably do this may be limited.

T4—Great Vessel and Cardiac Invasion

SVC Resections

Resection of the SVC is a common T4 structure that is approached surgically (Table 14.2) (28–35). The 5-year survival is approximately 20% to 25% (16,28,32), and the operative mortality is 10% to 14% (28,32,36). Recent studies suggest that both long-term survival (28–31%) and operative mortality (6–8%) has improved over time (16,28,37).

Multivariate analysis found the extent of surgery (pneumonectomy) and the extent of SVC resection (complete resection with graft replacement) to be negative prognostic factors (but not age, N status, R0 resection, neoadjuvant therapy) in a retrospective multicenter analysis of 109 patients from 1963 to 2000 (28). Another study of 39 patients undergoing SVC resection found the need for carinal resection and squamous histology to be the only negative prognostic factors (not N status, although

5-year survival was 20% vs. 38% with and without N2 involvement) (16). Several studies have found that the presence of N2 lymph nodes did not significantly affect survival (28,32,36). However, Suzuki et al. (32) found significantly worse survival (7% vs. 36%, $P < 0.05$) by multivariate analysis in 15 patients in whom the SVC was invaded by metastatic nodes as opposed to a primary tumor (but not the extent of SVC resection, R0 resection, T or N stage). In conclusion, one should be cautious in patients with extensive involvement of the SVC and adjacent structures.

Aortic Resections

Curative-intent aortic resections for NSCLC ranges from peeling off tumor with or without the adventitia to segmental resection and graft insertion (35,38). Simple removal of the adventitial layer of the aorta en bloc with the tumor is generally believed not to be equivalent to a complete resection. Only a few reports have reported on aortic resections either specifically (with 16, 16, and 5 patients) (38–40) or together with resection of other mediastinal organs (25–27,41,42). The latter studies do not provide sufficient detail about the patients with aortic involvement to draw conclusions.

Among those studies focusing specifically on aortic resection the overall 5-year survival was 25% to 50% (39,40). These studies did not employ invasive mediastinal staging routinely. The techniques of aortic reconstruction (e.g., the use of cardiopulmonary bypass [CPB]) were not substantially different between the two studies. The use

■ **Table 14.2** Surgery for T4$_{inv}$ with great vessel or cardiac invasion

Study	N With GV/CI	GV/CI: % of All Pts in Study	% Neoadjuvant CH	% Neoadjuvant RT	% R0 Resect	% Periop Mortal	% Adjuvant CH	% Adjuvant RT	% 5-Year Survival All	% 5-Year Survival R0	Invaded T4 Structures
Spaggiari (28)	109	100	20	8	73	12	16	30	21	—	SVC
Tsuchiya (29)	101	100	10	—	67	8	7	—	13	19	SVC, LA, AO, PA, PV
Wu (30)	46	100	22	—	100	0	100	19	—	22	LA, PV
Fukuse (31)	42	100	9	28	36	2	5	50	14	37	SVC, LA, AO[a]
Suzuki (32)	40	100	12	10	70	10	2	15	24	—	SVC
Bobbio (33)	23	100	yes[b]	yes[b]	83	9	yes[b]	yes[b]	10	—	SVC, LA
Doddoli (34)	23	79	10	3	86	7	45	55	28	—	SVC, LA, AO
Borri (35)	36	76	38	—	87	8	—	—	23	—	SVC, LA, AO
Average					75	7			19	26	

Inclusion criteria: Studies or series of T4 resections for NSCLC with ≥20 great vessel resections and with >75% of the total N undergoing great vessel resection published in peer reviewed journals from December, 1989, to December, 2009.

Great vessel invasion defined by involvement of the proximal (intrapericardial) pulmonary artery or vein, superior vena cava, left atrium, and aorta, and is irrespective of lymph node status.

[a] Also includes arch vessel involvement; [b] actual numbers not specified.

AO, aorta; CH, chemotherapy; GV/CI, great vessel or cardiac invasion; LA, left atrium; PA, intrapericardial pulmonary artery; Periop mortal, perioperative mortality; pts, patients; PV, intrapericardial pulmonary vein; p/ypN2, pN2 or ypN2 (after neoadjuvant treatment); R0 resect, complete resection; RT, radiotherapy; SVC, superior vena cava.

of neoadjuvant therapy varied from 20% to 62% with no clear conclusions able to be drawn, and the use of adjuvant therapy was not described.

Absence of N2 involvement appears to be associated with better survival. Ohta et al. (39) found a 5-year survival of 70% for N0 and 17% for six N2,3 patients. Klepetko et al. (40) reported that all three patients with N2 disease developed systemic metastases, although they survived 17, 26, and 27 months. Complete resection has also been associated with better survival (36% vs. 0%) (38). In series involving a subadventitial resection, the 5-year survival has been reported to be 0% (42).

Atrial Resection

Left atrial resection has generally been reported in combination with other types of T4 resections (Table 14.3) (16,25–27,31,34,35,41–47) without sufficient detail to define outcomes specifically for left atrial involvement. However, several studies (28–30,33) (44, 40, 23, and 15 patients) have reported specific outcomes, with a 5-year survival of 22% and an operative mortality of 0% to 13%. A better prognosis is associated with complete versus incomplete resection (5-year survival of 23% vs. 0%) (29). A worse prognosis is also associated with N2 versus N0 lymph node involvement (5-year survival 0% vs. 54%) (30). Another smaller study did not corroborate a significant difference for either of these factors (33).

The Need for CPB

The vast majority of resections of $T4_{Inv}$ tumors do not require the use of CPB, but occasionally it has been found necessary, especially for resections of the aorta and the pulmonary artery bifurcation (18,26,29,38,40,48). Using CPB during pulmonary resections appears to be safe; studies in which CPB is used specifically in the resection of NSCLC and not paired with a cardiac procedure requiring CPB have not demonstrated a higher morbidity related to CPB (38,39).

The incidence of N2 disease in patients undergoing resection of NSCLC with CPB is 28% (10/35) in larger studies (n > 5) of such patients (18,40,48). At the same time, most authors advocate excluding patients with N2 disease (18,39,40,48), perhaps because of poor outcomes. Some authors have included patients with N2 disease in the setting of neoadjuvant therapy (38,39).

Despite the locally advanced nature of lung cancers requiring resection with bypass, long-term survival has been reported (40,48). Given the limited number of patients having undergone resection with CPB, it is currently difficult to know which patients will benefit from these resections. Nevertheless, there may be a role in curative-intent treatment under specific circumstances that still need to be clarified.

T4—Other Structures (Esophagus, Vertebral Body)

Even proponents of surgery for T4 patients typically exclude those with esophageal involvement (8,9,49). Nevertheless, a few reports of full or partial esophageal resection en bloc with a primary lung cancer exist (26,27,35,41,42), but the data is too limited to draw conclusions.

Vertebral body involvement is typically associated with Pancoast tumors, discussed in another chapter. A recent study of 23 patients (74% Pancoast) reported a 3-year survival of 72% (50). An average of 3.5 vertebral bodies were resected, and an R0 resection was achieved in 83%. All patients underwent neoadjuvant therapy (chemoradiotherapy in 22 and chemotherapy in 1). Other series report similar results (51–53) in Pancoast tumors.

T4 Invasion With N2 Nodes ($T4_{Inv}$N2)

Data specifically focusing on patients with $T4_{Inv}$ N2M0 disease is summarized in Table 14.4 (8,15–18,20,26,30,35,45–47,54,55). The average 5-year survival of these patients is approximately 10%. The average survival is consistent with registry studies that have reported on resected patients (45). The extent of preoperative staging appears to have a mild effect; with more invasive staging, the percentage of patients with N2 disease is slightly lower (24% vs. 35%), and the survival slightly better (14% vs. 6%). The proportion receiving neoadjuvant therapy does not consistently affect the survival. A study that was too small to meet the inclusion criteria for the table reported a 5-year survival of 58% in seven patients undergoing complete resection (27). This study also had the lowest percentage of patients undergoing surgery, suggesting that perhaps by being more highly selective, better results could be achieved.

Several studies have demonstrated a significant difference in 5-year survival between the N0 and N2 patients by multivariate analysis (26,35,45), or at least a nonsignificant trend (28,34,39,42,56–58).

■ MULTIMODALITY THERAPY INCLUDING SURGERY FOR $T4_{Inv}$ AND N3

In the past 2 decades 16 prospective studies have been reported that accrued 20 or more patients to multimodality treatments including surgery in $T4_{Inv}$ or N3 patients (Table 14.5) (3,5–10,49,54,55,59–66). Six of these included only $T4_{Inv}$ and N3 patients, while the others included N2 patients and others as well. These studies have involved more patients with $T4_{Inv}$ than N3 disease. This is likely due to the logic of using the local modality of surgery for tumors that are locally invasive as opposed to those that have spread extensively to N3 nodes.

Only six of the prospective studies employed routine surgical staging, usually with cervical mediastinoscopy

Table 14.3 Surgery for a heterogeneous cohort of T4$_{inv}$ tumors

Study	Total N[a]	Structures Invaded and Resected (N)							% Neoadjuvant		% Adjuvant		% With p/ypN2	% 5-Year Survival
		T/C	SVC	LA	IPV	AO	ESO	VB	CH	RT	CH	RT		
Stamatis (41)	392	5	3	0	0	6	4	3	100	100	0	0	—	26
Macchiarini (43)	23	9	2	0	11	0	0	3	100	52	0	30	22	54[b]
Borri (35)	47	4	9	0	0	0	1	0	81	0	0	0	30	23
Yildizeli (16)	271	92	39	19	20	2	11	28	28	28	51	51	14	38
Martini (25)	102	20	10	8	1	20	6	2	10	12	5	46	—	19
Yang (26)	146	27	9	14	72	4	3	2	8	2	73	19	63	23
Doddoli (34)	25	6	17	5	0	1	0	0	0	0	52	64	38	28
Pitz (27)	89	35	13	15	31	17	12	2	0	0	4	53	35	19
Bernard (42)	77	7	8	19	30	8	8	6	0	0	0	52	41	21[b]
Fukuse (31)	42	0	13	14	0	15	0	0	9	28	5	50	52[c]	14
Average[d]													30	25
Registry/Database Studies														
IASLC 1990–2000 (44)	340												—	22
SEER 1992–2002 (45)	100												22[c]	20
CCR 1999–2003 (46)	1607												—	11[e]
SEER 1998–2003 (47)	8407												66[c,e]	9[e]
Subaverage[d]													22	21

Inclusion criteria: Studies that specifically included surgical resection of T4$_{inv}$ from December, 1989, to December, 2009 (still stage IIIB in the new 7th edition NSCLC staging system) with ≥20 total patients in the series.

[a] Total number in study, not necessarily the number with T4 invasion; [b] 3-year survival; [c] includes patients with N3 disease; [d] excluding values in parentheses; [e] vast majority of patients not resected.

AO, aorta; CH, chemotherapy; CCR, California Cancer Registry; ESO, esophagus; IASLC, International Association for the Study of Lung Cancer database; IPV, intrapericardial pulmonary vessels; LA, left atrium; RT, radiotherapy; SEER, Surveillance, Epidemiology and End Results database; SVC, superior vena cava; T/C, trachea or carina; VB, vertebral body.

■ **Table 14.4** Surgery for T4$_{inv}$N2 tumors

Study	Total N in Study	Preoperative Invasive Staging?	Invaded T4 Structure	Additional Treatment		% With p/ypN2	% 5-Year Survival p/ypN2 Patients
				% Neo adjuvant	% Adjuvant		
Grunenwald (8)	40	Majority-all	GV, Tr	90	—	20	12[a]
Hehr (54)	59	Majority-all	—[b]	77	—	25	14
De Perrot (18)	119	Majority-all	GV, Tr	19	32	26	15[a]
Subaverage						24	14
Friedel (55)	93	Some	H, Tr	90	≥24[c]	38[a]	19[a]
Borri (35)	47	Some-cN2	GV, H, Tr	81	—	30	8[d]
Rea (15)	49	Some-cN2	Tr	39	39	18	0
Yildizeli (16)	271	Some-cN2	GV, H, Tr, Eso	23	29	21	17[a]
Porhanov (20)	231	Some-cN2	Tr	19	16	22	7
Regnard (17)	65	Some-cN2	GV, H, Tr, Eso	17	28	35	5[d]
Subaverage						27	9
Yang (26)	146	None-minimal	GV, H, Tr/Car	8	—	63	13
Wu (30)	46	None-minimal	GV, H, Tr/Car	0	—	7	0
Subaverage						35	6
Average						**28**	**10**
Registry/Database Studies							
SEER (45)	1177		—[b]	10	47	22[a]	8[a]
SEER (47)	8407		—[b]	—	—	66[a,e]	7[a,e]
CCR (46)	1301		—[b]	—	—	62[a,e]	10[a,e]
Subaverage[f]						**22**	**8**

Inclusion criteria: Studies that specifically included 5-year survival data for surgical resection of T4$_{Inv}$ N2 disease from December, 1989, to December, 2009 with ≥40 total in the series.

[a] Includes patients with N3 disease that were not distinguished from those with N2 disease; [b] resected structures not specified; [c] estimated minimum due to incomplete data provided; [d] includes patients with <T4 status; [e] vast majority of patients not resected; [f] excluding values in parentheses.

CCR, California Cancer Registry; Eso, esophagus; GV, great vessels including the intrapericardial pulmonary vessels, superior vena cava, aorta; H, heart including left or right atrium; SEER, Surveillance, Epidemiology, End-Results registry; Tr, trachea/carina.

(6,49,54,60–62). This included the North American Intergroup study and five trials from Europe, especially Germany.

The majority of the prospective studies employed a platinum-based neoadjuvant chemotherapy regimen (one study used Gemcitabine and Docetaxel) (59). Three studies gave neoadjuvant chemoradiation (5,59,63). Approximately half of the studies gave two and the rest three cycles of chemotherapy; radiotherapy typically involved a total dose of 40 to 45 Gy, although in five studies this was given in a hyperfractionated schedule (twice daily).

Prospective studies during the past 20 years have consistently used neoadjuvant therapy (6–10,49,54,55,59–64). In fact, a Surveillance, Epidemiology and End Results (SEER) database analysis (45) revealed that neoadjuvant therapy has been increasing since 1992. On the other hand, retrospective reports of surgical therapy for T4/N3 patients (primarily T4) have usually involved surgery as the primary therapy. When neoadjuvant therapy has been

used, it was primarily in patients with N3 involvement. Similarly, it is primarily patients with pN2,3 disease that have been selected for adjuvant therapy, although its use is variable (26–28,30,33–35,38,42,45,50,57,67).

Approximately 2/3 of patients actually underwent surgery after neoadjuvant therapy, and approximately 60% had a complete resection. These rates vary moderately, but without a consistent pattern. It does not seem to be related to the extent of preoperative staging, the proportion of T4 or N3 patients, or the type of preoperative therapy given. Even the *European Organisation for Research and Treatment of Cancer* study, which was designed for initially unresectable patients, found that 55% of patients underwent surgery and 35% an R0 resection (61).

The average 5-year survival is 25% for the entire group (Table 14.5). Although there is variability in this outcome, there is no consistent pattern. The survival appeared to have no relationship to the proportion of T4 or N3 patients, the type of preoperative therapy given, the rate of resection or

■ Table 14.5 Prospective studies evaluating neoadjuvant therapy for patients with T4inv or N3 disease

Study	N (T4/N3 Pts)	% T4/N3 of All Pts in Study	Preoperative Regimen % T4	% N3	Cycles	CH	RT (Gy)	% Postoperative CH	RT	% Going to Surgery (of All Pts)	% R0 Resection (of All Pts)	% 5-Year Survival All	R0
Garrido (59)	67	49	49	0	3	GD	—	—	—	66	66	21 [a]	53
Rendina (5)	57	100	100	0	3	MVP	—	32 [b]	32 [b]	74	63	20	30
Galetta (9)	39	100	90	13 [c]	2	PF	50	97	97	56	54	23	38
Albain (60)	50	40	19	21	2	PE	45	22	22	74	63	24 [d]	—
Thomas (61)	166	64	47	21 [c]	3	PE	45 HF	0	72	59	32	31	42
Thomas (61)	182	69	53	22 [c]	3	PE	45 HF	0	19	54	37	39	45 [a]
Eberhardt (49)	42	45	20	25	3	PE	45 HF	—	—	59	45	29 [e]	46 [a]
Hehr (54)	38	65	54	25 [c]	3	CbPx	45 HF	—	—	63	54	—	41 [a]
Ichinose (10)	27	100	81	26 [c]	2	PUFT	40	81	89	93	78	56 [d]	67 [d]
Stupp (7)	46	100	78	28 [c]	3	PD	44	100	76	76	59	40	—
Thomas (62)	29	54	30	28 [c]	2	ICE	45 HF	—	22	69	59	26 [d]	—
Friedel (55)	78	84	68	36	2	PVd	36	—	24 [b]	64	53	24 [a]	39
Santo (63)	29	67	37	38 [b]	2	PG	—	70	30	37	30	—	—
Grunenwald (8)	40	100	75	47 [c]	2	PFV	42	98	98 [b]	73	60	19	35
Stamatis (6)	56	100	50	57 [c]	3	PE	45 HF	—	5	61	48	26	43
Aristu (64)	30	55	—	—	1–6	MVP	15 IORT	47 [f]	89 [f]	50	40	7	—
Average [g]		74	57	26						64	53	25	41
>50% T4 (5,7–10,54,55,59,61)										69	57	27	38
≤50% T4 (6,49,60–63,65,66)										61	49	27	46
<25% N3 (5,9,49,59–61,65,66)										64	52	27	42
≥25% N3 (6–8,10,54,55,62,63)										66	54	28	41
Variable invasive staging (5,7–10,55,59,63)										67	58	24	39
Routine invasive staging (6,49,54,60–62,65,66)										63	48	31	43
Preop HF RT (6,49,54,61,62)										61	49	31	44
Regular RT (7–10,55,60,65,66)										73	61	26	37
No RT (5,59,61,63)										59	48	24	42

Inclusion criteria: Studies of patients undergoing neoadjuvant therapy followed by curative-intent surgical therapy in ≥20 T4 or N3 patients published in peer-reviewed journals from December, 1989, to December, 2009.

[a] Includes stage IIIA patients; [b] minimum number estimated based upon description in publication; [c] includes T4N3 disease (together); [d] 3-year survival; [e] 4-year survival; [f] best estimate; [g] excluding values in parentheses.

CH, chemotherapy; HF, hyperfractionated; Gy, Gray; IORT, intraoperative radiotherapy; pts, patients; RT, radiotherapy.

Chemotherapy regimens: CbPx, carboplatin, paclitaxel; GD, gemcitabine, Docetaxol; ICE, ifosfamide, carboplatin, etoposide; MVP, mitomycin C, vinblastine, cisplatin; PD, cisplatin, docetaxel; PE cisplatin, etoposide; PF, cisplatin, 5-Fluorouracil; PG, cisplatin, gemcitabine; PVd, cisplatin, Vindesine; PUFT, cisplatin, Tegafur-Uracil.

complete resection, or adjuvant therapy. There appears to be a slight survival advantage for all patients in those studies that undertook routine preoperative invasive mediastinal staging, but this was not reflected in increased rates of R0 resection or survival of R0 patients. When a complete resection is achieved, the survival is approximately 40%. Again, there is no specific selection or treatment approach that seemed to correlate consistently between studies in predicting better or worse outcomes. Multivariate analysis has also not revealed any predictors of survival (7).

■ N3 DISEASE

Prospective trials that included patients with N3 disease are summarized in Table 14.5. In these studies, approximately 25% of the patients had N3 node involvement. The majority of these studies included only patients with contralateral N3 disease. Only three studies also included patients with supraclavicular N3 disease (8,10,60). Two of these studies involved only one and four N3 patients (8,10), whereas in the third study, the number of patients with supraclavicular node involvement was not specified (60,65).

The survival after neoadjuvant therapy and surgical resection of patients with N3 involvement is surprisingly good, although data is limited. The 5-year survival in those studies in Table 14.5 that have included a higher proportion of patients with N3 involvement is not clearly different than in studies involving predominantly $T4_{Inv}$ tumors. A 2-year survival of 25% was found in 27 N3 patients treated with neoadjuvant chemoradiotherapy and resection in a multicenter trial (60,65). Grunenwald et al. (8) reported a 17% 5-year survival in N3 patients. Stupp et al. (7) reported no difference in overall (40%) or event-free survival among patients with (n = 13) or without (n = 33) contralateral N3 disease. Another study observed a 5-year survival of 28% among 32 patients who had mediastinoscopy-proven N3 disease, even though only 44% underwent a complete resection following neoadjuvant chemoradiation therapy (6). In both of these latter two studies, a fairly high rate of pathologic complete response was observed after neoadjuvant chemoradiotherapy (13% and 25%), perhaps explaining the remarkably good results (6,7).

Prognostic factors have not been well studied. One study (Southwest Oncology Group [SWOG] 8805) has reported results by the type of N3 involvement: the 2-year survival was 35% with supraclavicular and 0% with contralateral N3 disease (60,65). A response to neoadjuvant therapy appears to be important (8); however, the 5-year survival was 12% with persistent N2,3 disease after neoadjuvant therapy and an R0 resection (8). On the other hand, survival was 0% with persistent N2,3 and an incomplete resection (8).

In summary, resection of patients with N3 involvement in the setting of neoadjuvant therapy does not appear to be futile. However, this should ideally be done in the context of a prospective trial in an experienced center.

■ ADDITIONAL TUMOR NODULES

General Approach

The clinical approach to a patient begins with a medical history and imaging. Data regarding pathologic findings and outcomes is clinically useful only if we can define these outcomes by characteristics that were available prior to resection. Unfortunately, the literature generally describes only features that are not known until after resection. This leaves a gap between what we know preoperatively and what might be found. It also reduces much of the available data to something that is largely of academic interest, because it is applicable only after the treatment decisions have been made (and carried out).

Additional solid, noncalcified pulmonary nodules occur in approximately 15% of patients with a potentially resectable lung cancer (68) It is crucial to recognize that the majority of such additional lesions are found to be benign (68–70). The experience with computed tomography (CT) screening for lung cancer also shows that the vast majority of nodules, especially if <8 mm, are benign (71,72). Therefore, additional lesions detected by imaging in patients with a newly diagnosed or suspected lung cancer should be assumed to be benign until proven otherwise. Finally, data also supports simple observation of additional foci of ground glass opacity when these are ≤8 mm (73–75).

However, if we know, or strongly suspect, an additional nodule to be malignant (e.g., by biopsy, growth, or positron emission tomography [PET] characteristics), we need to understand the nature of the lesion and its biologic behavior in order to make rational decisions about how to treat it. However, our understanding of biologic nature and behavior is rudimentary, especially when it comes to additional nodules (76–78). This creates another gap that is bridged primarily by speculation.

We have a reasonable understanding of the behavior of traditional solitary lung cancers that present as solid, often spiculated nodules. We assume that this is similar to the behavior of two lung cancers that arise independently in the same patient, either as synchronous or metachronous multiple primary lung cancers (MPLC). We also have a reasonably good understanding of the natural history when patients have widely disseminated lung cancer. We can imagine that at some point during dissemination there is only one distant metastatic site, although our understanding of the biologic processes and natural history of such oligometastatic lung cancers is poor, and it is probably not appropriate to extrapolate from the setting of multiple metastases. Finally, there are lung cancers that appear to have a predilection for multifocal involvement.

However, we have no conceptual framework for this, and therefore, this entity presents a particular problem.

Multifocal lung cancer generally arises from ground glass opacities, although they may become solid (79–82). They may be limited in number or multiple. They may be increasing in frequency, particularly in Asia, although it may be that an increased prevalence of CT scanning has merely led to an increased frequency of recognition. It is well accepted that bronchioloalveolar carcinoma (BAC) can present in a multifocal manner (83). The relationship between atypical adenomatous hyperplasia, BAC, and adenocarcinoma is not fully understood but a relationship is well accepted (84,85). It appears that multifocal disease has a decreased propensity for nodal and distant metastases (79–82,84), but a clear understanding is hampered by lack of a clear definition of multifocal disease (75).

The first reaction when confronted with multiple malignant nodules is to look to histology to define the nature of the cancers. However, this is immediately problematic because it requires resection; the histologic type identified by needle biopsy is erroneous in 30% of cases (86), and the ability to discern smaller nuances is poorly studied at best. A true understanding is difficult even with resected specimens; most second primary lung cancers as defined by Martini and Melamed criteria (87) have the same histologic type (4,70,88,89). This is logical, because the etiology of both cancers is likely the same (i.e., genetic predisposition and environmental exposures). Differentiation of adenocarcinomas by percentage of morphologic patterns (in resected specimens) has been proposed, but validation and definition of tumor behavior is needed (90). Definition of MPLCs by genetic characteristics has produced conflicting results so far (91–95). Thus, histology is of benefit in defining a relationship between additional foci of cancer in only a minority of cases involving resected specimens, and limited biopsies are of questionable value at best.

A practical approach to these difficulties is to examine the literature based on situations that can be reasonably well defined, albeit postoperatively. The management of patients must still take into account the chance that such a situation actually exists based on the preoperative information available. We will therefore discuss the management of additional foci of cancer in the same lobe (ipsilobar satellite or T3$_{Satell}$) and multiple primary "traditional" lung cancers (i.e., solid spiculated lesions) in patients with appropriate risk factors. A discussion of ipsilateral and contralateral additional foci of cancer follows, but is more difficult because it likely represents a mixture of biologic situations that are confounded by poorly characterized selection factors in the available literature.

Ipsilobar Satellite Nodule

The general approach to patients who are suspected of having an additional focus of cancer in the same lobe as a primary lung cancer, according to the American College of Chest Physicians (ACCP) lung cancer guidelines, is to proceed in the same manner as would be dictated by the primary lung cancer alone (70). No additional biopsy is recommended, and the staging evaluation (e.g., PET or invasive mediastinal staging) is the same as if the additional nodule was not present. The basis for this recommendation is the good outcome of patients who are managed in this manner, and because the additional nodule does not appear to substantially alter the risk of mediastinal or distant metastases. However, the level of evidence is graded as moderate to poor (70).

Data regarding ipsilobar satellite (T3$_{Satell}$) lesions is summarized in Table 14.6 (8,44,46,47,82,96–106). The 5-year survival for patients with same lobe satellite nodules is approximately 34% (range 20–48%). This figure is corroborated by results from population-based registries and large regional or international databases. This data involves patients primarily treated by surgical resection, regardless of nodal status or completeness of resection.

In general, studies have found a moderate decrease in survival with versus without a satellite nodule in each stage (ignoring the nodule in the stage classification) (44,47,98,99,105,107,108). This appears to be about a 10% to 15% decrease, although the magnitude of the difference is hard to define precisely. This is due to the limited number of studies, the long time periods involved, variability in survival results potentially stemming from small cohorts when divided by stage, and different editions of the stage classification system that was used. One of the more recent studies reported 5-year survival for stage I, II, and III disease (ignoring the additional nodule in the stage classification) of 64%, 31%, and 0%, respectively (Figure 14.1) (105).

Prognostic factors are not well defined. Nodal involvement appears to have a similar effect in patients with and without a same lobe satellite nodule (see previous paragraph). No difference in survival is seen whether there is one or several ipsilobar satellite nodules (105,109,110). Survival may be better in women (105).

Multiple Primary Lung Cancer

MPLC are readily distinguished when they are of different histologic types (or subtypes), but this occurs in a minority of MPLC. Traditionally, the empiric criteria of Martini and Melamed (87) have been used to define MPLC, but a modification is gaining recognition that shifts the interval for metachronous cancers to ≥4 years (4,70) and considers morphologic tumor subtyping (75,111). Approximately 1/3 of MPLCs are synchronous, and approximately 1/3 of these are found incidentally at the time of resection (4).

The survival of patients with synchronous (different lobe) MPLCs (either same or different histologic types) is highly variable, consistent with the difficulty of reliably classifying these tumors (Table 14.7) (4,70,81,88,89,111–127). The 5-year survival for all patients ranges from 0% to 70%, and the survival

■ **Table 14.6** Additional nodules in the same lobe

Study	N (Same Lobe)	% With Multiple Nodules	Continent	Survival (%) 2-Year	Survival (%) 5-Year
Nagai (96)	316	—	Asia	46	27
Okumura (8)	152	—	Asia	52	34
Okada (97)	51	—	Asia	52	30
Yano (98)	39	—	Asia	57	36
Shimizu (99)	37	—	Asia	41	27
Osaki (100)	36	—	Asia	46	27
Watanabe (101)	24 [a]	—	Asia	36	22
Yoshino (102)	22	—	Asia	34	34
Fukuse (103)	20	12	Asia	58	37
Oliaro (104)	39	49	Europe	49	20
Port (105)	53	19	N. Am	73	48
Battafarano (82)	27	—	N. Am	70	66[b]
Average[c]				51	31
Registry/Database Studies[d]					
IASLC 1990–2000 (44)	363	—	Global	50	28
CCR 1999–2003 (46)	422	—	N. Am	40	23
SEER 1999–2003 (106)	633	—	N. Am	44	35
SEER 1998–2003 (47)	2285	—	N. Am	43	24

Inclusion criteria: Studies of ≥20 patients with an additional nodule in the same lobe as the dominant primary lung cancer from December, 1989, to December, 2009.

[a] No distinction between same and different lobes, but text suggest most were same lobe; [b] 3-year survival; [c] excluding values in parentheses; [d] majority of patients in each study *were* resected.

CCR, California Cancer Registry; IASLC, International Association for the Study of Lung Cancer registry; N Am, North America; SEER, Surveillance, Epidemiology, End-Results registry.

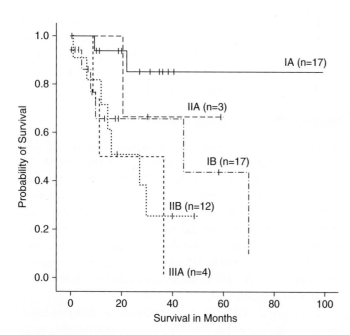

FIGURE 14.1 Overall survival based on the primary lesion's T and N status disregarding satellite nodule (6th edition stage classification). From Ref. 105 with permission.

of patients in whom both tumors are classified as stage I ranges from 0% to 79% (4,70). These data suggest that a great deal of caution is necessary in classifying two synchronous foci of cancer as two separate primary lung cancers. Therefore the ACCP recommends thorough distant imaging and invasive mediastinal staging in the face of MPLC. If no other sites of disease are found, resection of both lesions is reasonable, although the outcomes are variable and, overall, not that good.

Patients with metachronous MPLC exhibit slightly less variability in reported results (Table 14.7). However, the survival is clearly worse than in patients with only one lung cancer, with a 5-year survival of approximately 40% among those with two pathologic stage I cancers. The ACCP guidelines also recommends thorough investigation for distant and mediastinal disease in patients with metachronous MPLC before embarking on resection.

Ipsilateral Different Lobe Nodules

In recent years more series have been reported on patients with additional tumor nodules, and this has also been a focus of the International Association for the Study of Lung Cancer (IASLC) staging committee analysis. These are additional nodules of cancer of the same histologic

■ Table 14.7 Survival of patients with multiple primary lung cancers

Study	N	% Incidental[a]	% Resected	% Limited Resection[b]	% Operative Mortality	% 5-Year Survival All	Resected	pI
Synchronous								
Finley (111)	175	42	100[c]	27	1	52	52	64[d]
Trousse 07 (81)	125	—	100[c]	14	11	34	34	—
Riquet (112)	118	—	100[c]	16	5	26	26	—
Chang (113)	92	—	100[c]	11	1	35	35	—
Van Rens (114)	85	32	100[c]	13	14	20	20	23
van Bodegom (115)	64	—	50	34	—	—	—	24[e]
De Leyn (88)	36	—	100[c]	72	3	38	38	—
Deschamps (116)	36	42	100[c]	21	6	—	16	—
Vansteenkiste (117)	35	—	100[c]	23	9	33	33	—
Rosengart (118)	33	—	91	33	—	44	—	—
Ferguson (119)	28	18	68	47	0	0	0	0
Okada (120)	28	39	96[c]	7	0	70	—	79[e]
Antakli (121)	26	19	92	42	—	5	12	—
Ribet (122)	24	—	63	40	4	—	—	—
Average		32	90	28	5	32	27	38
Metachronous								
von Bodegom (115)	89	—	51	16	9	—	20	20[e]
Mathisen (123)	80	80	100[c]	61[f]	8[f]	33	—	—
Rosengart (118)	78	—	73	37	2	23	38	38
Battafarano (124)	69		100[c]	49	6	33	33	—
Lee (89)	58	—	100[c]	50	—	66	66	70
Ribet (122)	51	63	33	35	11	—	58	—
Deschamps (116)	44	86	100[c]	43	5	—	34	41
Verhagen (125)	40	90	83	18	15	18	—	27[e]
Antakli (121)	39	—	54	49	—	8	23	—
Adebonojo (126)	37	100	97	22	6	—	37	39
Okada (120)	29	—	100[c]	—	0	—	33	50[e]
Wu (127)	20	55	100[c]	30	—	—	42	—
Average		79	83	37	7	30	38	41

Inclusion criteria: Studies from 1980 to 2000 of ≥20 patients with synchronous or metachronous multiple primary lung cancers reporting survival data.
[a] Percentage found incidentally at time of resection (synchronous), or found by routine follow-up chest radiograph (metachronous); [b] Percentage of resected patients who underwent wedge resection or segmentectomy; [c] Surgical series with ≥90% of patients having been resected; [d] Stage Ia only; [e] Stage I and II; [f] Includes patients with synchronous multiple primary cancers (11%).
pI, pathologic stage I patients.

type, found synchronously with a primary lung cancer. It is unclear whether in recent years this is seen more commonly, is recognized more frequently, reflects an increased incidence of multifocal cancers, or is simply a nomenclature shift away from synchronous primary to additional nodule. Most series of additional nodules have excluded patients thought to have synchronous MPLC, but it is unclear how this distinction was made. Most likely MPLC were defined by different histology, but this ignores the fact that the majority of MPLC have had the same histologic type. However, a description of characteristics and outcomes of patients that is not linked to an etiologic definition (i.e., hematogenous metastasis, synchronous primary etc.) may be beneficial, because our understanding of the true etiology is limited at best. This is underscored by the fact that there is little difference in survival between patients with an additional nodule of the same or a different histologic type (4,82,88,89,110,111,116,118,123–126). BAC has often been excluded in studies of multiple nodules. This is because BAC is thought to represent a unique entity, and because studies of resection of multifocal BACs have demonstrated excellent long-term survival (128,129).

The average 5-year survival for ipsilateral, different lobe, additional nodules is only 13% (Table 14.8) (44,46,47,96,97,103,104,106,107). Many of the reports of additional nodules have come from Asia, suggesting, possibly, a different tumor etiology and different biologic behavior. It could also be due to an increased prevalence of CT screening. However, no differences in outcomes are apparent between continents. There is no data suggesting that a more limited resection in the face of a different lobe nodule accounts for the poor survival (4).

The long-term survival of patients with resected ipsilateral, different lobe, additional nodules is clearly less than for same lobe, satellite nodules. This is seen comparing Tables 14.6 and 14.8, and is consistent with other reviews (4). This is also observed in population-based registries (8% vs. 24% 5-year survival in the SEER database) (47). Individual studies have consistently shown worse survival for different lobe versus same lobe additional nodules, which is statistically significant in some (82,117) and a trend in others (probably due to sample size) (98,102–104,110).

Multivariate analysis has demonstrated worse survival with multiple versus single additional different lobe nodules, along with the mediastinal node status (109).

Ipsilateral Different Lobe Nodules With N2 Nodes (T4$_{Ipsi\,Nod}$N2)

Patients with ipsilateral nodules and N2 involvement have been placed in the IIIb stage group in the new lung cancer stage classification system (1). In the past 2 decades, six studies of >20 patients have evaluated outcomes for such patients (Table 14.9) (47,96,97,103,104,107,117), but only two have reported specifically on ipsilateral different lobe patients (T4$_{Ipsi\,Nod}$N2 M0) (96,104). Both found that any node involvement (N1 or N2) is associated with worse long-term survival than N0 patients (96,104). However, the impact of nodal involvement appears to be less for ipsilateral different lobe nodules than for same lobe satellite nodules, perhaps because of the already poor survival of patients with ipsilateral different lobe nodules.

■ MALIGNANT PLEURAL INVOLVEMENT

In North America, malignant pleural involvement from NSCLC is considered to be a contraindication to surgery. People cite poor results that are similar to stage IV patients treated with palliative chemotherapy as justification for this. However, there may be subsets of patients for whom a poor prognosis is not inevitable. Is a patient with a large effusion with radiographically apparent pleural nodules the same as one with no effusion and small pleural surface nodules visible only at surgery? Furthermore, the fact that essentially all patients in North America with malignant pleural involvement are treated with palliative measures only makes it hard to know whether the outcomes are similar to stage IV (distant metastasis) patients because the treatment is the same, or because the natural history of the disease state is the same.

Limited data suggest that some patients with malignant pleural involvement may have a reasonable outlook with aggressive curative-intent treatment. In the IASLC database, the 5-year survival of these patients was 11% when treated surgically (any node status and any type of resection) (44). Among those patients with malignant pleural involvement that underwent R0 resection (any node status), the 5-year survival was 24%, and for N0 patients with an R0 resection it is 31% (44). Similar results were reported by Naruke et al. (5-year survival of 16% after surgical resection with malignant pleural involvement) (130).

Which patients should be selected for curative-intent treatment is not clear. Different types of pleural involvement have not been clearly defined or studied. One study has suggested good outcomes with pleural involvement

■ Table 14.8 Additional ipsilateral (different lobe) nodules

Study	N (Diff Lobe)	% With Multiple Nodules	Continent	Survival (%) 2-Year	Survival (%) 5-Year
Nagai (96)	129	—	Asia	42	22
Okumura (107)	48	—	Asia	31	11
Okada (97)	38	—	Asia	49	23
Fukuse (103)	21	12	Asia	41	0
Oliaro (104)	35	49	Europe	49	10
Average				42	13
Registry/Database Studies					
IASLC 1990–2000 (44)	180		Global	40	22
CCR 1999–2003 (46)	745		N. Am	26[a]	9[a]
SEER 1999–2003 (106)	3010		N. Am	18[a]	7[a]
SEER 1998–2003 (47)	3019		N. Am	26[a]	8[a]

Inclusion criteria: Studies of ≥20 patients with an additional nodule in a different ipsilateral lobe as the dominant primary lung cancer from December, 1989, to December, 2009.

[a] Vast majority of patients not resected.

CCR, California Cancer Registry; IASLC, International Association for the Study of Lung Cancer registry; N Am, North America; SEER, Surveillance, Epidemiology, End-Results registry.

■ **Table 14.9** Surgery for T4$_{\text{Ipsi Nod}}$ N2 tumors

Study	Total N	% p/ypN2	Location in Ipsilateral Lobes	% Survival T4$_{\text{Ipsi Nod}}$ N2		Comments
				2-Year	5-Year	
Nagai (96)	128	41	Diff	29	10	N1 and N2 nodes with similar survival
Oliaro (104)	74	34	Diff	45 [a]	10	N status strongest survival predictor
Okumura (107)	200	24	Same & Diff	48	24	No differences in survival N0 vs. N1 vs. N2
Okada (97)	89	37	Same & Diff	46	7	N0/N1 better prognosis than N2/N3
Fukuse (103)	41	44	Same & Diff	28	13	Nodal status not predictive of outcome
Vansteenkiste (117)	35	22	Same & Diff	57	17	No differences in survival N0 vs. N1 vs. N2
Average [b]		34		42	13	
Registry/Database Studies SEER 1998–2003 (47)		66	Diff	16 [c,d]	2 [c,d]	

Inclusion criteria: Studies evaluating surgical resection for T4$_{\text{Ipsi Nod}}$ N2 specifically defined as ipsilateral, different lobe nodules from December, 1989, to December, 2009.

[a] 3-Year survival, not used in calculating average; [b] excluding values in parentheses; [c] includes N3 lymph nodes; [d] vast majority of patients not resected.

Diff, different lobe, but ipsilateral chest; SEER, Surveillance, Epidemiology, End-Results registry.

without an effusion (5-year survival of 19% after resection of the primary tumor and the pleural disease) (131). The same study also suggests that absence of nodal involvement is important (5-year survival of 58% after resection if N0, 8% if N1–3, $P < 0.01$) (131). The absence of N1 or N2 lymph node involvement in patients with pleural dissemination undergoing surgical resection has been shown to be associated with improved survival (2,132).

Which treatment is best is also not well defined. Several approaches have been used, including intrapleural, and neoadjuvant or adjuvant therapies (2,132–135).The 5-year survival in these studies ranges from 19% to 31% (131,132,135,136). Nevertheless, it is unclear if intrapleural and adjuvant chemotherapy improves survival (132,133).

Given the uncertainty of multiple aspects, curative-intent treatment of patients with malignant pleural involvement should be undertaken as part of a clinical trial in a major center. It would seem reasonable to explore this in patients without mediastinal node involvement, and perhaps with limited pleural involvement without a malignant effusion.

■ ISOLATED DISTANT METASTASES

NSCLC that is disseminated to distant sites is generally viewed as incurable, although palliative treatment often prolongs survival. However, it is well documented that some patients with a limited number of distant metastases (oligometastatic disease) have no further evidence of cancer once the primary and the metastasis are definitely treated (usually surgical resection), even after long (20-year) follow-up (3). Such results are usually reported in cancers with slower growth patterns than NSCLC. It should be noted that there are occasionally reasons to surgically remove an NSCLC metastasis for palliative reasons (3,137), but this chapter focuses only on curative-intent treatment. The brain and the adrenal gland, followed by the skin and soft tissue including muscle and extrathoracic lymph nodes are the most commonly reported sites involved in curative-intent metastasectomy.

General Series of Surgery in Patients with Isolated Distant Metastases

Several series have reported on surgical therapy of isolated metastatic disease from lung cancer, with remarkable median survivals of approximately 26 months and 5-year survival ranging from 32% to 86% (138–140). The organs involved have included extrathoracic lymph nodes, bones, kidney, gastrointestinal organs, and soft tissue structures including muscle and skin.

One prospective study has been reported (141). Eligible patients had solitary synchronous metastatic disease from NSCLC. The treatment consisted of surgical resection with pre- and postoperative chemotherapy (Mitomycin, Vinblastine, Cisplatin). Only 23 patients were enrolled, 20 received definitive therapy for their metastatic disease, 13 underwent complete resection of the primary lung tumor, and only 10 patients underwent complete resections of both the metastatic and primary focus. The substantial majority of these patients had isolated brain metastasis, but patients with adrenal, bone, spleen, and colon involvement were also included. The median survival was 11 months for the entire cohort (5-year survival was not reported). The study included many patients with N2 disease, and 50% of patients proceeding to resection had positive N2 lymph nodes (141). Given the general experience with patients with N2 nodes and isolated metastases (see next sections), inclusion of these patients was probably unwise.

Isolated Brain Metastasis

Approximately 20% to 40% of patients with lung cancer develop brain metastasis. Of these, 30% present with limited metastases, 25% of which are eligible for resection (3). Definitive treatment of a brain metastasis (resection or radiosurgery [RS]) and the primary tumor (typically lobectomy) can result in cure of patients with isolated brain metastases (3,142). Surgery and RS are considered equivalent in efficacy for brain metastases (3). These techniques should be considered complementary since some lesions are much more amenable to one technique or another. Clinical guidelines and a Cochrane review have documented equivalent outcomes (3,70,143,144). Generally the brain lesion is treated first, because of the often devastating consequences of untreated brain metastases.

Long-term (5-year) survival after definitive treatment of an isolated brain metastasis and a primary lung cancer is approximately 15% to 20%. A comparison between series suggests that survival is similar in patients with synchronous versus metachronous (>3 months) brain metastases (5-year survival 13% vs. 13%, Table 14.10) (145–153). Furthermore, comparisons within a series have found no statistically significant difference (152–155). At any rate, survival in both groups is sufficient to justify a curative-intent approach.

Involvement of mediastinal nodes portends the worst prognosis (Figure 14.2) (70,145,148–150,152,156–158). However, the difference is often not statistically significant. Nevertheless, given that resection of patients with N2 involvement in the absence of distant metastases is questionable, it seems better not to consider resection in patients with oligometastases. A good performance status may be a positive prognostic factor (148,151,159). Most of the recent studies suggest that adenocarcinoma histology is a positive factor (145,148,149,159) (but with some exceptions) (153). A higher T stage correlated with decreased survival in one study of synchronous brain metastases (145).

■ Table 14.10 Isolated brain metastases

Study	N	% Survival 2-Year	% Survival 5-Year
Synchronous presentation			
Bonnette (145)	103	28	11
Wronski (146)	86	14	8
Nakagawa (147)	60	10	—
Girard (148)	51	42	—
Granone (149)	30	47	14
Billing (150)	28	54	21
Average		**32**	**13**
Metachronous presentation			
Wronski (146)	145	29	17
Moazami (151)	91	10	6
Furak (152)	45	—	16
Mussi (153)	30	47	19
Nakagawa (147)	28	11	—
Average		**24**	**13**

Inclusion criteria: Studies of ≥20 patients reporting specific data for synchronous or metachronous brain metastases and curative-intent treatment from December, 1989, to December, 2009.

Administration of whole brain radiation (WBRT) after resection or RS for an isolated brain metastasis is widely practiced, although the data supporting this is less firm than the conviction that it is beneficial. The only randomized study (160) found no difference in survival, as did a case-matched study (161). Two of three multivariate analyses found no survival difference (146,162), but one (163) did in patients without extracranial metastases. Most of these studies included many patients with other metastases, in whom definitive treatment of the brain metastasis was a palliative procedure. Two retrospective comparison studies have found a survival benefit, both involving a majority of patients without extracranial metastases (148,154).

Studies of the effect of adjuvant WBRT on the rate of recurrent brain metastases have shown conflicting results. The only randomized study found the rate of brain recurrences to be significantly lower (18% vs. 70%, $P < 0.001$) after WBRT (160). A case-matched study found no difference (161). Two multivariate analyses found significantly lower brain relapse rates with WBRT (162,164). Individual studies have generally shown no difference (145,165,166), but some have (167). Most of these studies have included many patients with other metastatic sites. An analogy can be made to prophylactic cranial irradiation for patients with small cell lung cancer, where after years of controversy, a benefit was conclusively proven by meta-analysis to occur in those patients who had achieved good control of the disease at all sites. Thus, WBRT for patients with NSCLC after curative-intent treatment of oligometastatic disease makes some sense, although the data itself is somewhat conflicting.

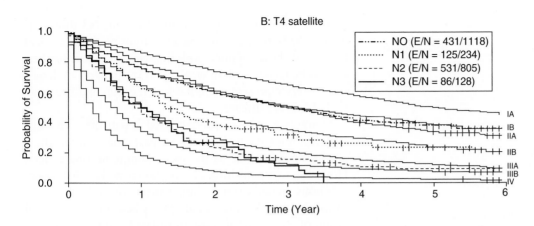

FIGURE 14.2 Survival following curative-intent resection of a brain metastasis by intrathoracic lymph node status. From Ref. 47 with permission.

In conclusion, curative-intent treatment of patients with isolated brain metastases is reasonable given the 5-year survival of 15% to 20%, although this appears to be underutilized. Other metastatic sites and N2,3 involvement should be carefully excluded. WBRT to reduce recurrences is reasonable, although the data supporting it is conflicting. The role of adjuvant chemotherapy is not proven, but reasonable, given a clearly established role in stage II and III patients.

Isolated Adrenal Metastasis

The second most common site for curative-intent metastasectomy is the adrenal gland. Curative-intent resection of an adrenal metastasis (and the primary lung caner) results in a 5-year survival of approximately 25% (Table 14.11) (3,168–179). This is similar to that of isolated brain metastases. The impression that it may be slightly better probably results from physicians being more selective in pursuing a curative strategy in the presence of an adrenal metastasis (at least many fewer

adrenal resections than brain resections/RS have been carried out).

Prognostic factors are incompletely defined due to the limited number of patients. A collective literature review and analysis suggested that nodal involvement was a key prognostic factor (Figure 14.3) (3,169). Several pooled analyses have found no difference between synchronous and metachronous metastases (3,168–170). An individual study (172) suggested that a disease-free interval of >6 months was a good prognostic factor.

Other Isolated Metastasis

A potentially curative approach in the case of other metastatic sites has been reported only rarely. Resection of a liver metastasis from lung cancer has been described twice with good long-term outcomes (>5 years) (180,181). Over the past 2 decades a fair number of resections for isolated metastasis to the pancreas have been reported (182–188). Despite these heroic efforts, though, the 5-year survival data is either poor or very

■ **Table 14.11** Adrenal metastasectomy				
Study	Total (N)	% Lung Cancer	% 5-Year Survival Lung Cancer Patients	Positive Prognostic Factors
Tanvetyanon (168)	110	100	25	None
Pham (169)	78	100	40	Negative intrathoracic nodes
Porte (170)	43	100	12	None
Mercier (171)	23	100	23	DFI >6 months
Lucchi (172)	14	100	36	None
Strong (173)	94	39	29	None
Wade (174)	47	30	26	None
Kim (175)	37	46	24[a]	R0 resection, DFI >6 months
Lo (176)	52	21	40[a,b]	None
Average[c]			25	

Inclusion criteria: Patients with adrenal metastasis undergoing curative-intent surgical therapy reported in publications with ≥10 patients with lung cancer from December, 1989, to December, 2009.

[a] Survival of entire cohort including nonlung cancer patients; [b] 2-year; [c] excluding values in parentheses.

Ca, cancer; DFI, Disease Free Interval from lung resection.

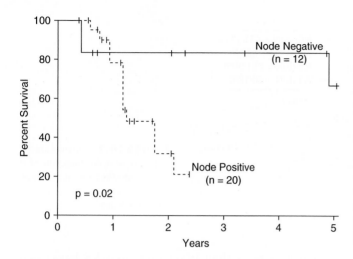

FIGURE 14.3 Survival following curative-intent resection of an adrenal metastasis by intrathoracic lymph node status. From Ref. 169 with permission.

limited leaving the role for pancreatic resections in this specific setting unclear. Resection of isolated lung cancer metastasis to the stomach (140), spleen (141,189), kidney(139), and colon(141) have been described, but no definite conclusions can be made. Generally, bone metastasis from lung cancer is associated with a median 6-month survival(190), but several patients have survived more than 5 years after resection of an isolated bone metastasis as well as the primary lung cancer (138,191). Resections of solitary skin, soft tissue, or muscle metastasis have been reported (192,193).

Collectively, substantial lymph node involvement or an uncontrolled primary lung cancer appears to preclude long-term survival. Other criteria to select patients with isolated metastatic sites for curative-intent treatment have not been well defined. In the metachronous setting, a disease-free interval of >6 months has been suggested to be beneficial (192,193). We suggest that, for either synchronous or metachronous situations, curative-intent resection of an isolated nonbrain metastasis be done after treatment with a course of chemotherapy (ideally with a response), and an observation period off treatment (>6 months). If no other sites of disease become apparent after an exhaustive search and after careful discussion in a multidisciplinary program, curative-intent treatment may be reasonable, albeit based on very limited data.

■ CONCLUSION

NSCLC involving T4, N3, or M1 disease is typically viewed as not being amenable to surgery. However, subsets of these patients have undergone resection with curative intent, and the data presented justify this. Surgery is probably most often considered for T4 tumors, particularly if

there appears to be no nodal involvement. N3 disease is approached surgically only in a few multimodality clinical trials, but these support exploring this approach further. It must be recognized, however, that the patients undergoing surgery represent a small selected group of all patients with T4 or N3 disease.

Surgery is more commonly used in patients with additional pulmonary foci of cancer, particularly when these are in the same lobe as the more dominant lung cancer. However, distinguishing an additional nodule from synchronous second primary lung cancers or multifocal lung cancer is difficult. Surgery can clearly be curative in a small group of patients that have an isolated distant metastasis involving the brain or adrenal gland.

■ REFERENCES

1. Detterbeck FC, Boffa DJ, Tanoue LT. The new lung cancer staging system. *Chest.* 2009;136(1):260–271.
2. Detterbeck FC, Jones DR. Surgery for stage IIIb non-small cell lung cancer. In: Detterbeck FC, Rivera MP, Socinski MA, Rosenman JG, eds. *Diagnosis and Treatment of Lung Cancer: an Evidence-Based Guide for the Practicing Clinician.* Philadelphia, PA: WB Saunders; 2001:283–289.
3. Detterbeck FC, Bleiweis MS, Ewend MG. Surgical treatment of stage IV non-small cell lung cancer. In: Detterbeck FC, Rivera MP, Socinski MA, Rosenman JG, eds. *Diagnosis and Treatment of Lung Cancer: an Evidence-Based Guide for the Practicing Clinician.* Philadelphia, PA: WB Saunders; 2001:326–338.
4. Detterbeck FC, Jones DR, Funkhouser Jr, WK. Satellite nodules and multiple primary cancers. In: Detterbeck FC, Rivera MP, Socinski MA, Rosenman JG, eds. *Diagnosis and Treatment of Lung Cancer: an Evidence-Based Guide for the Practicing Clinician.* Philadelphia, PA: WB Saunders; 2001:437–449.
5. Rendina EA, Venuta F, De Giacomo T, et al. Induction chemotherapy for T4 centrally located non-small cell lung cancer. *J Thorac Cardiovasc Surg.* 1999;117(2):225–233.
6. Stamatis G, Eberhardt W, Stüben G, Bildat S, Dahler O, Hillejan L. Preoperative chemoradiotherapy and surgery for selected non-small cell lung cancer IIIB subgroups: long-term results. *Ann Thorac Surg.* 1999;68(4):1144–1149.
7. Stupp R, Mayer M, Kann R, et al. Neoadjuvant chemotherapy and radiotherapy followed by surgery in selected patients with stage IIIB non-small-cell lung cancer: a multicentre phase II trial. *Lancet Oncol.* 2009;10(8):785–793.
8. Grunenwald DH, André F, Le Péchoux C, et al. Benefit of surgery after chemoradiotherapy in stage IIIB (T4 and/or N3) non-small cell lung cancer. *J Thorac Cardiovasc Surg.* 2001;122(4):796–802.
9. Galetta D, Cesario A, Margaritora S, et al. Enduring challenge in the treatment of nonsmall cell lung cancer with clinical stage IIIB: results of a trimodality approach. *Ann Thorac Surg.* 2003;76(6):1802–8; discussion 1808.
10. Ichinose Y, Fukuyama Y, Asoh H, et al. Induction chemoradiotherapy and surgical resection for selected stage IIIB non-small-cell lung cancer. *Ann Thorac Surg.* 2003;76(6):1810–4; discussion 1815.
11. Yamamoto K, Miyamoto Y, Ohsumi A, Imanishi N, Kojima F. Results of surgical resection for tracheobronchial cancer involving the tracheal carina. *Gen Thorac Cardiovasc Surg.* 2007;55(6):231–9; discussion 238.
12. Roviaro GC, Varoli F, Rebuffat C, et al. Tracheal sleeve pneumonectomy for bronchogenic carcinoma. *J Thorac Cardiovasc Surg.* 1994;107(1):13–18.

13. Roviaro G, Varoli F, Romanelli A, Vergani C, Maciocco M. Complications of tracheal sleeve pneumonectomy: personal experience and overview of the literature. *J Thorac Cardiovasc Surg.* 2001;121(2):234–240.

14. Roviaro G, Vergani C, Maciocco M, Varoli F, Francese M, Despini L. Tracheal sleeve pneumonectomy: long-term outcome. *Lung Cancer.* 2006;52(1):105–110.

15. Rea F, Marulli G, Schiavon M, et al. Tracheal sleeve pneumonectomy for non small cell lung cancer (NSCLC): short and long-term results in a single institution. *Lung Cancer.* 2008;61(2):202–208.

16. Yildizeli B, Dartevelle PG, Fadel E, Mussot S, Chapelier A. Results of primary surgery with T4 non-small cell lung cancer during a 25-year period in a single center: the benefit is worth the risk. *Ann Thorac Surg.* 2008;86(4):1065–75; discussion 1074.

17. Regnard JF, Perrotin C, Giovannetti R, et al. Resection for tumors with carinal involvement: technical aspects, results, and prognostic factors. *Ann Thorac Surg.* 2005;80(5):1841–1846.

18. de Perrot M, Fadel E, Mercier O, Mussot S, Chapelier A, Dartevelle P. Long-term results after carinal resection for carcinoma: does the benefit warrant the risk? *J Thorac Cardiovasc Surg.* 2006;131(1):81–89.

19. Dartevelle P. Extended operations for the treatment of lung cancer. *Ann Thorac Surg.* 1997;63:12–19.

20. Porhanov VA, Poliakov IS, Selvaschuk AP, et al. Indications and results of sleeve carinal resection. *Eur J Cardiothorac Surg.* 2002;22(5):685–694.

21. Mitchell JD, Mathisen DJ, Wright CD, et al. Resection for bronchogenic carcinoma involving the carina: long-term results and effect of nodal status on outcome. *J Thorac Cardiovasc Surg.* 2001;121(3):465–471.

22. Maeda M, Nakamoto K, Tsubota N, Okada T, Katsura H. Operative approaches for left-sided carinoplasty. *Ann Thorac Surg.* 1993;56(3):441–5; discussion 445.

23. Mathisen DJ, Grillo HC. Carinal resection for bronchogenic carcinoma. *J Thorac Cardiovasc Surg.* 1991;102(1):16–22; discussion 22.

24. Tsuchiya R, Goya T, Naruke T, Suemasu K. Resection of tracheal carina for lung cancer. Procedure, complications, and mortality. *J Thorac Cardiovasc Surg.* 1990;99(5):779–787.

25. Martini N, Yellin A, Ginsberg RJ, et al. Management of non-small cell lung cancer with direct mediastinal involvement. *Ann Thorac Surg.* 1994;58(5):1447–1451.

26. Yang HX, Hou X, Lin P, Rong TH, Yang H, Fu JH. Survival and risk factors of surgically treated mediastinal invasion T4 non-small cell lung cancer. *Ann Thorac Surg.* 2009;88(2):372–378.

27. Pitz CC, Brutel de la Rivière A, van Swieten HA, Westermann CJ, Lammers JW, van den Bosch JM. Results of surgical treatment of T4 non-small cell lung cancer. *Eur J Cardiothorac Surg.* 2003;24(6):1013–1018.

28. Spaggiari L, Magdeleinat P, Kondo H, et al. Results of superior vena cava resection for lung cancer. Analysis of prognostic factors. *Lung Cancer.* 2004;44(3):339–346.

29. Tsuchiya R, Asamura H, Kondo H, Goya T, Naruke T. Extended resection of the left atrium, great vessels, or both for lung cancer. *Ann Thorac Surg.* 1994;57(4):960–965.

30. Wu L, Xu Z, Zhao X, et al. Surgical treatment of lung cancer invading the left atrium or base of the pulmonary vein. *World J Surg.* 2009;33(3):492–496.

31. Fukuse T, Wada H, Hitomi S. Extended operation for non-small cell lung cancer invading great vessels and left atrium. *Eur J Cardiothorac Surg.* 1997;11(4):664–669.

32. Suzuki K, Asamura H, Watanabe S, Tsuchiya R. Combined resection of superior vena cava for lung carcinoma: prognostic significance of patterns of superior vena cava invasion. *Ann Thorac Surg.* 2004;78(4):1184–9; discussion 1184.

33. Bobbio A, Carbognani P, Grapeggia M, et al. Surgical outcome of combined pulmonary and atrial resection for lung cancer. *Thorac Cardiovasc Surg.* 2004;52(3):180–182.

34. Doddoli C, Rollet G, Thomas P, et al. Is lung cancer surgery justified in patients with direct mediastinal invasion? *Eur J Cardiothorac Surg.* 2001;20(2):339–343.

35. Borri A, Leo F, Veronesi G, et al. Extended pneumonectomy for non-small cell lung cancer: morbidity, mortality, and long-term results. *J Thorac Cardiovasc Surg.* 2007;134(5):1266–1272.

36. Shargall Y, de Perrot M, Keshavjee S, et al. 15 years single center experience with surgical resection of the superior vena cava for non-small cell lung cancer. *Lung Cancer.* 2004;45(3):357–363.

37. Spaggiari L, Leo F, Veronesi G, et al. Superior vena cava resection for lung and mediastinal malignancies: a single-center experience with 70 cases. *Ann Thorac Surg.* 2007;83(1):223–9; discussion 229.

38. Shiraishi T, Shirakusa T, Miyoshi T, et al. Extended resection of T4 lung cancer with invasion of the aorta: is it justified? *Thorac Cardiovasc Surg.* 2005;53(6):375–379.

39. Ohta M, Hirabayasi H, Shiono H, et al. Surgical resection for lung cancer with infiltration of the thoracic aorta. *J Thorac Cardiovasc Surg.* 2005;129(4):804–808.

40. Klepetko W, Wisser W, Bîrsan T, et al. T4 lung tumors with infiltration of the thoracic aorta: is an operation reasonable? *Ann Thorac Surg.* 1999;67(2):340–344.

41. Stamatis G, Eberhard W, Pöttgen C. Surgery after multimodality treatment for non-small-cell lung cancer. *Lung Cancer.* 2004;45(suppl 2):S107–S112.

42. Bernard A, Bouchot O, Hagry O, Favre JP. Risk analysis and long-term survival in patients undergoing resection of T4 lung cancer. *Eur J Cardiothorac Surg.* 2001;20(2):344–349.

43. Macchiarini P, Chapelier AR, Monnet I, et al. Extended operations after induction therapy for stage IIIb (T4) non-small cell lung cancer. *Ann Thorac Surg.* 1994;57(4):966–973.

44. Rami-Porta R, Ball D, Crowley J, et al.; International Staging Committee; Cancer Research and Biostatistics; Observers to the Committee; Participating Institutions. The IASLC Lung Cancer Staging Project: proposals for the revision of the T descriptors in the forthcoming (seventh) edition of the TNM classification for lung cancer. *J Thorac Oncol.* 2007;2(7):593–602.

45. Farjah F, Wood DE, Varghese TK Jr, Symons RG, Flum DR. Trends in the operative management and outcomes of T4 lung cancer. *Ann Thorac Surg.* 2008;86(2):368–374.

46. Ou SH, Zell JA. Validation study of the proposed IASLC staging revisions of the T4 and M non-small cell lung cancer descriptors using data from 23,583 patients in the California Cancer Registry. *J Thorac Oncol.* 2008;3(3):216–227.

47. William WN Jr, Lin HY, Lee JJ, Lippman SM, Roth JA, Kim ES. Revisiting stage IIIB and IV non-small cell lung cancer: analysis of the surveillance, epidemiology, and end results data. *Chest.* 2009;136(3):701–709.

48. Hasegawa S, Bando T, Isowa N, et al. The use of cardiopulmonary bypass during extended resection of non-small cell lung cancer. *Interact Cardiovasc Thorac Surg.* 2003;2(4):676–679.

49. Eberhardt W, Wilke H, Stamatis G, et al. Preoperative chemotherapy followed by concurrent chemoradiation therapy based on hyperfractionated accelerated radiotherapy and definitive surgery in locally advanced non-small-cell lung cancer: mature results of a phase II trial. *J Clin Oncol.* 1998;16(2):622–634.

50. Anraku M, Waddell TK, de Perrot M, et al. Induction chemoradiotherapy facilitates radical resection of T4 non-small cell lung cancer invading the spine. *J Thorac Cardiovasc Surg.* 2009;137(2):441–447.e1.

51. Grunenwald DH, Mazel C, Girard P, et al. Radical en bloc resection for lung cancer invading the spine. *J Thorac Cardiovasc Surg.* 2002;123(2):271–279.

52. Bilsky MH, Vitaz TW, Boland PJ, Bains MS, Rajaraman V, Rusch VW. Surgical treatment of superior sulcus tumors with spinal and brachial plexus involvement. *J Neurosurg.* 2002;97(3 suppl):301–309.

53. Bolton WD, Rice DC, Goodyear A, et al. Superior sulcus tumors with vertebral body involvement: a multimodality approach. *J Thorac Cardiovasc Surg.* 2009;137(6):1379–1387.

54. Hehr T, Friedel G, Steger V, et al. Neoadjuvant chemoradiation with paclitaxel/carboplatin for selected Stage III non-small-cell lung cancer: long-term results of a trimodality Phase II protocol. *Int J Radiat Oncol Biol Phys*. 2010;76(5): 1376–1381.

55. Friedel G, Hruska D, Budach W, et al. Neoadjuvant chemoradiotherapy of stage III non-small-cell lung cancer. *Lung Cancer*. 2000;30(3):175–185.

56. Spaggiari L, Regnard JF, Magdeleinat P, Jauffret B, Puyo P, Levasseur P. Extended resections for bronchogenic carcinoma invading the superior vena cava system. *Ann Thorac Surg*. 2000;69(1):233–236.

57. Spaggiari L, D' Aiuto M, Veronesi G, et al. Extended pneumonectomy with partial resection of the left atrium, without cardiopulmonary bypass, for lung cancer. *Ann Thorac Surg*. 2005;79(1):234–240.

58. Spaggiari L, Thomas P, Magdeleinat P, et al. Superior vena cava resection with prosthetic replacement for non-small cell lung cancer: long-term results of a multicentric study. *Eur J Cardiothorac Surg*. 2002;21(6):1080–1086.

59. Garrido P, González-Larriba JL, Insa A, et al. Long-term survival associated with complete resection after induction chemotherapy in stage IIIA (N2) and IIIB (T4N0–1) non small-cell lung cancer patients: the Spanish Lung Cancer Group Trial 9901. *J Clin Oncol*. 2007;25(30):4736–4742.

60. Albain KS, Rusch VW, Crowley JJ, et al. Concurrent cisplatin/etoposide plus chest radiotherapy followed by surgery for stages IIIA (N2) and IIIB non-small-cell lung cancer: mature results of Southwest Oncology Group phase II study 8805. *J Clin Oncol*. 1995;13(8):1880–1892.

61. Thomas M, Rübe C, Hoffknecht P, et al.; German Lung Cancer Cooperative Group. Effect of preoperative chemoradiation in addition to preoperative chemotherapy: a randomised trial in stage III non-small-cell lung cancer. *Lancet Oncol*. 2008;9(7):636–648.

62. Thomas M, Rübe C, Semik M, et al. Impact of preoperative bimodality induction including twice-daily radiation on tumor regression and survival in stage III non-small-cell lung cancer. *J Clin Oncol*. 1999;17(4):1185.

63. Santo A, Pedersini R, Pasini F, et al. A phase II study of induction chemotherapy with gemcitabine (G) and cisplatin (P) in locally advanced non-small cell lung cancer: interim analysis. *Lung Cancer*. 2001;34(suppl 4):S15–S20.

64. Aristu J, Rebollo J, Martínez-Monge R, et al. Cisplatin, mitomycin, and vindesine followed by intraoperative and postoperative radiotherapy for stage III non-small cell lung cancer: final results of a phase II study. *Am J Clin Oncol*. 1997;20(3): 276–281.

65. Rusch VW, Albain KS, Crowley JJ, et al. Neoadjuvant therapy: a novel and effective treatment for stage IIIb non-small cell lung cancer. Southwest Oncology Group. *Ann Thorac Surg*. 1994;58(2):290–4; discussion 294.

66. Rusch VW, Albain KS, Crowley JJ, et al. Surgical resection of stage IIIA and stage IIIB non-small-cell lung cancer after concurrent induction chemoradiotherapy. A Southwest Oncology Group trial. *J Thorac Cardiovasc Surg*. 1993;105(1):97–104; discussion 104.

67. Deeley TJ, Edwards JM. Radiotherapy in the management of cerebral secondaries from bronchial carcinoma. *Lancet*. 1968;1(7554):1209–1213.

68. Keogan MT, Tung KT, Kaplan DK, Goldstraw PJ, Hansell DM. The significance of pulmonary nodules detected on CT staging for lung cancer. *Clin Radiol*. 1993;48(2):94–96.

69. Kunitoh H, Eguchi K, Yamada K, et al. Intrapulmonary sublesions detected before surgery in patients with lung cancer. *Cancer*. 1992;70(7):1876–1879.

70. Shen KR, Meyers BF, Larner JM, Jones DR; American College of Chest Physicians. Special treatment issues in lung cancer: ACCP evidence-based clinical practice guidelines (2nd edition). *Chest*. 2007;132(3 suppl):290S–305S.

71. Swensen SJ, Jett JR, Hartman TE, et al. CT screening for lung cancer: five-year prospective experience. *Radiology*. 2005;235(1):259–265.

72. Pastorino U, Bellomi M, Landoni C, et al. Early lung-cancer detection with spiral CT and positron emission tomography in heavy smokers: 2-year results. *Lancet*. 2003;362(9384):593–597.

73. Kim H, Choi Y, Kim J, Shim Y, Kim K. Management of multiple pure ground-glass opacity lesions in patients with bronchioloalveolar carcinoma. *J Thorac Oncol*. 2009;in press.

74. Kim HK, Choi YS, Kim K, et al. Management of ground-glass opacity lesions detected in patients with otherwise operable non-small cell lung cancer. *J Thorac Oncol*. 2009;4(10):1242–1246.

75. Detterbeck FC. Synchronous, separate, and similar. *J Thorac Oncol*. 2010;5:150–152.

76. Lindell RM, Hartman TE, Swensen SJ, Jett JR, Midthun DE, Mandrekar JN. 5-year lung cancer screening experience: growth curves of 18 lung cancers compared to histologic type, CT attenuation, stage, survival, and size. *Chest*. 2009;136(6):1586–1595.

77. Detterbeck FC, Boffa DJ, Tanoue LT, Wilson LD. Details and difficulties regarding the new lung cancer staging system. *Chest*. 2010;137(5):1172–1180.

78. Detterbeck FC, Tanoue LT, Boffa DJ. Anatomy, biology and concepts, pertaining to lung cancer stage classification. *J Thorac Oncol*. 2009;4(4):437–443.

79. Travis WD, Garg K, Franklin WA, et al. Evolving concepts in the pathology and computed tomography imaging of lung adenocarcinoma and bronchioloalveolar carcinoma. *J Clin Oncol*. 2005;23(14):3279–3287.

80. Garfield DH, Cadranel JL, Wislez M, Franklin WA, Hirsch FR. The bronchioloalveolar carcinoma and peripheral adenocarcinoma spectrum of diseases. *J Thorac Oncol*. 2006;1(4):344–359.

81. Trousse D, Barlesi F, Loundou A, et al. Synchronous multiple primary lung cancer: an increasing clinical occurrence requiring multidisciplinary management. *J Thorac Cardiovasc Surg*. 2007;133(5):1193–1200.

82. Battafarano RJ, Meyers BF, Guthrie TJ, Cooper JD, Patterson GA. Surgical resection of multifocal non-small cell lung cancer is associated with prolonged survival. *Ann Thorac Surg*. 2002;74(4):988–93; discussion 993.

83. Arenberg D; American College of Chest Physicians. Bronchioloalveolar lung cancer: ACCP evidence-based clinical practice guidelines (2nd edition). *Chest*. 2007;132(3 suppl):306S–313S.

84. Travis W, Brambilla E, Noguchi M, *et al*. The new IASLC/ATS/ERS international multidisciplinary lung adenocarcinoma classification. In: 13th World Conference on Lung Cancer; 2009; San Francisco, CA.

85. Kerr KM. Pulmonary adenocarcinomas: classification and reporting. *Histopathology*. 2009;54(1):12–27.

86. Rivera MP, Detterbeck FC, Loomis DP. Epidemiology and classification of lung cancer. In: Detterbeck FC, Rivera MP, Socinski MA, Rosenman JG, eds. *Diagnosis and Treatment of Lung Cancer: an Evidence-Based Guide for the Practicing Clinician*. Philadelphia: WB Saunders; 2001:25–44.

87. Martini N, Melamed MR. Multiple primary lung cancers. *J Thorac Cardiovasc Surg*. 1975;70(4):606–612.

88. De Leyn P, Moons J, Vansteenkiste J, et al. Survival after resection of synchronous bilateral lung cancer. *Eur J Cardiothorac Surg*. 2008;34(6):1215–1222.

89. Lee JG, Lee CY, Kim DJ, Chung KY, Park IK. Non-small cell lung cancer with ipsilateral pulmonary metastases: prognosis analysis and staging assessment. *Eur J Cardiothorac Surg*. 2008;33(3):480–484.

90. Motoi N, Szoke J, Riely GJ, et al. Lung adenocarcinoma: modification of the 2004 WHO mixed subtype to include the major histologic subtype suggests correlations between papillary and micropapillary adenocarcinoma subtypes, EGFR mutations and gene expression analysis. *Am J Surg Pathol*. 2008;32(6): 810–827.

91. Wang X, Wang M, MacLennan GT, et al. Evidence for common clonal origin of multifocal lung cancers. *J Natl Cancer Inst.* 2009;101(8):560–570.

92. Hiroshima K, Toyozaki T, Kohno H, Ohwada H, Fujisawa T. Synchronous and metachronous lung carcinomas: molecular evidence for multicentricity. *Pathol Int.* 1998;48(11):869–876.

93. Huang J, Behrens C, Wistuba I, Gazdar AF, Jagirdar J. Molecular analysis of synchronous and metachronous tumors of the lung: impact on management and prognosis. *Ann Diagn Pathol.* 2001;5(6):321–329.

94. Dacic S, Ionescu DN, Finkelstein S, Yousem SA. Patterns of allelic loss of synchronous adenocarcinomas of the lung. *Am J Surg Pathol.* 2005;29(7):897–902.

95. Chang YL, Wu CT, Lin SC, Hsiao CF, Jou YS, Lee YC. Clonality and prognostic implications of p53 and epidermal growth factor receptor somatic aberrations in multiple primary lung cancers. *Clin Cancer Res.* 2007;13(1):52–58.

96. Nagai K, Sohara Y, Tsuchiya R, Goya T, Miyaoka E; Japan Lung Cancer Registration Committee. Prognosis of resected non-small cell lung cancer patients with intrapulmonary metastases. *J Thorac Oncol.* 2007;2(4):282–286.

97. Okada M, Tsubota N, Yoshimura M, Miyamoto Y, Nakai R. Evaluation of TMN classification for lung carcinoma with ipsilateral intrapulmonary metastasis. *Ann Thorac Surg.* 1999;68(2):326–30; discussion 331.

98. Yano M, Arai T, Inagaki K, Morita T, Nomura T, Ito H. Intrapulmonary satellite nodule of lung cancer as a T factor. *Chest.* 1998;114(5):1305–1308.

99. Shimizu N, Ando A, Date H, Teramoto S. Prognosis of undetected intrapulmonary metastases in resected lung cancer. *Cancer.* 1993;71(12):3868–3872.

100. Osaki T, Sugio K, Hanagiri T, et al. Survival and prognostic factors of surgically resected T4 non-small cell lung cancer. *Ann Thorac Surg.* 2003;75(6):1745–51; discussion 1751.

101. Watanabe Y, Shimizu J, Oda M, et al. Proposals regarding some deficiencies in the new international staging system for non-small cell lung cancer. *Jpn J Clin Oncol.* 1991;21(3):160–168.

102. Yoshino I, Nakanishi R, Osaki T, et al. Postoperative prognosis in patients with non-small cell lung cancer with synchronous ipsilateral intrapulmonary metastasis. *Ann Thorac Surg.* 1997;64(3):809–813.

103. Fukuse T, Hirata T, Tanaka F, Yanagihara K, Hitomi S, Wada H. Prognosis of ipsilateral intrapulmonary metastases in resected nonsmall cell lung cancer. *Eur J Cardiothorac Surg.* 1997;12(2):218–223.

104. Oliaro A, Filosso PL, Cavallo A, et al. The significance of intrapulmonary metastasis in non-small cell lung cancer: upstaging or downstaging? A re-appraisal for the next TNM staging system. *Eur J Cardiothorac Surg.* 2008;34(2):438–43; discussion 443.

105. Port JL, Korst RJ, Lee PC, Kansler AL, Kerem Y, Altorki NK. Surgical resection for multifocal (T4) non-small cell lung cancer: is the T4 designation valid? *Ann Thorac Surg.* 2007;83(2):397–400.

106. Zell JA, Ou SH, Ziogas A, Anton-Culver H. Survival improvements for advanced stage nonbronchioloalveolar carcinoma-type nonsmall cell lung cancer cases with ipsilateral intrapulmonary nodules. *Cancer.* 2008;112(1):136–143.

107. Okumura T, Asamura H, Suzuki K, Kondo H, Tsuchiya R. Intrapulmonary metastasis of non-small cell lung cancer: a prognostic assessment. *J Thorac Cardiovasc Surg.* 2001;122(1):24–28.

108. Deslauriers J, Brisson J, Cartier R, et al. Carcinoma of the lung. Evaluation of satellite nodules as a factor influencing prognosis after resection. *J Thorac Cardiovasc Surg.* 1989;97(4):504–512.

109. Okubo K, Bando T, Miyahara R, *et al.* Resection of pulmonary metastasis of non-small cell lung cancer. *J Thorac Oncol.* 2009;4:203–207.

110. Rostad H, Strand TE, Naalsund A, Norstein J. Resected synchronous primary malignant lung tumors: a population-based study. *Ann Thorac Surg.* 2008;85:204–209.

111. Finley DJ, Yoshizawa A, Travis W, et al. Predictors of outcomes after surgical treatment of synchronous primary lung cancers. *J Thorac Oncol.* 2010;5(2):197–205.

112. Riquet M, Cazes A, Pfeuty K, et al. Multiple lung cancers prognosis: what about histology? *Ann Thorac Surg.* 2008;86(3):921–926.

113. Chang YL, Wu CT, Lee YC. Surgical treatment of synchronous multiple primary lung cancers: experience of 92 patients. *J Thorac Cardiovasc Surg.* 2007;134(3):630–637.

114. van Rens MT, de la Rivière AB, Elbers HR, van Den Bosch JM. Prognostic assessment of 2,361 patients who underwent pulmonary resection for non-small cell lung cancer, stage I, II, and IIIA. *Chest.* 2000;117(2):374–379.

115. van Bodegom PC, Wagenaar SS, Corrin B, Baak JP, Berkel J, Vanderschueren RG. Second primary lung cancer: importance of long term follow up. *Thorax.* 1989;44(10):788–793.

116. Deschamps C, Pairolero PC, Trastek VF, Payne WS. Multiple primary lung cancers. Results of surgical treatment. *J Thorac Cardiovasc Surg.* 1990;99(5):769–77; discussion 777.

117. Vansteenkiste JF, De Belie B, Deneffe GJ, et al.; Leuven Lung Cancer Group. Practical approach to patients presenting with multiple synchronous suspect lung lesions: a reflection on the current TNM classification based on 54 cases with complete follow-up. *Lung Cancer.* 2001;34(2):169–175.

118. Rosengart TK, Martini N, Ghosn P, Burt M. Multiple primary lung carcinomas: prognosis and treatment. *Ann Thorac Surg.* 1991;52(4):773–8; discussion 778.

119. Ferguson MK, DeMeester TR, DesLauriers J, Little AG, Piraux M, Golomb H. Diagnosis and management of synchronous lung cancers. *J Thorac Cardiovasc Surg.* 1985;89(3):378–385.

120. Okada M, Tsubota N, Yoshimura M, Miyamoto Y. Operative approach for multiple primary lung carcinomas. *J Thorac Cardiovasc Surg.* 1998;115(4):836–840.

121. Antakli T, Schaefer RF, Rutherford JE, Read RC. Second primary lung cancer. *Ann Thorac Surg.* 1995;59(4):863–6; discussion 867.

122. Ribet M, Dambron P. Multiple primary lung cancers. *Eur J Cardiothorac Surg.* 1995;9(5):231–236.

123. Mathisen DJ, Jensik RJ, Faber LP, Kittle CF. Survival following resection for second and third primary lung cancers. *J Thorac Cardiovasc Surg.* 1984;88(4):502–510.

124. Battafarano RJ, Force SD, Meyers BF, et al. Benefits of resection for metachronous lung cancer. *J Thorac Cardiovasc Surg.* 2004;127(3):836–842.

125. Verhagen AF, Tavilla G, van de Wal HJ, Cox AL, Lacquet LK. Multiple primary lung cancers. *Thorac Cardiovasc Surg.* 1994;42(1):40–44.

126. Adebonojo SA, Moritz DM, Danby CA. The results of modern surgical therapy for multiple primary lung cancers. *Chest.* 1997;112(3):693–701.

127. Wu SC, Lin ZQ, Xu CW, Koo KS, Huang OL, Xie DQ. Multiple primary lung cancers. *Chest.* 1987;92(5):892–896.

128. Roberts PF, Straznicka M, Lara PN, et al. Resection of multifocal non-small cell lung cancer when the bronchioloalveolar subtype is involved. *J Thorac Cardiovasc Surg.* 2003;126(5):1597–1602.

129. Zell JA, Ou SH, Ziogas A, Anton-Culver H. Long-term survival differences for bronchiolo-alveolar carcinoma patients with ipsilateral intrapulmonary metastasis at diagnosis. *Ann Oncol.* 2006;17(8):1255–1262.

130. Naruke T, Tsuchiya R, Kondo H, Asamura H, Nakayama H. Implications of staging in lung cancer. *Chest.* 1997;112(4 suppl):242S–248S.

131. Shimizu J, Oda M, Morita K, et al. Comparison of pleuropneumonectomy and limited surgery for lung cancer with pleural dissemination. *J Surg Oncol.* 1996;61(1):1–6.

132. Ohta Y, Shimizu Y, Matsumoto I, Tamura M, Oda M, Watanabe G. Retrospective review of lung cancer patients with pleural dissemination after limited operations combined with parietal pleurectomy. *J Surg Oncol.* 2005;91(4):237–242.

133. Shigemura N, Akashi A, Ohta M, Matsuda H. Combined surgery of intrapleural perfusion hyperthermic chemotherapy and panpleuropneumonectomy for lung cancer with advanced pleural spread: a pilot study. *Interact Cardiovasc Thorac Surg.* 2003;2(4):671–675.

134. Kodama K, Doi O, Higashiyama M, Yokouchi H, Tatsuta M. Long-term results of postoperative intrathoracic chemothermotherapy for lung cancer with pleural dissemination. *Cancer.* 1993;72(2):426–431.

135. Fukuse T, Hirata T, Tanaka F, Wada H. The prognostic significance of malignant pleural effusion at the time of thoracotomy in patients with non-small cell lung cancer. *Lung Cancer.* 2001;34(1):75–81.

136. Yasumoto K, Nagashima A, Nakahashi H, Ishida T, Sugimachi K, Nomoto K. Effect of postoperative intrapleural instillations of interleukin-2 in patients with malignant pleurisy due to lung cancer. *Biotherapy.* 1993;6(2):133–138.

137. Patchell RA, Tibbs PA, Regine WF, et al. Direct decompressive surgical resection in the treatment of spinal cord compression caused by metastatic cancer: a randomised trial. *Lancet.* 2005;366(9486):643–648.

138. Luketich JD, Martini N, Ginsberg RJ, Rigberg D, Burt ME. Successful treatment of solitary extracranial metastases from non-small cell lung cancer. *Ann Thorac Surg.* 1995;60(6):1609–1611.

139. Ambrogi V, Nofroni I, Tonini G, Mineo TC. Skin metastases in lung cancer: analysis of a 10-year experience. *Oncol Rep.* 2001;8(1):57–61.

140. Hishida T, Nagai K, Yoshida J, et al. Is surgical resection indicated for a solitary non-small cell lung cancer recurrence? *J Thorac Cardiovasc Surg.* 2006;131(4):838–842.

141. Downey RJ, Ng KK, Kris MG, et al. A phase II trial of chemotherapy and surgery for non-small cell lung cancer patients with a synchronous solitary metastasis. *Lung Cancer.* 2002;38(2):193–197.

142. Hu C, Chang EL, Hassenbusch SJ 3rd, et al. Nonsmall cell lung cancer presenting with synchronous solitary brain metastasis. *Cancer.* 2006;106(9):1998–2004.

143. Bindal AK, Bindal RK, Hess KR, et al. Surgery versus radiosurgery in the treatment of brain metastasis. *J Neurosurg.* 1996;84(5):748–754.

144. Fuentes R, Bonfill X, Exposito J. Surgery versus radiosurgery for patients with a solitary brain metastasis from non-small cell lung cancer. *Cochrane Database Syst Rev.* 2006:CD004840.

145. Bonnette P, Puyo P, Gabriel C, et al.; Groupe Thorax. Surgical management of non-small cell lung cancer with synchronous brain metastases. *Chest.* 2001;119(5):1469–1475.

146. Wronski M, Arbit E, Burt M, Galicich JH. Survival after surgical treatment of brain metastases from lung cancer: a follow-up study of 231 patients treated between 1976 and 1991. *J Neurosurg.* 1995;83(4):605–616.

147. Nakagawa H, Miyawaki Y, Fujita T, et al. Surgical treatment of brain metastases of lung cancer: retrospective analysis of 89 cases. *J Neurol Neurosurg Psychiatr.* 1994;57(8):950–956.

148. Girard N, Cottin V, Tronc F, et al. Chemotherapy is the cornerstone of the combined surgical treatment of lung cancer with synchronous brain metastases. *Lung Cancer.* 2006;53(1):51–58.

149. Granone P, Margaritora S, D'Andrilli A, Cesario A, Kawamukai K, Meacci E. Non-small cell lung cancer with single brain metastasis: the role of surgical treatment. *Eur J Cardiothorac Surg.* 2001;20(2):361–366.

150. Billing PS, Miller DL, Allen MS, Deschamps C, Trastek VF, Pairolero PC. Surgical treatment of primary lung cancer with synchronous brain metastases. *J Thorac Cardiovasc Surg.* 2001;122(3):548–553.

151. Moazami N, Rice TW, Rybicki LA, et al. Stage III non-small cell lung cancer and metachronous brain metastases. *J Thorac Cardiovasc Surg.* 2002;124(1):113–122.

152. Furák J, Troján I, Szöke T, et al. Lung cancer and its operable brain metastasis: survival rate and staging problems. *Ann Thorac Surg.* 2005;79(1):241–7; discussion 241.

153. Mussi A, Pistolesi M, Lucchi M, et al. Resection of single brain metastasis in non-small-cell lung cancer: prognostic factors. *J Thorac Cardiovasc Surg.* 1996;112(1):146–153.

154. Burt M, Wronski M, Arbit E, Galicich JH. Resection of brain metastases from non-small-cell lung carcinoma. Results of therapy. Memorial Sloan-Kettering Cancer Center Thoracic Surgical Staff. *J Thorac Cardiovasc Surg.* 1992;103(3):399–410; discussion 410.

155. Getman V, Devyatko E, Dunkler D, et al. Prognosis of patients with non-small cell lung cancer with isolated brain metastases undergoing combined surgical treatment. *Eur J Cardiothorac Surg.* 2004;25(6):1107–1113.

156. Torre M, Quaini E, Chiesa G, Ravini M, Soresi E, Belloni PA. Synchronous brain metastasis from lung cancer. Result of surgical treatment in combined resection. *J Thorac Cardiovasc Surg.* 1988;95(6):994–997.

157. Modi A, Vohra HA, Weeden DF. Does surgery for primary non-small cell lung cancer and cerebral metastasis have any impact on survival? *Interact Cardiovasc Thorac Surg.* 2009;8(4):467–473.

158. Iwasaki A, Shirakusa T, Yoshinaga Y, Enatsu S, Yamamoto M. Evaluation of the treatment of non-small cell lung cancer with brain metastasis and the role of risk score as a survival predictor. *Eur J Cardiothorac Surg.* 2004;26(3):488–493.

159. Penel N, Brichet A, Prevost B, et al. Pronostic factors of synchronous brain metastases from lung cancer. *Lung Cancer.* 2001;33(2–3):143–154.

160. Patchell RA, Tibbs PA, Regine WF, et al. Postoperative radiotherapy in the treatment of single metastases to the brain: a randomized trial. *JAMA.* 1998;280(17):1485–1489.

161. Armstrong JG, Wronski M, Galicich J, Arbit E, Leibel SA, Burt M. Postoperative radiation for lung cancer metastatic to the brain. *J Clin Oncol.* 1994;12(11):2340–2344.

162. Flickinger JC, Kondziolka D, Lunsford LD, et al. A multi-institutional experience with stereotactic radiosurgery for solitary brain metastasis. *Int J Radiat Oncol Biol Phys.* 1994;28(4):797–802.

163. Smalley SR, Laws ER Jr, O'Fallon JR, Shaw EG, Schray MF. Resection for solitary brain metastasis. Role of adjuvant radiation and prognostic variables in 229 patients. *J Neurosurg.* 1992;77(4):531–540.

164. Smalley SR, Schray MF, Laws ER Jr, O'Fallon JR. Adjuvant radiation therapy after surgical resection of solitary brain metastasis: association with pattern of failure and survival. *Int J Radiat Oncol Biol Phys.* 1987;13(11):1611–1616.

165. Shiau CY, Sneed PK, Shu HK, et al. Radiosurgery for brain metastases: relationship of dose and pattern of enhancement to local control. *Int J Radiat Oncol Biol Phys.* 1997;37(2):375–383.

166. Young RF, Jacques DB, Duma C, et al. Gamma knife radiosurgery for treatment of multiple brain metastases: a comparison of patients with single versus multiple lesions. *Radiosurgery.* 1996;1:92–101.

167. DeAngelis LM, Mandell LR, Thaler HT, et al. The role of postoperative radiotherapy after resection of single brain metastases. *Neurosurgery.* 1989;24(6):798–805.

168. Tanvetyanon T, Robinson LA, Schell MJ, et al. Outcomes of adrenalectomy for isolated synchronous versus metachronous adrenal metastases in non-small-cell lung cancer: a systematic review and pooled analysis. *J Clin Oncol.* 2008;26(7):1142–1147.

169. Pham DT, Dean DA, Detterbeck FC. Adrenalectomy as the new treatment paradigm for solitary adrenal metastasis from lung cancer. In: The Society of Thoracic Surgeons Thirty-Seventh Annual Meeting, New Orleans, Louisiana 2001;158.

170. Porte H, Siat J, Guibert B, et al. Resection of adrenal metastases from non-small cell lung cancer: a multicenter study. *Ann Thorac Surg.* 2001;71(3):981–985.

171. Mercier O, Fadel E, de Perrot M, et al. Surgical treatment of solitary adrenal metastasis from non-small cell lung cancer. *J Thorac Cardiovasc Surg.* 2005;130(1):136–140.

172. Lucchi M, Dini P, Ambrogi MC, et al. Metachronous adrenal masses in resected non-small cell lung cancer patients: therapeutic implications of laparoscopic adrenalectomy. *Eur J Cardiothorac Surg.* 2005;27(5):753–756.

173. Strong VE, D'Angelica M, Tang L, et al. Laparoscopic adrenalectomy for isolated adrenal metastasis. *Ann Surg Oncol.* 2007;14(12):3392–3400.

174. Wade TP, Longo WE, Virgo KS, Johnson FE. A comparison of adrenalectomy with other resections for metastatic cancers. *Am J Surg.* 1998;175(3):183–186.

175. Kim SH, Brennan MF, Russo P, Burt ME, Coit DG. The role of surgery in the treatment of clinically isolated adrenal metastasis. *Cancer.* 1998;82(2):389–394.

176. Lo CY, van Heerden JA, Soreide JA, et al. Adrenalectomy for metastatic disease to the adrenal glands. *Br J Surg.* 1996;83(4):528–531.

177. Bretcha-Boix P, Rami-Porta R, Mateu-Navarro M, Hoyuela-Alonso C, Marco-Molina C. Surgical treatment of lung cancer with adrenal metastasis. *Lung Cancer.* 2000;27(2):101–105.

178. Porte HL, Roumilhac D, Graziana JP, et al. Adrenalectomy for a solitary adrenal metastasis from lung cancer. *Ann Thorac Surg.* 1998;65(2):331–335.

179. Pfannschmidt J, Schlolaut B, Muley T, Hoffmann H, Dienemann H. Adrenalectomy for solitary adrenal metastases from non-small cell lung cancer. *Lung Cancer.* 2005;49(2):203–207.

180. Kim KS, Na KJ, Kim YH, et al. Surgically resected isolated hepatic metastasis from non-small cell lung cancer: a case report. *J Thorac Oncol.* 2006;1(5):494–496.

181. Nagashima A, Abe Y, Yamada S, Nakagawa M, Yoshimatsu T. Long-term survival after surgical resection of liver metastasis from lung cancer. *Jpn J Thorac Cardiovasc Surg.* 2004;52(6):311–313.

182. Schwarz RE, Chu PG, Grannis FW Jr. Pancreatic tumors in patients with lung malignancies: a spectrum of clinicopathologic considerations. *South Med J.* 2004;97(9):811–815.

183. Medina-Franco H, Halpern NB, Aldrete JS. Pancreaticoduodenectomy for metastatic tumors to the periampullary region. *J Gastrointest Surg.* 1999;3(2):119–122.

184. Nakeeb A, Lillemoe KD, Cameron JL. The role of pancreaticoduodenectomy for locally recurrent or metastatic carcinoma to the periampullary region. *J Am Coll Surg.* 1995;180(2):188–192.

185. Le Borgne J, Partensky C, Glemain P, Dupas B, de Kerviller B. Pancreaticoduodenectomy for metastatic ampullary and pancreatic tumors. *Hepatogastroenterology.* 2000;47(32):540–544.

186. Pericleous S, Mukherjee S, Hutchins RR. Lung adenocarcinoma presenting as obstructive jaundice: a case report and review of literature. *World J Surg Oncol.* 2008;6:120.

187. Hiotis SP, Klimstra DS, Conlon KC, Brennan MF. Results after pancreatic resection for metastatic lesions. *Ann Surg Oncol.* 2002;9(7):675–679.

188. Seki M, Tsuchiya E, Hori M, et al. Pancreatic metastasis from a lung cancer. Preoperative diagnosis and management. *Int J Pancreatol.* 1998;24(1):55–59.

189. Lam KY, Tang V. Metastatic tumors to the spleen: a 25-year clinicopathologic study. *Arch Pathol Lab Med.* 2000;124(4):526–530.

190. Stanley KE. Prognostic factors for survival in patients with inoperable lung cancer. *J Natl Cancer Inst.* 1980;65(1):25–32.

191. Hirano Y, Oda M, Tsunezuka Y, Ishikawa N, Watanabe G. Long-term survival cases of lung cancer presented as solitary bone metastasis. *Ann Thorac Cardiovasc Surg.* 2005;11(6):401–404.

192. Pop D, Nadeemy AS, Venissac N, et al. Skeletal muscle metastasis from non-small cell lung cancer. *J Thorac Oncol.* 2009;4(10):1236–1241.

193. Mollet TW, Garcia CA, Koester G. Skin metastases from lung cancer. *Dermatol Online J.* 2009;15(5):1.

15 Stage IIIB and IV NSCLC: Primary Therapy

MILLIE DAS

HEATHER WAKELEE

■ INTRODUCTION

Lung cancer continues to be the leading cause of cancer death both worldwide and in the United States for both men and women. In the United States alone, the projected number of deaths from lung cancer in 2009 is 159,390 (1). Non–small cell lung cancer (NSCLC) comprises 80% to 85% of new cases of lung cancer and most commonly includes the histologic subtypes of adenocarcinoma, squamous cell carcinoma, and large cell carcinoma. Given that lung cancer is often diagnosed at an advanced stage, and has a high rate of relapse even in early stage, overall patient 5-year survival rates have remained low, currently about 15% overall (2). In 2009, the International Staging Committee of the International Association for the Study of Lung Cancer proposed changes in the 7th edition of the TNM staging classification based on differences in survival. According to the new stage grouping, T4 tumors by additional nodule(s) in the same lobe are reclassified as T3; M1 tumors by additional nodule(s) in another ipsilateral lobe are now T4; and T4 tumors by malignant pleural effusion are now M1a (with M1b representing distant metastasis). Notably, the proposed changes downstage T4N0–N1M0 tumors from stage IIIB to stage IIIA and change patients with a malignant effusion from IIIB (wet) to stage IVa (3).

Patients with stage IIIB disease comprise a heterogeneous group of patients who are often treated with multiple modalities with a low cure rate (4). Those with advanced-stage disease, including those with old stage IIIB (wet)—now IVa—and those with stage IV (IVa/IVb) disease, are generally considered incurable, but treatment with combination chemotherapy, particularly in the form of platinum doublets, has been shown to improve survival and quality of life (QOL) in comparison with best supportive care (BSC) (5). The American Society of Clinical Oncology (ASCO) supports the use of a platinum or non-platinum doublet as initial therapy for patients with newly diagnosed advanced-stage NSCLC who have a good performance status (PS) (6). More recently, targeted agents including bevacizumab and cetuximab have been shown to enhance chemotherapy, and epidermal growth factor receptor tyrosine kinase inhibitors (EGFR-TKIs) may be an alternative to first-line chemotherapy in a select group of patients with mutations in the EGFR gene (7). This chapter reviews the current data on the treatment of stage IIIB and IV NSCLC.

■ STAGE IIIB—A COMBINED MODALITY APPROACH

Patients with stage IIIB NSCLC are generally considered to be nonoperable, and radiation and chemotherapy are the standard treatment approach. Chemotherapy is felt to benefit stage IIIB patients by eradicating distant micrometastases, and improving local control as a radiosensitizer. Based on the high rate of distant metastases, early combined modality trials investigated the use of sequential chemotherapy, in which platinum-based chemotherapy precedes radiotherapy. Multiple randomized clinical trials have shown that combined modality approaches using cisplatin-based chemotherapy improve survival compared with radiotherapy alone in patients with surgically unresectable stage III disease (5,8,9). A meta-analysis of studies comparing cisplatin-containing induction therapy versus radiation alone showed a trend for longer survival for combination therapy, but the differences at 3 and 5 years were not significant (10).

More recently, both the Radiation Therapy Oncology Group (RTOG) and the West Japan Lung Cancer Group (WJLCG) have conducted trials directly comparing sequential and concurrent chemoradiotherapy regimens and have found improved survival with the concurrent approach (11,12). The RTOG trial involved 610 patients and compared induction versus concurrent cisplatin (100 mg/m^2) and vinblastine (5 mg/m^2). A third arm involved hyperfractionated (69.6 Gy) radiation with concurrent cisplatin and oral etoposide. The concurrent chemoradiation arms were superior to the sequential chemoradiotherapy in terms of median survival (17.0 months vs. 14.6 months, $P = 0.038$), but the hyperfractionated approach led to increased toxicity without an additional survival benefit (12). The WJLCG trial compared identical chemotherapy regimens (cisplatin 80 mg/m^2, vindesine 3 mg/m^2, and mitomycin 8 mg/m^2) given sequentially versus concurrently with 56 Gy of thoracic radiation. Approximately 80% of the patients in both arms received the planned treatment, and median survival was superior in the concurrent chemoradiotherapy arm (16.6 months vs. 13.3 months, $P < 0.04$) (11). A later phase III trial compared the WJLCG regimen of cisplatin, vindesine, and mitomycin with the third-generation regimen of cisplatin and docetaxel (40 mg/m^2 weekly for both) given concurrently with radiation and found that overall survival (OS) was superior with the cisplatin/docetaxel regimen. However, progression-free survival (PFS) was the same in each arm, suggesting that the older regimen may be associated with increased late toxicity (13). New chemoradiation regimens, including the combination of pemetrexed with cisplatin or carboplatin in full doses and the addition of cetuximab or bevacizumab to a platinum doublet, are being further explored in ongoing clinical trials. Cancer and Leukemia Group B (CALGB) 30407 is a phase II study currently underway in which patients with locally advanced unresectable NSCLC receive pemetrexed, carboplatin, and thoracic radiation with or without cetuximab. The treatment combination with cetuximab was found to be both feasible and fairly well tolerated, although preliminary results suggest that the addition of cetuximab does not appear to confer additional benefit as the cetuximab arm was noted to have PFS of 10.3 months (compared with 12.9 months) and median survival of 18.7 months (compared with 22.3 months) (14).

In an attempt to further reduce both the rate of local recurrence and distant metastases, the role of consolidation chemotherapy after combined chemoradiation has also been studied. In the Southwest Oncology Group (SWOG) 9019 trial, patients were treated with concurrent cisplatin, etoposide, and radiation followed by an additional two cycles of cisplatin/etoposide and were noted to have a median survival of 15 months and 3-year survival of 17% (15). The phase II SWOG 9504 trial treated patients with the identical SWOG 9019 concurrent cisplatin/etoposide/radiation regimen followed by three cycles of docetaxel instead of the additional cisplatin/etoposide (cisplatin 50 mg/m^2, d1 & 8 plus etoposide 50 mg/m^2 day 1–5, every 28 days for two cycles with concurrent thoracic radiation, 1.8–2 Gy fractions/day, total dose 61 Gy, followed by three cycles of docetaxel 75 mg/m^2). The results compared favorably with a median OS of 27 months and a 3-year survival of 37%, providing a basis for the development of a phase III trial investigating the consolidation approach (16). The Hoosier Oncology Group conducted a phase III trial comparing the concurrent chemotherapy/radiation portion of the SWOG 9019 with or without three

courses of docetaxel consolidation. Results from the phase III trial were not confirmatory, with no significant differences in OS seen between the two arms (median survival 21.6 months for consolidation docetaxel vs. 24.2 months for observation) (17). In addition, 28.8% of patients were hospitalized during treatment with docetaxel versus 8.1% on the observation arm, with a 5.5% treatment-related mortality observed in the docetaxel-treated patients. Thus significant controversy remains about the role of consolidation chemotherapy.

Building on the S9504 approach and the promising efficacy and mild toxicity associated with gefitinib, a maintenance/consolidation trial for stage III disease following definitive treatment per the S9504 regimen was developed by SWOG at the same time that the Hoosier Oncology Group trial was ongoing. In the phase III SWOG 0023 trial, patients who had received the SWOG 9504 core regimen without evidence of progression were randomized to receive gefitinib 250 mg per day or placebo until disease progression or intolerable toxicity, or for 5 years. Median survival for the gefitinib arm (n = 118) was 23 months compared with 35 months for the placebo arm (n = 125) ($P = 0.013$), indicating that gefitinib did not improve survival in the maintenance/consolidation setting in an unselected patient population (18). Additional cooperative group trials are underway in patients with locally advanced stage IIIA/B disease, including RTOG 0617, which is a randomized phase III trial evaluating standard-dose (60 Gy) versus high-dose (74 Gy) conformal radiotherapy with concurrent and consolidation carboplatin/paclitaxel with or without the addition of cetuximab (19).

Induction chemotherapy prior to chemoradiation has also been studied as a potential way to improve survival in patients with unresectable stage III disease. In the phase III CALGB 39801 trial, patients were randomized to receive either immediate chemoradiation (with carboplatin area under the curve [AUC] of 2 and paclitaxel 50 mg/m^2 each given weekly during 66 Gy chest XRT) or to receive two cycles of carboplatin AUC 6 and paclitaxel 200 mg/m^2 given every 21 days × two cycles followed by identical chemoradiation. Although the addition of induction chemotherapy to immediate concurrent chemoradiation was associated with a nonstatistically significant ($P = 0.154$) increase in median survival of 2.6 months, the median survival achieved in each of the treatment groups was low compared with other recent experiences in the literature for unclear reasons, though the chemotherapy agents used and the treatment schedule have been questioned. Given that these findings were not sufficient to reject the null hypothesis of no treatment difference between the two study arms, the final results did not support the use of induction chemotherapy followed by chemoradiation (20).

Concurrent chemotherapy and radiation is the standard of care for stage IIIB NSCLC. At this time, however, there is no consensus on the use of induction or consolidation chemotherapy, or on which chemotherapeutic agents to use. Many feel strongly about the need for full-dose chemotherapy during radiation as given in the SWOG cisplatin/etoposide and CALGB carboplatin/pemetrexed regimens, but not in the weekly carboplatin/paclitaxel regimens utilized in RTOG and other protocols. Others believe that two cycles of chemotherapy is inadequate and therefore consolidation chemotherapy remains critical. Ongoing studies will hopefully provide further answers to these questions as well as data on newer targeted agents and improved ways to individually tailor therapy.

Chemotherapy Doublets

Patients with metastatic NSCLC treated with BSC alone are noted to have a median survival of 4 to 5 months and 1-year survival rate of approximately 10% (21,22). Although it was long felt that chemotherapy did not benefit this subset of patients, a landmark meta-analysis in 1995 demonstrated a 1.5-month increase in median survival and 10% improvement in 1-year survival in patients with metastatic NSCLC treated with cisplatin-based chemotherapy (5). Subsequently, it was found that multiple doublet chemotherapy regimens, platinum-containing or not, conferred a survival advantage and improvement in QOL, with no significant difference in efficacy between the various doublets. The Eastern Cooperative Oncology Group (ECOG) E1594 phase 3 trial specifically compared four different platinum doublets, including paclitaxel/cisplatin, gemcitabine/cisplatin, docetaxel/cisplatin, and carboplatin/paclitaxel and found no differences in response rates (RR) or OS between the various doublet regimens (23). Based on the improved toxicity profile noted in multiple clinical trials, carboplatin/paclitaxel has become a widely adopted standard regimen in the United States (24–26).

Multiple phase III randomized trials have demonstrated that nonplatinum doublets can also be considered in the first-line setting, especially in those patients unable to tolerate platinum agents. The most common nonplatinum doublets consist of gemcitabine with a taxane. Alpha Oncology conducted a trial of 800 patients treated with either gemcitabine/carboplatin, gemcitabine/paclitaxel, or paclitaxel/carboplatin, and found no significant difference in efficacy between these regimens with a median survival time of approximately 8 months (27). Although a platinum doublet remains the standard, nonplatinum doublets can certainly be considered without hesitation when use of a platinum agent is prohibited.

Recently, there have been two phase III trials that have included pemetrexed as part of an initial platinum doublet in NSCLC. In both trials, pemetrexed/platinum was compared with gemcitabine/platinum with no difference in RRs or survival seen between arms overall, but with significantly decreased hematologic toxicity with pemetrexed

(28,29). As a result, pemetrexed/platinum has now emerged as an alternative choice for first-line therapy. Notably, a striking survival advantage on the pemetrexed arms was noted in both studies for patients with nonsquamous histology, and the drug is only approved in such patients. This survival difference may have to do with differential expression of thymidylate synthetase (TS). High levels of TS are associated with pemetrexed resistance and are more common in tumors of squamous cell histology (30).

Even after the decision to use a platinum doublet is made, the choice of platinum agent remains an area of controversy. The CISCA meta-analysis pooled nine trials for a total of 2,968 patients treated with a cytotoxic agent paired with either cisplatin or carboplatin (31). RRs were significantly higher with cisplatin-containing regimens (30% vs. 24%, $P < 0.001$) but OS was not (hazard ratio [HR] of death with carboplatin 1.07, 95% confidence interval [CI] 0.99–1.15, $P = 0.1$). Overall, only one of the trials favored carboplatin, and this trial was an outlier in terms of patient demographics and paired chemotherapy agent used. When the meta-analysis is done excluding this one trial, the OS HR improves to 1.11, 95% CI 1.01 to 1.21, favoring cisplatin. Although cisplatin was favored in OS, carboplatin was favored in toxicity profile. A subsequent meta-analysis also demonstrated improved RRs with cisplatin, but there was no corresponding significant survival benefit (32). Based on this data, it appears that cisplatin most likely has increased efficacy over carboplatin, but at a cost of increased toxicity, which must be carefully weighed for each individual patient.

■ DURATION OF THERAPY

The optimal duration of therapy remains unknown and many studies have explored the role of administering additional chemotherapy in an attempt to improve upon the outcomes of standard first-line treatment for advanced non–small cell lung cancer. Several randomized trials have demonstrated that extending first-line platinum-based chemotherapy beyond four cycles is associated with no survival benefit, but with added toxicity such as neuropathy (33). Based on the results of these studies, the current paradigm limits first-line chemotherapy to four to six cycles of a platinum doublet (6). Many studies have explored ways to administer additional chemotherapy after first-line treatment in order to provide an additional survival benefit without significant added toxicities (Table 15.1). For the purposes of this review, sequential/maintenance therapy refers to extending chemotherapy using a non–cross-reacting agent(s) for a defined number of cycles; alternating chemotherapy is the alternating administration of non–cross-resistant drugs for a defined number of cycles or until disease progression; and

■ **Table 15.1** Sequential and maintenance chemotherapy trials			
Study	**No. of Patients**	**Treatment**	**OS**
Smith et al. (34)	308	Mitomycin + vinblastine + cisplatin × 3 vs. 6 cycles	6 (× 3) vs. 7 months (× 6)
Socinski et al. (33)	230	Carboplatin + paclitaxel × 4 cycles vs. continuous until disease progression	6.6 vs. 8.5 mos; $P = 0.63$
Belani et al. (35)	130	Carboplatin + paclitaxel × 3 cycles → weekly paclitaxel vs. observation	60 weeks (observation) vs. 75 weeks (weekly paclitaxel)
Westeel et al. (36)	181	Mitomycin + ifosfamide + cisplatin × 4 cycles → vinorelbine × 6 mos vs. observation	No difference
Von Plessen et al. (37)	297	Carboplatin + vinorelbine × 3 vs. 6 cycles	28 (× 3) vs. 32 weeks (× 6); $P = 0.75$
Brodowicz et al. (38)	206	Carboplatin + gemcitabine × 4 cycles → gemcitabine vs. BSC	13 (Gem) vs. 11 months (BSC)
Park et al. (39)	314	Cisplatin + docetaxel OR cisplatin + paclitaxel OR cisplatin + gemcitabine × 4 vs. 6 cycles	No difference
Fidias et al. (40)	309	Carboplatin + gemcitabine × 4 cycles → immediate docetaxel vs. carboplatin + gemcitabine × 4 cycles → delayed docetaxel (at time of progression)	12.3 (immediate) vs. 9.7 months (delayed); $P = 0.08$
Belani et al. (41)	663	Platinum doublet × 4 cycles → pemetrexed vs. placebo	10.1 (placebo) vs. 13.0 months (Pem); $P = 0.06$
Cappuzzo et al: SATURN (42)	889	Platinum doublet × 4 cycles → erlotinib vs. placebo	11 months (placebo) vs. 12 months (erlotinib); HR 0.81; $P = 0.0088$
Miller et al: ATLAS (43)	370	Platinum doublet + bevacizumab → bevacizumab + erlotinib	NR
	373	Platinum doublet + bevacizumab → bevacizumab + placebo	

BSC, best supportive care; HR, hazard ratio; OS, overall survival.

extended/maintenance chemotherapy involves the prolongation of first-line chemotherapy with the administration of a drug included in the induction regimen for a defined time or until disease progression.

A meta-analysis that included 27 trials of sequential/maintenance chemotherapy in advanced NSCLC found that sequential/maintenance chemotherapy with a platinum-based doublet followed by a single agent is feasible in patients with good PS (44). A phase III trial conducted by Westeel et al. randomized patients responding to initial chemotherapy with mitomycin, ifosfamide, and cisplatin (MIC) to receive maintenance vinorelbine versus observation alone. Sequential/maintenance therapy did not improve survival, perhaps due to myelotoxicity-related discontinuations of treatment (21% of patients stopped treatment during maintenance vinorelbine) (36). Based upon this finding, and the relatively toxic initial therapy used in this study, subsequent trials focused on using other agents associated with less toxicity in the sequential/maintenance setting. Recently, Fidias et al. conducted a trial in which patients were randomized to receive immediate (sequential/maintenance) versus delayed (at time of progression) second-line treatment with docetaxel. The median PFS

was greater in the immediate docetaxel arm (5.7 mos) versus the delayed docetaxel arm (2.7 mos, $P = 0.0001$). Although not statistically significant, there was a trend toward improved median OS in the immediate docetaxel arm (12.3 mos) versus the delayed docetaxel arm (9.7 mos, $P = 0.0853$) (40). Likely much of the improved OS trend resulted from the fact that more patients were able to receive treatment in the immediate docetaxel arm due to significant symptomatic deterioration by the time patients reached disease progression in the delayed arm, rendering them unable to receive docetaxel therapy. When those actually receiving therapy on both arms were compared, the survival times were nearly identical.

A similar phase III trial randomized patients who completed four cycles of a platinum doublet and had at least stable disease to receive pemetrexed plus BSC versus placebo plus BSC (45). This study differed from the docetaxel trial in that it did not incorporate a delayed pemetrexed arm, and most patients (81%) on the placebo arm never received pemetrexed, though 67% did go on to receive some active second-line agent. Importantly, this study was statistically powered to detect an OS benefit for sequential/maintenance therapy. The study showed a large benefit in PFS (4 months in the pemetrexed arm vs. 2 months in the placebo arm, $P < 0.00001$) and preliminary OS data was also impressive with an HR of 0.79 ($P = 0.012$), again favoring pemetrexed over placebo (41). The survival benefit was more striking in patients with nonsquamous histology, and not significant in those with squamous histology. Based on these results, immediate second-line use of sequential/maintenance pemetrexed is now a Food and Drug Administration (FDA)-approved indication. Ongoing trials are needed to confirm the validity of sequential/maintenance treatment of patients with advanced NSCLC, but the sequential/maintenance approach is now a reasonable option for many patients who do not desire a chemotherapy holiday after completing four to six cycles of a platinum doublet. This is especially true for patients for whom there is concern of rapid disease progression. Similar work with the EGFR-TKI drug erlotinib has also been promising and will be presented later in this chapter. ECOG will be opening a randomized phase III trial looking at sequential/maintenance therapy with pemetrexed in two arms of a phase III trial (carboplatin/paclitaxel/bevacizumab for four cycles then randomization to pemetrexed vs. bevacizumab vs. both agents, E5508).

Various other trials have investigated the role of true maintenance (extended) chemotherapy in advanced NSCLC, that is, continuation of one of the first-line agents. In an underpowered phase II trial, patients who achieved at least a partial response after three cycles of carboplatin and paclitaxel were randomized to weekly paclitaxel versus observation, and those on the weekly chemotherapy extended/maintenance had a nonsignificant improvement in time to progression (TTP) (29 weeks vs. 38 weeks) and median survival (60 weeks vs. 75 weeks) compared with the observation arm (35). In a phase III trial by Brodowicz et al. (38), patients without progressive disease after initial therapy with carboplatin and gemcitabine were randomized to receive extended/maintenance therapy with gemcitabine plus BSC or BSC alone. There was a significant benefit seen in the extended/maintenance gemcitabine arm as compared with the BSC arm in terms of time to progressive disease (6.6 months vs. 5.0 months, $P < 0.001$), although the benefit in median survival (13.0 months vs. 11.0 months, $P = 0.195$) was not found to be statistically significant. Importantly, there was no negative impact on patient's individual QOL in the extended/maintenance gemcitabine arm. These results are consistent with retrospective analyses which showed that gemcitabine maintenance may delay patient-reported worsening of symptoms and suggested a strong correlation between time to worsening of symptoms and TTP (46).

The idea of extended/maintenance chemotherapy was utilized in a promising nonrandomized phase II trial in which patients received carboplatin/pemetrexed/bevacizumab for four cycles, then continued on pemetrexed/

bevacizumab until the time of progression (47). The median survival on this study was 14 months, and a phase III trial utilizing this regimen is ongoing. Finally, a recent meta-analysis involving 13 trials of sequential/maintenance and extended/maintenance chemotherapy showed that extending chemotherapy beyond a standard number of cycles was associated with a significant improvement in PFS and modest, yet statistically significant, improvement in OS (48). However this benefit was at the cost of increased adverse events and possible impairments in health-related QOL, emphasizing the need to weigh the overall benefits of chemotherapy against toxicity, inconvenience, and cost (49). The targeted agents bevacizumab and cetuximab were both developed utilizing an extended/maintenance approach, to be discussed later in this chapter.

Alternating chemotherapy has also been explored since the 1980s, as it was felt to avoid or limit cumulative toxicity seen with concomitant administration of the same drug combination. A Japanese trial compared three arms of treatment: vindesine and cisplatin (VP) versus mitomycin, vindesine, and cisplatin (MVP) versus etoposide and cisplatin alternating with vindesine and mitomycin (EP/VM) (50). The EP/VM arm had a significantly lower RR compared with the MVP arm (19% vs. 43%, $P < 0.01$). However, in further comparing the three arms of treatment, there were no significant differences in OS or toxicity, other than grade 3 to 4 thrombocytopenia which was higher in the MVP arm compared with the VP arm (22% vs. 5%, $P < 0.01$). A phase III trial conducted by Eagan et al. compared two arms of treatment: in the first arm, patients received alternating administration of cyclophosphamide, doxorubicin, and cisplatin (CAP) and mitomycin, lomustine, and methotrexate (MCM), up to the time of progression, while in the second arm, patients received CAP followed by MCM on progression (second-line MCM). There were no statistically significant differences in RR (39% in both arms), TTP (2.1 vs. 4.4 months), or OS (5.5 vs. 6.9 months) between the two treatment arms (51). More recently, alternating chemotherapy trials including third-generation agents have been conducted. Pérol et al. (52) evaluated a treatment alternating docetaxel with cisplatin plus vinorelbine in a phase II trial. The control arm of this noncomparative trial was cisplatin plus vinorelbine. The alternating chemotherapy arm did worse compared with the control arm displayed in terms of RR (10.8% vs. 25%), time to treatment failure (10.2 weeks vs. 17.3 weeks), and median survival (29.1 weeks vs. 39 weeks). Despite similar toxicities between the two arms, early treatment discontinuation as a result of toxicity was more frequent in the alternating arm (23.7% vs. 9.7%). Given these disappointing results, further evaluation of this regimen in a phase III trial was not pursued.

Alternating chemotherapy has also been studied with the administration of single-agent chemotherapy in three different phase II trials. Mattson et al. (53) investigated an alternating regimen of docetaxel and cisplatin at full doses, while Aguiar and colleagues studied a platinum-free regimen consisting of alternating weekly administration of paclitaxel and gemcitabine (54). Gridelli et al. (55) compared an alternating regimen of pemetrexed and gemcitabine with single-agent pemetrexed in a randomized study of elderly or poor PS patients. Preliminary data from these trials indicate feasibility of these regimens with RRs, toxicity, and survival comparing favorably with platinum-based chemotherapy, although additional confirmatory trials are required. Based on the trials of alternating chemotherapy published so far in the literature, it seems unlikely that an alternating chemotherapy regimen will prove superior to combination chemotherapy in advanced NSCLC patients with a good PS. In elderly or poor PS patients, alternating single-agent chemotherapy may prove to be an appropriate option pending further evaluation in phase III trials.

Molecular-Targeted Agents

While traditional chemotherapy targets some aspect of the DNA machinery, the newer "targeted" agents focus on other aspects of the biology of the cancer cell that distinguish them from normal tissues. There have been multiple trials combining platinum doublets with newer targeted agents in advanced NSCLC, the majority of which until recently were very disappointing (Table 15.2). In October 2006, however, bevacizumab became the first targeted agent to be approved by the U.S. Food and Drug Administration for use in combination with first-line chemotherapy in patients with advanced NSCLC. Approval was based on the ECOG 4599 phase III trial that studied carboplatin/paclitaxel with or without the anti–vascular endothelial growth factor (VEGF) monoclonal antibody bevacizumab in patients with recurrent or advanced NSCLC. Compared with the 392 patients receiving chemotherapy alone, the 381 patients receiving bevacizumab had a significantly higher RR (35% vs. 15%; $P < 0.001$), median PFS (6.2 months vs. 4.5 months; $P < 0.001$), and median OS (12.3 months vs. 10.3 months; $P = 0.003$) (56). However, the addition of bevacizumab to carboplatin/paclitaxel was associated with more treatment-related deaths, with 15 deaths in the bevacizumab arm (five due to pulmonary hemorrhage) versus two deaths in the chemotherapy-alone arm. Pulmonary hemorrhage occurred in patients treated with bevacizumab despite the fact that this study excluded patients felt to be at highest risk of

■ Table 15.2 Randomized phase III trials of targeted agents

Study	No. of Patients	Patient Selection	Treatment	RR	PFS	OS
Sandler et al. (56)	433	Unselected	Carboplatin/ paclitaxel	15% (n = 392)	4.5 months	10.3 months
	417		Bevacizumab/ carboplatin/ paclitaxel	35% (n = 381); $P < 0.0001$	6.2 months; $P < 0.001$	12.3 months; $P = 0.003$
Reck et al. (57)	345	Unselected	Cisplatin/ gemcitabine/ bevacizumab 7.5 mg/kg	34% (n = 332)	6.7 months; HR 0.75; $P = 0.0026$	13.6 months; HR 0.92 (95% CI 0.77–1.10)
	351		Cisplatin/ gemcitabine/ bevacizumab 15 mg/kg	30% (n = 332); $P = 0.002$	6.5 months; HR 0.82; $P = 0.0301$	13.4 months; HR 1.02 (95% CI 0.85–1.22)
Lynch et al. (58)	338	Unselected	Carboplatin/ taxane	17%	4.24 months	8.4 months
	338		Cetuximab/ carboplatin/ taxane	26% $P = 0.0066$	4.40 months; HR 0.902; $P = 0.2358$	9.7 months; HR 0.89; $P = 0.17$
Pirker et al. (59)	568	Unselected	Cisplatin/ vinorelbine	29%	4.8 months	10.1 months
	557		Cisplatin/ vinorelbine/ cetuximab	36%; $P = 0.012$	4.8 months	11.3 months
Mok et al. (7)	608	EGFR mutation	Carboplatin/ paclitaxel	47.3% (n = 61)		
	609		Gefitinib	71.2% (n = 94); $P < 0.001$	HR 0.48; $P < 0.001$	HR 0.78 (95% CI 0.50–1.20)

CI, confidence interval; EGFR, epidermal growth factor receptor; HR, hazard ratio; OS, overall survival; PFS, progression-free survival; RR, response rate.

bleeding, including patients with squamous cell histology, anticoagulant use, and a history of gross hemoptysis.

Another phase III trial, the Avastin in Lung Cancer (AVAiL) trial, evaluated cisplatin/gemcitabine (CG) with or without bevacizumab (57). A total of 1,043 patients were randomized to receive either placebo or bevacizumab 7.5 or 15 mg/kg every 3 weeks. Compared with placebo, an improvement in PFS was seen with the addition of bevacizumab at 7.5 mg/kg (HR 0.75; $P = 0.0026$) and 15 mg/kg (HR = 0.82; $P = 0.0301$), but no OS benefit was seen with bevacizumab at either dose (57). Serious adverse events were similar in the placebo plus CG and 7.5 mg/kg bevacizumab plus CG arms (35% in each arm), although were higher in the 15 mg/kg bevacizumab plus CG arm (44%). Encouragingly, there was no increase in arterial thrombotic events or venous thromboembolic events detected in patients receiving either dose of bevacizumab compared with placebo. Moreover, therapeutic anticoagulation was not found to increase bleeding risk in the patients receiving bevacizumab. The safety of bevacizumab in combination with other chemotherapy regimens (including carboplatin/gemcitabine and carboplatin/docetaxel) has recently been analyzed with the inclusion of patients with previously treated brain metastases and those who were on low molecular weight heparin or warfarin. Preliminary findings indicate that there have been no unexpected safety events, with a similar safety profile noted between the different chemotherapy combinations (60).

EGFR is another promising therapeutic target in NSCLC. Cetuximab is a monoclonal antibody (MoAb) to EGFR that has already been approved by the U.S. Food and Drug Administration for patients with refractory colon cancer and locally advanced head and neck cancer and recently has shown promising results in combination with chemotherapy in the first-line setting for patients with advanced NSCLC (61,62). BMS-099 randomized 338 patients to receive cetuximab/carboplatin/taxane and compared them with 338 patients receiving carboplatin/taxane alone (58). The Independent Radiologic Review Committee (IRRC) did not detect significant improvement in median PFS, although they did find improved RRs in the cetuximab-containing arm (26% vs. 17%, $P = 0.0066$). However, due to a discrepancy between IRCC and investigator assessment of PFS, the difference in RR could not be considered significant. The study showed a trend in OS favoring the cetuximab arm, but this failed to reach statistical significance. More recently, the phase III FLEX trial showed that the combination of cisplatin/vinorelbine and cetuximab was better than cisplatin/vinorelbine alone, with improvement in overall RRs (36% vs. 29%, $P = 0.010$) and OS (HR = 0.871, $P = 0.044$), though not in PFS (59). Based on these findings, cetuximab added to platinum-based chemotherapy may be considered an option as first-line chemotherapy for patients with EGFR-expressing NSCLC, but FDA approval is pending at this time.

Other targeted agents, including EGFR receptor TKIs, are also being investigated in combination with first-line chemotherapy doublets in advanced NSCLC. Erlotinib, an anti-EGFR TKI, when added to first-line chemotherapy in two separate trials was found not to show improvement in RR or OS compared with chemotherapy alone (63,64). However, a subset of patients, particularly those with no smoking history and Asians, seem to be particularly sensitive to the EGFR-TKIs. This finding led to the Iressa-Pan Asian Study (IPASS) which randomized selected patients (Asian never-smokers with advanced-stage adenocarcinomas) to receive gefitinib alone versus carboplatin/paclitaxel in the first-line setting. Superior PFS was demonstrated in patients receiving gefitinib (HR = 0.74, $P < 0.0001$); however, the curves cross in an interesting fashion and the PFS benefit with gefitinib is most pronounced in those patients with EGFR-mutation-positive tumors (HR = 0.48, $P < 0.0001$), whereas those without the mutation do significantly better with chemotherapy as first-line treatment. Similarly, while the OS was similar between the two groups in the overall population, analysis of OS according to mutation status revealed a HR of 0.78 (95% CI, 0.50–1.20) with gefitinib in the mutation-positive subgroup and a HR of 1.38 (95% CI, 0.92–2.09) in the mutation-negative subgroup (7). These results propose a potential paradigm shift in the approach to first-line treatment of patients with advanced NSCLC who harbor EGFR-activating mutations. This data also underscores the importance of performing EGFR mutational analyses before recommending first-line therapy with an EGFR-TKI. Additional trials with very similar results were conducted in Japan (65) and Korea (66) and are ongoing in Western populations to validate these results (67). Furthermore, there are clinical trials that are currently specifically recruiting patients with known EGFR mutations, including a study comparing erlotinib versus gemcitabine/carboplatin (68) as well as another investigating the novel agent BIBW 2992 (69) as first-line therapy in this special patient population.

The anti-VEGF TKIs are also being studied for use in the first-line setting. Cediranib (AZD2171) is an agent that targets multiple receptors including VEGFR-1, VEGFR-2, VEGFR-3, platelet derived growth factor receptor (PDGFR), and c-kit and has been found to be active in patients with advanced NSCLC in combination with standard first-line chemotherapy (70). The BR.24 phase II/III trial of carboplatin/paclitaxel with or without the addition of cediranib reported an increased RR of 38% versus 16%, as well as a trend for improved survival with the combination (HR = 0.78, $P = 0.11$) (71). However, increased toxicities were noted in this trial with cediranib being given at a dose of 30 mg, thereby leading to the similarly designed and ongoing BR.29 trial which investigates cediranib at the reduced dose of 20 mg. Sorafenib, another anti-VEGF TKI, inhibits RAF, VEGFR-1, VEGFR-2,

VEGFR-3, PDGFR-b, Flt-3, c-kit, and p38-a. A phase III trial that randomized patients with advanced NSCLC to receive carboplatin/paclitaxel with or without sorafenib failed to show a survival improvement and further demonstrated increased toxicities in patients receiving sorafenib, particularly in those with squamous histology (72). A similar phase III trial (NEXUS) was initiated and restricted to patients with nonsquamous histology, randomizing them to receive cisplatin/gemcitabine with or without sorafenib. Patient accrual was completed in February 2009 with results still pending at this time (73). Other investigations with the VEGFR-TKIs are ongoing in later stages of therapy.

Ongoing phase III trials are investigating the approach of using targeted agents in sequential/maintenance therapy of NSCLC. The SATURN study randomized patients who had completed four cycles of a platinum doublet without disease progression to receive erlotinib versus placebo until evidence of disease progression. Preliminary results indicate improved PFS in those patients receiving erlotinib maintenance therapy (HR = 0.71, $P < 0.0001$), which not surprisingly, is especially pronounced in those patients with positive EGFR-mutation status (HR = 0.10, $P < 0.0001$) (42). The ATLAS trial compares bevacizumab with or without erlotinib given after the completion of first-line treatment with chemotherapy plus bevacizumab for four cycles. In this case, PFS favors the bevacizumab plus erlotinib maintenance arm compared with the bevacizumab alone arm (HR = 0.72, $P = 0.001$) (43). However, the benefit in PFS was seen in the context of more grade 3 to 5 toxicities noted in the bevacizumab plus erlotinib arm (46.3% vs. 31.5%). An OS benefit was seen in both trials, though as both were randomized placebo-controlled studies, patients on the placebo arm did not necessarily go on to receive erlotinib as delayed therapy. As the treatment of advanced NSCLC continues to evolve particularly with the use of newer targeted agents, important phase III trials continue to be underway exploring various combination treatments to further improve both survival and QOL (Table 15.3).

■ **Table 15.3** Selected ongoing phase III trials of first-line treatment in non–small cell lung cancer

Trial	Treatment
EORTC-BREC	*Customized* chemotherapy to BRCA1
WJTOG 3605	Carboplatin/paclitaxel vs. carboplatin/S-1
NCIC BR.29	Carboplatin/paclitaxel ± cediranib (20 mg)
SYRINGES	Cisplatin + docetaxel ± enoxaparin
IFCT-GFPC 05.02	Observation vs. gemcitabine vs. erlotinib

■ SPECIAL PATIENT CONSIDERATIONS

Lung cancer remains primarily a disease of the elderly, with a median age at diagnosis of 68 years (74). When choosing a particular chemotherapeutic regimen, it is important to consider the toxicity profile of the agent, pharmacokinetics, organ function, as well as patient comorbidities and preferences. ASCO currently recommends first-line single-agent therapy for elderly patients, but this is not a universally accepted approach (6). The Elderly Lung Cancer Vinorelbine Italian Study Group conducted one of the first randomized clinical trials designed specifically for elderly patients with advanced NSCLC, comparing single-agent vinorelbine with BSC in patients 70 years of age or older (75). Treatment with vinorelbine improved median survival as compared with BSC (28 weeks vs. 21 weeks). Subsequently, the Multicenter Italian Lung Cancer in the Elderly Study (MILES) found that the combination of vinorelbine plus gemcitabine was not more effective than single-agent vinorelbine or gemcitabine in the treatment of elderly patients (76). Retrospective analyses of many cooperative-group phase III studies have shown that patients aged 70 years and older exhibit similar survival and QOL benefits to younger patients, thereby leading to the recommendation that platinum-based chemotherapy remains an appropriate treatment option for elderly patients with good PS (23,26,77,78). In addition, trials using targeted agents are being specifically evaluated in the elderly population, given the potential advantages of reduced toxicity and improved tolerability compared with standard therapies. Both erlotinib and sorafenib, a small molecule inhibitor of PDGFR and VEGF, are being investigated in older patients (79). The question of the use of bevacizumab in the elderly was raised by the ECOG 4599 trial, which found increased toxicity and no OS advantage in patients older than 70 years treated in the bevacizumab/chemotherapy arm compared with the chemotherapy-alone arm in a retrospective subgroup analysis (80).

Patients with poor PS, many of whom are also elderly, are also being specifically evaluated in clinical trials. The ECOG 1594 study reported poor median OS with doublet chemotherapy in patients with a PS of 2 compared with those with a PS of 0 (3.9 months vs. 10.8 months, $P < 0.001$), which led to exclusion of PS2 patients into the majority of the trial after an earlier interim look revealed the survival discrepancy (23). Interestingly, the poor outcomes noted in the patients with advanced PS was felt more to be related to the underlying disease process, rather than to increased treatment-related toxicities (81). Similar to the recommendation made for elderly patients, ASCO recommends that patients with a poor PS be treated with single-agent chemotherapy instead of doublet chemotherapy (6). A European Expert Panel, however, concludes that either single agents or doublet chemotherapy may be appropriate options (82). A recent study by Lilenbaum et al. (83) also concluded that patients with PS2 treated with first-line combination chemotherapy had a higher RR and longer TTP compared with those who received single-agent therapy, although OS did not appear significantly different.

Differential survival between men and women, with an advantage for women, has been found in multiple trials for all stages of NSCLC (84,85). More recently, in a subset analysis of the ECOG 1594 trial, women were found to have an improved median OS of approximately 2 months compared with men, and were also noted to have an increased rate of toxicity (86). There have also been differences in therapeutic outcomes noted among women treated with newer targeted agents, specifically with EGFR-TKIs.

In addition to sex differences in survival, there is emerging evidence for age/sex interactions and the role of estrogen in NSCLC. The presence of the estrogen receptor (ER) in lung tumor tissue is well established and suggests a role for estrogen signaling in the pathogenesis of NSCLC (87,88). High serum estradiol levels have been associated with worse survival among women with advanced NSCLC (89,90). The randomized Women's Health Initiative trial showed that the combined estrogen and progestin was found to significantly increase lung cancer mortality in postmenopausal women (91). A multivariate analysis of six recent trials including a total of 1,334 patients with advanced-stage NSCLC showed that older women (>60 years old) had a survival advantage compared with younger women, suggesting that differences in levels of estrogen and progesterone could be a potential explanation for these survival differences (92). These findings have led to efforts to further elucidate the underlying mechanisms associated with ER and lung carcinogenesis and to develop clinical trials targeting ERs in the treatment of NSCLC. Recently, the enhanced antitumor effect seen in the combined targeting of ER and EGFR (93) has led to the ongoing phase II trial of erlotinib/fulvestrant versus erlotinib alone in patients with advanced NSCLC (94).

■ FUTURE DIRECTIONS

Selecting treatment based upon an individual patient's molecular profile is an active area of research. Increasingly, clinicians are able to preselect patients who are felt to benefit from EGFR-TKI therapy based on EGFR mutation status. The IPASS trial specifically targeted chemo-naïve Asian females who are never- or light-smokers with adenocarcinoma to receive gefitinib, and demonstrated that the EGFR mutation status was the critical variable in deciding who to consider treating with first-line EGFR-TKI therapy (7). Histology is also proving to be important in predicting response to specific chemotherapeutic agents. A recent randomized phase III trial comparing the

OS between cisplatin/gemcitabine versus cisplatin/pemetrexed in chemotherapy-naïve patients with advanced NSCLC found that patients with adenocarcinoma had a significantly improved OS with cisplatin/pemetrexed compared with cisplatin/gemcitabine (HR 0.81, P = 0.03) (28). In addition, those patients with squamous histology displayed a trend toward improvement in OS with cisplatin/gemcitabine versus cisplatin/pemetrexed (10.8 months vs. 9.4 months, P = 0.05). These differences may be related to levels of TS and additional work is ongoing to determine whether TS levels or histology would be a better predictor of response to pemetrexed (30).

Other molecular markers are being identified to correlate with response to chemotherapy and survival. Excision repair cross-complementing gene 1 (ERCC1) is a DNA damage repair gene that plays a critical role in the repair of cisplatin damage to DNA. Lord et al. (95) evaluated ERCC1 expression in 56 patients with advanced NSCLC treated with gemcitabine and cisplatin and found that median OS was significantly longer in patients with low ERCC1 expression compared with patients with high expression (61.6 weeks vs. 20.4 weeks, P = 0.046). These findings led to a phase III trial that randomized patients to a control or genotypic arm. Patients in the control arm received cisplatin/docetaxel while patients in the genotypic arm were treated according to ERCC1 levels and received cisplatin/docetaxel if ERCC1 levels were low, or gemcitabine/docetaxel if ERCC1 levels were high. Out of a total 346 evaluable patients, those in the genotypic arm had a significantly higher RR compared with the control arm (51% vs. 39%, P = 0.02) (96). This study provided additional evidence that ERCC1 is a reliable biomarker for cisplatin sensitivity.

Similarly, ribonucleotide reductase M subunit 1 (RRM1) is an enzyme involved in DNA synthesis and is a molecular target of gemcitabine. A phase II trial confirming in vitro data found that tumoral levels of RRM1 expression were inversely correlated with magnitude of tumor shrinkage in patients treated with gemcitabine (97). In addition, RRM1 expression was found to correlate with expression of ERCC1, and high expression of both RRM1 and ERCC1 was found to be associated with a significant survival advantage (98). Recently, another phase II trial was designed to assess the feasibility and efficacy of a customized treatment approach utilizing ERCC1 and RRM1 mRNA expression levels obtained from tumor specimens of 53 patients. The molecular-analysis directed individual treatment (MADeIT) algorithm divided patients into four gene expression groups. Patients with low levels of both ERCC1 and RRM1 received carboplatin/gemcitabine, those with low RRM1 and high ERCC1 received gemcitabine/docetaxel, those with high RRM1 and low ERCC1 received docetaxel/carboplatin, and those with high RRM1 and high ERCC1 received vinorelbine/docetaxel. The RR was 42%, with overall and PFS noted to be 52% and 14% at 12 months, respectively (99). These encouraging results have led to a randomized phase III trial that is underway, comparing the customized approach with the standard arm of carboplatin/gemcitabine (100). Finally, Rosell and colleagues have proposed another gene expression signature, *BRCA1*, as a novel prognostic factor in resected stage IB–IIB NSCLC. They found that overexpression of *BRCA1* mRNA in resected specimens was strongly associated with poor survival, thereby suggesting that patients whose tumors have high *BRCA1* expression should be candidates for adjuvant chemotherapy (101). Prior studies have found that the absence of *BRCA1* results in high sensitivity to cisplatin, whereas its presence increases sensitivity to antimicrotubule agents (102). These findings have led to the ongoing BREC trial which is a multicenter, prospective phase III randomized pharmacogenetic study to evaluate treatment customized according to *BRCA1* assessment in patients with advanced NSCLC (103).

Another attractive and less conventional therapeutic approach involves immunotherapy in which strategies are being developed to harness the immune system to fight against the cancer. To date, more than 600 patients with lung cancer have been treated in over 25 pilot, phase I, or early phase II studies using 17 different vaccines, indicating that immunotherapy for lung cancer is both feasible and rational (104). Although many of the vaccine trials to date have been disappointing, there have been some promising results to warrant further investigation. A UK-based pharmaceutical company sponsored a phase III, nonplacebo-controlled trial in which 419 patients with stage III/IV NSCLC were randomized 1:1 to receive monthly injections of a heat-killed *Mycobacterium vaccae* (SRL 172) administered concurrently with six cycles of chemotherapy delivered on a 21-day schedule (105). Unfortunately, fewer than 50% of the subjects completed the prescribed series of vaccines, limiting the statistical power of the trial. However, the analysis based upon all of the patients who received the SRL 172 vaccine indicated that SRL 172 significantly improved patient QOL without affecting OS (223 days versus 225 days, $P = 0.65$). Interestingly, on further subset analysis, this benefit was only seen in those patients with adenocarcinoma, and was not seen in those with squamous cell cancer. Ongoing efforts are being made to further understand immune regulation in lung cancer in order to develop additional therapeutic options that can be studied and compared in future phase III trials.

■ CONCLUSIONS

- A combined modality approach with the use of concurrent chemoradiotherapy is the preferred treatment for patients with stage IIIB disease.

- A platinum-based doublet remains the standard first-line treatment for physically fit patients with advanced non–small cell lung cancer and no single regimen has stood out as the optimal regimen for all patients.
- The addition of the anti–vascular endothelial growth factor antibody bevacizumab should also be considered in selected patients, namely those with adenocarcinoma and no hemoptysis.
- The anti–epidermal growth factor receptor (EGFR) antibody cetuximab, also shows promise when added to first-line treatment.
- Currently, the oral EGFR–tyrosine kinase inhibitor (TKI) erlotinib is being studied as a first-line option for selected patients, specifically those with EGFR-activating mutations.
- The optimal duration of first-line chemotherapy remains unknown and there is increasing data to suggest a role for sequential or maintenance chemotherapy to delay progression and perhaps impact overall survival.
- Special patient populations, including patients with poor performance status, those who are elderly, and women, have unique considerations that must be taken into account when deciding upon a treatment plan.
- There is an increasing emphasis on tailoring selection of chemotherapy to optimize treatment for individual patients with this disease.

■ REFERENCES

1. Jemal A, Siegel R, Ward E, Hao Y, Xu J, Thun MJ. Cancer statistics, 2009. *CA Cancer J Clin.* 2009;59(4):225–249.
2. Horner MJ, Ries LAG, Krapcho M, et al. SEER Cancer Statistics Review, 1975–2006. Bethesda, MD: National Cancer Institute; 2006.
3. Rami-Porta R, Crowley JJ, Goldstraw P. The revised TNM staging system for lung cancer. *Ann Thorac Cardiovasc Surg.* 2009;15(1):4–9.
4. William WN Jr, Lin HY, Lee JJ, Lippman SM, Roth JA, Kim ES. Revisiting stage IIIB and IV non-small cell lung cancer: analysis of the surveillance, epidemiology, and end results data. *Chest.* 2009;136(3):701–709.
5. Chemotherapy in non-small cell lung cancer: a meta-analysis using updated data on individual patients from 52 randomised clinical trials. Non-small Cell Lung Cancer Collaborative Group. *BMJ* 1995;311(7010):899–909.
6. Pfister DG, Johnson DH, Azzoli CG, et al.; American Society of Clinical Oncology. American Society of Clinical Oncology treatment of unresectable non-small-cell lung cancer guideline: update 2003. *J Clin Oncol.* 2004;22(2):330–353.
7. Mok TS, Wu YL, Thongprasert S, et al. Gefitinib or carboplatin-paclitaxel in pulmonary adenocarcinoma. *N Engl J Med.* 2009;361(10):947–957.
8. Dillman RO, Herndon J, Seagren SL, Eaton WL Jr, Green MR. Improved survival in stage III non-small-cell lung cancer: seven-year follow-up of cancer and leukemia group B (CALGB) 8433 trial. *J Natl Cancer Inst.* 1996;88(17):1210–1215.

9. LeChevalier T, Arrigada R, Quoix E, et al. Radiotherapy alone versus combined chemotherapy and radiotherapy in non-resectable non-small cell lung cancer: first analysis of a randomized trial of 353 patients. *J Natl Cancer Inst.* 1991;83:417–423.

10. Marino P, Preatoni A, Cantoni A. Randomized trials of radiotherapy alone versus combined chemotherapy and radiotherapy in stages IIIa and IIIb nonsmall cell lung cancer. A meta-analysis. *Cancer.* 1995;76(4):593–601.

11. Furuse K, Fukuoka M, Kawahara M, et al. Phase III study of concurrent versus sequential thoracic radiotherapy in combination with mitomycin, vindesine, and cisplatin in unresectable stage III non-small-cell lung cancer. *J Clin Oncol.* 1999;17(9):2692–2699.

12. Curran WJ, Scott CB, Langer CJ, et al. Long-term benefit is observed in a phase III comparison of sequential vs. concurrent chemo-radiation for patients with unresected stage III NSCLC: RTOG 9410 [abstract 2499]. *Proc Am Soc Clin Oncol.* 2003;22.

13. Kiura K, Takigawa N, Segawa Y, et al. Randomized phase III trial of docetaxel and cisplatin combination chemotherapy versus mitomycin, vindesine, and cisplatin combination chemotherapy with concurrent thoracic radiation therapy for locally advanced non-small cell lung cancer [abstract 7515]. *J Clin Oncol.* 2008;26.

14. Govindan R, Bogart J, Wang X, Hodgson L, Kratzke R, Vokes EE. Phase II study of pemetrexed, carboplatin, and thoracic radiation with or without cetuximab in patients with locally advanced unresectable non-small cell lung cancer: CALGB 30407 [abstract 7505]. *J Clin Oncol.* 2009;27(15s).

15. Albain KS, Crowley JJ, Turrisi AT 3rd, et al. Concurrent cisplatin, etoposide, and chest radiotherapy in pathologic stage IIIB non-small-cell lung cancer: a Southwest Oncology Group phase II study, SWOG 9019. *J Clin Oncol.* 2002;20(16):3454–3460.

16. Gandara DR, Chansky K, Albain KS, et al.; Southwest Oncology Group. Consolidation docetaxel after concurrent chemoradiotherapy in stage IIIB non-small-cell lung cancer: phase II Southwest Oncology Group Study S9504. *J Clin Oncol.* 2003;21(10):2004–2010.

17. Hanna N, Neubauer M, Yiannoutsos C, et al.; Hoosier Oncology Group; US Oncology. Phase III study of cisplatin, etoposide, and concurrent chest radiation with or without consolidation docetaxel in patients with inoperable stage III non-small-cell lung cancer: the Hoosier Oncology Group and U.S. Oncology. *J Clin Oncol.* 2008;26(35):5755–5760.

18. Kelly K, Chansky K, Gaspar LE, et al. Updated analysis of SWOG 0023: a randomized phase III trial of gefitinib versus placebo maintenance after definitive chemoradiation followed by docetaxel in patients with locally advanced stage III non-small cell lung cancer [abstract 7513]. *J Clin Oncol.* 2007;25(18s).

19. High-dose or standard-dose radiation therapy and chemotherapy in treating patients with newly diagnosed stage III non-small cell lung cancer that cannot be removed by surgery. ClinicalTrialsgov [Website]: http://www.clinicaltrials.gov/ct2/show/NCT00533949 Accessed August 26, 2009.

20. Vokes EE, Herndon JE, Kelley MJ, et al. Induction chemotherapy followed by concomitant chemoradiotherapy (CT/XRT) versus CT/XRT alone for regionally advanced unresectable non-small cell lung cancer (NSCLC): initial analysis of a randomized phase III trial [abstract 7005]. *J Clin Oncol.* 2004;22(14s).

21. Molina JR, Adjei AA, Jett JR. Advances in chemotherapy of non-small cell lung cancer. *Chest.* 2006;130(4):1211–1219.

22. Spiro SG, Silvestri GA. One hundred years of lung cancer. *Am J Respir Crit Care Med.* 2005;172(5):523–529.

23. Schiller JH, Harrington D, Belani CP, et al.; Eastern Cooperative Oncology Group. Comparison of four chemotherapy regimens for advanced non-small-cell lung cancer. *N Engl J Med.* 2002;346(2):92–98.

24. Kelly K, Crowley J, Bunn PA Jr, et al. Randomized phase III trial of paclitaxel plus carboplatin versus vinorelbine plus cisplatin in the treatment of patients with advanced non–small-cell lung cancer: a Southwest Oncology Group trial. *J Clin Oncol.* 2001;19(13):3210–3218.

25. Scagliotti GV, De Marinis F, Rinaldi M, et al.; Italian Lung Cancer Project. Phase III randomized trial comparing three platinum-based doublets in advanced non-small-cell lung cancer. *J Clin Oncol.* 2002;20(21):4285–4291.

26. Fossella F, Pereira JR, von Pawel J, et al. Randomized, multinational, phase III study of docetaxel plus platinum combinations versus vinorelbine plus cisplatin for advanced non-small-cell lung cancer: the TAX 326 study group. *J Clin Oncol.* 2003;21(16):3016–3024.

27. Treat J. Incorporating novel agents with gemcitabine-based treatment of NSCLC. *Lung Cancer.* 2005;50(suppl 1):S8–S9.

28. Scagliotti GV, Parikh P, von Pawel J, et al. Phase III study comparing cisplatin plus gemcitabine with cisplatin plus pemetrexed in chemotherapy-naive patients with advanced-stage non-small-cell lung cancer. *J Clin Oncol.* 2008;26(21):3543–3551.

29. Grønberg BH, Bremnes RM, Fløtten O, et al. Phase III study by the Norwegian lung cancer study group: pemetrexed plus carboplatin compared with gemcitabine plus carboplatin as first-line chemotherapy in advanced non-small-cell lung cancer. *J Clin Oncol.* 2009;27(19):3217–3224.

30. Gandara D. Thymidylate synthase (TS) RNA expression in non-small cell lung cancer (NSCLC): implications for personalizing pemetrexed therapy [abstract D7.1]. In: 13th World Conference on Lung Cancer, San Francisco, USA, July 31–Aug 4, 2009.

31. Kubota K, Watanabe K, Kunitoh H, et al.; Japanese Taxotere Lung Cancer Study Group. Phase III randomized trial of docetaxel plus cisplatin versus vindesine plus cisplatin in patients with stage IV non-small-cell lung cancer: the Japanese Taxotere Lung Cancer Study Group. *J Clin Oncol.* 2004;22(2):254–261.

32. Ardizzoni A, Boni L, Tiseo M, et al.; CISCA (CISplatin versus CArboplatin) Meta-analysis Group. Cisplatin- versus carboplatin-based chemotherapy in first-line treatment of advanced non-small-cell lung cancer: an individual patient data meta-analysis. *J Natl Cancer Inst.* 2007;99(11):847–857.

33. Socinski MA, Schell MJ, Peterman A, et al. Phase III trial comparing a defined duration of therapy versus continuous therapy followed by second-line therapy in advanced-stage IIIB/IV non-small-cell lung cancer. *J Clin Oncol.* 2002;20(5):1335–1343.

34. Smith IE, O'Brien ME, Talbot DC, et al. Duration of chemotherapy in advanced non-small-cell lung cancer: a randomized trial of three versus six courses of mitomycin, vinblastine, and cisplatin. *J Clin Oncol.* 2001;19(5):1336–1343.

35. Belani CP, Barstis J, Perry MC, et al. Multicenter, randomized trial for stage IIIB or IV non-small-cell lung cancer using weekly paclitaxel and carboplatin followed by maintenance weekly paclitaxel or observation. *J Clin Oncol.* 2003;21(15):2933–2939.

36. Westeel V, Quoix E, Moro-Sibilot D, et al.; French Thoracic Oncology Collaborative Group (GCOT). Randomized study of maintenance vinorelbine in responders with advanced non-small-cell lung cancer. *J Natl Cancer Inst.* 2005;97(7):499–506.

37. von Plessen C, Bergman B, Andresen O, et al. Palliative chemotherapy beyond three courses conveys no survival or consistent quality-of-life benefits in advanced non-small-cell lung cancer. *Br J Cancer.* 2006;95(8):966–973.

38. Brodowicz T, Krzakowski M, Zwitter M, et al.; Central European Cooperative Oncology Group CECOG. Cisplatin and gemcitabine first-line chemotherapy followed by maintenance gemcitabine or best supportive care in advanced non-small cell lung cancer: a phase III trial. *Lung Cancer.* 2006;52(2):155–163.

39. Park JO, Kim SW, Ahn JS, et al. Phase III trial of two versus four additional cycles in patients who are nonprogressive after two cycles of platinum-based chemotherapy in non small-cell lung cancer. *J Clin Oncol.* 2007;25(33):5233–5239.

40. Fidias PM, Dakhil SR, Lyss AP, et al. Phase III study of immediate compared with delayed docetaxel after front-line therapy with gemcitabine plus carboplatin in advanced non-small-cell lung cancer. *J Clin Oncol.* 2009;27(4):591–598.

41. Belani CP, Brodowicz T, Ciuleanu TE, et al. Maintenance pemetrexed plus best supportive care (BSC) versus placebo plus

BSC: a phase III study in NSCLC [abstract 8000]. *J Clin Oncol.* 2009;27(18s).

42. Cappuzzo F, Ciuleanu T, Stelmakh L, et al. SATURN: a double-blind, randomized, phase III study of maintenance erlotinib versus placebo following nonprogression with first-line platinum-based chemotherapy in patients with advanced NSCLC [abstract 8001]. *J Clin Oncol.* 2009;27(15s).

43. Miller VA, O'Connor P, Soh C, Kabbinavar FF. A randomized, double-blind, placebo-controlled, phase IIIb trial (ATLAS) comparing bevacizumab (B) therapy with or without erlotinib (E) after completion of chemotherapy with B for first-line treatment of locally advanced, recurrent, or metastatic non-small cell lung cancer (NSCLC) [abstract LBA8002]. *J Clin Oncol.* 2009;27(18s).

44. Grossi F, Aita M, Follador A, et al. Sequential, alternating, and maintenance/consolidation chemotherapy in advanced non-small cell lung cancer: a review of the literature. *Oncologist.* 2007;12(4):451–464.

45. Ciuleanu TE, Brodowicz T, Belani CP, et al. Maintenance pemetrexed plus best supportive care (BSC) versus placebo plus BSC [abstract 8011]. *J Clin Oncol.* 2008;26(426s).

46. Peterson P, Zwitter M, Krzakowski M, et al. Delay in time to worsening of symptoms (TWS) of advanced non-small cell lung cancer (NSCLC) using gemcitabine (gem) maintenance therapy. *Proc Am Soc Clin Oncol.* 2006;24:399S.

47. Patel JD, Hensing TA, Rademaker F, et al. Pemetrexed and carboplatin plus bevacizumab with maintenance pemetrexed and bevacizumab as first-line therapy for advanced non-squamous non-small cell lung cancer (NSCLC) [abstract 8044]. *J Clin Oncol.* 2008;26(May 20 suppl).

48. Soon YY, Stockler MR, Askie LM, Boyer MJ. Duration of chemotherapy for advanced non-small-cell lung cancer: a systematic review and meta-analysis of randomized trials. *J Clin Oncol.* 2009;27(20):3277–3283.

49. Lustberg MB, Edelman MJ. Optimal duration of chemotherapy in advanced non-small cell lung cancer. *Curr Treat Options Oncol.* 2007;8(1):38–46.

50. Fukuoka M, Masuda N, Furuse K, et al. A randomized trial in inoperable non-small-cell lung cancer: vindesine and cisplatin versus mitomycin, vindesine, and cisplatin versus etoposide and cisplatin alternating with vindesine and mitomycin. *J Clin Oncol.* 1991;9(4):606–613.

51. Eagan RT, Frytak S, Richardson RL, et al. A randomized comparative trial of sequential versus alternating cyclophosphamide, doxorubicin, and cisplatin and mitomycin, lomustine, and methotrexate in metastatic non-small-cell lung cancer. *J Clin Oncol.* 1988;6(1):5–8.

52. Pérol M, Léna H, Thomas P, et al. Phase II randomized multicenter study evaluating a treatment regimen alternating docetaxel and cisplatin-vinorelbine with a cisplatin-vinorelbine control group in patients with stage IV non-small-cell lung cancer: GFPC 97.01 study. *Ann Oncol.* 2002;13(5):742–747.

53. Mattson K, Vansteenkiste J, Stupp R, et al. Phase II study of docetaxel alternating with cisplatin in chemotherapy-naïve patients with advanced non-small cell lung cancer. *Anticancer Drugs.* 2000;11(1):7–13.

54. Aguiar D, Aguiar J, Bohn U. Alternating weekly administration of paclitaxel and gemcitabine: a phase II study in patients with advanced non-small-cell lung cancer. *Cancer Chemother Pharmacol.* 2005;55(2):152–158.

55. Gridelli C, Kaukel E, Gregorc V, et al. Single-agent pemetrexed or sequential pemetrexed/gemcitabine as front-line treatment of advanced non-small cell lung cancer in elderly patients or patients ineligible for platinum-based chemotherapy: a multicenter, randomized, phase II trial. *J Thorac Oncol.* 2007;2(3):221–229.

56. Sandler A, Gray R, Perry MC, et al. Paclitaxel-carboplatin alone or with bevacizumab for non-small-cell lung cancer. *N Engl J Med.* 2006;355(24):2542–2550.57.   Reck M, von Pawel J, Zatloukal P, et al. Phase III trial of cisplatin plus gemcitabine with either placebo or bevacizumab as first-line therapy for nonsquamous non-small-cell lung cancer: AVAiL. *J Clin Oncol.* 2009;27(8):1227–1234.

58. Lynch TJ, Patel T, Dreisbach L. A randomized multicenter phase III study of cetuximab in combination with taxane/carboplatin versus taxane/carboplatin alone as first-line treatment for patients with advanced/metastatic non-small cell lung cancer (NSCLC) [abstract B3–03]. *J Thorac Oncol.* 2007;2(S340).

59. Pirker R, Pereira JR, Szczesna A, et al.; FLEX Study Team. Cetuximab plus chemotherapy in patients with advanced non-small-cell lung cancer (FLEX): an open-label randomised phase III trial. *Lancet.* 2009;373(9674):1525–1531.

60. Polikoff J, Hainsworth JD, Fehrenbacher L, et al. Safety of bevacizumab (Bv) therapy in combination with chemotherapy in subjects with non-small cell lung cancer (NSCLC) treated on ATLAS [abstract 8079]. *J Clin Oncol.* 2008;26(May 20 suppl).

61. Cunningham D, Humblet Y, Siena S, et al. Cetuximab monotherapy and cetuximab plus irinotecan in irinotecan-refractory metastatic colorectal cancer. *N Engl J Med.* 2004;351(4):337–345.

62. Bonner JA, Harari PM, Giralt J, et al. Radiotherapy plus cetuximab for squamous-cell carcinoma of the head and neck. *N Engl J Med.* 2006;354(6):567–578.

63. Herbst RS, Prager D, Hermann R, et al.; TRIBUTE Investigator Group. TRIBUTE: a phase III trial of erlotinib hydrochloride (OSI-774) combined with carboplatin and paclitaxel chemotherapy in advanced non-small-cell lung cancer. *J Clin Oncol.* 2005;23(25):5892–5899.

64. Gatzemeier U, Pluzanska A, Szczesna A, et al. Phase III study of erlotinib in combination with cisplatin and gemcitabine in advanced non-small-cell lung cancer: the Tarceva Lung Cancer Investigation Trial. *J Clin Oncol.* 2007;25(12):1545–1552.

65. Kobayashi K, Inoue A, Maemondo M, et al. First-line gefitinib versus first-line chemotherapy by carboplatin (CBDCA) plus paclitaxel (TXL) in non-small cell lung cancer (NSCLC) patients (pts) with EGFR mutations: a phase III study (002) by North East Japan Gefitinib Study Group [abstract 8016]. *J Clin Oncol.* 2009;27(15s).

66. Lee JS, Park K, Kim SW, et al. A randomized phase III study of gefitinib (IRESSA) versus standard chemotherapy (gemcitabine plus cisplatin) as a first-line treatment for never-smokers with advanced or metastatic adenocarcinoma on the lung [abstract PRS4]. In: 13th World Conference on Lung Cancer, San Francisco, USA, July 31-Aug 4, 2009.

67. Phase III study (Tarceva) vs chemotherapy to treat advanced non-small cell lung cancer (NSCLC) in patients with mutations in the TK domain of EGFR. ClinicalTrialsgov [Website]: http://www.clinicaltrials.gov/ct2/show/NCT00446225 Accessed August 26, 2009.

68. Erlotinib versus gemcitabine/carboplatin in chemo-naive stage III/IV non-small cell lung cancer patients with epidermal growth factor receptor (EGFR) exon 19 or 21 mutation. ClinicalTrialsgov [Website]: http://www.clinicaltrials.gov/ct2/show/NCT00874419 Accessed August 26, 2009.

69. BIBW 2992 versus chemotherapy as first line treatment in NSCLC with EGFR mutation. ClinicalTrialsgov [Website]: Accessed: http://www.clinicaltrials.gov/ct2/show/NCT00949650 Accessed August 26, 2009.

70. Wedge SR, Kendrew J, Hennequin LF, et al. AZD2171: a highly potent, orally bioavailable, vascular endothelial growth factor receptor-2 tyrosine kinase inhibitor for the treatment of cancer. *Cancer Res.* 2005;65(10):4389–4400.

71. Goss GD, Arnold A, Shepherd FA, et al. Randomized, double-blind trial of carboplatin and paclitaxel with either daily oral cediranib or placebo in advanced non-small-cell lung cancer: NCIC clinical trials group BR24 study. *J Clin Oncol.* 2010;28(1):49–55.

72. Hanna NH, von Pawel J, Reck M, Scagliotti G. Carboplatin/paclitaxel with/without sorefenib in chemonaiive patients with stage IIIB-IV non-small cell lung cancer (NSCLC): interim analysis results from a randomized phase III trial (ESCAPE). *J Thorac Oncol.* 2008;11(268s).

73. Scagliotti G, von Pawel J, Reck M, et al. Sorafenib plus carboplatin/paclitaxel in chemonaiive patients with stage IIIB-IV non-small cell lung cancer: interim analysis results from the phase III, randomized, double-blind, placebo-controlled, ESCAPE (Evaluation of Sorafenib, Carboplaitn and Paclitaxel Efficacy in NSCLC) trial. *J Thorac Oncol.* 2008;4(S97).

74. Ramsey SD, Howlader N, Etzioni RD, Donato B. Chemotherapy use, outcomes, and costs for older persons with advanced non-small-cell lung cancer: evidence from surveillance, epidemiology and end results-Medicare. *J Clin Oncol.* 2004;22(24):4971–4978.

75. Effects of vinorelbine on quality of life and survival of elderly patients with advanced non-small-cell lung cancer. The Elderly Lung Cancer Vinorelbine Italian Study Group. *J Natl Cancer Inst.* 1999;91(1):66–72.

76. Gridelli C, Perrone F, Gallo C, et al.; MILES Investigators. Chemotherapy for elderly patients with advanced non-small-cell lung cancer: the Multicenter Italian Lung Cancer in the Elderly Study (MILES) phase III randomized trial. *J Natl Cancer Inst.* 2003;95(5):362–372.

77. Lilenbaum RC, Herndon JE 2nd, List MA, et al. Single-agent versus combination chemotherapy in advanced non-small-cell lung cancer: the cancer and leukemia group B (study 9730). *J Clin Oncol.* 2005;23(1):190–196.

78. Langer CJ, Manola J, Bernardo P, et al. Cisplatin-based therapy for elderly patients with advanced non-small-cell lung cancer: implications of Eastern Cooperative Oncology Group 5592, a randomized trial. *J Natl Cancer Inst.* 2002;94(3):173–181.

79. Gridelli C, Rossi A, Mongillo F, Bareschino M, Maione P, Ciardiello F. A randomized phase II study of sorafenib/gemcitabine or sorafenib/erlotinib for advanced non-small-cell lung cancer in elderly patients or patients with a performance status of 2: treatment rationale and protocol dynamics. *Clin Lung Cancer.* 2007;8(6):396–398.

80. Ramalingam SS, Dahlberg SE, Langer CJ, et al.; Eastern Cooperative Oncology Group. Outcomes for elderly, advanced-stage non small-cell lung cancer patients treated with bevacizumab in combination with carboplatin and paclitaxel: analysis of Eastern Cooperative Oncology Group Trial 4599. *J Clin Oncol.* 2008;26(1):60–65.

81. Sweeney CJ, Zhu J, Sandler AB, et al. Outcome of patients with a performance status of 2 in Eastern Cooperative Oncology Group Study E1594: a Phase II trial in patients with metastatic nonsmall cell lung carcinoma. *Cancer.* 2001;92(10):2639–2647.

82. Gridelli C, Ardizzoni A, Le Chevalier T, et al. Treatment of advanced non-small-cell lung cancer patients with ECOG performance status 2: results of an European Experts Panel. *Ann Oncol.* 2004;15(3):419–426.

83. Lilenbaum R, Villaflor VM, Langer C, et al. Single-agent versus combination chemotherapy in patients with advanced non-small cell lung cancer and a performance status of 2: prognostic factors and treatment selection based on two large randomized clinical trials. *J Thorac Oncol.* 2009;4(7):869–874.

84. Finkelstein DM, Ettinger DS, Ruckdeschel JC. Long-term survivors in metastatic non-small-cell lung cancer: an Eastern Cooperative Oncology Group Study. *J Clin Oncol.* 1986;4(5):702–709.

85. Albain KS, Crowley JJ, LeBlanc M, Livingston RB. Survival determinants in extensive-stage non-small-cell lung cancer: the Southwest Oncology Group experience. *J Clin Oncol.* 1991;9(9):1618–1626.

86. Wakelee HA, Wang W, Schiller JH, et al.; for the Eastern Cooperative Oncology Group. Survival differences by sex for patients with advanced non-small cell lung cancer on Eastern Cooperative Oncology Group trial 1594. *J Thorac Oncol.* 2006;1(5):441–446.

87. Stabile LP, Davis AL, Gubish CT, et al. Human non-small cell lung tumors and cells derived from normal lung express both estrogen receptor alpha and beta and show biological responses to estrogen. *Cancer Res.* 2002;62(7):2141–2150.

88. Mollerup S, Jørgensen K, Berge G, Haugen A. Expression of estrogen receptors alpha and beta in human lung tissue and cell lines. *Lung Cancer.* 2002;37(2):153–159.

89. Ganti AK, Sahmoun AE, Panwalkar AW, Tendulkar KK, Potti A. Hormone replacement therapy is associated with decreased survival in women with lung cancer. *J Clin Oncol.* 2006;24(1):59–63.

90. Stabile LP, Siegfried JM. Estrogen receptor pathways in lung cancer. *Curr Oncol Rep.* 2004;6(4):259–267.

91. Chlebowski RT, Schwartz A, Wakelee H, et al. Non-small cell lung cancer and estrogen plus progestin use in postmenopausal women in the Women's Health Initiative randomized clinical trial [abstract CRA1500]. *J Clin Oncol.* 2009;27(804s).

92. Albain KS, Unger J, Gotay CC, et al. Toxicity and survival by sex in patients with advanced non-small cell lung carcinoma (NSCLC) on modern Southwest Oncology Group (SWOG) trials [abstract 7549]. *J Clin Oncol.* 2007;25(396s).

93. Stabile LP, Lyker JS, Gubish CT, Zhang W, Grandis JR, Siegfried JM. Combined targeting of the estrogen receptor and the epidermal growth factor receptor in non-small cell lung cancer shows enhanced antiproliferative effects. *Cancer Res.* 2005;65(4):1459–1470.

94. Garon EB, Sadeghi S, Kabbinavar FF, et al. Interim safety analysis of a phase II study of erlotinib (E) alone or combined with fulvestrant (F) in previously treated patients with advanced non-small cell lung cancer (NSCLC). *J Clin Oncol.* 2008;26(15s):19091.

95. Lord RV, Brabender J, Gandara D, et al. Low ERCC1 expression correlates with prolonged survival after cisplatin plus gemcitabine chemotherapy in non-small cell lung cancer. *Clin Cancer Res.* 2002;8(7):2286–2291.

96. Cobo M, Isla D, Massuti B, et al. Customizing cisplatin based on quantitative excision repair cross-complementing 1 mRNA expression: a phase III trial in non-small-cell lung cancer. *J Clin Oncol.* 2007;25(19):2747–2754.

97. Bepler G, Kusmartseva I, Sharma S, et al. RRM1 modulated *in vitro* and *in vivo* efficacy of gemcitabine and platinum in non-small-cell lung cancer. *J Clin Oncol.* 2006;24(29):4731–4737.

98. Zheng Z, Chen T, Li X, Haura E, Sharma A, Bepler G. DNA synthesis and repair genes RRM1 and ERCC1 in lung cancer. *N Engl J Med.* 2007;356(8):800–808.

99. Simon G, Sharma A, Li X, et al. Feasibility and efficacy of molecular analysis-directed individualized therapy in advanced non-small-cell lung cancer. *J Clin Oncol.* 2007;25(19):2741–2746.

100. Phase III of RRM1 & ERCC1 directed customized chemotherapy for the treatment of patients with NSCLC. ClinicalTrialsgov [Website]: http://www.clinicaltrials.gov/ct2/show/NCT00499109 Accessed August 26, 2009.

101. Rosell R, Skrzypski M, Jassem E, et al. BRCA1: a novel prognostic factor in resected non-small-cell lung cancer. *PLoS ONE.* 2007;2(11):e1129.

102. Quinn JE, Kennedy RD, Mullan PB, et al. BRCA1 functions as a differential modulator of chemotherapy-induced apoptosis. *Cancer Res.* 2003;63(19):6221–6228.

103. Multicenter, predictive, prospective, phase III, open, randomized pharmacogenetic study in patients with advanced lung carcinoma (BREC). ClinicalTrialsgov [Website]: http://www.clinicaltrials.gov/ct2/show/NCT00617656 Accessed August 26, 2009.

104. Hirschowitz EA, Yannelli JR. Immunotherapy for lung cancer. *Proc Am Thorac Soc.* 2009;6(2):224–232.

105. O'Brien ME, Anderson H, Kaukel E, et al.; SR-ON-12 Study Group. SRL172 (killed Mycobacterium vaccae) in addition to standard chemotherapy improves quality of life without affecting survival, in patients with advanced non-small-cell lung cancer: phase III results. *Ann Oncol.* 2004;15(6):906–914.

16

Stage IIIB and IV NSCLC: Recurrent Disease

ENRIQUETA FELIP

TERESA MORÁN

BARTOMEU MASSUTI

RAFAEL ROSELL

◼ INTRODUCTION

Non–small cell lung cancer (NSCLC) accounts for 80% of all lung cancer cases and is the leading cause of cancer mortality. The majority of NSCLC patients present with advanced, unresectable disease, which remains incurable. In advanced NSCLC patients with progression after first-line chemotherapy, docetaxel has shown superiority to best supportive care in terms of survival and quality of life. In a phase III trial, second-line treatment with pemetrexed demonstrated overall survival comparable with docetaxel with a more manageable toxicity profile. In chemotherapy-refractory, advanced NSCLC patients, erlotinib improved survival when compared with placebo. The INTEREST trial established noninferior survival of gefitinib compared with docetaxel in previously treated NSCLC patients. These agents appear to have similar efficacy in terms of response and overall survival, but have significantly different toxicity profiles.

Epidermal growth factor receptor (EGFR) mutations are associated with a higher and longer-lasting response following treatment with EGFR tyrosine-kinase inhibitors (TKIs) in both chemotherapy-naïve and pretreated NSCLC patients. Patients with EGFR mutations should therefore receive EGFR TKIs at some point during evolution of the disease.

Recently, several new agents have shown activity in clinical trials in pretreated NSCLC patients and are expected to be integrated into treatment approaches to recurrent disease in the immediate future.

The present review focuses on a number of targeted agents/chemotherapy drugs. First to be addressed will be those drugs that are now standard of care in patients with recurrent disease, and second, we will focus on drugs being evaluated in ongoing clinical trials.

◼ DOCETAXEL

Docetaxel was the first drug approved for second-line NSCLC treatment. In second-line treatment, the Fossella et al. (1) and Shepherd et al. (2) randomized trials reported improvements in 1-year survival, and in quality of life with docetaxel when compared with ifosfamide, vinorelbine, or best supportive care alone. The docetaxel dose recommended in this setting was 75 mg/m^2 every 3 weeks. Due to the fact that febrile neutropenia was observed in 12% to 16% of patients using this schedule, subsequent randomized trials analyzed the appropriateness of the weekly docetaxel schedule. A pooled analysis comparing docetaxel weekly versus 3-weekly found similar survival rates between the schedules and a nonsignificant reduction in febrile neutropenia for the weekly regimen (3).

◼ PEMETREXED

In a randomized phase III trial, the efficacy and toxicity of pemetrexed was compared with that of docetaxel in relapsed NSCLC patients (4). Until that trial, docetaxel was the only approved cytotoxic chemotherapy in second-line NSCLC treatment. Eligible patients had a performance status of 0 to 2, previous treatment with one prior chemotherapy regimen for advanced disease, and adequate organ function. In this noninferiority study, both pemetrexed and docetaxel were given on day 1 of a 21-day cycle. Patients in the pemetrexed arm received folate and B12 supplementation. Five hundred seventy-one eligible patients were randomized to receive either pemetrexed or docetaxel. Prerandomization stratification factors included performance status, disease stage, number of previous chemotherapy regimens, response to most recent chemotherapy, whether the patient had ever received either platinum or paclitaxel therapy, treatment site, and baseline homocysteine level. Following disease progression, poststudy chemotherapy was allowed. The results of this study are summarized in Table 16.1. Response rates were 9.1% and 8.8%, and median survival times were 8.3 months and 7.9 months in the pemetrexed

■ **Table 16.1** Efficacy results of the phase III second-line trial comparing pemetrexed to docetaxel

	Pemetrexed (n = 283)	Docetaxel (n = 288)	HR; P Value
Median overall survival	8.3 months	7.9 months	HR = 0.99; $P = -0.93$
1-year survival rate	29.7%	29.7%	–
Median progression-free survival	2.9 months	2.9 months	–
Time to progressive disease	3.4 months	3.5 months	–
Overall response rate	9.1%	8.8%	–

HR, hazard ratio.

and docetaxel arms, respectively. Median progression-free survival was 2.9 months for each arm and the 1-year survival rate for each arm was 29.7%. The docetaxel arm had higher incidence of grade 3 or 4 neutropenia (40% vs. 5%), neutropenic fever (13% vs. 2%), and neuropathy (8% vs. 3%) than the pemetrexed arm. Thus, pemetrexed produced similar results and was better tolerated than docetaxel in the treatment of pretreated NSCLC patients.

In a retrospective analysis of the aforementioned phase III study comparing pemetrexed versus docetaxel in second-line setting, the authors presented the finding that docetaxel had statistically better survival than pemetrexed in the squamous cell subgroup, whereas pemetrexed had statistically better survival than docetaxel in the combined nonsquamous subgroup (5). These results agree with those reported in the first-line study comparing cisplatin/gemcitabine with cisplatin/pemetrexed (6).

Weiss et al. (7) performed a subset analysis of the aforementioned randomized phase III trial of pemetrexed versus docetaxel to analyze whether the elderly population benefits from second-line cytotoxic chemotherapy. Eighty-six of 571 patients (15%) were 70 years or older, similar to rates of the elderly observed in the first-line setting. Elderly patients receiving pemetrexed (n = 47) or docetaxel (n = 39) had a median survival of 9.5 months and 7.7 months compared with 7.8 months and 8.0 months for younger patients receiving pemetrexed (n = 236) or docetaxel (n = 249), respectively. Elderly patients treated with pemetrexed had a longer time to progression and a longer survival than their counterparts treated with docetaxel (not statistically significant). Febrile neutropenia was less frequent in the elderly patients treated with pemetrexed (2.5%) than in those receiving docetaxel (19%; $P = 0.025$).

Pujol et al. (8) performed a retrospective risk-benefit analysis of survival without grade 3 to 4 toxicity, defined as the time to the first occurrence of Common Toxicity Criteria grade 3 or 4 toxicity or death, in the above prospective phase III study comparing pemetrexed with docetaxel. In this analysis, pemetrexed demonstrated a statistically significant longer survival without grade 3 or 4 toxicity compared with docetaxel (hazard ratio [HR] 0.60; $P < 0.0001$). A supportive analysis based on selected

grade 3 or 4 toxicities (neutropenia lasting >5 days, febrile neutropenia, infection with neutropenia, anemia, thrombocytopenia, fatigue, nausea, vomiting, diarrhea, stomatitis, and neurosensory events) also demonstrated an advantage for pemetrexed (HR 0.53; $P < 0.0001$). This analysis of survival without grade 3 or 4 toxicities suggests a benefit-to-risk profile that favors pemetrexed over decetaxel in the second-line treatment of nonsquamous NSCLC patients.

Cullen et al. (9) published a study in which they compared a high dose of pemetrexed (900 mg/m^2) with the standard dose (500 mg/m^2), each given once every 21 days, in advanced NSCLC patients with disease progression after treatment with a platinum-containing regimen. The primary objective of this study was survival. In this trial, 629 patients were accrued, of which 588 were eligible for inclusion, 295 received the standard pemetrexed dose, and 293 received the higher pemetrexed dose. No differences were detected between the high dose and the standard dose of pemetrexed in terms of survival, progression-free survival, or response rate. Overall survival in the two arms was similar (median survival of standard dose of 6.7 months compared with 6.9 months for patients who received the higher dose). Patients in the higher dose arm had slightly higher toxicity. Thus, the standard pemetrexed dose in second-line therapy should remain at 500 mg/m^2.

Smit et al. (10) recently published the results of a randomized phase II trial comparing pemetrexed with pemetrexed/carboplatin in patients experiencing relapse after platinum-based chemotherapy. A total of 240 patients were enrolled and median time to progression was 4.2 months for patients treated with pemetrexed/carboplatin and 2.8 months for those treated with pemetrexed. Subgroup analyses found adenocarcinoma to be associated with favorable outcome.

A recently published meta-analysis included individual patient data from randomized trials comparing single-agent with doublet chemotherapy as second-line treatment of advanced NSCLC (11). Eight eligible trials were identified. In this meta-analysis, doublet chemotherapy as second-line treatment significantly increases response rate and progression-free survival, but was found to be more toxic and did not improve overall survival compared with single-agent chemotherapy.

■ ERLOTINIB

Erlotinib is approved for treating advanced NSCLC patients who progress after 1 or 2 prior regimens. A phase II trial using erlotinib (150 mg/day) was performed in 57 previously treated advanced NSCLC patients who had an available tumor biopsy sample with >10% of cancer cells positive for EGFR expression (12). The objective response rate was 12.3%; 39% of patients had stable disease and 49% progressed. In this study, response did not correlate with EGFR level expression. The median duration of response was 19.7 weeks, the median progression-free survival was 9 weeks, the median overall survival was 8.4 months, and the 1-year survival rate was 40%. Rash was reported in 67% of patients and diarrhea in 56%. Incidence and severity of rash correlated with improved survival.

The National Cancer Institute of Canada conducted a randomized placebo-controlled trial of erlotinib in patients with advanced NSCLC following failure of first-line or second-line chemotherapy (13). A total of 731 patients were randomized 2:1 to receive oral erlotinib 150 mg, or placebo, daily. Patients' characteristics were well balanced between the two arms. The overall response to erlotinib was 8.9%. Significant improvements were observed in the time of deterioration of patient-reported cough ($P = 0.04$), dyspnea ($P = 0.01$), and pain ($P = 0.02$). The most frequent toxicities were rash (76%, 9% grade 3 or 4) and diarrhea (55%, 6% grade 3 or 4). Skin rash was associated with favorable survival and objective tumor response in erlotinib-treated patients. There was no apparent hematologic toxicity associated with erlotinib therapy. Eye disorders were more frequent in the erlotinib group than in the placebo group (27% vs. 9%). Only 5% of patients discontinued erlotinib, due to toxicity compared with 2% of patients on placebo. Overall survival for patients who received erlotinib was 6.7 months, compared with 4.7 months for patients who were treated with placebo (HR 0.73; $P = 0.001$). Results of the BR.21 trial are summarized in Table 16.2.

In the exploratory univariate analyses, the favorable effect of erlotinib on survival was maintained in most groups. However, the greatest survival prolongation was seen in two subsets of patients: never-smokers and those with EGFR mutation-positive tumors.

■ GEFITINIB

Two phase II trials in patients with previously treated advanced NSCLC suggested that gefitinib was efficacious and less toxic than chemotherapy (14,15). Gefitinib was analyzed in a placebo-controlled phase III study as second-line or third-line treatment (16). A total of 1,692 patients who were refractory or intolerant to their latest chemotherapy were randomly assigned to either gefitinib or placebo. In this study, median survival did not differ significantly between the groups in the overall study population (5.6 months for gefitinib and 5.1 months for placebo). Preplanned subgroup analyses showed significantly longer survival in the gefitinib group for never-smokers and patients of Asian origin.

In the INTEREST trial, gefitinib was compared with docetaxel in patients with advanced NSCLC who had been pretreated with platinum-based chemotherapy (17). A total of 1,466 patients were included and the noninferiority of gefitinib compared with docetaxel was confirmed for overall survival.

■ EGFR TKIS IN RECURRENT NSCLC PATIENTS WITH EGFR MUTATIONS

There is, at present, clear evidence to suggest that in patients with advanced NSCLC, activating mutations in the EGFR gene confer hypersensitivity to the TKIs gefitinib and erlotinib. Almost 90% of lung cancer–specific EGFR mutations comprise a leucine-to-arginine substitution at position 858 (L858R) and deletion mutants in exon 19 that affect the conserved sequence LREA (delE746-A750). These mutations cause constitutive activation of the EGFR tyrosine-kinase domain by destabilizing its autoinhibited conformation, which is normally maintained in the absence of ligand stimulation. Several studies have shown that EGFR mutations are independent predictors of response and progression-free survival in patients treated with EGFR TKIs. In all these studies, EGFR mutations

---

■ Table 16.2 Clinical results of BR.21 trial

Treatment	No. of Patients	Response Rate (%)	Median Progression-free Survival (months)	Median Overall Survival (months)	1-Year Survival (%)
Erlotinib	488	8.9	2.2	6.7	31
Placebo	243	<1%	1.8	4.7	22

were found to be more frequent in women, patients with adenocarcinomas, never-smokers, and East Asians.

In Spain, lung cancer samples from 2,105 patients from 129 institutions were prospectively screened for EGFR mutations, from April 2005 through November 2008; patients with EGFR mutations were eligible for erlotinib treatment. EGFR mutations were found in 350 of the 2,105 patients (16.6%) (18). Mutations were more frequently found in women, in never-smokers, and in those with adenocarcinoma. The mutations observed were deletion in exon 19 in 62.2% of the patients and L858R in 37.8% of patients. Median progression-free survival for EGFR-mutated patients receiving erlotinib as second-line therapy was 13.0 months, with an overall survival of 28.0 months—an improvement over previously reported findings in lung cancer patients. These results highlight the idea that EGFR-mutant lung cancer is a different type of NSCLC. This and other studies clearly support the role of EGFR TKIs in patients with EGFR mutations (18–21). At present, the most favorable sequence of these agents (in first-line or second-line) is yet to be established.

■ NEW DRUGS IN RECURRENT ADVANCED NSCLC

Chemotherapy Agents

Patupilone (EPO906; Epothilone B)

This is a novel microtubule stabilizer active in NSCLC. In a phase I trial in NSCLC patients, patupilone every 3 weeks was found to be safe and well tolerated and showed antitumor activity (22). A phase II trial using patupilone in previously treated NSCLC patients has finished recruitment.

Paclitaxel poliglumex

This is a water-soluble paclitaxel polymer. A phase I trial determined the safety, maximum tolerated dose, pharmacokinetics, and toxicities associated with the administration of paclitaxel poliglumex given on either 3-weekly or 2-weekly schedules. Dose-limiting toxicities were neutropenia and neuropathy. A phase III trial comparing paclitaxel poliglumex with docetaxel as second-line treatment found overall survival to be similar between arms (23).

Vinflunine

This is a novel vinca alkaloid. A multicentre phase II trial was designed to determine the efficacy of single-agent vinflunine in advanced NSCLC patients previously treated with a platinum-based regimen and yielding a response rate of 7.9% (24). Disease control was achieved in a

further 58% of patients. Median progression-free survival was 2.6 months and median survival was 7 months.

A phase III study in platinum pretreated patients compared vinflunine versus docetaxel (25). A total of 547 patients were included and the study concluded that vinflunine shows efficacy equivalent to docetaxel in second-line NSCLC chemotherapy. Low, manageable, but different toxicity profiles were observed in both arms.

Targeted Agents

Vandetanib

This is an oral aniliquinazoline derivative that has a dual inhibitor effect on the vascular endothelial growth factor receptor (VEGFR)-2 and the EGFR. Preclinical studies have demonstrated that vandetanib administration results in dose-dependent inhibition of lung tumor growth in human xenograft models. Preclinical data also suggest that vandetanib may be active in erlotinib-resistant NSCLC xenograft tumors. Vandetanib-related side effects included rash, fatigue, diarrhea, and asymptomatic Q-T interval prolongation.

Vandetanib has been analyzed in randomized trials in pretreated NSCLC patients. In a phase II randomized study, vandetanib was compared with gefitinib in 168 previously treated patients (26). A statistically significant improvement in time to progression was observed for vandetanib compared with gefitinib (11 vs. 8.1 weeks, $P = 0.013$).

In a further phase II randomized trial, 127 previously treated NSCLC patients received vandetanib (100 or 300 mg) or placebo, in combination with docetaxel (75 mg m^2) (27). Results showed a median time to progression of 18.7 weeks for docetaxel/vandetanib at 100 mg, 17 weeks for docetaxel/vandetanib at 300 mg, and 12.0 weeks for docetaxel/placebo.

A phase III study analyzing vandetanib/docetaxel versus docetaxel alone in second-line treatment (ZODIAC trial) concluded that the addition of vandetanib to docetaxel showed a statistically significant improvement in progression-free survival (28).

In second-line therapy in advanced NSCLC patients, vandetanib/pemetrexed was compared with pemetrexed (29). A total of 534 patients were included in the trial and although the combination of vandetanib/pemetrexed demonstrated evidence of clinical benefit in pretreated NSCLC patients, the study did not meet the primary endpoint of statistically significant progression-free survival prolongation with vandetanib/pemetrexed versus pemetrexed alone.

In a phase III study vandetanib was compared with erlotinib in advanced NSCLC patients after failure of at least one prior cytotoxic chemotherapy (ZEST trial) (30). The primary objective was to show superiority in progression-free survival for vandetanib versus erlotinib.

A total of 1,240 patients were included. The study did not meet its primary objective of demonstrating progression-free survival prolongation with vandetanib versus erlotinib. However, vandetanib and erlotinib showed equivalent efficacy for progression-free survival and overall survival in a preplanned noninferiority analysis.

Sorafenib

This is a multikinase inhibitor that inhibits the kinase activity of both C-Raf and B-Raf and targets the VEGFR family (VEGFR-2 and VEGFR-3) and the platelet-derived growth factor receptor family (PDGFR-βand stem cell factor receptor [KIT]). Sorafenib showed preclinical activity against NSCLC cell lines. The recommended sorafenib dose for phase II studies was 400 mg twice daily. Gatzemeier et al. (31) performed a phase II trial that evaluated sorafenib in patients with relapsed or refractory NSCLC. In this study, stable disease was observed in 59% of evaluable patients. Although there were no partial responses, tumor shrinkage was observed in 29% of patients. Patients with stable disease had a median progression-free survival of 23.7 weeks, whereas all evaluable patients had a median progression-free survival of 11.9 weeks and median overall survival of 29.3 weeks. The most frequent drug-related adverse events observed included diarrhea (40%), hand-foot skin reaction (37%), and fatigue (27%).

In a randomized discontinuation phase II study, patients with at least two prior chemotherapy regimens received sorafenib for 2 months (32). Patients with stable disease after the 2 months of sorafenib treatment were randomized to placebo or sorafenib, and the authors found longer median progression-free survival in those patients receiving sorafenib.

Sunitinib

It is an oral, multitargeted receptor TKI targeting VEGFRs, PDGFR, fms-like tyrosine-kinase 3, and KIT. Socinski et al. (33) published the results of a multicenter phase II trial evaluating the activity of sunitinib in refractory NSCLC. Patients received sunitinib at 50 mg per day for 4 weeks followed by 2 weeks off treatment. In this study, 63 patients were treated with sunitinib. Seven partial responses were observed (11.1%), and stable disease was seen in an additional 18 patients (29%). Grade 3 or 4 toxicities included fatigue/asthenia (21%) and hypertension (5%). Two patients died from lung hemorrhage, and one from cerebral bleeding. The pulmonary bleedings occurred in two squamous cell carcinoma patients. A progression-free survival of 12.0 weeks and median overall survival of 23.4 weeks were reported. In this multicenter phase II trial in previously treated advanced NSCLC, sunitinib was found to have promising single-agent activity. A phase III trial is at present evaluating sunitinib in combination with

erlotinib versus erlotinib alone in 956 patients in second- or third-line setting.

Cetuximab

Cetuximab (C225) is a chimeric human-mouse monoclonal antibody that targets the EGFR. Cetuximab has a high affinity for the extracellular ligand binding domain of the EGFR, leading to receptor internalization, inhibition of phosphorylation, and subsequent blockage of downstream signaling.

In previously treated NSCLC patients, single-agent cetuximab produced an objective response in three of 66 eligible patients (4.5%) and a median survival of 8.1 months. Toxicities were mild, with only 6% of patients experiencing grade 3 or 4 rash (34).

In a phase II trial, the docetaxel/cetuximab combination was tested in chemotherapy-refractory NSCLC patients (35). Response was observed in 20% of patients and stable disease in 36.4%. The median time to disease progression was 104 days and median overall survival was 7.5 months. The docetaxel/cetuximab combination was well tolerated.

BIBW 2992

This is a potent, irreversible, oral, new-generation TKI. This agent is a dual inhibitor of EGFR and HER2 and is active against tumors overexpressing EGFR with the secondary T790M point mutation, which confers resistance to the first-generation EGFR inhibitors, gefitinib and erlotinib (36). In phase I/II trials, BIBW-2992 was effective in patients with solid tumors, including those with NSCLC with activating EGFR mutations, and was generally well tolerated (37). BIBW-2992 is now being analyzed in phase II and III trials in NSCLC patients.

Lapatinib

Lapatinib (GW572016) is an oral, reversible small-molecule inhibitor of EGFR and HER2. In vitro and in vivo studies have shown that lapatinib inhibits the growth of human tumor cell lines with overexpression of EGFR and HER2, and in tumor xenograft models. Lapatinib has shown to abrogate catalytic activity by reducing the tyrosine phosphorylation of EGFR and HER2 receptors and the subsequent activation of downstream effectors of proliferation and cell survival, such as extracellular signal-regulated kinases (Erk1/2) and AKT.

In a phase I trial in heavily pretreated patients, lapatinib was well tolerated at doses ranging from 500 to 1,600 mg given once daily. The most common side effects were diarrhea and rash. Skin toxicity was not correlated to clinical response.

A randomized phase II trial compared two schedules of lapatinib (1,500 mg once a day or 500 mg twice a day) as first-line therapy for patients with advanced NSCLC (38). The preliminary safety results showed that both doses and schedules of lapatinib were well tolerated and the most common adverse events were diarrhea, nausea, and rash (39).

A recently presented phase I study, analyzed the combination of lapatinib/pemetrexed in the second-line treatment of advanced NSCLC (40). Eighteen patients were treated; the combination was well tolerated and encouraging activity was seen with three patients having partial response.

Bortezomib

This is a proteasome inhibitor affecting the ubiquitin-proteasome pathway and resulting in cell-cycle disruption, inhibition of transcription factors, and antiangiogenic effects, which ultimately affect tumor growth and proliferation. Bortezomib has demonstrated preclinical activity in NSCLC tumor cell lines as a single agent and in combination with other chemotherapy agents. A randomized phase II study of bortezomib alone and bortezomib in combination with docetaxel in 155 previously treated advanced NSCLC patients showed disease control rates of 29% in bortezomib-alone arm and 54% in bortezomib/docetaxel arm (41). Median time to progression was 1.5 months in bortezomib-alone arm and 4.0 months in bortezomib/docetaxel arm. No differences in median survival were observed between the two arms.

The Southwest Oncology group recently published the results of a phase II trial of bortezomib/gemcitabine/carboplatin in 114 chemonaive advanced NSCLC patients (42). The toxicity profile of this regimen was favorable. Response was observed in 23% of patients. Progression-free survival and median survival times were 5 months and 11 months, respectively, and 1-year survival was 46%.

Enzastaurin

Enzastaurin (LY317615) is a synthetic acyclic bisindolylmaleimide specifically targeting the protein kinase C β through its competitive binding to the ATP-binding site of the serine/threonine kinase. In vitro and in vivo studies have shown that enzastaurin is active against several human cancer cell lines, including colorectal cancer and NSCLC.

In a phase I trial in patients with advanced solid tumors, enzastaurin was well tolerated at doses up to 700 mg/day (43). The maximum tolerated dose was not identified and the 525-mg option once daily was chosen as the recommended dose for phase II trials, since it produced an optimal steady-state concentration for clinical efficacy. No objective responses were observed, but 21 patients achieved stable disease.

A phase II trial analyzed enzastaurin as second- or third-line NSCLC treatment (44). Fifty-five patients were enrolled; median progression-free survival was 1.8 months,

6 months progression-free survival rate was 13%, and median overall survival was 8.4 months.

■ PERSPECTIVES

In recent years substantial progress has been made in the search for therapeutic options for advanced NSCLC. Several randomized trials concurred on the evidence of the efficacy of second- and third-line treatments. Ongoing randomized trials are testing the role of targeted agents and new chemotherapy drugs in advanced NSCLC patients with recurrent disease.

One of the strategies currently under investigation with the aim of prolonging survival in NSCLC patients is maintenance treatment with either a chemotherapy agent or a targeted agent after first-line chemotherapy. According to currently available data, maintenance treatment with a different agent is perhaps the most promising strategy. If this "early second-line" approach is established in advanced NSCLC, the role of second- and third-line therapies should be redefined.

■ REFERENCES

1. Fossella FV, DeVore R, Kerr RN, et al. Randomized phase III trial of docetaxel versus vinorelbine or ifosfamide in patients with advanced non-small-cell lung cancer previously treated with platinum-containing chemotherapy regimens. The TAX 320 Non-Small Cell Lung Cancer Study Group. *J Clin Oncol.* 2000;18(12):2354–2362.
2. Shepherd FA, Dancey J, Ramlau R, et al. Prospective randomized trial of docetaxel versus best supportive care in patients with non-small-cell lung cancer previously treated with platinum-based chemotherapy. *J Clin Oncol.* 2000;18(10):2095–2103.
3. Di Maio M, Perrone F, Chiodini P, et al. Individual patient data meta-analysis of docetaxel administered once every 3 weeks compared with once every week second-line treatment of advanced non-small-cell lung cancer. *J Clin Oncol.* 2007;25(11):1377–1382.
4. Hanna N, Shepherd FA, Fossella FV, et al. Randomized phase III trial of pemetrexed versus docetaxel in patients with non-small-cell lung cancer previously treated with chemotherapy. *J Clin Oncol.* 2004;22(9):1589–1597.
5. Peterson P, Park K, Fossella FV, et al. 12th World Conference on Lung Cancer. Is pemetrexed more effective in adenocarcinoma and large cell lung cancer than in squamous cell carcinoma? A retrospective analysis of a phase III trial of pemetrexed vs docetaxel in previously treated patients with advanced non-small cell lung cancer (NSCLC) (abstract P2–328). 12th World Conference on Lung Cancer; September 2–6, 2007; Seoul, Korea.
6. Scagliotti G-V, Parikh P, von Pawel J, et al. Phase III study comparing cisplatin plus gemcitabine with cisplatin plus pemetrexed in chemotherapy-naive patients with advanced-stage non-small-cell lung cancer. *J Clin Oncol.* 2008;26(21):3543–3551.
7. Weiss GJ, Langer C, Rosell R, et al. Elderly patients benefit from second-line cytotoxic chemotherapy: a subset analysis of a randomized phase III trial of pemetrexed compared with docetaxel in patients with previously treated advanced non-small-cell lung cancer. *J Clin Oncol.* 2006;24(27):4405–4411.

8. Pujol JL, Paul S, Chouaki N, et al. Survival without common toxicity criteria grade ¾ toxicity for pemetrexed compared with docetaxel in previously treated patients with advanced non-small cell lung cancer (NSCLC): a risk-benefit analysis. *J Thorac Oncol.* 2007;2(5):397–401.

9. Cullen MH, Zatloukal P, Sörenson S, et al. A randomized phase III trial comparing standard and high-dose pemetrexed as second-line treatment in patients with locally advanced or metastatic non-small-cell lung cancer. *Ann Oncol.* 2008;19(5):939–945.

10. Smit EF, Burgers SA, Biesma B, et al. Randomized phase II and pharmacogenetic study of pemetrexed compared with pemetrexed plus carboplatin in pretreated patients with advanced non-small-cell lung cancer. *J Clin Oncol.* 2009;27(12):2038–2045.

11. Di Maio M, Chiodini P, Georgoulias V, et al. Meta-analysis of single-agent chemotherapy compared with combination chemotherapy as second-line treatment of advanced non-small-cell lung cancer. *J Clin Oncol.* 2009;27(11):1836–1843.

12. Pérez-Soler R, Chachoua A, Hammond LA, et al. Determinants of tumor response and survival with erlotinib in patients with non–small-cell lung cancer. *J Clin Oncol.* 2004;22(16):3238–3247.

13. Shepherd FA, Rodrigues Pereira J, Ciuleanu T, et al.; National Cancer Institute of Canada Clinical Trials Group. Erlotinib in previously treated non-small-cell lung cancer. *N Engl J Med.* 2005;353(2):123–132.

14. Fukuoka M, Yano S, Giaccone G, et al. Multi-institutional randomized phase II trial of gefitinib for previously treated patients with advanced non-small-cell lung cancer (The IDEAL 1 Trial) [corrected]. *J Clin Oncol.* 2003;21(12):2237–2246.

15. Kris MG, Natale RB, Herbst RS, et al. Efficacy of gefitinib, an inhibitor of the epidermal growth factor receptor tyrosine kinase, in symptomatic patients with non-small cell lung cancer: a randomized trial. *JAMA.* 2003;290(16):2149–2158.

16. Thatcher N, Chang A, Parikh P, et al. Gefitinib plus best supportive care in previously treated patients with refractory advanced non-small-cell lung cancer: results from a randomised, placebo-controlled, multicentre study (Iressa Survival Evaluation in Lung Cancer). *Lancet.* 2005;366(9496):1527–1537.

17. Kim ES, Hirsh V, Mok T, et al. Gefitinib versus docetaxel in previously treated non-small-cell lung cancer (INTEREST): a randomised phase III trial. *Lancet.* 2008;372(9652):1809–1818.

18. Rosell R, Moran T, Queralt C, et al.; Spanish Lung Cancer Group. Screening for epidermal growth factor receptor mutations in lung cancer. *N Engl J Med.* 2009;361(10):958–967.

19. Taron M, Ichinose Y, Rosell R, et al. Activating mutations in the tyrosine kinase domain of the epidermal growth factor receptor are associated with improved survival in gefitinib-treated chemorefractory lung adenocarcinomas. *Clin Cancer Res.* 2005;11(16):5878–5885.

20. Sequist LV, Martins RG, Spigel D, et al. First-line gefitinib in patients with advanced non-small-cell lung cancer harboring somatic EGFR mutations. *J Clin Oncol.* 2008;26(15):2442–2449.

21. Molina-Vila MA, Bertran-Alamillo J, Reguart N, et al. A sensitive method for detecting EGFR mutations in non-small cell lung cancer samples with few tumor cells. *J Thorac Oncol.* 2008;3(11):1224–1235.

22. Sánchez JM, Mellemgaard A, Perry M, et al. Efficacy and safety of patupilone in non-small cell lung cancer (NSCLC): a phase I/II trial (abstract). *Proc Am Soc Clin Oncol.* 2006;18:7104.

23. Paz-Ares L, Ross H, O'Brien M, et al. Phase III trial comparing paclitaxel poliglumex vs docetaxel in the second-line treatment of non-small-cell lung cancer. *Br J Cancer.* 2008;98(10):1608–1613.

24. Bennouna J, Breton JL, Tourani JM, et al. Vinflunine—an active chemotherapy for treatment of advanced non-small-cell lung cancer previously treated with a platinum-based regimen: results of a phase II study. *Br J Cancer.* 2006;94(10):1383–1388.

25. Krzakowski M, Douillard J, Ramlau R, et al. Phase III study of vinflunine versus docetaxel in patients (pts) with advanced non-small-cell lung cancer (NSCLC) previously treated with platinum-containing regimen (abstract). *Proc Am Soc Clin Oncol.* 2007;25:7511.

26. Natale RB, Bodkin D, Govindan R, et al. Vandetanib versus gefitinib in patients with advanced non-small-cell lung cancer: results from a two-part, double-blind, randomized phase ii study. *J Clin Oncol.* 2009;27(15):2523–2529.

27. Heymach JV, Johnson BE, Prager D, et al. Randomized, placebo-controlled phase II study of vandetanib plus docetaxel in previously treated non small-cell lung cancer. *J Clin Oncol.* 2007;25(27):4270–4277.

28. Herbst RS, Sun Y, Korfee S, et al. Vandetanib plus docetaxel versus docetaxel as second-line treatment for patients with advanced non-small cell lung cancer (NSCLC): a randomized, double-blind phase III trial (ZODIAC) (abstract). *Proc Am Soc Clin Oncol.* 2009;27:8003CRA.

29. De Boer R, Arrieta O, Gottfried M, et al. Vandetanib plus pemetrexed versus pemetrexed as second-line therapy in patients with advanced non-small cell lung cancer (NSCLC): a randomized, double-blind phase III trial (ZEAL) (abstract). *Proc Am Soc Clin Oncol.* 2009;27:8010a.

30. Natale RB, Thongprasert S, Greco FA, et al. Vandetanib versus erlotinib in patients with advanced non-small cell lung cancer (NSCLC) after failure of at least one prior cytotoxic chemotherapy: a randomized, double-blind phase III trial (ZEST) (abstract). *Proc Am Soc Clin Oncol.* 2009;27:8009a.

31. Gatzemeier U, Blumenschein G, Fossella F, et al. Phase II trial of single-agent sorafenib in patients with advanced non-small cell lung carcinoma (abstract). *Proc Am Soc Clin Oncol.* 2006; 18:7002.

32. Schiller JH, Lee JW, Hanna NH, Traynor AM, Carbone DP. A randomized discontinuation phase II study of sorafenib versus placebo in patients with non-small cell lung cancer who have failed at least two prior chemotherapy regimens: E2501 (abstract). *Proc Am Soc Clin Oncol.* 2008;26:8014a.

33. Socinski MA, Novello S, Brahmer JR, et al. Multicenter, phase II trial of sunitinib in previously treated, advanced non-small-cell lung cancer. *J Clin Oncol.* 2008;26(4):650–656.

34. Hanna N, Lilenbaum R, Ansari R, et al. Phase II trial of cetuximab in patients with previously treated non-small-cell lung cancer. *J Clin Oncol.* 2006;24(33):5253–5258.

35. Kim ES, Mauer AM, William WN Jr, et al. A phase 2 study of cetuximab in combination with docetaxel in chemotherapy-refractory/resistant patients with advanced nonsmall cell lung cancer. *Cancer.* 2009;115(8):1713–1722.

36. Li D, Ambrogio L, Shimamura T, et al. BIBW2992, an irreversible EGFR/HER2 inhibitor highly effective in preclinical lung cancer models. *Oncogene.* 2008;27(34):4702–4711.

37. Bean J, Riely GJ, Balak M, et al. Acquired resistance to epidermal growth factor receptor kinase inhibitors associated with a novel T854A mutation in a patient with EGFR-mutant lung adenocarcinoma. *Clin Cancer Res.* 2008;14(22):7519–7525.

38. Burris HA 3rd, Hurwitz HI, Dees EC, et al. Phase I safety, pharmacokinetics, and clinical activity study of lapatinib (GW572016), a reversible dual inhibitor of epidermal growth factor receptor tyrosine kinases, in heavily pretreated patients with metastatic carcinomas. *J Clin Oncol.* 2005;23(23):5305–5313.

39. Ross JS, Blumenschein GR, Dowlati A, et al. Preliminary safety results of a phase II trial comparing two schedules of lapatinib (GW572016) as first line therapy for advanced or metastatic non-small cell lung cancer (abstract). *Proc Am Soc Clin Oncol.* 2005;16:7099.

40. Ramlau R, Thomas M, Plummer R, et al. Phase I study of lapatinib, a dual-tyrosine kinase inhibitor, and pemetrexed in the second-line treatment of advanced or metastatic non-small cell lung cancer (abstract). *Proc Am Soc Clin Oncol.* 2009;27:19027e.

41. Fanucchi MP, Fossella FV, Belt R, et al. Randomized phase II study of bortezomib alone and bortezomib in combination with docetaxel in previously treated advanced non-small-cell lung cancer. *J Clin Oncol.* 2006;24(31):5025–5033.

42. Davies AM, Chansky K, Lara PN Jr, et al.; Southwest Oncology Group. Bortezomib plus gemcitabine/carboplatin as first-line treatment of advanced non-small cell lung cancer: a phase II Southwest Oncology Group Study (S0339). *J Thorac Oncol.* 2009;4(1):87–92.

43. Carducci MA, Musib L, Kies MS, et al. Phase I dose escalation and pharmacokinetic study of enzastaurin, an oral protein kinase C beta inhibitor, in patients with advanced cancer. *J Clin Oncol.* 2006;24(25):4092–4099.

44. Oh Y, Herbst RS, Burris H, et al. Enzastaurin, an oral serine/threonine kinase inhibitor, as second- or third-line therapy of non-small-cell lung cancer. *J Clin Oncol.* 2008;26(7):1135–1141.

17 Conformal Radiotherapy for Non–Small Cell and Small Cell Lung Cancer: Primary, Metastatic, and Recurrent Disease

CHARLOTTE DAI KUBICKY

JOHN M. HOLLAND

■ INTENSITY-MODULATED RADIATION THERAPY FOR LOCOREGIONALLY ADVANCED NON–SMALL CELL LUNG CARCINOMA

Intensity-modulated radiation therapy (IMRT) can deliver a more conformal dose of radiation than three-dimensional conformal radiation (3D-CRT) potentially resulting in better sparing of normal tissues, increased dose to the tumor, and enhancement of the therapeutic ratio.

Radiation therapy has long been used in an attempt to manage locoregionally advanced lung cancer. Even when combining radiation therapy with chemotherapy, results to date have been unsatisfactory. Overall survival rates are low, thus revealing the limitation of thoracic radiation and suboptimal local control. Le Chevalier et al. (1) evaluated radiotherapy alone versus radiotherapy combined with vindesine, cyclophosphamide, cisplatin, and lomustine chemotherapy. In this study, using 2.5 Gy fractions to a total dose of 65 Gy, local control was assessed by bronchoscopy and found to be lacking: only 15% after both chemotherapy and radiation.

Escalation of radiation dose may be a way to improve outcomes for stage III non–small cell lung cancer (NSCLC). Radiobiologically, the concept of dose response is appealing and there is data supporting its use in lung cancer. Bradley et al. (2) reported results from Radiation Therapy Oncology Group (RTOG) 9311, a phase I–II dose-escalation study utilizing 3D-CRT for inoperable NSCLC. Stratifying dose escalation based on total volume of lung receiving >20 Gy (V20), radiation dose was safely escalated to 83.8 Gy for patients with lung V20 <25% and to 77.4 Gy for patients with V20 between 25% and 36% using 2.15 Gy fractions. Escalation to 90.3 Gy was found to be too toxic with two treatment-related deaths. In reviewing the topic of dose escalation, Bradley (3) concluded that

"when concurrent chemotherapy and 3D-CRT are used, the maximum tolerated dose of radiation is reduced, and current indications suggest the maximum tolerated dose in this setting is in the range of 70 to 74 Gy." Newlin et al. (4) reported improved cause-specific survival and overall survival when using doses of 65 Gy or higher for unresectable squamous cell carcinoma of the lung.

Limiting successful dose escalation to tumor is, of course, the dose of radiation to critical normal thoracic organs including the heart, esophagus, and especially the lung. The sensitivity of the lung to radiation can be a particular challenge to dose escalation. The primary clinical toxicities are radiation pneumonitis and fibrosis. Various dosimetric and clinical factors have been associated with the development of radiation pneumonitis in a retrospective review of 223 patients receiving concurrent chemotherapy and 3D-CRT (5). On univariate analysis, many factors including lung volume, gross tumor volume (GTV), mean lung dose, and relative V5 through V65 (in increments of 5 Gy) were significantly associated with the development of grade 3 or higher pneumonitis. However, on multivariate analysis, relative V5 (rV5) was the most significant factor associated with the development of pneumonitis. When the volume of lung receiving 5 Gy was more than 42%, pneumonitis developed in 38% compared with only 3% if the rV5 was 42% or less.

With its more conformal dose distribution, IMRT-based treatment planning and delivery should allow for better sparing of normal tissues including uninvolved lung, thus leading to a diminished incidence of radiation pneumonitis. Comparing 3D-CRT with IMRT in the treatment of inoperable NSCLC, Grills et al. (6) found a benefit when using IMRT over 3D-CRT in lymph node–positive patients. When considering normal-tissue tolerances, IMRT was found capable of delivering doses 25% to 30% more than 3D-CRT in node-positive patients. Investigators at M.D. Anderson have been active in researching IMRT for locoregionally advanced NSCLC. Murshed et al. (7) reviewed 41 patients with advanced-stage NSCLC previously planned via 3D-CRT. IMRT plans were designed to

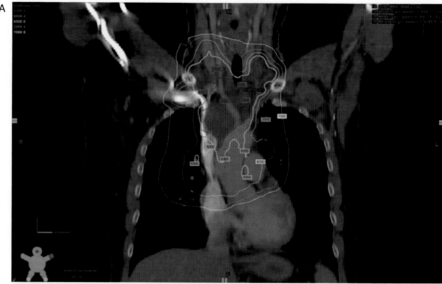

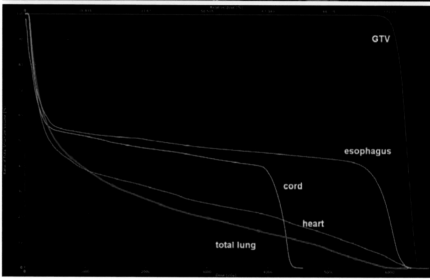

FIGURE 17.1 (A) Coronal display of isodose lines covering a locoregionally advanced non–small cell lung cancer (NSCLC) with bilateral supraclavicular adenopathy using intensity-modulated radiation therapy (IMRT). The red isodose line represents 6,500 cGy, the pink 6,000 cGy, the blue 4,500 cGy, the orange 2,000 cGy, and the white represents the 1,000 cGy isodose line. (B) Dose volume histogram (DVH) for this locoregionally advanced NSCLC treated with IMRT. Despite the bilateral supraclavicular nodal disease, the spinal cord maximum dose is good (<46 Gy) and the volume of normal lung irradiated is reasonable (V20 27%, V5 50%). GTV coverage is fair with V60 97%.

deliver 63 Gy to 95% of the planning target volume (PTV) using nine coplanar beams of 6 MV photons. With IMRT, the median absolute reduction in the percent lung volume receiving >10 and >20 Gy was 7% and 10%, respectively. This was felt to translate into a projected 10% reduction in clinical radiation pneumonitis. Using IMRT also led to reductions in the volumes of esophagus and heart receiving >40 Gy. IMRT plans did result in a slight increase in the maximal dose to the spinal cord and the amount of lung volume receiving >5 Gy. In a prospective study of an additional 10 NSCLC patients, Liu et al. (8) compared 3D-CRT with nine-beam IMRT and found an 8% median reduction in the volume of lung receiving >20 Gy using IMRT. Further reductions in the >5 Gy and >10 Gy volumes were more challenging with IMRT but felt to be achievable when fewer than nine beams were utilized. Christian et al. (9) also found improved dosimetry using IMRT over 3D-CRT in 10 patients with localized NSCLC. Here, IMRT plans utilizing nine coplanar beams were found to provide significantly improved percentages

of the PTV covered by the 90% isodose line and decreased amount of lung volume receiving >20 Gy compared with 3D-CRT or IMRT plans using fewer coplanar beams.

Yom et al. (10) reviewed the development of treatment-related pneumonitis in 151 NSCLC patients treated at M.D. Anderson with concurrent chemotherapy and IMRT. Most of these patients had "large, fixed tumors when acceptable 3D-CRT plans were difficult to achieve." Four-dimensional (4D) computed tomography (CT) scanning was used to account for respiration-induced tumor motion. Using this 4D CT imaging, the GTV was expanded to include tumor excursion during all phases of the respiratory cycle. An 8-mm margin was added to this GTV to create a clinical tumor volume (CTV). An additional 10 mm was added to the CTV to account for treatment uncertainties to create the PTV.

For most patients in this review, 63 Gy was delivered to the PTV with 180 cGy daily fractions. Lung dose objectives were set to limit the relative volume of lung treated to doses above 5, 10, and 20 Gy to less than 65%, 50%,

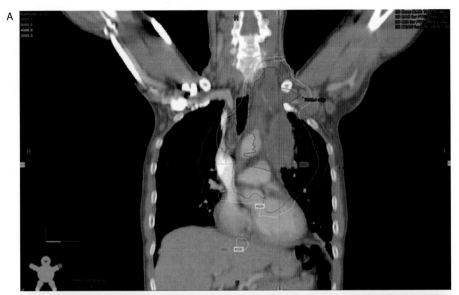

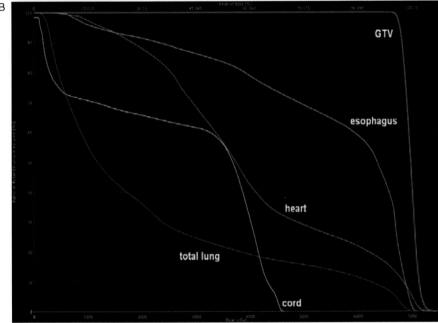

FIGURE 17.2 (A) Coronal display of iso-dose lines covering an advanced non–small cell lung cancer (NSCLC) with left supraclavicular and right mediastinal adenopathy using intensity-modulated radiation therapy (IMRT). The red isodose line represents 6,500 cGy, the pink 6,000 cGy, the yellow 4,500 cGy, and the green represents the 2,000 cGy isodose line. (B) DVH for this advanced NSCLC treated with IMRT. The dose to the GTV is higher (V67 99%). The spinal cord maximum dose is good (<47 Gy). However, the dose to other volumes is greater: esophagus (V60 59%) and lung (V20 36%, V5 78%).

and 35%, respectively. Most patients were treated with five or six coplanar 6 MV photon beams. Amifostine, a daily preradiation treatment intravenously administered cytoprotectant, was used in 16 patients with particularly large PTVs and lung V20 >35%.

Comparing pneumonitis outcomes in 222 patients with similar clinical-stage NSCLC treated with concurrent chemotherapy and 3D-CRT, the IMRT patients had a lower rate of developing ≥grade 3 pneumonitis. Even though the IMRT population had larger GTVs than the 3D-CRT group, the rate of pneumonitis at 12 months was 8% versus 32% in the 3D-CRT population. IMRT resulted in lower volumes of lung receiving ≥20 Gy compared with the 3D-CRT patients ($P < 0.001$). However, in this series, IMRT did not lower the volume of lung receiving >10 Gy or >5 Gy. The relative amount of normal lung volume (rV) receiving 5 Gy was greater with IMRT (63%)

than with 3D-CRT (57%), $P = 0.011$. In fact, four of five IMRT patients developing high-grade pneumonitis had rV5 values more than 70%. The 12-month incidence of grade ≥3 pneumonitis for IMRT patients with rV5 ≤70% was only 2%. This rate of pneumonitis rose to 21% in the 22 patients with an rV5 >70%.

One approach to lower the rV5 is to try to reduce the beam angles and field segments along with less monitor units. Liu et al. (11) at M.D. Anderson have evaluated beam angle combinations to find the best angles to limit the number of beams. Using this beam angle optimization, the authors found that plans with seven or even five beams could achieve similar dosimetric quality to those plans using nine equal-spaced beam angles with fewer field segments and lower monitor units.

Of course, as important as limiting dose to normal lung may be, one of the appeals of IMRT is the potential

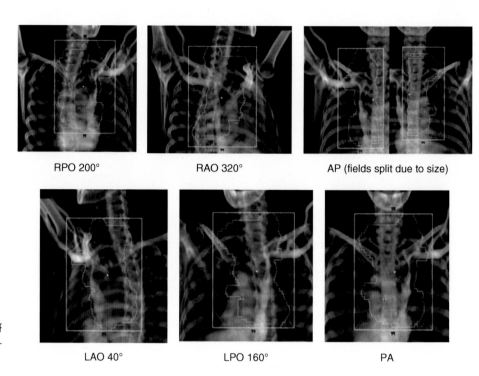

RPO 200°   RAO 320°   AP (fields split due to size)

LAO 40°   LPO 160°   PA

FIGURE 17.3 Beams eye views of six coplanar fields for a lung intensity-modulated radiation therapy plan.

for dose escalation in NSCLC. Schwarz et al. (12) performed a study on 10 NSCLC patients quantifying the amount of dose escalation possible by allowing dose heterogeneity within the treatment target and by using IMRT planning and delivery. By doing so, they found the overall dose could be escalated "as high as 35%" even for large and concave tumors. Further, they report no increase in the volume of lung receiving radiation "even doses to 5 Gy."

As exciting as IMRT with photons may prove to be, maybe the future belongs to protons. Zhang et al. (13) have performed a "virtual clinical study" comparing IMRT with intensity-modulated proton therapy (IMPT) in 10 selected patients with stage IIIB disease. These patients were chosen due to the extensive nature of their disease and were felt to be IMRT–dose limited at 60–63 Gy using constraints of lung volume receiving 20 Gy <35% and total mean lung dose <20 Gy. By using IMPT, there was improved sparing of lung, heart, esophagus, and spinal cord and dose could be escalated from the 63 Gy used in IMRT up to 83.5 Gy.

Respiratory motion can present challenges when using IMRT to increase precision for lung cancer radiotherapy. Compared with 3D-CRT, IMRT has steeper dose gradient and highly conformal dose distribution. A small shift in target position could result in a significant change in dose received by the intended target. Furthermore, a typical IMRT plan has multiple beam segments from each angle, treating only a partial target volume at any given time. Respiratory tumor motion can result in deviation from the planned dose distribution. Recognizing this concern, the Advanced Technology Consortium (http://atc.wustl.edu/

home/about/html) has developed guidelines when incorporating IMRT for thoracic malignancies (14). These recommendations have been communicated by the National Cancer Institute (NCI) to all clinical trial cooperatives. Special care must be taken during the planning CT to avoid motion effect. Several different techniques can be used including 4D CT, spirometry, abdominal compression, and inspiration/expiration scans on a fast CT scanner able to image the entire volume in one scan sequence for each phase of breathing. Onboard imaging to document positioning of normal tissues and targets is recommended. The International Commission of Radiation Units Report No. 50 established general guidelines for radiation target volumes for lung cancer. They include GTV, CTV, and PTV. In 1999, the guidelines were amended to include internal target volume (ITV) to account for tumor motion (15,16). We will discuss the definition of these target volumes and ways to optimize them using various imaging tools for radiation treatment planning.

GTV is defined as visible tumor by any imaging modality. It is traditionally defined on CT, by using the pulmonary window for the primary tumor and the mediastinal window for mediastinal tumor extension and positive lymph nodes. Lymph nodes more than 1 cm in the short axis are considered positive. Recently, utilization of positron emission tomography (PET)/CT has had a significant impact in radiotherapy treatment planning. PET/CT is particularly helpful in distinguishing primary tumors from atelectasis and identifying positive mediastinal or hilar lymph nodes. A positive PET or PET/CT in the mediastinum requires pathologic confirmation. Endobronchial ultrasound–fine-needle aspiration (EBUS-FNA), or endoscopic ultrasound–fine needle aspiration (EUS-FNA), or mediastinoscopy, or video-assisted surgical mediastinal evaluation is necessary to obtain greater certainty of mediastinal involvement. Further information on this subject can be found in chapters dealing with surgery and with lung cancer staging. A number of studies have demonstrated that incorporation of PET or PET/CT significantly altered radiation treatment volume, resulting in more accurate GTV delineation (17). Reduction of target volume also allows further dose escalation without increasing normal-tissue toxicity.

CTV is defined as the anatomic region of microscopic disease around GTV. An elegant pathologic analysis by Giraud et al. showed that in order to account for 95% of microscopic disease extension, a margin of 8 mm is needed for adenocarcinoma and 6 mm for squamous cell carcinoma (18). Assuming the radiographic border of tumor is the same as that observed on gross examination, many centers are now routinely performing 8-mm expansion to obtain CTV. The expansion should be nonuniform, following the natural path of spread, and should not cross over anatomic boundaries such as the airway, heart, chest wall, vertebral bodies, unless otherwise indicated on imaging.

In 1999, ICRU 62 introduced the concept of internal margin and ITV to specifically address respiratory and tumor motion. It accounts for "variations in size, shape, and position of the CTV in relation to anatomical reference points." Geographic miss due to respiratory motion is an important cause of local failure after radiotherapy. To accurately account for or suppress tumor motion several different techniques can be used, including 4D CT, inspiration/expiration scans, abdominal compression, respiratory gating, and real-time tumor tracking. Following is a brief description of each technique. Some of the techniques will be discussed in detail in the chapter on stereotactic body radiation therapy.

During a 4D CT simulation, CT images are acquired over consecutive phases of the respiratory cycle. Each image is then registered to one of the 10 phases of the cycle. By overlaying the images from all 10 phases, motion envelope of the tumor can be traced, covering all possible positions of the tumor during a respiratory cycle. This technique is suitable for patients with regular and reproducible respiration. Additional coaching may be needed to enforce breathing regularity and hence minimize internal margins. When 4D CT is not available, another approach is to have the patient hold his/her breath twice during simulation, once at the end of expiration and once at the end of inspiration. Both sets of CT images are acquired and registered to the same patient positioning references. GTV and CTV then are delineated for each. The two sets of GTVs and CTVs are superimposed to form ITV.

Abdominal compression is a widely used method to limit diaphragmatic movement and decrease ITV. A number of studies have shown improved overall tumor motion or superior-inferior motion using this technique (19).

Potential drawbacks of abdominal compression are patient discomfort, inability to comply with the procedure, or changes in respiratory status or abdominal girth, causing day-to-day variability in the level of compression.

Respiratory gating is a technique to decrease ITV and reduce the volume of irradiated normal tissue. In gated radiotherapy, the beam is turned on only during a certain phase of the respiratory cycle, generally the end of expiration. Respiration is monitored using external markers placed on the patient's chest, which are assumed to move similarly to the tumor. This is suitable for patients who can breathe regularly and reproducibly. Potential drawbacks of this approach are prolonged treatment time and a lack of direct imaging of tumor position during treatment.

Another method to decrease ITV is to continuously synchronize radiation treatment delivery with target movement. Real-time tracking is more commonly used in stereotactic radiosurgery where a much higher dose per fraction and a steeper dose gradient is delivered, compared with conventional radiation. Treatment volume must be limited to minimize doses to normal tissue. A good example is Cyberknife Synchrony system (Accuray Inc, Sunnyvale, CA), where a linear accelerator is mounted on a robotic arm. This is coupled with in-room stereoscopic x-ray imaging device that continuously obtains real-time positioning of the tumor or of previously placed fiducial markers. The robotic arm then adjusts and synchronizes treatment delivery with respiratory-induced tumor motion throughout the cycle. Similar technology using robotic treatment couch for synchronized radiation delivery is being developed. This technology will be discussed in detail in a later chapter on stereotactic body radiation therapy.

When tumor motion is accounted for by ITV, PTV is obtained by adding a margin around ITV to allow for daily setup errors. PTV should be determined for each individual patient, based on immobilization and setup techniques used. Daily onboard imaging using either cone-beam CT or orthogonal pairs is highly recommended to verify baseline organ positions and to minimize day-to-day setup error.

To date, most practitioners have limited their use of IMRT in lung cancer to patients with exceptionally bulky disease or tumors with bilateral supraclavicular or hilar adenopathy. In such cases, IMRT's improved conformality has definite appeal. While IMRT may allow for less volume of lung receiving 20 Gy compared with 3D-CRT, there remain serious questions on its ability to limit the amount of lung receiving 5 Gy. This rV5 may be a problem in limiting the development of clinical pneumonitis especially when using IMRT planning with standard nine angle beam arrangements. Still, as technical advancements are made, dose escalation has become possible. Clinicians are hopeful that IMRT notwithstanding the lack of any head-to-head comparison with 3D-CRT in prospective phase III clinical trial setting, with improved target coverage and increased radiation dose to the tumor, will lead to improved outcomes for patients with locoregionally advanced NSCLC.

■ CONFORMAL RADIATION IN THE RETREATMENT OF RECURRENT OR PERSISTENT NSCLC

Unfortunately, local and regional recurrence after definitive thoracic radiotherapy remains a clinically significant problem in NSCLC. Often, these failures are symptomatic causing hemoptysis and obstruction. Radiation oncologists are then presented with the challenge of delivering further meaningful therapy to a volume including normal tissues of lung, esophagus, heart, and spinal cord that have already received high doses of radiation. Fortunately, the literature supports the ability to use reirradiation in this situation.

Montebello et al. (20) retrospectively reviewed 30 patients who had received a median dose of 60 Gy over 6 weeks at initial therapy. The median time from initial treatment to recurrence was 12 months. Symptomatic response to reirradiation was seen in 70% with toxicities including esophagitis (20%) and pneumonitis (3%). The authors concluded that reirradiation using doses "in the range of 2000–3000 cGy in 2 to 3 weeks appears safe and effective in reirradiating recurrent bronchogenic carcinoma."

Kramer et al. (21) continued on this concept of palliative reirradiation for recurrent NSCLC but used a hypofractionated approach with two fractions of 8 Gy separated by 1 week. Median time from initial radiotherapy to reirradiation was 17 months (range 6–72 months). Symptoms of hemoptysis and superior vena cava obstruction were relieved in all patients but this therapy was less effective in relieving cough (67%) and dyspnea (35%). The median duration of the palliative benefit using this brief course was 4 months. Toxicities included 5/28 (18%) suffering fatal hemoptysis and one death from bronchoesophageal fistula (4%).

Okamoto et al. (22) evaluated the safety and efficacy of dose escalation in reirradiation for locally recurrent lung cancer after prior radiotherapy. In this series of 34 patients recurring after a median prior dose of 60 Gy, 18 patients received "radical treatment" of 50 to 70 Gy with the goal of achieving a cure or at least meaningful prolongation of life. An additional 16 patients received "symptomatic treatment" with doses limited to that "which could relieve each symptom." The median interval between the initial radiotherapy to reirradiation was 23 months (range 5–87 months). All treatment was delivered via parallel-opposed fields with limited volumes. For radical retreatment, the volume included only the detected measurable recurrent tumor. For symptomatic therapy, the volume was further limited to only "the affected region." Overall response rates were good: 78% after radical therapy and 75% after symptomatic therapy. Radical treatment resulted in a survival rate of 51% at 2 years (compared with no survivors in the symptomatic therapy group). After reirradiation, grade 3 pneumonitis occurred in seven patients (21%) and grade 3 esophagitis occurred in two patients (6%). No case of myelopathy was associated with reirradiation. Here, "radical" reirradiation for select patients was shown to result in meaningful survival at 2 years.

Tada et al. (23) confirmed that reirradiation with doses of 50 to 60 Gy could be utilized. These authors found a 2-year survival rate of 11%. Patients with time intervals between radiotherapeutic courses of more than 18 months had better outcomes and were felt to be particularly good candidates for reirradiation. However, patients with poor performance status (ECOG 3) did not do well with a median survival time of only 1 month.

Wu et al. (24) utilized 3D-CRT for their reirradiation of locoregionally recurrent lung cancer in a prospective phase I–II trial. Here, 23 patients received a median dose of 66 Gy during their first course of radiotherapy. Reirradiation was performed utilizing 3D-CRT. A margin of 1.5 to 2 cm was extended from the GTV to generate a PTV. No elective nodal radiation was performed. Spinal cord dose was restricted to <25 Gy for the second radiation course. Multiple noncoplanar field arrangements were often used, with generally four to five fields or a dynamic arc technique employed. The median time interval from initial radiotherapy to reirradiation was 13 months. The median reirradiation dose was 51 Gy (range: 46–60 Gy). The 1- and 2-year survival rates following reirradiation were 59% and 21%, respectively. No grade 3 esophagitis or pneumonitis has been observed. Grade 2 or 3 pulmonary fibrosis did develop in 26%. Overall, the authors conclude that "high doses of reirradiation by 3D-CRT can be given safely and successfully to this group of patients with locally recurrent lung carcinoma."

Finally, Beavis et al. (25) have utilized an IMRT approach for lung cancer reirradiation. In this case report, the authors used constraints based upon prior dose to the spinal cord and the heart and found improved target coverage using IMRT. Using a "simple" four-field IMRT plan, they were able to provide 100% coverage of the PTV by the 95% isodose line while a conventional plan resulted in only 77% coverage.

In conclusion, high-dose lung reirradiation using conformal techniques is possible. Doses of 50 to 60 Gy can be utilized safely with appropriate dose limits to the spinal cord, lung, and heart. Radiation volumes should be limited, and there is no clear role for elective nodal radiation. Appropriate patients should have reasonable performance status. Patients with longer intervals between radiation courses may particularly benefit from high-dose conformal reirradiation.

■ CONFORMAL RADIOTHERAPY FOR SMALL CELL LUNG CANCER

Small cell lung cancer (SCLC) accounts for approximately 13% of all lung cancers diagnosed in the United States each year (26). Traditionally, they have been classified as limited-stage and extensive-stage, according to the *Veterans Administration Lung Cancer Study Group*. Limited-stage is defined as disease that can be encompassed within one tolerable radiation portal, which includes primary tumor within one hemithorax, mediastinal lymph nodes, and ipsilateral supraclavicular fossa. Extensive-stage includes disease outside of those regions. However, whether contralateral hilar and supraclavicular lymph nodes are considered extensive-stage is an area of controversy. In a recent Surveillance, Epidemiology, and End Results analysis, about 40% of SCLCs were limited-stage (26).

The use of chemotherapy has significantly improved the outcome of patients with SCLC. Because small cell carcinoma by nature is a systemic disease, in limited-stage disease, whether local control in the thorax can have an impact on overall survival was questioned. At least 16 randomized trials were conducted trying to address this question. Among them, some showed a small survival benefit with the addition of thoracic radiation to chemotherapy, while others showed no benefit or even a survival detriment. However, most of the trials lack the statistical power to detect a 5% to 10% difference in survival at 5 years. To clarify this issue, two meta-analyses were conducted and both were published in 1992 (27,28). Warde and Payne (27) performed a meta-analysis of 11 randomized trials comparing chemotherapy alone versus chemotherapy and thoracic radiation. Radiation improved 2-year survival by 5.4% (95% confidence interval [CI], 1.1–9.7%) and intrathoracic tumor control by 25.3% (95% CI, 16.5–34.1%). This improvement in disease control was associated with a small increase of treatment-related death 1.2% (95% CI, –0.6% to 3.0%). Pignon et al. (28) conducted a meta-analysis of 2,140 patients from 13 randomized clinical trials that compared chemotherapy alone versus chemotherapy combined with thoracic radiation. Radiation improved 3-year overall survival by 5.4% ± 1.4%. The survival benefit was the greatest in patients younger than 55 years. Results of these two meta-analyses clearly established the role of thoracic radiation in the treatment of limited-stage SCLC.

■ TIMING OF RADIATION

Although there was a well-demonstrated overall survival benefit of thoracic radiation, when radiation should be administered remained a question. The randomized trials included in the meta-analyses incorporated concurrent, alternating, and sequential radiation. Among those administering concurrent radiation, some were initiated with the first cycle of chemo, while others were with subsequent cycles. In the meta-analysis by Pignon et al. (28), indirect comparisons of early versus late and sequential versus nonsequential radiotherapy approaches did not reveal any optimal strategies.

The NCI of Canada conducted a phase III trial comparing early versus late radiation (29). Three hundred and eight patients with limited-stage small cell carcinoma were randomized to initiating radiation with the second cycle of chemotherapy versus the sixth cycle of chemotherapy. Chemotherapy was cyclophosphamide, doxorubicin, and vincristine alternating with cisplatin and etoposide. In both arms, radiation was 40 Gy in 1.5 Gy fractions over 3 weeks. Early radiation resulted in a significant improvement of progression-free survival (26% vs. 19%, $P = 0.04$), overall survival (39.7% vs. 21.5%, $P = 0.008$) at 3 years, and a lower incidence of relapse in the brain ($P = 0.006$). Interestingly, the complete response rates were not different between the early (69.3%) and the late radiation arm (55.6%), neither were the rates of local recurrence ($P = 0.28$). Patients who received early radiation had higher incidence of esophagitis. These findings suggest the importance of early radiation in systemic disease control.

The Japan Clinical Oncology Group conducted a phase III study of concurrent versus sequential thoracic radiotherapy in combination with cisplatin and etoposide (30). Radiation was 45 Gy (1.5 Gy twice daily) over 3 weeks in both arms. Two hundred and thirty-one patients with limited-stage disease were randomized to either starting radiation with the first cycle of chemotherapy versus after the last cycle. Concurrent radiotherapy improved median survival from 27.2 months to 19.7 months ($P = 0.097$), and 5-year overall survival from 18.3% to 23.7%.

De Ruysscher et al. (31) identified treatment time as the single most important predictor of outcome. In a meta-analysis of four randomized trials, they examined the influence of time, defined as start of any treatment to the end of radiotherapy (SER), on treatment outcome. They showed that SER less than 30 days was associated with significant improvement in 5-year survival. A similar observation has been made in definitive treatment of head and neck cancer using concurrent chemoradiotherapy, where prolonged treatment breaks correlate with poor local control and survival. The findings suggest accelerated repopulation, and development of radio- and chemoresistant clones may play an important role in treatment failures. Therefore, intensifying treatment upfront with concurrent radiation during the early phase of chemotherapy is crucial in achieving good disease control.

■ DOSE AND FRACTIONATION

What is the optimal dose and fractionation of radiation? Small cell carcinomas are known to be highly radio- and chemosensitive. In vitro studies of SCLC cell lines showed remarkable sensitivity to radiation, even at low doses. The dose-response curves for small cell lack a shoulder, suggesting that exponential cell killing occurs even at low doses. On the other hand, late-responding tissue including most normal tissues in the thorax display a shoulder, suggesting more tissue sparing at low doses. For these reasons, a hyperfractionated and accelerated radiation scheme was developed for small cell carcinomas in order to take advantage of exponential cell kill and at the same time reducing permanent damage to the normal tissues (32).

Based on some promising results of a pilot study, Turrisi et al. (33) conducted a randomized phase III study (RTOG 8815, Intergroup 0096) of concurrent chemotherapy with two radiation regimens. Chemotherapy consisted of four cycles of VP-16 and cisplatin. The first two cycles were administered concurrently with radiation, followed by two additional cycles. Patients were randomized to either 45 Gy in 25 fractions (1.8 Gy once daily) or 45 Gy in 30 fractions (1.5 Gy twice daily). For the twice-daily radiation, radiation portals were AP/PA in the am and pm during week 1, AP/PA in the am and off-cord oblique angles in the pm during week 2 and 3 to spare to the spinal cord. Radiation target included the gross tumor, as defined by chest CT, bilateral mediastinal, and ipsilateral hilar nodes. Irradiation of uninvolved supraclavicular fossa was not permitted. Patients with complete response were offered prophylactic cranial irradiation. At 5 years, twice-daily radiation significantly improved overall survival from 16% to 26%. Grade 3 and 4 esophagitis was significantly higher in the twice-daily radiation group (32% vs. 16%). This study established the current standard of care of concurrent chemotherapy and twice-daily radiotherapy.

■ DOSE ESCALATION

In the Turrisi study, it is often argued that 45 Gy given in 1.8 Gy daily fractions was radiobiologically inferior compared with 45 Gy given in 1.5 Gy twice-daily fractions. It remains unclear if twice-daily radiation is truly superior to once-daily radiation when given at a biologically equivalent dose. In addition, twice-daily radiation can be logistically difficult at many centers and the risk of esophagitis is particularly high. Moreover, even in the winning arm of the study, local failure rate was unacceptably high at 36% (33). For these reasons, studies have been designed to investigate alternative dosing and fractionation schedules that may be more effective.

Choi et al. (34) conducted phase I dose-escalation studies to determine the maximum tolerated dose of twice-daily radiotherapy and once-daily radiotherapy with concurrent PCE/PE chemotherapy (cisplatin, cyclophosphamide, etoposide/cisplatin, etoposide). Chemotherapy consisted of three cycles of PCE, followed by two cycles of PE. Radiation was administered at the start of the fourth cycle of chemotherapy. 45 Gy in 30 fractions (1.5 Gy twice daily) over 3 weeks was determined to be the maximum tolerated dose for twice-daily radiation. For once-daily radiation, 70 Gy in 35 fractions (2 Gy once daily) over 7 weeks was the maximum tolerated dose. This was based on 29% and 33% incidence of grade 4 or 5 esophagitis and 43% and 50% incidence of grade 4 granulocytopenia, for twice-daily and once-daily radiation, respectively.

RTOG 0241 (35) is a phase I study of escalating doses of irinotecan with fixed doses of cisplatin in combination with twice-daily radiation to 45 Gy or once-daily radiation to 70 Gy. Early analysis of the results showed that dose-limiting toxicity was seen at 50 mg/m² irinotecan and 70 Gy with grade 4 diarrhea and esophagitis.

RTOG 9712 (36) tested an alternative strategy for dose escalation. It is a phase I trial designed to determine the maximum tolerated dose of thoracic radiation using a concomitant boost approach. Radiation was once daily 1.8 Gy to 36 Gy to a large field, followed by 1.8 Gy twice daily to a reduced volume for the last 3, 5, 7, 9, and 11 treatment days, for a total dose of 50.4, 54, 57.6, 61.2, and 64.8 Gy, respectively. Chemotherapy was cisplatin and etoposide, with concurrent thoracic radiotherapy for two cycles, starting on day 1, followed by two adjuvant cycles. A total dose of 61.2 Gy in 34 fractions was determined to be the maximum tolerated dose. Treatment outcome was excellent at this dose, with 82% survival at 18 months.

Based on the promising results of RTOG 9712, a phase II study RTOG 0239 (37) was designed to further evaluate the efficacy of this concomitant boost approach. 61.2 Gy, the maximum tolerated dose determined by RTOG 9712, was used as the total radiation dose in this trial. Radiation was delivered to a large field to 30.6 Gy in 1.8 Gy daily fractions, followed by 1.8 Gy twice daily (AP/PA to the large field in am, boost field in pm) for eight fractions, followed by 1.8 Gy twice-daily off-cord boost fields for the final 10 fractions. Total dose to the large field was 36 Gy. Chemotherapy was administered in a similar fashion as RTOG 9712. Seventy-two patients were accrued, 71 were eligible. Two-year local control and overall survival were 80% and 37%, respectively. The incidence of acute severe esophagitis was acceptable at 18%.

With two promising strategies of dose escalation, a randomized trial was opened. RTOG 0538/Cancer And Leukemia Group B 30610 is an ongoing phase III trial comparing three radiation regimens, 45 Gy in 1.5 Gy twice-daily fractions (winning arm INT 0096), 70 Gy once daily (RTOG 0241), and 61.2 Gy with concomitant boost (RTOG 0239). The trial was activated in March 2008 and results are eagerly awaited.

■ RADIATION VOLUME

An obvious way to achieve dose escalation without significantly increasing normal-tissue toxicity is to reduce target volume. In non–small cell lung carcinoma, omitting elective nodal irradiation has not resulted in increased nodal failures(2,38–40). Rosenzweig et al. reported a 6% elective nodal failure rate in NSCLC. Emami et al. evaluated infield progression and overall survival of patients in relation to adequacy of nodal coverage in four large RTOG trials. They found that neither infield progression nor 2-year survival was affected by coverage in the uninvolved mediastinum, contralateral hilum, or ipsilateral supraclavicular fossa.

Can we reduce the volume of radiation and toxicity by omitting elective lymph node irradiation in small cell carcinoma? Ruysscher et al. conducted a phase II trial of omitting elective node irradiation in patients with limited-disease SCLC. Target delineation was based on the pretreatment CT scan. Only the primary tumor and enlarged lymph nodes were included. In the 27 patients enrolled, 3 (11%) developed nodal failure outside of radiation field. All three failures were in the nonirradiated ipsilateral supraclavicular fossa, which is not normally covered in the radiation volume (41).

Whether or not we can omit elective nodal irradiation in small cell lung carcinoma remains controversial. The original Turrisi study required coverage of the bilateral mediastinal and ipsilateral hilum (33). However, due to the need for dose escalation and radiation volume reduction, recent RTOG trials have moved away from elective nodal irradiation. With improvement of functional imaging technologies and incorporation of PET/CT and minimally invasive mediastinal assessing technologies, we may be able to identify "occult" lymph nodes and more accurately define target volume. Two small prospective studies have shown that use of PET altered disease staging in 8.3% and 17% of cases (42,43). One showed that PET identified unsuspected lymph node metastasis in 25% of patients (43), although no pathologic confirmation was obtained. Rigorous use of PET and EUS/EBUS endobronchial assessment and, as necessary, mediastinoscopy and/or video-assisted mediastinal surgical staging may eventually obviate the need for elective nodal irradiation in small cell carcinomas.

■ PROPHYLACTIC CRANIAL IRRADIATION

Brain metastasis is extremely common in SCLC. About 10% of patients have brain metastasis at diagnosis; the incidence rises to more than 50% by 2 years (44). As local and systemic disease control improves with combination chemoradiotherapy, brain metastasis as the first site of failure becomes a significant problem. A number of randomized trials have demonstrated the benefit of prophylactic cranial irradiation in reducing brain metastasis. However, no clear overall survival benefit was demonstrated by individual trials.

Aupérin et al. (44) conducted a meta-analysis of 987 patients from seven randomized clinical trials, comparing the outcomes with and without prophylactic cranial irradiation, after a complete response to initial therapy. Prophylactic cranial irradiation was shown to improve overall survival by 5.4% at 3 years (from 15.3% to 20.7%, $P < 0.01$) and decrease the incidence of brain metastasis by 46% ($P < 0.001$).

In the meta-analysis, Aupérin et al. also investigated radiation dose through indirect comparisons. Larger doses of radiation correlated with lower incidence of brain metastasis. The relative risks of developing brain metastasis were 76% after 8 Gy in 1 fraction, 52% after 24 to 25 Gy in 8 to 12 fractions, 34% with 30 Gy in 10 fractions and 36 to 40 Gy in 18 to 20 fractions ($P = 0.02$), suggesting a potential dose-response relationship (44).

To further test of dose-response relationship and to determine the optimal dose and fractionation schedule of prophylactic cranial irradiation, RTOG 0212/EORTC 22–03-08004/IFCT 99–01/PCI 99–01 compared standard dose of 25 Gy in 10 fractions with a higher dose of 36 Gy in conventional fractions (18 daily fractions of 2 Gy) or accelerated hyperfractionation (24 twice-daily fractions of 1.5 Gy). There was no significant difference in the 2-year incidence of brain metastasis, but a lower overall survival was found in the high-dose group, compared with the low dose group (37% vs 42%, $P = 0.05$). Therefore, 25 Gy in 10 fractions became the standard of care for prophylactic cranial irradiation for SCLC.

What is the role of prophylactic cranial irradiation in extensive-stage SCLC? The majority of patients in the meta-analysis were of limited-stage disease. About 16% had extensive-stage disease. Whether prophylactic cranial irradiation can improve survival in this group of patients was investigated by the EORTC (45) in a phase III randomized trial. Two hundred and eighty-six patients with extensive-stage SCLC who have had a response to chemotherapy were randomized to undergo prophylactic cranial irradiation versus no further therapy. Prophylactic cranial irradiation improved median survival from 5.4 months to 6.7 months ($P = 0.003$) and 1-year survival from 13.3% to 27.1%.

In summary, prophylactic cranial irradiation should be offered to patients with either limited-stage or extensive-stage disease who have a complete or partial response to initial chemotherapy or chemoradiotherapy. Prophylactic cranial irradiation should not be offered to patients with very poor performance status or cognitive function. A short interval between chemoradiotherapy and prophylactic cranial irradiation is preferred. 25 Gy in 10 daily fractions is the current standard of care.

■ SUMMARY AND NEW DIRECTIONS

Use of IMRT in locoregionally advanced NSCLC has becoming increasingly common. In patients with bulky disease, or bilateral supraclavicular or hilar adenopathy, IMRT offers superior dose distribution comparing with 3D-CRT. In some cases, IMRT is the only way we can achieve a desirable dose to the target. While IMRT may allow for less volume of lung receiving 20 Gy compared with 3D-CRT, there remain serious questions on its ability to limit the amount of lung receiving 5 Gy. Role of increased V5 in radiation pneumonitis or other long-term pulmonary complications required further investigations. When using IMRT, respiratory motion mitigation techniques are necessary to ensure accuracy of treatment, to prevent geographic misses, and to minimize normal-tissue toxicity. Reirradiation to 50 to 60 Gy using conformal techniques is possible with appropriate dose limits to the spinal cord, lung, and heart. Reirradiation volumes should be limited. Patients with longer intervals between radiation courses may particularly benefit from high-dose conformal reirradiation. Furthermore, emerging technology such as IMPT may play a role in the treatment of locally advanced NSCLC.

Randomized trials and meta-analyses have helped make great advances in the treatment of SCLC. In limited-stage disease, definitive chemoradiotherapy has been shown to improve survival compared with chemotherapy alone. Further studies demonstrated a benefit of concurrent over sequential and early over late radiotherapy. Because of the high prevalence of brain metastasis, prophylactic cranial irradiation is recommended for all SCLC patients who either have a complete or partial response to initial chemoradiotherapy or chemotherapy. The standard dose for prophylactic cranial irradiation is 25 Gy in 10 fractions. Future efforts are aimed at optimizing radiation delivery through dose escalation without increasing normal-tissue toxicity. One ongoing clinical trial is comparing different strategies of dose escalation and fractionation, twice daily to 45 Gy versus once daily to 70 Gy versus concomitant boost to 61.2 Gy. Incorporation of functional imaging, such as PET/CT may enhance staging accuracy, improve target delineation, and ultimately effect local control. PET/CT followed by pathologic confirmation may help identify "occult" lymph node metastasis, and may eventually obviate the need for elective nodal irradiation. Even though early investigations are encouraging, further studies are needed to establish the role of PET/CT in the management of SCLC. Lastly, new combination chemotherapy regimens or targeted biologics are being investigated for improved efficacy of systemic control.

■ REFERENCES

1. Le Chevalier T, Arriagada R, Quoix E, et al. Radiotherapy alone versus combined chemotherapy and radiotherapy in nonresectable non-small-cell lung cancer: first analysis of a randomized trial in 353 patients. *J Natl Cancer Inst.* 1991;83(6):417–423.

2. Bradley J, Graham MV, Winter K, et al. Toxicity and outcome results of RTOG 9311: a phase I-II dose-escalation study using three-dimensional conformal radiotherapy in patients with inoperable non-small-cell lung carcinoma. *Int J Radiat Oncol Biol Phys.* 2005;61(2):318–328.

3. Bradley J. A review of radiation dose escalation trials for non-small cell lung cancer within the Radiation Therapy Oncology Group. *Semin Oncol.* 2005;32(2 suppl 3):S111–S113.

4. Newlin HE, Iyengar M, Morris CG, Olivier K. Unresectable squamous cell carcinoma of the lung: an outcomes study. *Int J Radiat Oncol Biol Phys.* 2009;74(2):370–376.

5. Wang S, Liao Z, Wei X, et al. Analysis of clinical and dosimetric factors associated with treatment-related pneumonitis (TRP) in patients with non-small-cell lung cancer (NSCLC) treated with concurrent chemotherapy and three-dimensional conformal radiotherapy (3D-CRT). *Int J Radiat Oncol Biol Phys.* 2006;66(5):1399–1407.

6. Grills IS, Yan D, Martinez AA, Vicini FA, Wong JW, Kestin LL. Potential for reduced toxicity and dose escalation in the treatment of inoperable non-small-cell lung cancer: a comparison of intensity-modulated radiation therapy (IMRT), 3D conformal radiation, and elective nodal irradiation. *Int J Radiat Oncol Biol Phys.* 2003;57(3):875–890.

7. Murshed H, Liu HH, Liao Z, et al. Dose and volume reduction for normal lung using intensity-modulated radiotherapy for advanced-stage non-small-cell lung cancer. *Int J Radiat Oncol Biol Phys.* 2004;58(4):1258–1267.

8. Liu HH, Wang X, Dong L, et al. Feasibility of sparing lung and other thoracic structures with intensity-modulated radiotherapy for non-small-cell lung cancer. *Int J Radiat Oncol Biol Phys.* 2004;58(4):1268–1279.

9. Christian JA, Bedford JL, Webb S, Brada M. Comparison of inverse-planned three-dimensional conformal radiotherapy and intensity-modulated radiotherapy for non-small-cell lung cancer. *Int J Radiat Oncol Biol Phys.* 2007;67(3):735–741.

10. Yom SS, Liao Z, Liu HH, et al. Initial evaluation of treatment-related pneumonitis in advanced-stage non-small-cell lung cancer patients treated with concurrent chemotherapy and intensity-modulated radiotherapy. *Int J Radiat Oncol Biol Phys.* 2007;68(1):94–102.

11. Liu HH, Jauregui M, Zhang X, Wang X, Dong L, Mohan R. Beam angle optimization and reduction for intensity-modulated radiation therapy of non-small-cell lung cancers. *Int J Radiat Oncol Biol Phys.* 2006;65(2):561–572.

12. Schwarz M, Alber M, Lebesque JV, Mijnheer BJ, Damen EM. Dose heterogeneity in the target volume and intensity-modulated radiotherapy to escalate the dose in the treatment of non-small-cell lung cancer. *Int J Radiat Oncol Biol Phys.* 2005;62(2):561–570.

13. Zhang X, Li Y, Pan X, et al. Intensity-modulated proton therapy reduces the dose to normal tissue compared with intensity-modulated radiation therapy or passive scattering proton therapy and enables individualized radical radiotherapy for extensive stage IIIB non-small-cell lung cancer: a virtual clinical study. *Int J Radiat Oncol Biol Phys.* 2010;77:357–366.

14. Palta JR, Deye JA, Ibbott GS, Purdy JA, Urie MM. Credentialing of institutions for IMRT in clinical trials. *Int J Radiat Oncol Biol Phys.* 2004;59(4):1257–1259; author reply 1259.

15. International Commission on Radiation Units and Measurements. Prescribing, recording, and reporting photon beam therapy. Report No 50. Bethesda, MD 1993.

16. International Commission on Radiation Units and Measurements. Prescribing, recording, and reporting photon beam therapy. Report No 62. Bethesda, MD 1999.

17. Nestle U, Kremp S, Grosu AL. Practical integration of [18F]-FDG-PET and PET-CT in the planning of radiotherapy for non-small cell lung cancer (NSCLC): the technical basis, ICRU-target volumes, problems, perspectives. *Radiother Oncol.* 2006;81(2): 209–225.

18. Giraud P, Antoine M, Larrouy A et al. Evaluation of microscopic tumor extension in non-small cell lung cancer for three-dimensional conformal radiotherapy planning. *Int J Radiat Oncol Biol Phys.* 2000: 48(4):1015-1024

19. Heinzerling JH, Anderson JF, Papiez L, et al. Four-dimensional computed tomography scan analysis of tumor and organ motion at varying levels of abdominal compression during stereotactic treatment of lung and liver. *Int J Radiat Oncol Biol Phys.* 2008;70(5):1571–1578.

20. Montebello JF, Aron BS, Manatunga AK, Horvath JL, Peyton FW. The reirradiation of recurrent bronchogenic carcinoma with external beam irradiation. *Am J Clin Oncol.* 1993;16(6):482–488.

21. Kramer GW, Gans S, Ullmann E, van Meerbeeck JP, Legrand CC, Leer JW. Hypofractionated external beam radiotherapy as retreatment for symptomatic non-small-cell lung carcinoma: an effective treatment? *Int J Radiat Oncol Biol Phys.* 2004;58(5): 1388–1393.

22. Okamoto Y, Murakami M, Yoden E, et al. Reirradiation for locally recurrent lung cancer previously treated with radiation therapy. *Int J Radiat Oncol Biol Phys.* 2002;52(2):390–396.

23. Tada T, Fukuda H, Matsui K, et al. Non-small-cell lung cancer: reirradiation for loco-regional relapse previously treated with radiation therapy. *Int J Clin Oncol.* 2005;10(4):247–250.

24. Wu KL, Jiang GL, Qian H, et al. Three-dimensional conformal radiotherapy for locoregionally recurrent lung carcinoma after external beam irradiation: a prospective phase I-II clinical trial. *Int J Radiat Oncol Biol Phys.* 2003;57(5):1345–1350.

25. Beavis AW, Abdel-Hamid A, Upadhyay S. Re-treatment of a lung tumour using a simple intensity-modulated radiotherapy approach. *Br J Radiol.* 2005;78(928):358–361.

26. Govindan R, Page N, Morgensztern D, et al. Changing epidemiology of small-cell lung cancer in the United States over the last 30 years: analysis of the surveillance, epidemiologic, and end results database. *J Clin Oncol.* 2006;24(28):4539–4544.

27. Warde P, Payne D. Does thoracic irradiation improve survival and local control in limited-stage small-cell carcinoma of the lung? A meta-analysis. *J Clin Oncol.* 1992;10(6):890–895.

28. Pignon JP, Arriagada R, Ihde DC, et al. A meta-analysis of thoracic radiotherapy for small-cell lung cancer. *N Engl J Med.* 1992;327(23):1618–1624.

29. Murray N, Coy P, Pater JL, et al. Importance of timing for thoracic irradiation in the combined modality treatment of limited-stage small-cell lung cancer. The National Cancer Institute of Canada Clinical Trials Group. *J Clin Oncol.* 1993;11(2):336–344.

30. Takada M, Fukuoka M, Kawahara M, et al. Phase III study of concurrent versus sequential thoracic radiotherapy in combination with cisplatin and etoposide for limited-stage small-cell lung cancer: results of the Japan Clinical Oncology Group Study 9104. *J Clin Oncol.* 2002;20(14):3054–3060.

31. De Ruysscher D, Pijls-Johannesma M, Bentzen SM, et al. Time between the first day of chemotherapy and the last day of chest radiation is the most important predictor of survival in limited-disease small-cell lung cancer. *J Clin Oncol.* 2006;24(7):1057–1063.

32. Turrisi AT 3rd, Glover DJ, Mason BA. A preliminary report: concurrent twice-daily radiotherapy plus platinum-etoposide chemotherapy for limited small cell lung cancer. *Int J Radiat Oncol Biol Phys.* 1988;15(1):183–187.

33. Turrisi AT 3rd, Kim K, Blum R, et al. Twice-daily compared with once-daily thoracic radiotherapy in limited small-cell lung cancer treated concurrently with cisplatin and etoposide. *N Engl J Med.* 1999;340(4):265–271.

34. Choi NC, Herndon JE 2nd, Rosenman J, et al. Phase I study to determine the maximum-tolerated dose of radiation in standard daily and hyperfractionated-accelerated twice-daily radiation schedules with concurrent chemotherapy for limited-stage small-cell lung cancer. *J Clin Oncol.* 1998;16(11):3528–3536.

35. Langer CJ, Swann S, Werner-Wasik M, et al. Phase I study of irinotecan (Ir) and cisplatin (DDP) in combination with thoracic radiotherapy (RT), either twice daily (45Gy) or once daily (70Gy), in patients with limited (Ltd) small cell lung carcinoma (SCLC): early analysis of RTOG 0241 [abstract 7058]. *J Clin Oncol.* 2006;24(18S, June 20 suppl).

36. Komaki R, Swann RS, Ettinger DS, et al. Phase I study of thoracic radiation dose escalation with concurrent chemotherapy for patients with limited small-cell lung cancer: Report of Radiation Therapy Oncology Group (RTOG) protocol 97–12. *Int J Radiat Oncol Biol Phys.* 2005;62(2):342–350.

37. Komaki R, Paulus R, Ettinger DS, et al. A phase II study of accelerated high-dose thoracic radiation therapy (AHTRT) with concurrent chemotherapy for limited small cell lung cancer: RTOG 0239 [abstract 7527]. *J Clin Oncol.* 2009;27:15S.

38. Senan S, Burgers S, Samson MJ, et al. Can elective nodal irradiation be omitted in stage III non-small-cell lung cancer? Analysis of recurrences in a phase II study of induction chemotherapy and involved-field radiotherapy. *Int J Radiat Oncol Biol Phys.* 2002;54(4):999–1006.

39. Rosenzweig KE, Sim SE, Mychalczak B, Braban LE, Schindelheim R, Leibel SA. Elective nodal irradiation in the treatment of non-small-cell lung cancer with three-dimensional conformal radiation therapy. *Int J Radiat Oncol Biol Phys.* 2001;50(3): 681–685.

40. Emami B, Mirkovic N, Scott C, et al. The impact of regional nodal radiotherapy (dose/volume) on regional progression and survival in unresectable non-small cell lung cancer: an analysis of RTOG data. *Lung Cancer.* 2003;41(2):207–214.

41. De Ruysscher D, Bremer RH, Koppe F, et al. Omission of elective node irradiation on basis of CT-scans in patients with limited disease small cell lung cancer: a phase II trial. *Radiother Oncol.* 2006;80(3):307–312.

42. Fischer BM, Mortensen J, Langer SW, et al. A prospective study of PET/CT in initial staging of small-cell lung cancer: comparison with CT, bone scintigraphy and bone marrow analysis. *Ann Oncol.* 2007;18(2):338–345.

43. Bradley JD, Dehdashti F, Mintun MA, Govindan R, Trinkaus K, Siegel BA. Positron emission tomography in limited-stage small-cell lung cancer: a prospective study. *J Clin Oncol.* 2004;22(16):3248–3254.

44. Aupérin A, Arriagada R, Pignon JP, et al. Prophylactic cranial irradiation for patients with small-cell lung cancer in complete remission. Prophylactic Cranial Irradiation Overview Collaborative Group. *N Engl J Med.* 1999;341(7):476–484.

45. Slotman B, Faivre-Finn C, Kramer G, et al.; EORTC Radiation Oncology Group and Lung Cancer Group. Prophylactic cranial irradiation in extensive small-cell lung cancer. *N Engl J Med.* 2007;357(7):664–672.

18 Stereotactic Radiation Therapy for Primary, Metastatic, and Recurrent Disease

SIMON S. LO

NINA A. MAYR

ROBERT D. TIMMERMAN

■ INTRODUCTION

The standard treatment for stage I ($T_{1-2}N_0M_0$) non–small cell lung cancer (NSCLC) is anatomical resection with lobectomy or pneumonectomy which results in a 5-year overall survival rate of 60% to 70% (1–4). However, for patients with early-stage NSCLC who are deemed not to be good surgical candidates as a result of concurrent medical conditions, nonanatomical surgical or nonsurgical treatment options are offered. Some medically operable patients with stage I NSCLC may decline surgical intervention. The nonsurgical options include observation, conventional fractionated radiation therapy (CFRT), radiofrequency ablation (RFA), and stereotactic body radiation therapy (SBRT). With observation, over half of the patients will eventually die from their NSCLC, and nonsurgical treatment of the primary tumor can potentially improve survival (5). In a published population study using the Surveillance, Epidemiology, and End Results (SEER) database, observation of stage I NSCLC resulted in 5- and 10-year survival rates of 14% and 8%, respectively (6). CFRT has been used for the treatment of medically inoperable early-stage NSCLC for the past few decades with an overall survival rate of 15% to 30% (7–10). Modern series escalating the dose of CFRT utilizing 3-dimensional conformal radiation therapy showed improved outcomes (10). However, it has not achieved sufficient local control rates to be considered the first-line treatment for medically inoperable stage I NSCLC. This is covered in a separate chapter of this book on Conformal Radiation Therapy.

RFA is an emerging modality for the treatment of medically inoperable stage I NSCLC. However, in most series, the follow-up times were relatively short. Furthermore, RFA is an invasive procedure requiring general anesthesia. The risks include a pneumothorax rate of 15% to 63% and a pleural effusion rate of 3% to 21% (11–16). SBRT has emerged as a novel treatment modality utilizing sophisticated image guidance, motion assessment and control, and an oligofractionated regimen of five or fewer ablative dose-range radiation treatments for localized primary or metastatic tumors. With the accumulation of a 15-year experience, for the treatment of medically inoperable early-stage NSCLC and metastatic and recurrent lung cancer, SBRT appears safe and efficacious.

■ HISTORICAL DEVELOPMENT OF SBRT

Intracranial stereotactic radiosurgery (SRS) was pioneered by Swedish neurosurgeon Lars Leksell who challenged the radiobiologic dogma of the use of CFRT. SRS such as from a Gamma Knife unit entails the delivery of a single ablative radiation dose to a target using a secure immobilization, image guidance, and delivery of radiation with extremely steep gradients toward normal tissues. In contrast, CFRT treats large volumes of normal tissue that surrounds the target. Radiation delivered in individual ablative doses is extremely effective in the treatment of brain metastasis (17).

In contrast, for noncranial tumors, immobilization of the target may be challenging, such as with lung tumors where respiratory excursion must be considered in planning. In the early 1990s, Ingmar Lax and Henric Blomgren from the Karolinska Institute of Sweden constructed a stereotactic body frame that immobilized and dampened the motion of noncranial targets. With the use of this body frame, they treated patients with localized tumors using highly conformal techniques that mimicked SRS (18). The highly conformal isodose distribution around the target volume with rapid falloff was created utilizing multiple noncoplanar and nonopposing beams with each of these beams carrying a much lower weighting than with conformal fractionated radiation therapy. As a result, the target dose at the convergence of those beams can be significantly escalated. As a result of the promising outcomes observed with the use of SBRT, colleagues from the Karolinska Institute subsequently treated more patients including patients with early-stage cancer (18–20). At approximately the same time, Japanese investigators used

SRS-like treatments for noncranial tumors, mostly lung tumors. Uematsu and colleagues developed methods to deliver multiple focus beams of radiation for noncranial targets, mimicking SRS (21,22).

Subsequently, various groups from Europe and Japan and Indiana University further refined the approach to SBRT and began conducting prospective trials on liver and lung tumors (23–31). The use of SBRT to treat noncranial primary and metastatic tumors is being intensely studied and the results are forthcoming.

■ RADIOBIOLOGY OF SBRT

Wolbarst et al. described a conceptual three-dimensional model where normal tissue is composed of small individual functional subunits (FSUs). Within each FSU, there is a small population of regenerative clonogenic cells along with the well-differentiated functional cells. The clonogenic cells can replenish well-differentiated functional cells that may be injured or die (1,2,32). FSUs can either be structurally defined as in lung and liver or structurally undefined as in spinal cord, airway, and esophagus. The lung, for example, has a lot of redundancy; destruction of a number of FSUs does not impair respiratory function. Furthermore, within each structurally defined FSU, after radiation exposure to an infra-threshold dose of radiation, the radiation-damaged area can potentially be repaired by the migration of the clonogenic cells within the FSU. However, if an FSU receives a suprathreshold dose, all the clonogenic cells within the FSU will be killed and the whole FSU will become nonfunctional (1,2,32). Given the fact that the FSUs are structurally defined in lung parenchyma, the clonogenic cells cannot migrate across from one FSU (i.e., one alveolus) to a neighbor as such migration would be blocked by the basement membrane. The resulting pulmonary dysfunction is related to the loss of functional lung volume exposed to a dose exceeding the threshold dose. According to this model, any extra dose delivered to the same volume will not increase the pulmonary dysfunction for the given volume (1,18). With the use of proper planning, individual ablative radiation doses can be delivered to a lung tumor with a very steep dose gradient beyond the planning treatment volume (PTV), limiting the the amount of normal lung exposed. Given that many early-stage lung cancer patients treated with SBRT have poor pulmonary reserve, SBRT could improve the therapeutic ratio.

Traditionally, the linear quadratic (LQ) model has been used to predict cell killing by fractionated radiation. There are two components in the LQ model, one that is directly proportional to the dose and the other that is proportional to the dose squared. It has been proposed that at ablative doses using SBRT, the LQ model will probably overestimate cell killing (33). Alternative models have been used to predict the effect of ablative radiation doses. Park et al. have constructed a universal survival curve (USC) by combining the LQ and the multitarget models to better predict the ablative radiation dose from SBRT. The USC can be used to compare the dose fractionation schemes of both CFRT and SBRT and provides an empirically and a clinically well-justified rationale for SBRT (33). Using a generalized LQ formula, Wang et al. (34) bridged the radiotherapy regimens from CFRT to hypofractionated high dose rate brachytherapy and radiosurgery. It should be remembered that these formulae are estimates of the in vivo tumor survival after radiation delivery, something that is biologically dependent upon multiple factors that cannot possibly be accurately determined by a simplified mathematical formula.

At the molecular level mechanisms of injury may be different between CFRT and SBRT. Tissue microvasculature has a role in regulating tumor response to radiation. After exposure of mouse MCA129 fibrosarcoma and B16 melanoma cells to single doses of 15 to 20 Gy, vascular endothelial apoptosis occurred 1 to 6 hours after irradiation followed by cell death 2 to 3 days later (35,36). The process was mediated through the acid sphingomyelinase pathway, was not present in CFRT. In addition, an ablative radiation dose of 15 to 25 Gy increases T-cell priming, leading to reduction or eradication of the primary tumor or distant metastasis in a CD8 T-cell dependent fashion (37).

■ TECHNICAL ASPECTS OF SBRT

Lung SBRT entails the delivery of individual effective ablative doses to the target limiting dose to surrounding normal tissue. To achieve all these goals, a combination of accurate target delineation, robust immobilization, assessment and control of respiratory motion, proper computer dosimetric planning, and image-guidance capability is necessary.

Target Delineation

Since SBRT only targets the local tumor, accurate nodal staging is very important. 18-Fluorodeoxyglucose–positron emission tomography (FDG-PET) (18), especially when fused with computerized tomography (CT), is a highly recommended tool for staging NSCLC. In the Radiation Therapy and Oncology Group (RTOG) 0236 protocol of SBRT for medically inoperable NSCLC, patients with mediastinal or hilar lymph nodes ≤1 cm in size and absent uptake on PET were deemed having

N0 disease. However, there is now significant information about the inaccuracy of PET-CT to stage the mediastinum that warrants further clinical evaluation such as with endoscopic ultrasound (EUS) and endobronchial ultrasound (EBUS) and mediastinoscopy and/or video-assisted mediastinal assessment (see chapters on radiologic imaging and surgery).

The gross tumor volume (GTV) is usually contoured based on the lung windows on a contrast-enhanced treatment planning CT (1,2). Typically, blood vessels and atelectasis are excluded from the GTV (1). When a four-dimensional (4D) CT or a combination of free-breathing, deep-inspiration, and deep-expiration CTs is used, an internal target volume is created (38–40). An additional margin that accounts for setup variation is then given to create a PTV. The practice of clinical target volume (CTV) is variable among different institutions or trial groups. In the Indiana University and RTOG 0236 trials, a CTV expansion was not performed whereas at M.D. Anderson Cancer Center, a CTV expansion of 8 mm is performed (28,41,42). If a 4D CT is not used, it is crucial to ascertain that the amount of GTV excursion, as determined by fluoroscopy, does not exceed the confines of the PTV. The typical PTV expansion used is 10 mm craniocaudally and 5 mm radially (2,41).

Immobilization and Respiratory Motion Control

To accomplish consistent and reproducible immobilization, devices such as stereotactic body frames, vacuum pillows, and thermal plastic restraints have been used.

Alternatively, frameless systems such as the CyberKnife, Novalis, and other radiation delivery systems employ frequent reassessments of target position so that corrections might be applied. The type of motion control used is not as crucial as the treatment team's training and experience with the procedure and proper quality assurance programs to ensure accuracy of patient setup and delivery. Comfortable positioning during the lengthy treatment sessions is one of the most important aspects to ascertain accurate patient positioning during treatment delivery.

As in other noncranial targets, lung tumors are moving targets as a result of respiratory motion. Control of organ motion is a prerequisite for SBRT and different techniques have been used for respiratory control. These techniques can be divided into three broad categories, namely dampening, gating, and tracking (1,2).

Dampening of target motion is accomplished using abdominal compression or breath-holding techniques (1,2). Abdominal compression, achieved by the use of an abdominal compression plate, which is usually built into the stereotactic bodyframe, limits the diaphragmatic excursion resulting in limitation of lung tumor motion.

When active or passive breath-holding techniques are used to control respiratory motion of the lung tumor, the radiation beam is turned on when the breath is held with the proper tidal volume. When gating or tracking techniques are used, a surrogate marker with a highly reproducible relationship with the lung tumor, such as a fiducial marker, is typically needed. When gating is used, the fixed radiation beam is turned on at a particular phase of the respiratory cycle, which is assessed in real-time (1,2). When tracking is used, the radiation beam follows the moving lung tumor with the use of a fiducial marker implanted within the tumor (1,2).

Treatment Devices

Different commercially available treatment delivery units can be used to deliver SBRT. One common feature is the image-guidance capability, which enables verification of the position of the lung tumor immediately prior to treatment. This will then enhance the setup accuracy, which is crucial to avoid a "geographic miss" and the delivery of a higher-than-expected dose to critical structures.

Treatment devices such as the Varian Trilogy and the Elekta Synergy units have an integrated gantry mounted kV cone beam CT and treatment head that allow for near real-time image guidance to allow for pretreatment verification of tumor position. The Siemens Primus and Oncor units utilize an integrated megavolt (MV) cone beam CT for image guidance. The Siemens Primaotom unit provides a CT-on-rail linked to a linear accelerator sharing the same couch-top (43,44).

The CyberKnife (Accuray, Sunnyvale, CA) is a frameless radiosurgical system equipped with a robotic-arm-mounted compact linear accelerator that is directed toward the tumor volume with image guidance. The robotic arm provides six degrees of freedom compared with three in most regular linear accelerators. Real-time tracking during treatment delivery is accomplished using two orthogonal ceiling-mounted x-ray cameras. Implant fiducial markers are used for target localization and real-time treatment delivery in SBRT for lung tumors (43,44).

The TomoTherapy HiArt System (TomoTherapy, Madison, Wisconsin, USA) delivers intensity modulated radiation therapy (IMRT) throughout continuous 360° rotations using a binary multileaf collimator when the treatment couch moves continuously during treatment delivery (43,44). Radiation detectors are located opposite the MLC rendering MV CT for image guidance prior to treatment possible. Because of the inherent configuration of the device, all the beams delivered are coplanar.

The Novalis radiosurgery system (BrainLAB, Germany) is a specialized linear accelerator dedicated to the stereotactic delivery of radiation therapy. Highly conformal beam shaping is facilitated by its 2.5 mm high definition leaves. The ExacTrac positioning system allows for automatic six-dimensional fusion of reference digitally reconstructed radiographs generated by the treatment planning system with stereoscopic x-ray images taken at the treatment machine, and this will detect and identify any setup error or target deviation and will allow for corrections with robotic table movement. The Novalis Tx unit also has a gantry mounted kV cone beam CT that allows for near real-time image guidance.

Regardless of the treatment unit used, the most important elements to deliver high quality treatments for SBRT are the training and experience of the SBRT treatment team and the quality assurance procedure in the treatment center. There is no obvious difference in the treatment outcomes attributed to the difference of treatment units for SBRT for early-stage NSCLC and other disease sites.

Physics and Dosimetry

The use of treatment planning CT is necessary for simultaneous visualization of patient anatomy in three dimensions and fiducial markers for stereotactic targeting. If a 4D CT is used, the amount of lung tumor excursion can be quantified, and this information can be accounted for in the process of target delineation.

Dependent upon the treatment unit used, the treatment planning techniques can vary significantly. For instance, when a TomoTherapy unit is used, IMRT is delivered throughout the continuous 360-degree rotation of the linear accelerator and all the beams are coplanar; when a CyberKnife unit is used, inverse planning is performed using multiple isocenters. However, in most circumstances, 3D conformal radiation therapy treatment planning is used. Regardless of the technique used, the goals of a SBRT plan are to achieve adequate coverage of the gross tumor within the high-dose zone and a very steep dose gradient beyond the PTV. To accomplish these goals, multiple (typically 10–12) noncoplanar and nonopposing highly collimated beams are used (1,2,18). The typical beam orientation will create an even radiation-dose falloff in all directions beyond the PTV (Figure 18.1). However, in cases where the tumor is close to critical structures such as the spinal cord, esophagus, heart, ipsilateral brachial

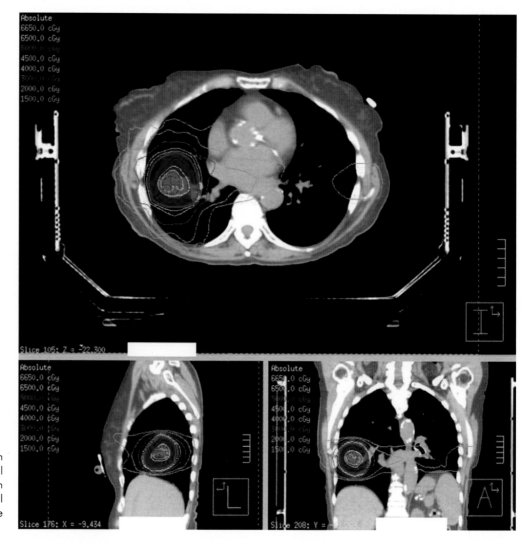

FIGURE 18.1 This is an example of a highly conformal plan used in SBRT; there is an even falloff of radiation in all directions; the prescribed dose was 10 Gy × 5 (50 Gy).

plexus, and proximal airways, or an area with history of prior radiation therapy, beam orientation and weighting are modified to steer the isodose curves away from those areas (1). Unlike CFRT where heterogeneity dose levels are avoided, a "hot spot" inside the PTV is allowed, as in Gamma Knife–based SRS, in SBRT. In terms of beam energy selection, 6-MV photons are usually preferred although higher energy, such as 18 MV, beams may be used in cases where the PTV is very close to the skin and lowering of the skin dose is necessary to avoid serious skin toxicities (1).

Since the lung parenchyma has a much lower electronic density relative to soft tissue, isodose computation without heterogeneity correction will result in significant discrepancy between the computer plan and the actual dose delivered (18). A treatment planning system with algorithms that allow for accurate calculation of tissue heterogeneity effect is highly desirable. Unfortunately, the quality of algorithms for different treatment planning systems is highly variable. The utilization of a suboptimal heterogeneity correction algorithm may cause greater inaccuracies of dose representation at the edge of the PTV compared with the use of no heterogeneity correction (18,45). Colleagues at Indiana University compared Monte Carlo calculations with actual treatment plans without heterogeneity correction and found that the dose to the PTV margin and the resultant beam monitor units were quite similar although there were significant discrepancies in the PTV and lungs (18). In a study from Vanderbilt University, the SBRT plans of 10 patients were generated using pencil beam convolution (PBC) without heterogeneity corrections and were then recalculated using PBC with modified Bartho heterogeneity corrections and anisotropic analytic algorithm (AAA) using identical beams and monitor units. Comparison to Monte Carlo dose calculations showed that AAA could accurately predict the dose distribution in the lungs and at the lung–soft tissue interface for a 6-MV beam but not for a 10-MV beam (46). Using AAA as a reference, the real PTV dose coverage calculated using PBC without heterogeneity correction was closer to the prescribed dose compared with using PBC with modified Bartho heterogeneity corrections. However, there were still significant discrepancies (≤10%) in PTV dose coverage between AAA and PBC without heterogeneity corrections.

The most important parameters in the evaluation of the quality if an SBRT plan are the conformality index, the high-dose spillage, and the *low*-dose spillage (1,18). The maximum point doses to serial critical structures, such as the spinal cord and esophagus, and their dose-volume histograms are also important parameters in cases where the PTV is in close proximity to those structures. The conformality index is defined as the ratio of the volume of the prescription isodose shell to the PTV. Since individual ablative doses of radiation is delivered to the area encompassed by the prescription isodose shell, it is important to limit the amount of lung tissue included in the prescription isodose shell by limiting the conformality index to below 1.2 to avoid excessive collateral damage to the lung parenchyma (1,18). High-dose spillage takes into account the location and the volume of normal tissue receiving an ablative dose of radiation and must be avoided in serial structures such as the spinal cord and the esophagus. Low-dose spillage can affect the organ more globally, similar to the damage caused by large-field CFRT.

SELECTION OF PATIENTS FOR SBRT

Since SBRT targets only the local tumor, accurate staging is crucial to avoid understaging of patients with NSCLC. If SBRT is being considered for patients with presumably stage I NSCLC, it is important to ascertain that there are no associated hilar or mediastinal adenopathies, or distant metastasis. Positron emission tomography (PET) with 2-fluoro-2-deoxyglucose (FDG-PET) has been used in the staging of NSCLC, specifically to confirm the nodal status and to rule out distant metastasis prior to recommending SBRT. Patients with hilar or mediastinal lymph nodes that are ≤1 cm and FDG-PET negative should not be assumed to be without mediastinal or hilar involvement. Technologies such as EUS and EBUS can be used to provide greater certainty. Mediastinoscopy and video-assisted surgical assessment of the mediastinum may be necessary. Furthermore, if any hilar or mediastinal lymph nodes are >1 cm or show FDG-PET positivity, tissue biopsies are necessary to exclude nodal metastasis. In patients with metastatic or recurrent NSCLC, FDG-PET can help rule out more extensive disease that would render them ineligible for SBRT. Since SBRT involves the delivery of individual ablative doses of radiation, the target lung tumor to be treated must be easily delineated on treatment planning CT. In terms of size limit, a maximum diameter of 5 to 7 cm is typically used.

CLINICAL OUTCOMES

Early-Stage (Stage I) NSCLC

SBRT was first utilized for the treatment of early-stage NSCLC in Sweden and Japan. Excellent local tumor control was achieved. Uematsu et al. treated 50 patients (21 medically inoperable) with SBRT delivering 50 to 60 Gy in 5 to 10 fractions. Eighteen patients also received conventional fractionated radiotherapy of 40 to 60 Gy to the chest prior to SBRT. The crude local control rate was 94% with a median follow-up of 36 months (22). The

3-year overall survival and cause-specific rates were 66% (86% in the 29 patients with operable disease) and 88%, respectively. Nagata et al. treated 40 patients with lung tumors (31 had T1–3N0M0 primary NSCLC) with SBRT to a dose of 10 to 12 Gy × 4 (40–48 Gy). With a median follow-up of 19 months, all the 16 patients with T1N0M0 NSCLC treated to a dose of 12 Gy × 4 achieved local tumor control (47). Onishi et al. performed a retrospective study pooling data of 245 patients with early-stage NSCLC (T1, n = 155; T2, n = 90) from multiple Japanese institutions treated with SBRT. The dose regimens were 18 to 75 Gy in 1 to 22 fractions. The median calculated biologic effective dose (BED) was 108 Gy (range, 57–180 Gy). At a median follow-up interval of 24 months, the local progression rate was 8.1% for BED ≥100 Gy and 26.4% for BED <100 Gy (48). The corresponding 3-year overall survival rates for BED ≥100 Gy and BED <100 Gy for medically operable patients were 88.4% and 69.4%, respectively (48).

Zimmermann et al. reported their preliminary results with the treatment of 30 patients with stage I medically inoperable NSCLC with SBRT. The dose schedules used were 24 to 37.5 in three to five fractions (12.5 Gy × 3 in most cases). The crude local control rate was 93% at a median follow-up of 18 months (49). From the same group, 68 patients with medically inoperable stage I NSCLC were treated to a dose of 37.5 Gy in three to five fractions. The 1-, 2-, and 3-year actuarial local control was 96%, 88%, and 88%, respectively, at a median follow-up of 17 months (50). Local, regional, and distant recurrences occurred in 6%, 6%, and 16% of patients, respectively. The 1- and 3-year overall survival rates were 83% and 51%, respectively. Nyman et al. reported their mature results of SBRT for medically inoperable stage I NSCLC in 45 patients treated to a dose of 15 Gy × 3 (45 Gy). At a median follow-up of 43 months, 80% of the patients achieved local tumor control (51). Twenty percent and 4.4% of patients developed distant and regional recurrence, respectively. The 3- and 5-year overall survival rates were 55% and 30%, respectively. Baumann et al. performed a pooled analysis of 138 patients with medically inoperable NSCLC treated with SBRT. The prescribed dose was 30 to 48 Gy in two to four fractions (15 Gy × 3 in most cases). At a median follow-up of 33 months, the local control rate was 88%. Twenty-five percent of the patients developed distant metastasis. The 3- and 5-year overall survival rates were 52% and 26%, respectively (52). Equivalent dose in two Gy fractions >55.6 Gy was associated with better survival. Lagerwaard et al. reported the treatment outcomes of 206 patients with stage I NSCLC (81% medically inoperable) treated with risk-adapted SBRT using regimens including 20 Gy × 3, 12 Gy × 5, and 7.5 Gy × 8. Pathologic diagnosis was available in 31% of the tumors. There were seven (3.5%) local failures with two (1%) of them isolated failure. At a median follow-up of 12 months, the 1-year, 2-year, and median overall survival were 81%, 64%, and

34 months (53). The crude regional failure rate was 9% (4% with isolated regional failure). The 1- and 2-year distant progression-free survival rates were 85% and 77%, respectively. Ng et al. reported the outcomes of 20 patients with medically inoperable stage I NSCLC treated with SBRT to doses ranging from 45 Gy to 54 Gy in three to four fractions. At a median follow-up interval of 21 months, the 2-year local control and cancer-specific survival rates were 94.7 and 77.6%, respectively (54). Other retrospective SBRT series using various dose regimens showed similar high local tumor control rates (1).

There have been several prospective studies and trials on the use of SBRT for Stage I NSCLC, mainly medically inoperable. In the phase I dose-escalation trial of SBRT for medically inoperable NSCLC conducted at Indiana University, 47 patients were enrolled. Patients with T_1 and T_2 tumors were studied in a dose-escalating fashion; the starting radiation dose was 8 Gy × 3 (24 Gy) and seven subsequent escalating dose levels were tested. The dose increment was 2 Gy per treatment. The maximum tolerated dose (MTD) has not been reached for T_1 and T_2 tumors smaller than 5 cm in size even when the prescribed dose was escalated to 20 to 22 Gy × 3 (60–66 Gy). For patients with tumors measuring 5 to 7 cm in size, the escalation to 24 Gy × 3 (72 Gy) was associated with significant toxicities (42). Ten out of 47 patients developed local failure 3 to 31 months after SBRT. Nine out of 10 patients who developed recurrence received doses of 16 Gy × 3 or lower. Building upon the results of the phase-I trial, a phase II SBRT trial was performed utilizing 20 Gy × 3 (60 Gy) for T_1 tumors and 22 Gy × 3 (66 Gy) for T_2 tumors. The median follow-up of the 70 patients enrolled was 50.2 months. The 3-year Kaplan-Meier local control was 88.1% (25). Nodal and distant recurrence occurred in 8.6% and 12.9% of the patients, respectively. The 3-year and median overall survival were 42.7% and 32.4 months, respectively. The 3-year cancer-specific survival was 81.7%. The median survival time for patient with T_1 tumors and those with T_2 tumors were 30.7 months and 24.5 months, respectively. There was no significant difference in overall survival between patients with peripheral and those with central tumors. Nagata et al. from Japan conducted a phase I/II trial of SBRT for stage I NSCLC utilizing a dose regimen of 12 Gy × 4 (48 Gy). Thirty-two patients with stage IA and 13 patients with stage IB disease were enrolled in the trial. Both operable and medically inoperable patients were eligible. The crude local control rate was 90% with median follow-up times of 30 and 22 months for patients with stage IA and IB disease, respectively (23). The tumor response was 100% with complete response occurring in 16% of the tumors. Nodal recurrence occurred in three and zero patients with stage IA and stage IB disease, respectively. Five patients with stage IA disease and four patients with stage IB disease developed distant metastases. Grade 3 or higher pulmonary toxicities were not observed. Koto et al. enrolled 31 patients (19 with T1 and 12 with T2 tumors), of which 20 were medically inoperable, in another phase II study of SBRT for stage I NSCLC from Japan. The radiation regimen used was 15 Gy × 3 (45 Gy); 7.5 Gy × 8 (60 Gy) was used in patients with tumors located close to organ-at-risk. At a median follow-up interval of 32 months, the 3-year local control rates were 77.9% and 40% for T1 and T2 tumors, respectively (26). The 3-year overall and cause-specific survival rates were 71.7% and 83.5%, respectively.

In a phase II trial from Scandinavia, Baumann et al. enrolled 57 patients with medically inoperable stage I NSCLC. The radiation-dose regimen was 15 Gy × 3 (45 Gy) prescribed at the 67% isodose line. With a median follow-up of 35 months, the actuarial local control at 3 years was 92% (24). The 1-, 2-, and 3-year overall survival rates were 86%, 65%, and 60%, respectively. The corresponding cancer-specific survival rates were 93%, 88%, and 88%. The 3-year progression-free survival rate was 52%. Ricardi et al. from Italy reported the final results of a phase II SBRT trial which enrolled 62 patients, 43 with T1 and 19 with T2 tumors, with stage I NSCLC. The radiation regimen was 15 Gy × 3 (45 Gy). At a median follow-up of 28 months, the 3-year local control, cancer-specific survival, and overall survival rates were 87.8%, 72.5%, and 57.1% (27). Eight of the 20 deaths were non-cancer related. In a study from M.D. Anderson Cancer Center, thirteen patients with stage I centrally or superiorly located NSCLC enrolled in a phase I/II trial were treated with SBRT to doses ranging from 10 Gy to 12.5 Gy per fraction × 4 (40–50 Gy). At a median follow-up of 17 months, all the patients treated with 50 Gy achieved local control (28). Mediastinal nodal and distant metastasis occurred in 7.7% and 15.4% of patients, respectively.

Most recently, mature results of the RTOG 0236 trial were reported. A total of 59 patients with peripherally located medically inoperable stage I NSCLC were accrued and 55 (44 with T1 and 11 with T2 disease) were evaluable. The actual prescribed dose was 18 Gy × 3 fractions. The 3-year local tumor control was 97.6% at a median follow-up of 34.4 months (55). Three patients had recurrence in the involved lobe which was included in their definition of local control. Two patients developed locoregional recurrence and the locoregional rate was 87.2%. The 3-year distant metastasis rate was 22.1% and the 3-year disease-free survival and overall survival were 48.3% and 55.8% (55). Grade 3 and 4 adverse events occurred in 13 (24%) and 2 (4%) patients, respectively.

In most studies, excellent local control was achieved using various radiation-dose regimens (Figure 18.2). Isolated nodal recurrence is uncommon. Table 18.1 summarizes the treatment outcomes of selected studies and prospective trials. The radiation-dose regimen used in Indiana University trial was more aggressive than the regimens used in other trials and retrospective studies, but similar local tumor control rates were reported. Data from the Indiana University phase-II trial showed that patients with centrally located tumors had an 11-fold increased risk of severe toxicity (46% vs. 17% for patients with peripheral tumors) when a radiation-dose regimen of 20 to 22 Gy × 3 (60–66 Gy) was used (57). Similar significant toxicities have not been observed in trials and studies using more protracted regimens such as 12 Gy × 4 (48 Gy) as used in the Japanese phase II trial (23,28). Given these observations, it would be prudent to consider using more protracted dose regimens for patients with centrally located tumors. The RTOG 0813 trial is a phase I/II study of SBRT for centrally located medically inoperable stage I NSCLC utilizing five fractions and is currently enrolling patients.

Metastatic NSCLC

In lung cancer, the use of SBRT to treat symptomatic and asymptomatic metastatic lesions for palliation and cure is under investigation. In a University of Chicago retrospective study of 38 NSCLC stage IIIB/IV patients treated with chemotherapy only, 50% of patients had stable or progressive disease solely in the original sites without new metastatic lesions (58). In another study from University of Colorado, the pattern of failure after first-line systemic therapy for advanced NSCLC was examined. The sites of disease at maximal response were evaluated for theoretical SBRT eligibility based on institutional criteria. All

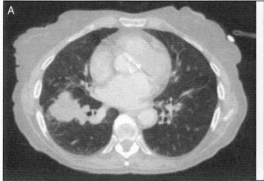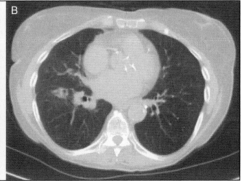

FIGURE 18.2 This patient was treated with SBRT for medically inoperable stage I non–small cell lung cancer; a dose of 10 Gy × 5 (50 Gy) was selected because of the central location of the tumor (A); the plan was demonstrated in Figure 18.1; significant tumor shrinkage was demonstrated after 3 months (B).

■ Table 18.1 Treatment outcomes of selected studies of SBRT for stage I or early-stage NSCLC

Series	Type	Disease	No. of Patients	Dose	Follow-up (months)	Outcomes
Uematsu (22)	Retrospective	Stage I	50	50–60 Gy in 5–10 fxs to isocenter (18 pts also had external beam RT) (40–60 Gy in 20–33 fxs)	36	LC: 94% (crude) OS: 66% (3 years) for all pts and 86% for operable pts CSS: 88% (3 years)
Nagata (47)	Retrospective	Stage IA	16	12 Gy × 4 (48 Gy)	19	LC: 100% (crude)
Onishi (48)	Retrospective	Stage I	245	18–75 Gy in 1–22 fxs to isocenter	24	LC: 91.9% for BED ≥100 and 73.6% for BED <100 OS: 88.4% for BED ≥100 and 69.4% for BED <100 at 3 years
Zimmermann (50)	Retrospective	Medically inoperable stage I	68	24–40 Gy in 3–5 fxs to 60%	17	LC: 96%, 88%, and 88% at 1, 2 and 3 years OS: 53% (3 years) CaSS: 96%, 82%, and 73% at 1, 2 and 3 years
Nyman (51)	Retrospective	Medically inoperable stage I	45	15 Gy × 3 fxs to periphery of PTV	43	LC: 80% (crude) OS: 55% and 30% at 3 and 5 years DF:20% RF: 4.4%
Baumann (56)	Retrospective	Medically inoperable stage I	138	30–48 Gy in 2–4 fxs (mostly 15 Gy × 3 fxs) at 65%	33	LC: 88% OS: 52% and 26 % at 3 years and 5 years LCaSS: 66% and 40% at 3 and 5 years DF: 25%
Lagerwaard (53)	Retrospective	Stage I	206	20 Gy × 3 (60 Gy), 12 Gy × 5 (60 Gy) and 7.5 Gy × 8 (60 Gy)	12	LC: 97% (crude) OS: 81% and 64% at 1 and 2 years DSS: 83% and 68% at 1 and 2 years RPFS: 94% and 83% at 1 and 2 years DPFS: 85% and 77% at 1 and 2 years RF: 9%
Ng (54)	Retrospective	Medically inoperable stage I	20	45–54 Gy in 3–4 fxs to 85% or 90%	21	LC: 94.7% (2 years) CaSS: 77.6% (2 years)

Study	Phase	Patient population	No. of patients	Dose/fractionation	BED	Outcomes
Fakiris (25)	Phase II	Medically inoperable stage I	70	T1: 20 Gy × 3 fxs T2: 22 Gy × 3 fxs	50.2	LC: 88.1% (3 years) OS: 42.7% (3 years) CaSS: 81.7% (3 years) RF: 8.6% DF: 12.8%
Nagata (23)	Phase I/II	Stage I	45	12 Gy × 4 (48 Gy) to isocenter	IA: 30 IB: 22	LC: 90% (crude) OS: 83% for T1 and 72% for T2 at 3 years DFS: 72% for T1 and 71% for T2 at 3 years RF: 15.6% for T1 and 30.8% for T2 DF: 9.4% for T1 and 0 for T2
Koto (26)	Phase II	Stage I	31	15 Gy × 3 (45 Gy) and 7.5 Gy × 8 (60 Gy)	32	LC: 77.9% for T1 and 40% for T2 at 3 years OS: 71.7% (3 years) CSS: 83.5% (3 years)
Ricardi (27)	Phase II	Stage I	62	15 Gy × 3 fxs	28	LC: 87.8% (3 years) CSS: 72.5% (3 years) OS: 57.1% (3 years)
Chang (28)	Phase I/II	Stage I, centrally and superiorly located	13	40–50 Gy in 4 fxs	12	LC: 100% (crude) RF: 7.7% DF: 15.4%
Baumann (24)	Phase II	Medically inoperable stage I	57	15 Gy × 3 fxs to 67%	35	LC: 92% (3 years) OS: 86%, 65%, and 60% at 1, 2, and 3 years CaSS: 93%, 88%, and 88% at 1, 2, and 3 years PFS: 52% (3 years)
Timmerman (55)	Phase II	Medically inoperable stage I	55	20 Gy × 3 (Actual dose 18 Gy × 3)	34.4	LC: 97.6% (3 years) DFS: 48.3% (3 years) OS: 55.8% (3 years)

BED, biologic effective dose; CaSS, cancer-specific survival; CSS, cause-specific survival; DF, distant failure; DFS, disease-free survival; DPFS, distant progression-free survival; DSS, disease-specific survival; fxs, fractions; LC, local control; LCaSS, lung cancer–specific survival; NSCLC, non–small cell lung cancer; OS, overall survival; PFS, progression-free survival; PTV, planning treatment volume; RF, regional failure; RPFS, regional progression-free survival; RT, radiation therapy; SBRT, stereotactic body radiation therapy.

patients were followed until they developed extracranial progression. Sixty-four patients met the eligibility criteria and 34 were SBRT-eligible (59). Among SBRT-eligible patients, 68% developed local only, 14% distant only, and 18% combined local and distant extracranial failure (59). These studies suggest that there is a subset of patients with limited metastases from NSCLC who may benefit from systemic therapy with local therapy to consolidate tumor response.

There is a large body of experience in the use of SBRT for lung, liver, and spinal metastases but not specifically pertaining to NSCLC histology. Overall, excellent local control rates were observed with relatively short-term follow-up (60).

Lung Metastasis

There are several retrospective and prospective studies on the use of SBRT for lung metastasis of various histologies including NSCLC (60). The reported local control rates range from 63% to 98% among different studies with most of them demonstrating local control above 85% (29,60,61). Ernst-Stecken reported the results of a prospective dose-escalating phase I/II trial of SBRT for lung tumors in 21 patients, three of whom had primary NSCLC, with 39 tumors (6 metastatic NSCLC). The dose was escalated from 35 Gy in five fractions to 40 Gy in five fractions. Complete response, partial response, and stable disease were observed in 51%, 33%, and 3% of the lung tumors, respectively (61). In a recently reported multi-institutional phase I/II trial of SBRT for patients with one to three lung metastases, the radiation dose was safely escalated from 16 Gy × 3 (48 Gy) to 20 Gy × 3 (60 Gy) without dose-limiting toxicity. After the completion of the phase I portion, a dose of 20 Gy × 3 (60 Gy) was used in the phase II portion of the trial. Thirty-eight patients (five had metastatic NSCLC) with 63 lesions were enrolled in the study. No grade 4 toxicities were observed. The 1- and 2-year actuarial local control rates were 100% and 96%, respectively, for the 50 evaluable tumors (29). Median survival was 19 months.

Liver Metastasis

Retrospective and prospective studies in the literature on SBRT for liver metastasis of various histologies including NSCLC showed good local control rate with short-term follow-up (30,60,62–64). A single-dose SBRT of 14 to 26 Gy was given to primary and metastatic liver tumors in a dose-escalation study from Germany. No dose-limiting toxicities or radiation-induced liver disease was observed after SBRT to 56 liver metastases, four from NSCLC. The 18-month actuarial local control was 67% for all tumors and 81% for tumors treated to a dose of 20 Gy or higher (62). In a Canadian phase I risk-adapted dose-escalation study of SBRT for

liver metastases where 70 patients, two with metastatic NSCLC, with 143 tumors were treated with dose regimens of 27.7 to 60 Gy (median 41.8 Gy) in six fractions, no dose-limiting toxicities were observed. At a median follow-up of 10.8 months, the 1-year local control was 71% (64). In a multi-institutional phase I/II trial of SBRT for liver metastases where 47 patients, 10 with metastatic NSCLC, with 63 lesions were treated with SBRT, the radiation dose was escalated from 12 Gy × 3 (36 Gy) to 20 Gy × 3 (60 Gy) in the phase I portion of the study without causing dose-limiting toxicities. The 1- and 2-year actuarial local control rates were 95% and 92%, respectively, for the 49 evaluable tumors and 100% and 100%, respectively for tumors measuring 3 cm or less (30). The median survival time was 20.5 months.

Spinal Metastasis

A large body of experience with the use of SBRT for spinal metastasis of various histologies including NSCLC has emerged (60,65–68). Overall, the reported local control rates were excellent with relatively short follow-up (65,67). Based on the pooled data from the literature, local control rates for unirradiated patients, postoperative patients, reirradiated patients, and mixed patients were 87%, 94%, 96%, and 87% (67). In a phase I/II study where 63 patients, 7 with metastatic NSCLC, with 74 spinal metastases were treated with SBRT to a dose of 30 Gy in five fractions or 27 Gy in three fractions, at a median follow-up time of 21.3 months, the local control rate was 77%, and the 1-year progression-free rate was 84% (68).

Recurrent NSCLC

In patients with recurrent NSCLC after conventional radiation therapy, reirradiation with conventional techniques is not feasible given the significantly increased risk of complications. SBRT provides a viable means of salvage treatment for recurrent NSCLC. Compared with data on SBRT for stage I NSCLC, data on recurrent NSCLC is limited. In a series from University of Pittsburgh, 12 patients with recurrent NSCLC were treated with CyberKnife-based SBRT to a dose of 60 Gy in three fractions. With a median follow-up of 12 months (including 26 and 13 patients with stage I NSCLC and solitary lung metastasis), the local control rate was 92% (69). The 1-year overall survival was 67%. In a study from M.D. Anderson Cancer Center, 14 patients with isolated recurrence of NSCLC in lung parenchyma were treated with SBRT to a dose of 40 to 50 Gy in four fractions. None of the patients treated to a dose of 50 Gy in four fractions developed local recurrence. However, four (28.6%) of patients developed grade 2 pneumonitis (28). No other severe complications were observed. In a retrospective study from the same institution, 42 patients who had prior chest radiotherapy received SBRT for recurrent, metastatic, or secondary lung parenchymal cancer (personal communication with Dr Joe Chang from M.D. Anderson Cancer Center). The dose was 10 to 12.5 Gy × 4 (40–50 Gy). At a median follow-up time of 11.8 months, infield local control rate was 95% and 1-year overall survival rate was 86%. The most common site of failure was the chest, but outside the SBRT field (52%). Dyspnea occurred in 40% of patients, and 14% required increased oxygen supplementation. No grade 4 or 5 toxicities were observed. In another study, Salazar et al. reported the treatment outcomes of 13 patients with recurrent NSCLC treated with SBRT to a dose of 40 Gy in four fractions. Only three (23%) patients were alive at analysis (70). The remaining patients died of disease or intercurrent conditions.

■ EVALUATION OF TREATMENT RESPONSE

CT of the chest is for the primary means of monitoring patients who undergo SBRT. The parenchymal changes after SBRT are different from those seen with CFRT. Radiation-induced lung injury manifests as mass-like consolidation or dense fibrosis potentially difficult to differentiate from persistent or recurrent tumor. This can potentially cause confusion in the evaluation of treatment response when the area of dense consolidation overlaps the original tumor (71–74). Matsuo et al. reported that mass-like consolidation was observed after SBRT for lung tumors after doses of 10 to 12 Gy × 4 to 5 fractions (40–60 Gy) in 68% of the lung tumors treated at a median of 5 months (range 2–9 months). With further follow-up, 89% of the mass consolidations were deemed to be radiation-induced lung injury in that no further enlargement of those lesions was observed after 12 months or longer (71). This was in contrast to local recurrences where the mass consolidation continued to enlarge after 12 months. Takeda et al. reported that after SBRT for localized NSCLC using a dose regimen of 10 Gy × 5 (50 Gy), 20 (40%) out of 50 patients developed abnormal opacities suspicious for recurrence. However, only 3 (6%) patients were finally confirmed to have recurrence; and 14 (28%) were deemed to have fibrosis and be free of recurrence (74).

For stage I NSCLC, FDG-PET with or without fusion with CT has been used to follow patients after SBRT. Apart from the evaluation of local response to SBRT, concurrent nodal or distant recurrence can be evaluated concurrently. Given the problems associated with the evaluation of treatment response using chest CT, FDG-PET, which has superior sensitivity and specificity, is frequently used to evaluate post-SBRT treatment response. In a retrospective

evaluation of the use of FDG-PET in 28 SBRT-treated NSCLC patients, there were four who developed moderate hypermetabolic activity in the site of the original tumor without evidence of local recurrence (75). In a companion prospective study to the Indiana University phase II trial, 14 SBRT-treated NSCLC patients using a regimen of 20 to 22 Gy × 3 (60–66 Gy) were followed with FDG-PET. With median follow-up of 30.2 months, no patients experienced local failure. The median tumor maximum standardized uptake values (SUV(max)) pre-SBRT, and then at 2 weeks, 6 months, and 12 months was 8.70, 6.04, 2.80, and 3.58, respectively (76).Patients with low pre-SBRT SUV were more likely to develop initial 2-week increase in SUV; patients with high pre-SBRT SUV frequently had decrease in SUV 2 weeks after treatment. Six (43%) of 13 patients with primary tumor SUV(max) >3.5 at 12 months after SBRT remained without evidence of local disease failure on further follow-up (76). Based on the observations of these studies, routine use of serial FDG-PET for post-SBRT follow-up of stage I NSCLC is not recommended. However, FDG-PET does have a role in suspected recurrence, although a rise in SUV(max) does not confirm recurrence. The role of FDG-PET in post-SBRT surveillance must be better defined before any recommendations can be made.

■ TOXICITIES

Overall, SBRT is well tolerated even in patients with chronic obstructive pulmonary disease (56). Poor baseline pulmonary function does not portend a poor survival or treatment-related poorer pulmonary function after SBRT (77). However, various types of toxicities have been reported in different retrospective and prospective studies of SBRT for stage I NSCLC. In the dose-escalating phase I study including both peripherally and centrally located tumors, the MTD was reached at 24 Gy × 3 (72 Gy) for patients with tumors >5 cm, three (60%) of the five patients developed ≥grade 3 that included radiation pneumonitis and tracheal stenosis (42). Other complications reported in the trial were pericardial effusion, dermatitis, distal pneumonia, bronchitis, and hypoxia. In a preliminary report of the Indiana University phase II trial of SBRT for medically inoperable NSCLC utilizing a regimen of 20 to 22 Gy × 3 (60–66 Gy), Timmerman et al. (57) discovered that 83% of patients developed grade 1 to 2 toxicities, including fatigue, musculoskeletal discomfort, and radiation pneumonitis, which typically occurred within 1 to 2 months of SBRT and resolved by 3 to 4 months after treatment. Compared with patients with peripherally located tumors, those with centrally located tumors had an 11-fold increased risk of severe toxicities (46% compared with 17%). Similar toxicities have not been observed in a phase I/II trial of SBRT for lung metastasis using a similar dose regimen, the Scandinavian phase II trial of SBRT for medically inoperable stage I NSCLC using a regimen of 15 Gy × 3 (45 Gy), and other trials of SBRT for stage I NSCLC using more protracted regimens (23,24,28,29). Because of the findings of the study from Indiana University, patients with centrally located tumors were excluded from the RTOG 0236 trial, which used a dose regimen of 20 Gy × 3 (60 Gy). Based on the data available so far, it would be prudent to avoid using the regimen of 20 Gy × 3 in patients with centrally located tumors, and a more protracted regimen is recommended.

Other late complications include esophagitis, esophageal strictures, massive hemoptysis, severe skin toxicity, chronic chest wall pain, rib fractures, and brachial plexopathy (1,42,57,78–81). The esophagus and the large blood vessels are located in the mediastinum/hilar regions, and the risk of injury to those structures is higher when a centrally located lung tumor is treated. The esophagus and the great vessels are located in close proximity in the mediastinum/hilar regions and the risk of injury to those structures is higher when a centrally located lung tumor is treated. During treatment planning the esophagus and large blood vessels should be contoured. Late complications such as skin toxicity, chronic chest wall pain, and rib fractures may occur in patients with peripheral tumors. Planning techniques to minimize skin toxicity include allowing a 0.5-cm concentric ring beneath the skin surface, the use of a large number of beams, and high energy for the beams

entering through the portion of the chest wall next to the tumor, and the use of a more protracted regimen may help decrease the risk of severe skin complications (82). Chest wall pain and/or rib fractures are related to the volume of chest wall receiving 30 Gy in three to five fractions (79). One approach to reduce the risk is to consider the chest wall as organ-at-risk during treatment planning minimizing the dose received at that location. For apical tumors, the ipsilateral brachial plexus is at risk. There is little data in the literature on the brachial plexus tolerance in the SBRT dose range. A retrospective study from Indiana University examined brachial plexus toxicity in medically inoperable apical stage I NSCLC patients treated with SBRT. The risk of brachial plexopathy increased if the dose exceeded 26 Gy in three to four fractions (81). Table 18.2 summarizes the dose constraints used by RTOG trials in SBRT for medically operable or inoperable stage I/II NSCLC.

■ **SUMMARY**

Based on the large body of experience with the use of SBRT for the treatment of medically inoperable stage I NSCLC and the mature results from some prospective trials, SBRT has become an important part of the armamentarium for treatment of NSCLC. Using a three-fraction SBRT regimen, the treatment of centrally located tumors may cause an unacceptably high likelihood of severe complications and should be avoided. A more protracted SBRT regimen

■ **Table 18.2** Dose constraints used by RTOG				
Organ	1 Fraction	3 Fractions	4 Fractions	5 Fractions
Spinal cord	14 Gy (max.)	21.9 Gy (max.)	26 (max.)	30 Gy (max.)
	10 Gy (<0.35 cc)	18 Gy (<0.35 cc)	20.8 (<0.35 cc)	23 Gy (<0.35 cc)
	7 Gy (<1.2 cc)	12.3 Gy (<1.2 cc)	13.6 (<1.2 cc)	14.5 Gy (<1.2 cc)
Esophagus	15.4 Gy (max.)	25.2 Gy (max.)	30 Gy (max.)	35 Gy (max.)
	11.9 Gy (<5 cc)	17.7 Gy (<5 cc)	18.8 Gy (<5 cc)	19.5 Gy (<5 cc)
Ipsilateral brachial plexus	17.5 Gy (max.)	24 Gy (max.)	27.2 Gy (max.)	30.5 Gy (max.)
	14 Gy (<3 cc)	20.4 Gy (<3 cc)	23.6 (<3 cc)	27 Gy (<3 cc)
Heart/pericardium	22 Gy (max.)	30 Gy (max.)	34 Gy (max.)	38 Gy (max.)
	16 Gy (<15 cc)	24 Gy (<15 cc)	28 Gy (<15 cc)	32 Gy (<15 cc)
Trachea and large bronchus	20.2 Gy (max.)	30 Gy (max.)	34.8 Gy (max.)	40 Gy (max.)
	10.5 Gy (<4 cc)	15 Gy (<4 cc)	15.6 Gy (<4 cc)	16.5 Gy (<4 cc)
Skin	26 Gy (max.)	33 Gy (max.)	36 Gy (max.)	39.5 Gy (max.)
	23 Gy (<10 cc)	30 Gy (<10 cc)	33.2 Gy (<10 cc)	36.5 Gy (<10 cc)
Great vessels, nonadjacent wall	37 Gy (max.)	45 Gy (max.)	49 Gy (max.)	53 Gy (max.)
	31 Gy (<10 cc)	39 Gy (<10 cc)	43 Gy (<10 cc)	47 Gy (<10 cc)
Rib	30 Gy (max.)	36.9 Gy (max.)	40 Gy (max.)	43 Gy (max.)
	22 Gy (<1 cc)	28.8 Gy (<1 cc)	32 Gy (<1 cc)	35 Gy (<1 cc)
Stomach	12.4 Gy (max.)	22.2 Gy (max.)	27.2 Gy (max.)	32 Gy (max.)
	11.2 Gy (<10 cc)	16.5 Gy (<10 cc)	17.6 Gy (<10 cc)	18 Gy (<10 cc)

Maximum dose defined as the highest dose to a volume of >0.035 cc.
max., maximum; PTV, planning treatment volume.

should be used. Excellent local tumor can be achieved with different dose regimens. Mediastinal and hilar nodal failure is uncommon but distant failure with or without nodal failure remains problematic. Post-SBRT surveillance can be challenging given the confusing CT and FDG-PET findings.

■ FUTURE DIRECTIONS

RTOG is currently conducting three SBRT trials for stage I or early-stage NSCLC—a phase II trial of SBRT for operable stage I/II NSCLC (RTOG 0618), a phase I/II trial of SBRT for centrally located stage I medically inoperable NSCLC (RTOG 0813), and a phase II trial comparing different dose regimens (34 Gy × 1 vs. 12 Gy × 4) for medically inoperable peripherally located stage I NSCLC (RTOG 0915). Japanese Clinical Oncology Group (JCOG) 0403 trial is currently enrolling patients with stage IA (T1N0M0) operable or medically inoperable NSCLC to be treated with SBRT using a regimen of 12 Gy × 4 (48 Gy).

A separate dose-escalating trial for medically inoperable or "unfit" stage IB (T2N0M0) NSCLC (JCOG 0702) will escalate the total dose from 12 Gy × 4 (48 Gy) to 16.5 Gy × 4 (66 Gy). Long-term outcomes from these trials can further define the role of SBRT in the management of medically inoperable or operable stage I NSCLC. Long-term toxicities and consequently dose constraints of various organs-at-risk will also be better defined. Although excellent local control is readily achievable with SBRT, distant metastasis remains problematic. The combination of SBRT with effective systemic or biologic agents should be explored to further improve the survival outcomes.

■ REFERENCES

1. Lo SS, Fakiris AJ, Papiez L, et al. Stereotactic body radiation therapy for early-stage non-small-cell lung cancer. *Expert Rev Anticancer Ther.* 2008;8(1):87–98.
2. Timmerman RD, Kavanagh BD, Cho LC, Papiez L, Xing L. Stereotactic body radiation therapy in multiple organ sites. *J Clin Oncol.* 2007;25(8):947–952.
3. Mountain CF. A new international staging system for lung cancer. *Chest.* 1986;89(4 suppl):225S–233S.
4. Naruke T, Goya T, Tsuchiya R, Suemasu K. Prognosis and survival in resected lung carcinoma based on the new international staging system. *J Thorac Cardiovasc Surg.* 1988;96(3):440–447.
5. McGarry RC, Song G, des Rosiers P, Timmerman R. Observation-only management of early stage, medically inoperable lung cancer: poor outcome. *Chest.* 2002;121(4):1155–1158.
6. Wisnivesky JP, Bonomi M, Henschke C, Iannuzzi M, McGinn T. Radiation therapy for the treatment of unresected stage I-II non-small cell lung cancer. *Chest.* 2005;128(3):1461–1467.
7. Gauden S, Ramsay J, Tripcony L. The curative treatment by radiotherapy alone of stage I non-small cell carcinoma of the lung. *Chest.* 1995;108(5):1278–1282.
8. Hayakawa K, Mitsuhashi N, Furuta M, et al. High-dose radiation therapy for inoperable non-small cell lung cancer without mediastinal involvement (clinical stage N0, N1). *Strahlenther Onkol.* 1996;172(9):489–495.
9. Sibley GS. Radiotherapy for patients with medically inoperable Stage I nonsmall cell lung carcinoma: smaller volumes and higher doses–a review. *Cancer.* 1998;82(3):433–438.
10. Fang LC, Komaki R, Allen P, Guerrero T, Mohan R, Cox JD. Comparison of outcomes for patients with medically inoperable Stage I non-small-cell lung cancer treated with two-dimensional vs. three-dimensional radiotherapy. *Int J Radiat Oncol Biol Phys.* 2006;66(1):108–116.
11. Ambrogi MC, Lucchi M, Dini P, et al. Percutaneous radiofrequency ablation of lung tumours: results in the mid-term. *Eur J Cardiothorac Surg.* 2006;30(1):177–183.
12. Dupuy DE, DiPetrillo T, Gandhi S, et al. Radiofrequency ablation followed by conventional radiotherapy for medically inoperable stage I non-small cell lung cancer. *Chest.* 2006;129(3):738–745.
13. Fernando HC, De Hoyos A, Landreneau RJ, et al. Radiofrequency ablation for the treatment of non-small cell lung cancer in marginal surgical candidates. *J Thorac Cardiovasc Surg.* 2005;129(3):639–644.
14. Lanuti M, Sharma A, Digumarthy SR, et al. Radiofrequency ablation of medically inoperable stage I non-small cell lung cancer. *J Thorac Cardiovasc Surg.* 2009;137(1):160–166.
15. Pennathur A, Luketich JD, Abbas G, et al. Radiofrequency ablation for the treatment of stage I non-small cell lung cancer in high-risk patients. *J Thorac Cardiovasc Surg.* 2007;134(4):857–864.
16. Lencioni R, Crocetti L, Cioni R, et al. Response to radiofrequency ablation of pulmonary tumours: a prospective, intention-to-treat, multicentre clinical trial (the RAPTURE study). *Lancet Oncol.* 2008;9(7):621–628.
17. Lo SS, Chang EL, Suh JH. Stereotactic radiosurgery with and without whole-brain radiotherapy for newly diagnosed brain metastases. *Expert Rev Neurother.* 2005;5(4):487–495.
18. Timmerman RD, Kavanagh BD. Stereotactic body radiation therapy. *Curr Probl Cancer.* 2005;29(3):120–157.
19. Blomgren H, Lax I, Näslund I, Svanström R. Stereotactic high dose fraction radiation therapy of extracranial tumors using an accelerator. Clinical experience of the first thirty-one patients. *Acta Oncol.* 1995;34(6):861–870.
20. Blomgren H, Lax I, Goranson H, et al. Radiosurgery for tumors in the body: clinical experience using a new method. *J Radiosurg.* 1998;1:63–74.
21. Uematsu M, Shioda A, Tahara K, et al. Focal, high dose, and fractionated modified stereotactic radiation therapy for lung carcinoma patients: a preliminary experience. *Cancer.* 1998;82(6):1062–1070.
22. Uematsu M, Shioda A, Suda A, et al. Computed tomography-guided frameless stereotactic radiotherapy for stage I non-small cell lung cancer: a 5-year experience. *Int J Radiat Oncol Biol Phys.* 2001;51(3):666–670.
23. Nagata Y, Takayama K, Matsuo Y, et al. Clinical outcomes of a phase I/II study of 48 Gy of stereotactic body radiotherapy in 4 fractions for primary lung cancer using a stereotactic body frame. *Int J Radiat Oncol Biol Phys.* 2005;63(5):1427–1431.
24. Baumann P, Nyman J, Hoyer M, et al. Outcome in a prospective phase II trial of medically inoperable stage I non-small-cell lung cancer patients treated with stereotactic body radiotherapy. *J Clin Oncol.* 2009;27(20):3290–3296.
25. Fakiris AJ, McGarry RC, Yiannoutsos CT, et al. Stereotactic body radiation therapy for early-stage non-small-cell lung carcinoma: four-year results of a prospective phase II study. *Int J Radiat Oncol Biol Phys.* 2009;75(3):677–682.
26. Koto M, Takai Y, Ogawa Y, et al. A phase II study on stereotactic body radiotherapy for stage I non-small cell lung cancer. *Radiother Oncol.* 2007;85(3):429–434.

27. Ricardi U, Filippi AR, Guarneri A, et al. Stereotactic body radiation therapy for early stage non-small cell lung cancer: results of a prospective trial. *Lung Cancer.* 2010;68(1):72–77.

28. Chang JY, Balter PA, Dong L, et al. Stereotactic body radiation therapy in centrally and superiorly located stage I or isolated recurrent non-small-cell lung cancer. *Int J Radiat Oncol Biol Phys.* 2008;72(4):967–971.

29. Rusthoven KE, Kavanagh BD, Burri SH, et al. Multi-institutional phase I/II trial of stereotactic body radiation therapy for lung metastases. *J Clin Oncol.* 2009;27(10):1579–1584.

30. Rusthoven KE, Kavanagh BD, Cardenes H, et al. Multi-institutional phase I/II trial of stereotactic body radiation therapy for liver metastases. *J Clin Oncol.* 2009;27(10):1572–1578.

31. Tse RV, Hawkins M, Lockwood G, et al. Phase I study of individualized stereotactic body radiotherapy for hepatocellular carcinoma and intrahepatic cholangiocarcinoma. *J Clin Oncol.* 2008;26(4):657–664.

32. Wolbarst AB, Chin LM, Svensson GK. Optimization of radiation therapy: integral-response of a model biological system. *Int J Radiat Oncol Biol Phys.* 1982;8(10):1761–1769.

33. Park C, Papiez L, Zhang S, Story M, Timmerman RD. Universal survival curve and single fraction equivalent dose: useful tools in understanding potency of ablative radiotherapy. *Int J Radiat Oncol Biol Phys.* 2008;70(3):847–852.

34. Wang JZ, Mayr NA, Yuh WTC. A generalized linear-qudratic formula for high-dose-rate brachytherapy and radiosurgery. *Int J Radiat Oncol Biol Phys.* 2007;69(3):S619–S620.

35. Garcia-Barros M, Paris F, Cordon-Cardo C, et al. Tumor response to radiotherapy regulated by endothelial cell apoptosis. *Science.* 2003;300(5622):1155–1159.

36. Fuks Z, Kolesnick R. Engaging the vascular component of the tumor response. *Cancer Cell.* 2005;8(2):89–91.

37. Lee Y, Auh SL, Wang Y, et al. Therapeutic effects of ablative radiation on local tumor require CD8+ T cells: changing strategies for cancer treatment. *Blood.* 2009;114(3):589–595.

38. Underberg RW, Lagerwaard FJ, Cuijpers JP, Slotman BJ, van Sörnsen de Koste JR, Senan S. Four-dimensional CT scans for treatment planning in stereotactic radiotherapy for stage I lung cancer. *Int J Radiat Oncol Biol Phys.* 2004;60(4):1283–1290.

39. Guckenberger M, Wilbert J, Krieger T, et al. Four-dimensional treatment planning for stereotactic body radiotherapy. *Int J Radiat Oncol Biol Phys.* 2007;69(1):276–285.

40. Wang L, Feigenberg S, Chen L, Pasklev K, Ma CC. Benefit of three-dimensional image-guided stereotactic localization in the hypofractionated treatment of lung cancer. *Int J Radiat Oncol Biol Phys.* 2006;66(3):738–747.

41. Timmerman R, Papiez L, McGarry R, et al. Extracranial stereotactic radioablation: results of a phase I study in medically inoperable stage I non-small cell lung cancer. *Chest.* 2003;124(5):1946–1955.

42. McGarry RC, Papiez L, Williams M, Whitford T, Timmerman RD. Stereotactic body radiation therapy of early-stage non-small-cell lung carcinoma: phase I study. *Int J Radiat Oncol Biol Phys.* 2005;63(4):1010–1015.

43. Chang BK, Timmerman RD. Stereotactic body radiation therapy: a comprehensive review. *Am J Clin Oncol.* 2007;30(6):637–644.

44. Lo SS, Cardenes HR, Teh BS, et al. Stereotactic body radiation therapy for nonpulmonary primary tumors. *Expert Rev Anticancer Ther.* 2008;8(12):1939–1951.

45. Haedinger U, Krieger T, Flentje M, Wulf J. Influence of calculation model on dose distribution in stereotactic radiotherapy for pulmonary targets. *Int J Radiat Oncol Biol Phys.* 2005;61(1):239–249.

46. Ding GX, Duggan DM, Lu B, et al. Impact of inhomogeneity corrections on dose coverage in the treatment of lung cancer using stereotactic body radiation therapy. *Med Phys.* 2007;34(7):2985–2994.

47. Nagata Y, Negoro Y, Aoki T, et al. Clinical outcomes of 3D conformal hypofractionated single high-dose radiotherapy for one or two lung tumors using a stereotactic body frame. *Int J Radiat Oncol Biol Phys.* 2002;52(4):1041–1046.

48. Onishi H, Araki T, Shirato H, et al. Stereotactic hypofractionated high-dose irradiation for stage I nonsmall cell lung carcinoma: clinical outcomes in 245 subjects in a Japanese multiinstitutional study. *Cancer.* 2004;101(7):1623–1631.

49. Zimmermann FB, Geinitz H, Schill S, et al. Stereotactic hypofractionated radiation therapy for stage I non-small cell lung cancer. *Lung Cancer.* 2005;48(1):107–114.

50. Zimmermann FB, Geinitz H, Schill S, et al. Stereotactic hypofractionated radiotherapy in stage I (T1–2 N0 M0) non-small-cell lung cancer (NSCLC). *Acta Oncol.* 2006;45(7):796–801.

51. Nyman J, Johansson KA, Hultén U. Stereotactic hypofractionated radiotherapy for stage I non-small cell lung cancer–mature results for medically inoperable patients. *Lung Cancer.* 2006;51(1):97–103.

52. Baumann P, Nyman J, Lax I, et al. Factors important for efficacy of stereotactic body radiotherapy of medically inoperable stage I lung cancer. A retrospective analysis of patients treated in the Nordic countries. *Acta Oncol.* 2006;45(7):787–795.

53. Lagerwaard FJ, Haasbeek CJ, Smit EF, Slotman BJ, Senan S. Outcomes of risk-adapted fractionated stereotactic radiotherapy for stage I non-small-cell lung cancer. *Int J Radiat Oncol Biol Phys.* 2008;70(3):685–692.

54. Ng AW, Tung SY, Wong VY. Hypofractionated stereotactic radiotherapy for medically inoperable stage I non-small cell lung cancer–report on clinical outcome and dose to critical organs. *Radiother Oncol.* 2008;87(1):24–28.

55. Timmerman R, Paulus R, Galvin J, et al. Stereotactic body radiation therapy for inoperable early stage lung cancer. *JAMA.* 2010;303(11):1070–1076.

56. Baumann P, Nyman J, Hoyer M, et al. Stereotactic body radiotherapy for medically inoperable patients with stage I non-small cell lung cancer - a first report of toxicity related to COPD/CVD in a non-randomized prospective phase II study. *Radiother Oncol.* 2008;88(3):359–367.

57. Timmerman R, McGarry R, Yiannoutsos C, et al. Excessive toxicity when treating central tumors in a phase II study of stereotactic body radiation therapy for medically inoperable early-stage lung cancer. *J Clin Oncol.* 2006;24(30):4833–4839.

58. Mehta N, Mauer AM, Hellman S, et al. Analysis of further disease progression in metastatic non-small cell lung cancer: implications for locoregional treatment. *Int J Oncol.* 2004;25(6):1677–1683.

59. Rusthoven KE, Hammerman SF, Kavanagh BD, Birtwhistle MJ, Stares M, Camidge DR. Is there a role for consolidative stereotactic body radiation therapy following first-line systemic therapy for metastatic lung cancer? A patterns-of-failure analysis. *Acta Oncol.* 2009;48(4):578–583.

60. Lo SS, Fakiris AJ, Teh BS, et al. Stereotactic body radiation therapy for oligometastases. *Expert Rev Anticancer Ther.* 2009;9(5):621–635.

61. Ernst-Stecken A, Lambrecht U, Mueller R, Sauer R, Grabenbauer G. Hypofractionated stereotactic radiotherapy for primary and secondary intrapulmonary tumors: first results of a phase I/II study. *Strahlenther Onkol.* 2006;182(12):696–702.

62. Herfarth KK, Debus J, Lohr F, et al. Stereotactic single-dose radiation therapy of liver tumors: results of a phase I/II trial. *J Clin Oncol.* 2001;19(1):164–170.

63. Méndez Romero A, Wunderink W, Hussain SM, et al. Stereotactic body radiation therapy for primary and metastatic liver tumors: A single institution phase i-ii study. *Acta Oncol.* 2006;45(7):831–837.

64. Lee MT, Kim JJ, Dinniwell R, et al. Phase I study of individualized stereotactic body radiotherapy of liver metastases. *J Clin Oncol.* 2009;27(10):1585–1591.

65. Lo SS, Chang EL, Yamada Y, Sloan AE, Suh JH, Mendel E. Stereotactic radiosurgery and radiation therapy for spinal tumors. *Expert Rev Neurother.* 2007;7(1):85–93.

66. Sahgal A, Chuang C, Larson D. Proximity of spinous/paraspinous radiosurgery metastatic targets to the spinal cord versus risk of local failure. *Int J Radiat Oncol Biol Phys.* 2007;69:S243.

67. Sahgal A, Larson DA, Chang EL. Stereotactic body radiosurgery for spinal metastases: a critical review. *Int J Radiat Oncol Biol Phys.* 2008;71(3):652–665.

68. Chang EL, Shiu AS, Mendel E, et al. Phase I/II study of stereotactic body radiotherapy for spinal metastasis and its pattern of failure. *J Neurosurg Spine.* 2007;7(2):151–160.

69. Coon D, Gokhale AS, Burton SA, Heron DE, Ozhasoglu C, Christie N. Fractionated stereotactic body radiation therapy in the treatment of primary, recurrent, and metastatic lung tumors: the role of positron emission tomography/computed tomography-based treatment planning. *Clin Lung Cancer.* 2008;9(4): 217–221.

70. Salazar OM, Sandhu TS, Lattin PB, et al. Once-weekly, high-dose stereotactic body radiotherapy for lung cancer: 6-year analysis of 60 early-stage, 42 locally advanced, and 7 metastatic lung cancers. *Int J Radiat Oncol Biol Phys.* 2008;72(3):707–715.

71. Matsuo Y, Nagata Y, Mizowaki T, et al. Evaluation of mass-like consolidation after stereotactic body radiation therapy for lung tumors. *Int J Clin Oncol.* 2007;12(5):356–362.

72. Aoki T, Nagata Y, Negoro Y, et al. Evaluation of lung injury after three-dimensional conformal stereotactic radiation therapy for solitary lung tumors: CT appearance. *Radiology.* 2004;230(1):101–108.

73. Takeda T, Takeda A, Kunieda E, et al. Radiation injury after hypofractionated stereotactic radiotherapy for peripheral small lung tumors: serial changes on CT. *AJR Am J Roentgenol.* 2004;182(5):1123–1128.

74. Takeda A, Kunieda E, Takeda T, et al. Possible misinterpretation of demarcated solid patterns of radiation fibrosis on CT scans as tumor recurrence in patients receiving hypofractionated stereotactic radiotherapy for lung cancer. *Int J Radiat Oncol Biol Phys.* 2008;70(4):1057–1065.

75. Hoopes DJ, Tann M, Fletcher JW, et al. FDG-PET and stereotactic body radiotherapy (SBRT) for stage I non-small-cell lung cancer. *Lung Cancer.* 2007;56(2):229–234.

76. Henderson MA, Hoopes DJ, Fletcher JW, et al. A pilot trial of serial 18F-fluorodeoxyglucose positron emission tomography in patients with medically inoperable stage I non-small-cell lung cancer treated with hypofractionated stereotactic body radiotherapy. *Int J Radiat Oncol Biol Phys.* 2010;76(3):789–795.

77. Henderson M, McGarry R, Yiannoutsos C, et al. Baseline pulmonary function as a predictor for survival and decline in pulmonary function over time in patients undergoing stereotactic body radiotherapy for the treatment of stage I non-small-cell lung cancer. *Int J Radiat Oncol Biol Phys.* 2008;72(2):404–409.

78. Hoppe BS, Laser B, Kowalski AV, et al. Acute skin toxicity following stereotactic body radiation therapy for stage I non-small-cell lung cancer: who's at risk? *Int J Radiat Oncol Biol Phys.* 2008;72(5):1283–1286.

79. Dunlap NE, Cai J, Biedermann GB, et al. Chest Wall Volume Receiving >30 Gy Predicts Risk of Severe Pain and/or Rib Fracture After Lung Stereotactic Body Radiotherapy. *Int J Radiat Oncol Biol Phys.* 2010, 76(3):796–801.

80. Voroney JP, Hope A, Dahele MR, et al. Chest wall pain and rib fracture after stereotactic radiotherapy for peripheral non-small cell lung cancer. *J Thorac Oncol.* 2009;4(8):1035–1037.

81. Forquer JA, Fakiris AJ, Timmerman RD, et al. Brachial plexopathy from stereotactic body radiotherapy in early-stage NSCLC: dose-limiting toxicity in apical tumor sites. *Radiother Oncol.* 2009;93(3):408–413.

82. Lo SS, Fakiris AJ, Wang JZ, Mayr NA. In regard to Hoppe et al. (Int J Radiat Oncol Biol Phys 2008;72:1283–1286). *Int J Radiat Oncol Biol Phys.* 2009;74(3):977; author reply 8.

Special Circumstances

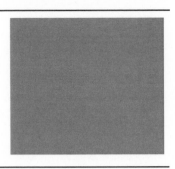

Special Circumstances

19 Tracheobronchial Cancers: Nd:YAG Laser Resection, Brachytherapy, and Photodynamic Ablation

HENRI G. COLT

INTRODUCTION

Bronchoscopic treatment of airway tumors is an important aspect of cancer care. Of the nearly 200,000 people diagnosed with lung cancer annually in the United States, it is estimated that approximately 30% present with airway obstruction and 35% will die from complications of loco-regional disease (1). In addition, advanced stage cancers may cause decreased quality of life, shortness of breath, hypoxemia, and postobstructive pneumonia from obstructing airway lesions or extrinsic compression. Most cases referred for bronchoscopic procedures are, in fact, cases of advanced disease with impending respiratory failure from airway obstruction. The interventional bronchoscopist must attempt to re-establish airway patency, prolong life, and restore quality of life. Goals of care must be carefully weighed, however, against procedure-related risks, and the operator must choose carefully among a variety of available treatment modalities to best serve the patient. Sometimes, patients might be best served by advising supportive care or removal from mechanical ventilation, especially in patients with advanced cancer when restoration of airway patency is unsuccessful. In many instances, multimodality treatments are warranted, and it is the interventional bronchoscopist's responsibility to assure that patients receive timely radiation and/or chemotherapy. In many instances, patients can safely undergo these treatments with greater comfort after airway patency has been restored. Finally, in patients with early lung cancer who are not felt to be surgical candidates, bronchoscopic treatments may provide disease-free survival, and therefore, close collaboration with an experienced oncologic and surgical service is mandatory to assure a team approach to medical decision-making. The purpose of this review is to describe indications for bronchoscopic treatment of airway cancers, describe basic techniques of rigid bronchoscopic debulking, laser with or without airway stent insertion, brachytherapy, and photodynamic therapy (PDT), and to describe some of the benefits of bronchoscopic treatment regarding level of care, quality of life, symptom control, and survival.

■ RIGID AND FLEXIBLE BRONCHOSCOPY

The workhorse for the interventional bronchoscopist is the rigid bronchoscope. This rigid stainless steel tube was originally used to remove foreign bodies and was "discovered" by the great Gustave Killian, a German Otorhinolaryngologist in 1897. Although the rigid tube fell into near oblivion after the introduction of the flexible fiberoptic bronchoscope in the 1970s, several modifications of the rigid tube, made to facilitate ventilation and laser resection, led to a resurgence of its use in the 1980s and 1990s. Today, it remains an essential instrument for tumor debulking, laser photocoagulation and vaporization, and silicone airway stent insertion (2). Rigid debulking is done using the beveled edge of the rigid bronchoscope to core out tumor while safeguarding the integrity of normal airway wall as much as possible. The rigid tube can thus be used to remove tumor, but also to compress a bleeding mucosa to assure clot formation. In obstructing tumors, the rigid tube can also be moved beyond the obstruction in order to assure ventilation prior to debulking, by pushing the tumor aside. Care must be taken to remain within the axis of the airway lumen, avoid mediastinal perforation, and to remember that the beveled edge of the bronchoscope is, after all, a relatively sharp and potentially dangerous instrument and thus must be used with caution to avoid inadvertent damage to airway mucosa, cartilage, and of course the larynx, lips, and gums during intubation and rigid bronchoscopic resection.

The flexible bronchoscope, usually with video, can be used as a stand-alone instrument for interventional procedures, and is also used in addition to the rigid tube (Figure 19.1). Bronchial toilet, suctioning of blood and secretions, and careful inspection of more distal bronchial segments is carried out before and after bronchoscopic

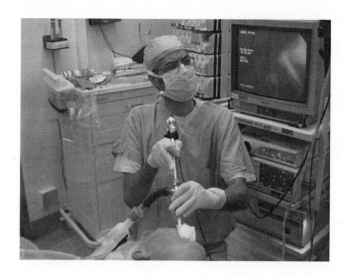

FIGURE 19.1 Rigid and flexible bronchoscopy performed under general anesthesia.

resection and stenting. The flexible scope was introduced by Shigeto Ikeda of Japan in the spring of 1964 and rapidly became the miracle instrument through which physicians could visualize the lumen and mucosa of the tracheobronchial tree, perform biopsies, obtain specimens of lung parenchyma, diagnose respiratory tract infections, remove tumors or inflammatory granulation tissue, insert self-expandable metal or covered metal stents, detect early lung cancer using autofluorescence techniques, inspect the airways of patients with primary cancers such as colon, kidney, breast, lymphoma, or melanoma to detect airway metastases, and treat early lung cancers using, for example, PDT (3).

■ INDICATIONS FOR BRONCHOSCOPIC TREATMENT

Combined therapeutic approaches, including potential use of chemotherapy and radiation therapy, are often advocated in addition to bronchoscopic management strategies for patients with primary or metastatic airway cancers. Combined approaches can also be used to enable patients with newly diagnosed, limited-stage cancer with airway involvement who undergo lung sparing open surgical resections (4). The majority of the indications for bronchoscopic treatments, however, are related to palliative care of symptomatic central airway obstruction involving the trachea and bronchial trees. Most procedures are limited to restoring airway patency in the main and lobar bronchi, and only infrequently are segmental bronchial resections performed. In these instances of segmental airway obstruction, however, PDT and brachytherapy might be particularly beneficial, especially when tumor does not extend far beyond the airway wall.

Signs and symptoms of central airway disease include atelectasis, postobstructive pneumonia, hemoptysis,

hypoxemia, cough, and dyspnea related to intraluminal exophytic airway obstruction, reduction of airway lumen from extrinsic compression by tumor and lymph nodes, or postsurgical changes. Indications for bronchoscopic treatment may also be found in patients with other tumors that can compress or invade the airway. These include esophageal and thyroid tumors and primary airway tumors other than primary lung cancer, such as carcinoid tumors, adenoid cystic carcinomas, and even lymphomas that infiltrate airway mucosa and cause intraluminal disease as well as extrinsic compression. Tumors may be large, centrally located mass-type lesions obstructing airway lumen, but may also arise from distal lung parenchyma or from beyond the airway wall, extending into the lumen, and be associated with necrosis, bleeding, cartilaginous destruction, or distortion of anatomic landmarks (enlarged carina, deviations of normal bronchial anatomy). In many instances, tumors may also be infiltrating with significant submucosal swelling. This is often the case of small cell lung cancer, in which case bronchoscopic therapies, such as stents inserted in the larger airways, may prove beneficial until systemic therapies result in restoration of airway patency and decreased mucosal infiltration, especially of the smaller segmental airways.

Circumstances during which patients are referred for bronchoscopic procedures are variable. Most are referred in extremis, when emergency admission from airway distress, atelectasis, unresolving pulmonary infiltrates, hemoptysis, or impending respiratory failure prompts bronchoscopic or computed tomographic evaluation that detects airway obstruction. Many patients may have already been admitted to the hospital or intensive care unit, and some may already have been intubated and placed on mechanical ventilation. Others are referred after diagnostic bronchoscopy has discovered an airway tumor partially or totally obstructing the airway lumen. In these cases, bronchoscopic intervention, if available, can be attempted, rather than emergency external-beam radiation therapy, in order to immediately improve the patient's ventilatory status so that the patient is better able to tolerate subsequent chemotherapy or external-beam radiation treatments. In this and other settings, the procedure is also warranted to improve quality of life and prolong survival until the patient succumbs from the effects of other comorbidities.

Bronchoscopic treatment, however, is not reserved for palliation of symptoms in patients with advanced disease. Some patients may be referred after the diagnosis of early superficial lung cancer, radiologically occult tumors, or carcinoma in situ (5). In these cases, in fact, long-term survival secondary to bronchoscopic treatments has been demonstrated in surgically unfit patients, as well as after additional treatment modalities such as steriotactic radiation, radiofrequency ablation, cryotherapy, and PDT in both early and later disease (6).

■ LASER RESECTION

Laser resection applies to the use of laser energy delivered through flexible optical fibers (Figure 19.2). The main type of laser used for bronchoscopic resection is the Neodynium:yttrium aluminum garnet (Nd:YAG) laser with its 1,064-nm wavelength. During laser application, light energy is transmitted through the optical fiber to the target tissues, where some of the energy is absorbed, while other energy is transmitted through the tissue, or scattered, and reflected by tissues. While light is that portion of the electromagnetic spectrum that is visible to the human eye and results from the spontaneous emission and random and diffuse distribution of photons through space, laser energy corresponds to light amplification stimulated emission of radiation (LASER). Some wavelengths are clearly visible, such as a red (helium neon at 632 nm) or blue wavelength (400–500 nm). Color often depends on what energy is absorbed and what is reflected, recognizing that objects that reflect no visible light are black. Nonvisible wavelengths include the ultraviolet (100–400 nm), near infrared (700–1,400 nm), and mid infrared (1,400–20,000 nm). Laser energy causes tissue disruption using either heat, kinetic, or chemical energies.

Tissue effect is usually the result of the wavelength used, tissue color (Nd:YAG energy is rapidly absorbed by darker pigments), laser power, and power density (power/surface area). When using the Nd:YAG laser with its 1,064-nm wavelength, tissue effects are the result of heat. As energy is applied, tissues are heated to more than 100°C, as a core of tissue is affected. Thermal energy is absorbed, conducted away from the initial target area, and scattered around and into adjacent tissues. The Nd:YAG laser is often referred to as a "what you see is not what you get" laser, because many tissue effects are actually occurring deep within the tissues, up to 10 mm, in fact, below the tissue surface. Tissues are first devascularized using the thermal effect of the laser, resulting in deep laser photocoagulation that causes vasoconstriction. Additional applications of laser energy, or when tissue surfaces are dark and rapidly absorb the 1,064 laser light wavelength, cause charring and subsequent vaporization. Because of deep tissue penetration, and because the 1,064-nm wavelength is readily absorbed by dark pigment (such as blood), perforation of vessels well below the tissue surface is possible. Also, one might expect late tissue necrosis because of devascularization of a large target area. Collateral damage of normal adjacent tissues should be avoided by limiting resection to abnormal tissues and keeping scatter to minimum.

After photocoagulation, obstructing tissues can be mechanically debulked using forceps or the beveled edge of the stainless steel rigid bronchoscope (7). In order to avoid excessive bleeding during resection, deep devascularization

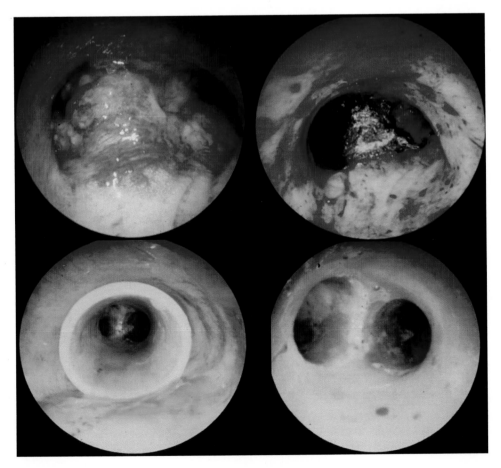

FIGURE 19.2 Laser resection performed to reshape widened main carina involved by tumor. A silicone Y-stent has been placed to restore and maintain airway patency to the left and right main bronchi.

is warranted. Suction catheters are used through the rigid tube to remove smoke, blood, and tissue debris. A high level of manual dexterity is required allowing the rigid bronchoscopist to work both with and through the 10- to 12-mm diameter rigid tube in order to adequately debulk tumor and control airway bleeding. Procedures are almost always performed under general anesthesia (8) and of course require a careful evaluation of patient comorbidities, anesthesia risks, and the patient's goals and values as they pertain to emergency and subsequent longer term cancer care (9).

■ AIRWAY STENT INSERTION

Tracheobronchial stents are prostheses made of silicone, metal, or a combination of both, inserted bronchoscopically in order to prop open the obstructed airway (10). Used in conjunction with resectional therapies, or, as in the case of pure extrinsic compression caused by narrowing of airway lumen, stents restore airway patency, improve breathing, and facilitate clearance of airway secretions. Stents can also be used to palliate symptoms from tracheoesophageal or bronchopleural fistula. Several factors usually need to be considered before patients with cancer and airway obstruction are "stented". This is, in part, because stents are not ideal and often are associated with adverse events including stent migration and obstruction by recurrent tumor growth or granulation tissue, as well as fracture from compressive tumor (usually only in metal stents). Overall, however, stents are often life-saving and life-prolonging, allowing interventional bronchoscopists to alleviate airway obstruction even in the setting of respiratory failure, and enabling physicians to remove patients from mechanical ventilation or to reduce level of care in critically/terminally ill patients (11–13).

Stents have no adverse effect on radiation therapy, brachytherapy, or chemotherapy. If airway caliber improves after systemic therapies, silicone stents can be removed, whereas metal stents are usually permanent. Surveillance bronchoscopy, although its use is often debated, may not be necessary unless patients develop symptoms suggestive of a stent-related complication such as new onset of dyspnea, cough, hemoptysis, or atelectasis on radiographic studies (14). Stents can remain in place for many years, or may be removed if tumors shrink as a result of systemic therapy. Stents, therefore, provide an excellent therapeutic bridge allowing patients to undergo systemic therapy with less shortness of breath, anxiety, and greater overall comfort.

Many physicians and patients fear the potential complications of airway stent insertion. Such fears are unfounded, especially in patients with airway malignancies. While it is true that stents require some maintenance,

such as daily nebulizer treatments using saline solution to enhance lubrification and facilitate clearance of airway secretions, stents are usually not noticed, and patients do not feel the stent inside their airway. When complications do occur, including stent migration, obstruction by secretions, or obstruction by granulation tissue or tumor regrowth, they are usually controlled by repeat flexible or rigid bronchoscopy with or without stent revision. In some cases, stents can be downsized or upsized depending on the underlying anatomy. In other cases, they can be removed altogether. Even in the terminal phases of malignancy, stents can improve symptoms and avoid death by suffocation. Should a patient with an indwelling stent develop life-threatening shortness of breath, intubation is usually possible using an uncuffed #6 endotracheal tube. Many stents are visible on chest radiograph, but emergent flexible bronchoscopy in patients with potential stent-related complications will provide diagnosis. A medical alert document (downloadable from www.bronchoscopy.org) can be given to patients, providing them with specific instructions in case of potential stent-related adverse events.

■ PHOTODYNAMIC THERAPY

PDT requires the administration of an intravenous tumor-specific photosensitizing agent that is selectively retained by neoplastic tissues, and activated using monochromatic light laser energy (640-nm wavelength) administered during flexible bronchoscopy (15). The subsequent production of reactive oxygen singlets causes tumor necrosis and tissue sloughing, which then requires follow-up bronchoscopy for removal 1 or 2 days after the initial application (Figure 19.3). PDT causes in vivo thrombosis of tumor vasculature and local edema. There is selective retention of the photosensitizer by tumor cells, and any related necrosis usually spares cartilage and the collagen matrix. Tissue effects are, for the most part, dependent on the light energy delivered (usually a total of 200–400 joules), power output, and the duration of energy delivery. The effectiveness of PDT often depends on the depth of mucosal penetration. The usual depth of penetration is about 5 mm for a 630-nm laser wavelength. By using cylindrical fibers, greater dosimetry is possible than when using simple end-on fibers. Tissues can thus be irradiated in a circumferential fashion, making PDT extremely useful, on occasion, for restoring airway patency in cases of lobar and segmental obstruction without extensive extramural extension.

PDT has been approved for use in early lung cancer patients and carcinoma in situ, as well as for palliation of obstructing central airway lesions from non–small cell lung cancer (16–19). In patients with airway obstruction, PDT has been shown to be effective. Moghissi et al. (20),

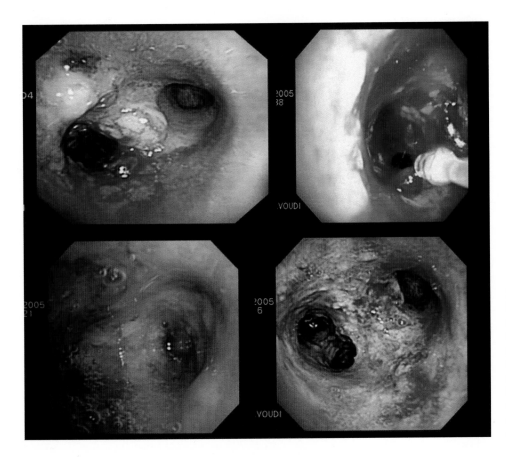

FIGURE 19.3 Exophytic segmental bronchial obstruction before, during, and after photodynamic therapy. A cylindrical probe was used to deliver photoradiation, resulting in necrotic tissue slough and temporary airway obstruction. Slough was removed by flexible bronchoscopy resulting in restored segmental airway patency and removal of tumor involving minor carina.

for example, showed that when PDT was used to treat 100 patients with airway obstruction, airway patency improved by 68% with corresponding increases in forced vital capacity and forced expiratory volume in 1 second. Median survival following PDT was better compared with other treatment modalities.

Contraindications include allergy to porphyrin and porphyria, as well as lesions where substantial worsening of any underlying necrosis might cause fistulas or erosion into major blood vessels. One major disadvantage of PDT is the need for patients to avoid exposure to sunlight for up to 6 weeks after applications. Because the effect of PDT is not immediate, PDT is infrequently used in the emergency setting. In addition, the photosensitivity associated with PDT is such that it may not be ideal for patients with limited life expectancies who wish to remain as physically active outdoors as much as possible during their remaining weeks or months of life. Another potential disadvantage of PDT is its cost, with doses of photosensitizer often exceeding several thousand dollars.

There are also many drug interactions that must be taken into consideration when choosing a patient for PDT. Photosensitizers such as Photofrin may cause porphyria, hypersensitivity reactions, and have synergistic additive interactions with ionizing radiation and chemotherapeutic agents such as Adriamycin and mitomycin. An attenuation of the effects of PDT might be noted in patients using non-steroidal anti-inflammatory drugs and steroids (21,22).

Clinical contraindications to PDT include chances for overdose risk caused by profound light sensitivity, unstable respiratory status, unavoidable sunlight or intense lighting, risk of fatal massive hemoptysis, central tumors with blood vessel invasion, existing or high risk for fistula formation, inability to work with the PDT team or inability to adequately understand instructions, and lack of access to emergency or scheduled flexible bronchoscopy for removal of tissue slough.

■ BRACHYTHERAPY

Endobronchial brachytherapy uses intraluminal radiation therapy to treat tumors within the airway lumen. The word brachy means "short" in Greek and denotes both the distance of the radiation source from the tissue being treated as well as the duration of therapy. Early on in the evolution of this treatment modality, radiation seeds were directly implanted into the tumor (aka interstitial brachytherapy). More recently, brachytherapy is performed by placing the radiation source within the airway. Improvements in after loading techniques using iridium-192 for high-dose-rate brachytherapy (HDR) on an outpatient basis, for example, creates minimal risk to health-care personnel and has resulted in methods that allow high-dose tumor irradiation with a rapid falloff of radiation effect outside the target area.

Of course, external-beam radiation therapy can be used for patients with central airway obstruction. However, it is only moderately effective. In their study of 330 patients, Slawson and Scott (23) found external-beam radiation therapy effective for palliating hemoptysis in 84% of patients and superior vena cava syndrome in 86% of patients, but improved atelectasis caused by airway obstruction in only 23% of patients.

Usually, brachytherapy is reserved for patients who have already received maximum external-beam radiation, although it can also be used as a stand-alone treatment modality in selected instances of segmental obstruction, or in association with other bronchoscopic treatments such as laser resection or electrocautery. Recent evidence suggests that brachytherapy is, in fact, best used as a complimentary treatment modality, and when associated with systemic therapies, external-beam radiation, or bronchoscopic therapies, results in better relief of dyspnea and other symptoms than brachytherapy alone (24–26).

Brachytherapy requires the bronchoscopic insertion of a catheter into the area of interest, and is best applied when there is minimal or no extramural extension of tumor. A target area several centimeters long can be irradiated using either HDR or low-dose (LDR) techniques depending on institutional preferences and equipment availability. Radiation planning is usually done by radiation oncology. For LDR, an arbitrary cumulative dose of 3,000 cGy at a radius of 10 mm in the trachea, and 5 mm in the bronchi, is commonly used. Traditionally, this technique requires hospitalization in order to administer a typical treatment session using fractions of 200 to 1,200 cGy/hour, with each session lasting 1 to 4 hours. HDR delivers more than 1,000 to 1,200 cGy/hour. Dose and fractionation vary widely from 15 Gy in one fraction to five fractions of 4 Gy each. A typical regimen delivers 500 cGy at 10 mm, with an average of three fractions at weekly intervals, and a total dose of 1,500 cGy, although fractions of up to 1,000 cGy have also been used. Because each treatment fraction lasts between 3 and 30 minutes, therapy can be provided in the ambulatory setting.

The catheter is usually placed bronchoscopically. It is inserted through the working channel of the flexible bronchoscope, often after initial placement of a guide-wire. The catheter is positioned about 2 cm beyond the estimated distal end of the target area and anchored within the segmental bronchus. Sometimes fluoroscopy can be used to assist in guidance, but this is not absolutely necessary. Once in place, the catheter is secured at the nostril, where its position is often marked with indelible ink and the external length from the tip of the nostril is measured in order to identify catheter migration. This can be especially important when patients need to be moved to the radiation oncology department (rather than performing the bronchoscopy in the department itself). The irradiation length is marked using external tags, or color codes on the catheter with a reference site externally. Prescription depths for after loading are calculated by the radiation oncologist and reflect the changing caliber of the TB tree, the location of the catheter, and the need to treat mucosal as well as peribronchial disease. A small margin prolonging the field of radiation is usually calculated in order to allow for small catheter movements within the target area.

While there are few head-to-head comparison trials of low-dose-rate versus HDR brachytherapy, restoration of some airway patency and symptomatic improvement is usually reported in more than 70% of patients (27,28). In one prospective study (29), Huber looked at the effect of brachytherapy in addition to external-beam radiation and noted a trend toward better local control in the brachytherapy and radiation therapy group, especially for those patents with squamous cell carcinoma ($P = 0.007$ in subgroup analysis).

Brachytherapy is usually contraindicated in tumors that invade major arteries or structures within the mediastinum. Complications include radiation bronchitis in up to 10% of patients and hemoptysis in 7% of patients. Other complications include bronchial stenosis and bronchopleural or bronchoesophageal fistula (30,31). There appears to be no identifiable predictors of fatal hemoptysis, but radiation injury is particularly likely in areas where the catheter is in contact with the bronchial wall, and when Nd:YAG laser therapy is done in addition to brachytherapy (32).

■ RESULTS OF BRONCHOSCOPIC INTERVENTION INCLUDING PALLIATIVE LASER RESECTION, PHOTODYNAMIC THERAPY, AND ENDOSCOPIC TREATMENT OF EARLY LUNG CANCER

Palliative bronchoscopic interventions for patients with obstructing airway cancers are, for the most part, and in experienced hands, safe and fraught with few procedure-related complications. Several studies during the past 20 years have, in fact, demonstrated survival benefit, improved dyspnea scores, and improved quality of life scores directly related to bronchoscopic treatment (33–35). Patients who undergo successful reestablishment of airway patency usually survive longer then those who have continued partial obstruction or in whom attempts at restoring airway patency are unsuccessful. Pulmonary function has been shown to improve by as much as 300 ml, Karnofsky scores often improve from 40 to 60, but median survival after stent insertion is about 5 months. This reinforces the fact that patients are either referred late in the course of their disease or that life-threatening symptoms of airway obstruction occur as terminal or near-terminal events, that can, however, be palliated in order to provide improved comfort, diminished breathlessness, and increased ability to interact with family and friends (36).

In patients with superficial early lung cancer and carcinoma in situ, potentially curative bronchoscopic treatment should also be considered. PDT may be a valuable adjunct, especially in patients who are not surgical candidates, as demonstrated from a study in which 13 publications pertaining to a total of 523 patients was reviewed, revealing greatest long-term survival (70% to 5 years) among patients with TIS tumors and stage I lung cancer (19). In patients with radiographically occult lung cancer not eligible for surgical resection, bronchoscopic application of electrocautery has also been used to assure long-term survival without tumor recurrence (37).

■ CONCLUSION

In summary, bronchoscopic therapy using debulking techniques, laser resection, airway stents, brachytherapy, and other modalities such as electrocautery and cryo-ablation not covered in this paper, is warranted to improve symptoms, enhance quality of life, and increase survival in patients with malignant central airway obstruction. Despite the lack of evidence comparing results with those of laser resection and stent insertion in patients with advanced disease, PDT is also, in fact, an effective and valuable lung cancer treatment modality. In patients with early-stage lung cancer within the proximal airways, especially with early superficial cancers and carcinoma in situ or those that refuse surgery or who are poor surgical risks or have multiple synchronous cancers in the airway, PDT may also be particularly beneficial.

■ REFERENCES

1. Cox JD, Yesner R, Mietlowski W, Petrovich Z. Influence of cell type on failure pattern after irradiation for locally advanced carcinoma of the lung. *Cancer.* 1979;44(1):94–98.
2. Becker HD, Marsh BR. History of the rigid bronchoscope. *Prog Respir Res.* 2000;30:2–15.
3. Miyazawa T. History of the flexible bronchoscope. *Prog Respir Res.* 2000;30:16–21.
4. Kato H, Konaka C, Ono J, et al. Preoperative laser photodynamic therapy in combination with operation in lung cancer. *J Thorac Cardiovasc Surg.* 1985;90(3):420–429.
5. Sutedja TG, Codrington H, Risse EK, et al. Autofluorescence bronchoscopy improves staging of radiographically occult lung cancer and has an impact on therapeutic strategy. *Chest.* 2001;120(4):1327–1332.
6. Pasic A, Brokx HA, Vonk Noordegraaf A, Paul RM, Postmus PE, Sutedja TG. Cost-effectiveness of early intervention: comparison between intraluminal bronchoscopic treatment and surgical resection for T1N0 lung cancer patients. *Respiration.* 2004;71(4):391–396.
7. Colt HG. Bronchoscopic laser resection in thoracic neoplasia. In Aisner, Arriagadaa, Green, Martin, Perry, eds. *Comprehensive Textbook of Thoracic Oncology.* Baltimore MD: Williams and Wilkins; 1996:925–939.
8. Perrin G, Colt HG, Martin C, Mak MA, Dumon JF, Gouin F. Safety of interventional rigid bronchoscopy using intravenous anesthesia and spontaneous assisted ventilation. A prospective study. *Chest.* 1992;102(5):1526–1530.
9. Colt HG. Functional evaluation before and after interventional bronchoscopy. In Bolliger CT, Mathur PN, eds. *Interventional Bronchoscopy, Textbook.* Basel, Switzerland: Karger Publisher. *Prog Respir Res.* 2000;30:55–64.
10. Dineen KM, Jantz MA, Silvestri GA. Tracheobronchial stents. *J Bronchol.* 2002;9:127–137.
11. Colt HG, Harrell JH. Therapeutic rigid bronchoscopy allows level of care changes in patients with acute respiratory failure from central airways obstruction. *Chest.* 1997;112(1):202–206.
12. Shaffer JP, Allen JN. The use of expandable metal stents to facilitate extubation in patients with large airway obstruction. *Chest.* 1998;114(5):1378–1382.
13. Colt HG, Murgu SD. Closure of pneumonectomy stump fistula using custom Y and cuff-link-shaped silicone prostheses. *Ann Thorac Cardiovasc Surg.* 2009;15(5):339–342.
14. Matsuo T, Colt HG. Evidence against routine scheduling of surveillance bronchoscopy after stent insertion. *Chest.* 2000;118(5):1455–1459.
15. Levine DJ, Angel LF. Role of the interventional pulmonologist. *Clin Pulm Med.* 2006;13:128–141.
16. Dougherty TJ, Marcus SL. Photodynamic therapy. *Eur J Cancer.* 1992;28A(10):1734–1742.
17. LoCicero J 3rd, Metzdorff M, Almgren C. Photodynamic therapy in the palliation of late stage obstructing non-small cell lung cancer. *Chest.* 1990;98(1):97–100.
18. McCaughan JS Jr, Williams TE. Photodynamic therapy for endobronchial malignant disease: a prospective fourteen-year study. *J Thorac Cardiovasc Surg.* 1997;114(6):940–6; discussion 946.
19. Moghissi K, Dixon K. Is bronchoscopic photodynamic therapy a therapeutic option in lung cancer? *Eur Respir J.* 2003;22(3):535–541.
20. Moghissi K, Dixon K, Stringer M, Freeman T, Thorpe A, Brown S. The place of bronchoscopic photodynamic therapy in advanced unresectable lung cancer: experience of 100 cases. *Eur J Cardiothorac Surg.* 1999;15(1):1–6.
21. Allison RR, Downie GH, Cuenca R, et al. Photosensitizers in clinical PDT. *Photodiag Photodyna Ther.* 2004;1:27–42.
22. Huang Z, Xu H, Meyers AD, et al. Photodynamic therapy for treatment of solid tumors–potential and technical challenges. *Technol Cancer Res Treat.* 2008;7(4):309–320.
23. Slawson RG, Scott RM. Radiation therapy in bronchogenic carcinoma. *Radiology.* 1979;132(1):175–176.
24. Langendijk H, de Jong J, Tjwa M, et al. External irradiation versus external irradiation plus endobronchial brachytherapy in inoperable non-small cell lung cancer: a prospective randomized study. *Radiother Oncol.* 2001;58(3):257–268.
25. Anacak Y, Mogulkoc N, Ozkok S, Goksel T, Haydaroglu A, Bayindir U. High dose rate endobronchial brachytherapy in combination with external beam radiotherapy for stage III non-small cell lung cancer. *Lung Cancer.* 2001;34(2):253–259.
26. Gollins SW, Burt PA, Barber PV, Stout R. Long-term survival and symptom palliation in small primary bronchial carcinomas following treatment with intraluminal radiotherapy alone. *Clin Oncol (R Coll Radiol).* 1996;8(4):239–246.
27. Lo TC, Girshovich L, Healey GA, et al. Low dose rate versus high dose rate intraluminal brachytherapy for malignant endobronchial tumors. *Radiother Oncol.* 1995;35(3):193–197.
28. Kvale PA, Selecky PA, Prakash UB; American College of Chest Physicians. Palliative care in lung cancer: ACCP evidence-based clinical practice guidelines (2nd edition). *Chest.* 2007;132(3 suppl):368S–403S.

29. Huber RM, Fischer R, Hautmann H, Pöllinger B, Häussinger K, Wendt T. Does additional brachytherapy improve the effect of external irradiation? A prospective, randomized study in central lung tumors. *Int J Radiat Oncol Biol Phys.* 1997;38(3): 533–540.

30. Suh JH, Dass KK, Pagliaccio L, et al. Endobronchial radiation therapy with or without neodymium yttrium aluminum garnet laser resection for managing malignant airway obstruction. *Cancer.* 1994;73(10):2583–2588.

31. Hennequin C, Tredaniel J, Chevret S, et al. Predictive factors for late toxicity after endobronchial brachytherapy: a multivariate analysis. *Int J Radiat Oncol Biol Phys.* 1998;42(1):21–27.

32. Ofiara L, Roman T, Schwartzman K, Levy RD. Local determinants of response to endobronchial high-dose rate brachytherapy in bronchogenic carcinoma. *Chest.* 1997;112(4):946–953.

33. Bolliger CT, Sutedja TG, Strausz J, Freitag L. Therapeutic bronchoscopy with immediate effect: laser, electrocautery, argon plasma coagulation and stents. *Eur Respir J.* 2006;27(6):1258–1271.

34. Detterbeck FC, Jones DR, Morris DE. Palliative treatment of lung cancer. In: *Diagnosis and Treatment of Lung Cancer.* Philadelphia PA: Saunders pub; 2001: 419–436.

35. Vergnon JM, Huber RM, Moghissi K. Place of cryotherapy, brachytherapy and photodynamic therapy in therapeutic bronchoscopy of lung cancers. *Eur Respir J.* 2006;28(1):200–218.

36. Wahidi MM, Herth FJ, Ernst A. State of the art: interventional pulmonology. *Chest.* 2007;131(1):261–274.

37. Vonk-Noordegraaf A, Postmus PE, Sutedja TG. Bronchoscopic treatment of patients with intraluminal microinvasive radiographically occult lung cancer not eligible for surgical resection: a follow-up study. *Lung Cancer.* 2003;39(1):49–53.

SUMANTA KUMAR PAL

KAREN RECKAMP

20 Targeted Pathways in NSCLC and SCLC

■ INTRODUCTION

Comparisons of standard chemotherapeutic regimens for lung cancer have left oncologists in a state of equipoise. As one example, the Eastern Cooperative Oncology Group (ECOG) led a pivotal trial in which 1,155 patients with advanced non–small cell lung cancer (NSCLC) were randomized to one of four platinum-containing doublets (1). In this study, each therapeutic arm yielded nearly equivalent response rates (RR) and survival. While cytotoxics remain an integral component of lung cancer treatment, recent advances in targeted therapy have led to substantial improvements in therapeutic outcome. Oncologists are now faced with the challenge of implementing these biologic agents, each with unique clinical application and a distinct panel of associated toxicities. Herein, we provide a framework of both clinical and translational data to aid in this process.

■ ANTIANGIOGENIC THERAPIES

Conceptualization of the link between tumor angiogenesis and tumor proliferation is frequently attributed to Judah Folkmann, with his theoretic and biologic work published in 1971(2). Evolution of this preclinical work led to the identification of the vascular endothelial growth factor (VEGF) ligands, VEGF-A, VEGF-B, VEGF-C, VEGF-D, and placental growth factor (PlGF) (3). These ligands carry affinity for VEGF receptor 1 (VEGFR-1) and VEGFR-2; binding of the latter leads to increased tumor growth presumably through enhanced tumor-related angiogenesis (Figure 20.1) (4).

Monoclonal Antibodies: Bevacizumab

Treatment with bevacizumab, a monoclonal antibody with specificity for VEGF, represents an antiangiogenic strategy that has been implemented in a wide spectrum of malignancies, including colon cancer, breast cancer, glioblastoma multiforme, and ovarian cancer (6–9). A plethora of data also suggest a role for the agent in the setting of NSCLC. A randomized phase II trial of carboplatin and paclitaxel alone or in combination with bevacizumab was conducted in treatment-naïve patients (10). Notably, patients receiving bevacizumab with chemotherapy received a dose of either 7.5 mg/kg or 15 mg/kg every 3 weeks. The addition of bevacizumab (at 15 mg/kg) to carboplatin and paclitaxel led to an improvement in RR (31.5% vs. 18%) and median overall survival (OS; 17.7 vs. 14.9 months). An important observation in this study was an association between major hemoptysis and squamous histology in bevacizumab recipients. These adverse events informed the design of subsequent phase III trials of the antiangiogenic, in which patients with squamous histology were excluded.

Following the aforementioned phase II trial, the first published randomized, phase III study of bevacizumab in NSCLC randomized patients to carboplatin and paclitaxel alone or in combination with bevacizumab at 15 mg/kg (ECOG 4599) (11). Chemotherapy was administered to patients with advanced or recurrent NSCLC every 3 weeks for a total of six cycles, and bevacizumab was administered every 3 weeks until evidence of disease progression or intolerable adverse effects. With a total of 878 assessable patients, median OS in the bevacizumab arm was significantly longer than that in the control arm (12.3 vs. 10.3 months, $P = 0.003$). Furthermore, the outcome of the bevacizumab-treated population marked the first observation of median survival in excess of 1 year in a phase III trial for NSCLC. Preliminary biomarker analyses suggest that various single nucleotide polymorphisms in genes encoding moieties related to angiogenic pathways may predict response to bevacizumab therapy. These moieties include VEGF, epidermal growth factor, intercellular adhesion molecule-1, and WNK1 (12). Interestingly, hypertension (an adverse event frequently attributed to bevacizumab) may actually be a predictor of response to therapy as well. In landmark analyses of ECOG 4599, OS from the median time of onset of hypertension (1.9 months) was improved in patients who experienced hypertension as compared

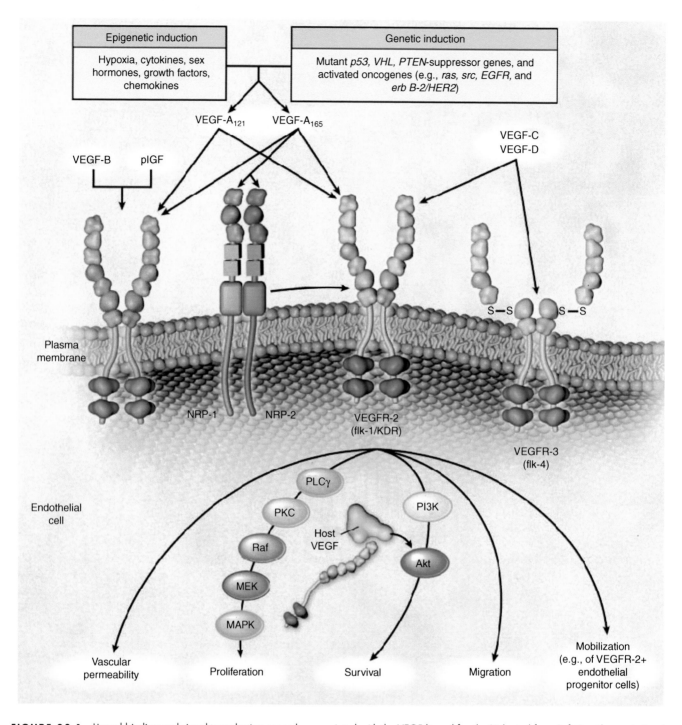

FIGURE 20.1 Ligand binding and signal transduction cascades associated with the VEGF ligand family. (Adapted from Ref. 5, with permission.)

with those who did not (14.0 vs. 11.3 months, P = not significant) (13).

A reasonable question emerging from ECOG 4599 was whether other platinum-based doublets in combination with bevacizumab had similar efficacy for the treatment for NSCLC. To this end, the AVAiL trial was a placebo-controlled, phase III effort in which patients were treated with either cisplatin and gemcitabine (with placebo) or the same chemotherapy regimen in combination

with low-dose (7.5 mg/kg) or high-dose (15 mg/kg) bevacizumab (14). The trial enrolled 1,043 patients, and at the time of most recent publication, the duration of follow-up was insufficient for a comparison of OS—only approximately half of the required deaths had been observed at the time of the final progression-free survival (PFS) analysis (356 out of 709). Notably, OS represented the initial primary endpoint of the study; this was replaced with PFS in a subsequent amendment (15). As compared with placebo, it was determined that PFS was prolonged in bevacizumab-treated patients in both the high-dose group (6.7 vs. 6.1 months, $P = 0.003$) and low-dose group (6.5 vs. 6.1 months, $P = 0.03$). OS was similar in both groups.

Other platinum-based doublets in combination with bevacizumab hold substantial promise. A phase II trial of cisplatin and docetaxel in combination with bevacizumab is underway, with two complete responses (CRs) and one partial response (PR) in four assessable patients thus far (16). Additionally, encouraging phase III data for the combination of carboplatin and pemetrexed in NSCLC with adenocarcinoma histology have spurred trials using this regimen with biologic therapies (17). In a phase II trial of carboplatin, pemetrexed, and bevacizumab, an objective RR of 55% was observed (18). Median time to progression (TTP) and OS in this study were 7.8 months and 14.1 months, respectively. Notably, in this trial design, both bevacizumab and pemetrexed were continued until the time of progression. A phase III trial comparing a similar three-drug regimen to carboplatin and pemetrexed alone is currently underway (19).

Use of cancer therapy in select patient populations is often accompanied by unique toxicities and efficacy data. To this end, subset analyses have been performed in trials using bevacizumab in several subgroups of patients with advanced NSCLC. A subset analysis of older adults enrolled in ECOG 4599 was reported, comparing patients of 70 years or older with younger cohorts (20). In 224 patients over the age of 70 (representing 26% of the enrolled patients overall), there was a nonstatistically significant trend toward higher RR (29% vs. 17%, $P = 0.067$) and PFS (5.9 vs. 4.9 months, $P = 0.063$) with the addition of bevacizumab to carboplatin and paclitaxel. However, there appeared to be no difference in OS with the three-drug regimen as compared with carboplatin and paclitaxel alone (11.3 vs. 12.1 months, respectively; $P = 0.4$). As compared with younger patients, an increased incidence of grade 3-to-5 neutropenia, bleeding, and proteinuria was observed in older adults. Importantly, these results were derived from an unplanned, retrospective analysis; it will be critical to prospectively analyze the benefit of bevacizumab therapy in older adults. Efforts have also been directed toward exploring differences in benefit from bevacizumab across gender. A comprehensive review of phase II and III clinical trials of bevacizumab therapy in both metastatic colorectal cancer and advanced NSCLC seems to suggest no lack of benefit from bevacizumab therapy in females (21).

Other studies have assessed the toxicities related to bevacizumab therapy when applied in specific clinicopathologic settings. The phase II PASSPORT study assessed the role of bevacizumab in combination with first- or second-line systemic therapy in nonsquamous NSCLC and brain metastases. In this study, prior therapy for brain metastases with either localized or whole-brain radiation was allowed. With 65 patients enrolled at the time of the most recent report, no central nervous system hemorrhages had been observed (22). As per the authors of this analysis, these data strongly suggest the safety of bevacizumab in this setting.

Small Molecule Tyrosine Kinase Inhibitors

Sunitinib

A distinct strategy to abrogate proangiogenic signaling is targeting of the intracellular tyrosine kinase domain of VEGF receptors. Various small molecules have been developed with affinity for VEGFR-1 and VEGFR-2; frequently, these agents are nonspecific and bind structurally related moieties. One example of this is sunitinib malate, which binds the VEGF family of receptors in addition to fetal liver tyrosine kinase receptor 3 (FLT-3), stem cell factor receptor (SCF receptor, or KIT), platelet-derived growth factor-α (PDGFR-α) and PDGFR-β (23,24). Phase I data for the agent identified manageable toxicity a dose of 50 mg oral daily (4 weeks on, 2 weeks off), with activity seen in patients with renal cell carcinoma (RCC) and several other tumor types (25). Consistent with these observations, sunitinib has been shown to prolong OS in the setting of metastatic RCC (26). Data for sunitinib in the setting of lung cancer is not as mature, but is evolving. A phase II study of sunitinib monotherapy in advanced NSCLC patients who had failed platinum-based chemotherapy demonstrated a median PFS of 12.0 weeks and a median OS of 23.4 weeks (27). The overall RR observed in this study (11.1%) was comparable to that seen with other agents approved for second-line therapy of advanced NSCLC, including docetaxel, erlotinib, and pemetrexed (28–30). Currently, trials are in progress to assess the combination of sunitinib with platinum-based chemotherapy. As one example, phase I data is available for the combination of sunitinib with cisplatin and gemcitabine (31). With data available for 13 patients, a combination of sunitinib at 37.5 mg daily (2 weeks on, 1 week off) with cisplatin and gemcitabine (at 80 mg/m^2 and 1,000 mg/m^2 intravenously every 3 weeks, respectively) appears to be safe and tolerable.

Sorafenib

Sorafenib represents a distinct multikinase inhibitor originally designed to inhibit the Raf family of signal transduction mediators. However, like sunitinib, the agent has affinity for multiple moieties, including KIT, FLT-3, VEGFR-2, VEGFR-3, and PDGFR-β (32). Preclinical models suggest that sorafenib delays tumor growth in NSCLC xenograft models when used in combination with gefitinib, cisplatin, or vinorelbine. A front-line "window of opportunity" study conducted by the North Central Cancer Treatment Group treated patients with sorafenib at a dose of 400 mg oral twice daily (33). The study was ultimately closed prematurely due to inadequate efficacy, with only one confirmed PR observed in the first 20 patients. Ultimately, however, after enrollment of 25 patients, an overall RR of 12% was observed, with a median OS of 8.8 months. Given RR similar to other approved second-line therapies for NSCLC, the authors of this study encouraged further assessment of sorafenib in this setting (28–30). Sorafenib has been further assessed in a double-blind phase II randomized discontinuation study (34). In this unique schema, NSCLC patients who had at least two prior chemotherapy regimens and progressing disease all received sorafenib. In a second "step," patients who responded continued on sorafenib, patients who progressed discontinued use, and patients who had stable disease were randomized to either sorafenib or placebo. Of 342 patients enrolled in the first step of the study, 97 were subsequently randomized in the second step. Median PFS on the sorafenib and placebo arms in 83 evaluable patients were 3.8 and 2.0 months, respectively (P = 0.01), leading the study authors to posit that sorafenib may be effective in a group of slowly growing tumors. Phase III data on sorafenib monotherapy is not available at this time. Notably, the phase III ESCAPE trial evaluating the combination of carboplatin and paclitaxel alone or with sorafenib in NSCLC was closed early when an interim analysis revealed that the trial would not meet its primary endpoint of improved OS (35). A press release associated with the ESCAPE suggested that higher mortality was observed in the subset of squamous cell carcinoma (SCC) patients treated with the three-drug regimen as opposed to carboplatin and paclitaxel alone.

Vandetanib

Vandetanib is a multikinase inhibitor with affinity for both VEGFR-2 and EGFR, and has shown activity in preclinical xenograft models of NSCLC (36). Separate studies in multiple tumor types suggest that antagonism of VEGFR-2–mediated signaling by the agent is largely responsible for its antitumor activity (37). A randomized, double-blind phase IIa dose-finding study of vandetanib in Japanese NSCLC patients suggested that doses between 100 and 300 mg oral daily were safe and tolerable, and yielded appreciable RR (38). The agent has also been assessed in combination with cytotoxic chemotherapy. A separate randomized phase II study has assessed the combination of vandetanib with chemotherapy (39). In this trial, patients were assigned 2:1:1 to receive vandetanib alone, vandetanib in combination with carboplatin and paclitaxel, or carboplatin and paclitaxel alone. The vandetanib monotherapy arm was discontinued after the agent failed to improve PFS as compared with carboplatin and paclitaxel in a planned interim analysis. Median PFS with the addition of vandetanib to carboplatin and paclitaxel was minimally prolonged (24 vs. 23 weeks, P = 0.098); no difference in OS was observed. Importantly, correlative

studies from this trial have suggested important biomarkers for activity; low levels of hepatocyte growth factor and interleukin-2 (IL-2) receptor were predictive of benefit from vandetanib alone, but were not predictive in chemotherapy-containing arms (40).

A separate randomized phase II trial of docetaxel alone or in combination with vandetanib in NSCLC patients who had failed first-line platinum-based chemotherapy demonstrated an improvement in PFS with the addition of vandetanib at 100 mg oral daily (18.7 vs. 12.0 weeks, P = 0.037) (41). Notably, addition of a higher level of vandetanib did not yield a statistically significant PFS improvement (17.0 vs. 12.0 weeks, P = 0.23). A phase III effort in advanced NSCLC used a similar design, randomizing 694 patients to vandetanib with docetaxel and 697 patients to placebo with docetaxel (42). Patients in this study had received prior first-line therapy, and had good performance status (ECOG PS 0–1). Addition of vandetanib to docetaxel resulted in an improved PFS as compared to placebo with docetaxel (hazard ratio [HR] 0.79, 98% confidence interval [CI] 0.70–0.90; P < 0.001). A nonstatistically significant trend toward improved OS was also observed with vandetanib therapy (HR 0.91, 98% CI 0.78–1.07; P = 0.196). Though nausea, rash, and neutropenia occurred more frequently with vandetanib, the rate of nausea, vomiting, and anemia were actually improved.

A distinct phase III dataset for vandetanib is derived from the ZEAL trial, comparing pemetrexed with vandetanib to pemetrexed with placebo in patients with advanced NSCLC (43). A total of 534 patients were enrolled on this trial, with a median follow-up of 9.0 months at the time of a preliminary analysis. The trial failed to show improvement in PFS with the addition of vandetanib; however, use of the agent did enhance overall RR (19.1% vs. 7.9%, P < 0.001). Interestingly, there appeared to be evidence of reduced toxicity with the addition of vandetanib therapy. Single agent vandetanib has also been assessed in a phase III trial; the ZEST trial randomized patients with one to two prior chemotherapy regimens to receive either vandetanib or erlotinib (44). A total of 1,240 patients were enrolled. A preplanned noninferiority analysis for PFS and OS demonstrated the equivalency of both agents. An increase in the incidence of several toxicities occurred with vandetanib as compared with erlotinib, namely diarrhea and hypertension. Rash, as anticipated, was more common with erlotinib. Interestingly, these data contrast with a randomized phase II experience comparing vandetanib with gefitinib (45). In this trial, patients with advanced NSCLC who had failed first-line platinum-based chemotherapy were allocated to receive either daily vandetanib (n = 83) or gefitinib (n = 85) until disease progression. Though no difference in OS was detected, vandetanib prolonged PFS as compared with gefitinib (HR = 0.69, 95% CI 0.50–0.96; P = 0.013).

Pazopanib

Pazopanib is a second-generation small molecule tyrosine kinase inhibitor with affinity for several receptors: VEGFR-1, VEGFR-2, VEGFR-3, PDGFR-α, PDGF-β, and KIT (46). Like the aforementioned small molecule antiangiogenics, pazopanib has shown preclinical activity in models of NSCLC. A neoadjuvant trial of single agent pazopanib for stage I/II NSCLC suggested appreciable antitumor activity at a dose of 800 mg oral daily; 20 out of 26 patients evaluated (87%) had a decrease in tumor volume at the time of surgery (after receiving 2–6 weeks of therapy) (47). Correlative analyses of 19 paired samples from this study suggest that pazopanib therapy is associated with a decrease in soluble VEGFR-2 ($P < 0.001$) (48). Furthermore, increases in numerous cytokines and angiogenic factors were observed, particularly PIGF.

■ EGFR-TARGETING THERAPIES

The ErbB family of proteins includes four cell surface receptors: HER1 (or EGFR), HER2, HER3, and HER4 (Figure 20.2). EGFR has been identified as a therapeutic target in NSCLC, given the fact that it is frequently

overexpressed in this disease process (50). Furthermore, data from retrospective analyses suggest that ErbB family receptor expression may be related to survival in NSCLC (51). Similar to antiangiogenic therapy, two broad classes of therapeutics have evolved—monoclonal antibodies and small molecule tyrosine kinase inhibitors.

Monoclonal Antibodies: Cetuximab

A disease-specific phase I trial in patients with head and neck SCC and NSCLC has been conducted for the combination of cetuximab with cisplatin (52). In this study, 9 out of 13 patients (69%) treated with cetuximab at 50 mg/m² received 12 weeks of therapy, and 2 patients experienced a PR. Several phase II studies have further assessed the combination of platinum-based chemotherapy and cetuximab in the setting of NSCLC. One such trial assigned previously untreated patients to receive carboplatin/paclitaxel and cetuximab (53). With 53 patients enrolled, an RR of 57% was observed with an estimated OS of 13.8 months. The most commonly encountered grade ≥3 toxicity was neutropenia (38%), followed by skin rash (28%). A total of three other phase II trials have been performed with a carboplatin/taxane and cetuximab regimen, all reported median OS in the rate of 11.0 to 13.8 months (54–56). These encouraging

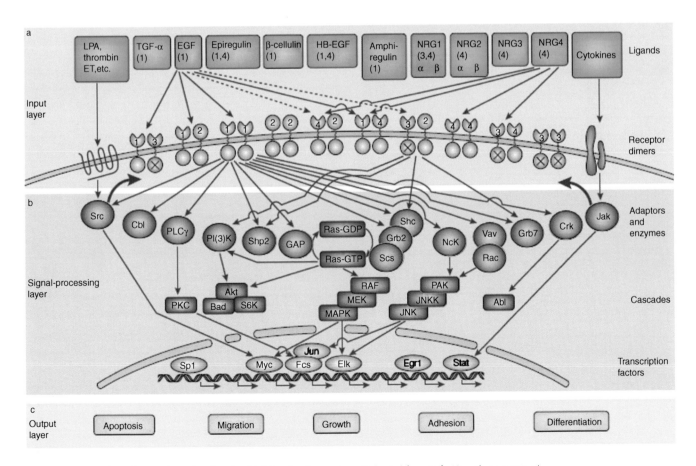

FIGURE 20.2 Signal cascades related to the ErbB family of receptors. (Adapted from Ref. 49, with permission.)

data led to a phase III study (BMS-099) comparing carbo-platin and taxane alone (paclitaxel or docetaxel at the inves-tigator's discretion) to the same regimen with cetuximab. In this trial, a total of 676 patients were randomized. There was a nonstatistically significant trend toward improved OS with the addition of cetuximab (9.7 vs. 8.4 months, 95% CI 0.75–1.05; $P = 0.17$), and a statistical improvement in PFS (4.4 vs. 3.8 months; HR = 0.79, $P = 0.0036$).

Data from the combination of cisplatin and vinorel-bine with cetuximab appear to be more promising. In a randomized phase II study of cisplatin/vinorelbine alone or in combination with cetuximab, a total of 86 patients were enrolled (57). Both RR and median OS were improved with the addition of cetuximab to chemotherapy (35% vs. 28% and 8.3 vs. 7.3 months, respectively). These data led to a larger phase III effort utilizing a similar schema (58). In the FLEX trial, a total of 1,175 patients were random-ized. The addition of cetuximab significantly prolonged median OS (10.5 vs. 9.1 months, $P = 0.003$). Notably, this improvement in OS was observed without any difference in PFS (4.8 months in both groups). In the confines of this study, cetuximab represents an approach with benefit in SCC subtypes of NSCLC. In 347 such patients, survival was improved from 8.9 months to 10.2 months, albeit with a CI crossing over 1.0 (HR 0.794, 95% CI 0.626–1.007). The combination of cetuximab with cisplatin and vinore-lbine led to higher rates of grade ≥3 febrile neutropenia than with chemotherapy alone (22% vs. 15%, $P < 0.05$); there was also a higher frequency of grade ≥3 acne-like rash (10% vs. <1%, $P < 0.05$) and diarrhea (5% vs. 2%, $P < 0.05$).

Mirroring the aforementioned experience with beva-cizumab, a number of trials have emerged to test cetux-imab with other platinum-based doublets. A phase I/IIa study of cetuximab in combination with carboplatin and gemcitabine in patients with advanced NSCLC reported 10 PRs in 35 assessable patients (28.6%); median OS was 11.1 months (59). The same regimen is being assessed in a phase II/III study (GemTaxIV), comparing cetuximab in combination with either carboplatin/gemcitabine or gem-citabine followed by docetaxel in patients with treatment-naïve advanced NSCLC (60). Available safety data from 142 patients enrolled thus far suggested that cetuximab did not add significantly to known chemotherapy toxicity. Efficacy data from this study is eagerly awaited.

Various cut-points have been utilized for eligibility criteria in clinical trials of cetuximab, ranging from no requirement for testing to 1% to 10% EGFR-staining by immunohistochemistry (IHC) (58, 61). A focus of cur-rent research has been prediction of cetuximab response using clinicopathologic factors. As one example, speci-mens from a phase II selection trial comparing sequen-tial or concurrent carboplatin/paclitaxel with cetuximab for advanced NSCLC were assessed for EGFR amplifi-cation via fluorescence in situ hybridization (FISH) (62).

A total of 76 samples were assessable; response was numerically higher in patients with FISH-positive tumors (45% vs. 26%), but this did not reach statistical sig-nificance ($P = 0.14$). However, a comparison of disease control rate (characterized as the total rate of CRs, PRs, and stable disease) was improved in those patients with EGFR FISH-amplification (81% vs. 55%, $P = 0.02$). Furthermore, patients with FISH-positive tumors had a prolonged median PFS (6 vs. 3 months, $P = 0.0008$) and median OS (15 vs. 7 months, $P = 0.04$). Though prospec-tive validation of these findings is warranted, these are encouraging data to suggest the role of EGFR FISH as a predictor of clinical response to cetuximab. *KRAS* muta-tional status has also emerged as a potential biomarker of cetuximab response, with strong supporting data in the setting of colorectal cancer (63). From correlative analyses accompanying the FLEX trial, however, it does not appear that *KRAS* mutational status predicts the efficacy of the combination of cetuximab and chemotherapy in NSCLC (64). Interestingly, a similar correlative analysis accom-panied the report of BMS-099, comparing carboplatin/taxane doublet therapy with or without cetuximab (65). With samples available for roughly one third of the study population, approximately 17% of specimens assessed had *KRAS* mutation. Analyses by treatment showed no differ-ential effect on PFS, OS, or RR based on *KRAS* status.

Since the initial phase III data for cetuximab in col-orectal cancer, much attention has also been turned to the role of rash as a predictor of cetuximab response (61). To this end, an EGFR-inhibition-related rash (EIRR) rating scale has been developed to better characterize associated lesions. The EIRR rating scale has been validated prospec-tively in patients with advanced NSCLC, using enrollees in a trial comparing cetuximab and pemetrexed versus cetuximab followed by pemetrexed at the time of progres-sion (66). We now await assessment of this scale prospec-tively for association with treatment outcome.

Cetuximab with Radiation

The impetus to assess cetuximab in combination with radiation therapy comes from positive data in the setting of head and neck SCC, where the combination of these modalities leads to an improvement in locoregional con-trol and median OS as compared with radiation alone (67). Several studies are ongoing to address the combina-tion. In the phase I SCRATCH trial, patients with stage III NSCLC are treated with weekly cetuximab and concomi-tant radiotherapy after receiving platinum-based induc-tion therapy (68). With experience to date reported for 12 patients, only nine completed the complete schedule. Of concern, one patient died from broncho-pneumonia during treatment. Two other patients declined further treatment because of grade 3 lethargy and grade 2 skin reaction, respectively. Nonetheless, eight patients who completed therapy have survived to greater than 1 year. A similar phase II effort is underway (the NEAR study, combining radiation with cetuximab therapy with a targeted accrual of 30 patients with stage III NSCLC) (69).

The largest experience of combined radiation and cetuximab in lung cancer to date is derived from the Cancer and Leukemia Group B 30407 trial, a randomized phase II effort in which patients are either assigned to carboplatin/pemetrexed alone (arm A) or with cetuximab (arm B). Thoracic radiation (70 Gy) is administered concurrently, and all patients receive four cycles of consolidation therapy with pemetrexed alone following four cycles of the initial systemic therapy. With data for 106 patients reported, the cetuximab-containing regimen appears to be fairly well tolerated. In Arm B, 7% of patients experienced grade ≥3 febrile neutropenia and 23% experience grade ≥3 skin toxicity. Interestingly, a numerically smaller proportion of patients experienced esophagitis (35% vs. 22%) and fatigue (22% vs. 18%) with cetuximab therapy as compared without (70).

Neoadjuvant Cetuximab

Limited data is available at present to guide the use of cetuximab in the neoadjuvant setting. Preliminary results have been reported from a phase II pilot study in which patients with stage IB-IIIA NSCLC are treated with cisplatin, gemcitabine, and cetuximab (71). With 16 patients recruited to date, six PRs, four SDs, and one case of progressive disease (PD) have been observed. Skin rash was present in every patient enrolled; the most common grade 3 or 4 toxicities were neutropenia (73%) and thrombocytopenia (45%). Importantly, two grade 4 cardiovascular toxicities were observed in patients with substantial cardiac comorbidities. The trial is ongoing, and data from associated biomarker studies (a significant benefit of neoadjuvant trial design) may aid in selecting patients appropriate for this treatment.

Small Molecule Tyrosine Kinase Inhibitors

Erlotinib

Erlotinib is a highly specific small molecule inhibitor of the tyrosine kinase domain of EGFR. In a phase II experience, 57 patients with advanced NSCLC previously treated with platinum-based chemotherapy were assigned to erlotinib therapy (150 mg oral daily) (72). An objective RR of 12.3% was observed, and response did not appear to be related to the number of prior chemotherapeutic regimens received. A median OS of 8.4 months was determined, and Cox modeling suggested predictors of response. Importantly, results of immunohistochemical staining for EGFR were not correlated with survival.

The aforementioned data established the framework for a larger phase III effort examining the clinical utility of erlotinib in NSCLC. The National Cancer Institute of Canada Clinial Trials Group (NCIC-CTG) BR.21 trial

was a randomized, placebo-controlled effort in which patients with stage IIIB or IV NSCLC (who had received ≤2 prior chemotherapy regimens) were assigned in a 2:1 ratio to receive either erlotinib or placebo (29). A comparison to placebo was deemed reasonable in light of the fact that previous data had shown no benefit to third-line therapy as compared with supportive care (73). A total of 731 patients were enrolled on NCIC-CTG BR.21 and included in the final efficacy analysis. Although not externally validated, RRs were improved in the erlotinib-treated group (8.9% vs. <1%, P < 0.001). Median OS in the erlotinib-treated group was superior to that in the placebo group (6.7 vs. 4.7 months, P < 0.01). A total of 19% of patients receiving erlotinib required dose reductions, secondary to rash (12%) and diarrhea (5%) in the majority of cases. Quality of life (using tools to assess cough, dyspnea, and pain) appeared to be improved with erlotinib therapy.

Subgroup analysis from NCIC-CTG BR.21 yielded numerous hypothesis-generating results. Cox regression suggested an association between longer survival and Asian origin (P = 0.01), adenocarcinoma histology (P = 0.004), and never-smoker status (P = 0.048 as compared with current or past smoking) (29). In a companion study, molecular correlates were assessed in available tissue specimens (74). These analyses included EGFR expression by IHC (325 patients), EGFR mutation by polymerase chain reaction (197 patients), and EGFR gene amplification (221 patients). On univariate analysis, it appeared that higher EGFR expression and amplification (assessed by IHC and FISH, respectively) both correlated with survival. Multivariate analysis, however, suggested that neither parameter was associated with survival—instead, two clinical parameters identified in the parent study (adenocarcinoma histology and never-smoker status) and EGFR expression correlated with response. Clinicopathologic data from these extensive studies have been compiled to generate a prognostic index for patients treated with erlotinib; this foray still requires prospective validation (75).

Data from NCIC-CTG BR.21 provide insight related to the benefit of erlotinib in certain high-risk groups. A separately reported analysis comparing patients younger and older than 70 years suggested that older adults had no significant difference in PFS or OS benefit from erlotinib therapy, despite receiving a lesser relative dose-intensity (64% vs. 82% receiving >90% of the planned dose, P < 0.001) (76). Furthermore, quality of life gains associated with erlotinib therapy appear to be preserved in the older population. However, patients over the age of 70 were more likely to have grade ≥3 toxicity (35% vs. 18%, P < 0.001) and discontinue treatment due to treatment-related toxicities (12% vs. 3%, P < 0.001). Perhaps the most compelling data related to erlotinib use in the older adults is derived from a prospective, phase II trial of erlotinib monotherapy in patients of 70 years or older (77).

Among 88 patients enrolled, median TTP was 3.5 months and median OS was 10.9 months. Rash and diarrhea occurred in 79% and 69% of the trial population, respectively. EGFR mutations were detected in 9 of 43 patients assessed, and correlated strongly with TTP and OS.

In poor PS patients, there is additional prospective data to guide therapy with erlotinib. In a randomized phase II design, NSCLC patients with PS of 2 were assigned to receive either erlotinib or carboplatin/paclitaxel as first-line therapy. Median OS was actually improved with chemotherapy (6.5 vs. 9.7 months, P = 0.018). However, selection criteria such as gender, tumor histology, smoking status, and the presence or absence of skin rash did seem to predict erlotinib benefit. These data indicate that in poor PS patients, chemotherapy is the preferred first-line treatment. Ultimately, selection criteria may help identify subgroups that benefit from erlotinib (78).

More recently, erlotinib has demonstrated efficacy as maintenance therapy following platinum-based chemotherapy. In the SATURN trial, 1,949 patients with advanced NSCLC who had received four cycles of platinum-based chemotherapy were randomized to receive either erlotinib (150 mg oral daily) or placebo (79). The primary endpoint of the trial was PFS, with a unique coprimary endpoint of PRs in patients with EGFR IHC(+) tumors. The trial met both endpoints, with an HR for PFS of 0.71 (95% CI 0.62–0.82, P < 0.0001) and 0.69 (95% CI 0.58–0.82, P < 0.0001) in both groups, respectively. The regimen appeared to be well tolerated, resulting in primarily grade 1 or 2 toxicities. Further biomarker data suggested that patients benefitted irrespective of EGFR FISH or EGFR intron 1 CA repeat status (80).

Given the success of erlotinib monotherapy, efforts have been made to combine this treatment with distinct modalities. Several reports of combinations of cytotoxic chemotherapy with erlotinib are available; the results are largely disappointing. A phase I trial of erlotinib and vinorelbine in advanced NSCLC patients (both treatment naïve and refractory) was terminated after accrual of 12 patients; no responses were observed, and 25% of the enrolled patients developed febrile neutropenia. Two much larger efforts from randomized trials have revealed also negative results. The Tarceva Lung Cancer Investigation Trial randomized 1,172 patients to either erlotinib or placebo, in addition to cisplatin/gemcitabine chemotherapy (81). No differences in OS were observed between erlotinib- and placebo-treated arms (43 vs. 44.1 weeks, respectively; HR 1.06). Similarly, TTP, RR, and quality of life did not differ between arms. Erlotinib with cisplatin/gemcitabine was well tolerated, but did lead to an increase in the frequency of rash and diarrhea. The TRIBUTE trial utilized a similar randomization, with the exception of substituting carboplatin/paclitaxel for cisplatin/gemcitabine (82). With 1,059 assessable patients, there was no difference in median OS (10.6 months for erlotinib

vs. 10.5 months with placebo, P = 0.95). One encouraging subset analysis from this trial included never-smokers, who did appear to possess a survival advantage with erlotinib therapy (22.5 vs. 10.1 months). Never-smokers therefore represent a demographic that may be further explored in future trials of chemotherapy with erlotinib.

Similar to combination with chemotherapy, various combinations of erlotinib with radiation therapy have been attempted. A phase I trial of combining erlotinib with chemoradiotherapy for unresectable stage III NSCLC enrolled a total of 34 patients (83). Patients received either erlotinib, cisplatin/etoposide, and radiotherapy followed by docetaxel (arm A), or induction carboplatin/paclitaxel followed by erlotinib, carboplatin/paclitaxel, and radiotherapy (arm B). The study authors commented that survival data yielded from the study was disappointing, with a median OS of 10.2 months and 13.7 months on arm A and arm B, respectively. The Galican Lung Cancer Study Group examined the role of erlotinib as maintenance therapy after chemoradiation (84). In a phase II effort, 28 patients with stage III NSCLC were enrolled after receipt of standard concurrent chemoradiotherapy. In a preliminary analysis, the majority of patients appeared to have no evidence of PD while receiving erlotinib maintenance. Finally, erlotinib has also been tested in combination with whole-brain radiotherapy (WBRT) (85). In a phase I trial, 13 patients with untreated NSCLC brain metastases received concurrent and maintenance erlotinib with WBRT. The regimen appears to be well tolerated. Interestingly, all disease progression noted in this trial occurred in an extracranial distribution; no intracranial progression was noted during erlotinib therapy.

Gefitinib

Like erlotinib, gefitinib selectively inhibits EGFR-stimulated tumor proliferation in preclinical models (86). Randomized, phase II data from the IDEAL-2 trial (conducted in the U.S.) compared two dose levels of gefitinib monotherapy in patients with advanced NSCLC that had failed two prior chemotherapy regimens (87). A total of 216 patients were randomized; radiographic PRs were observed in 12% of patients receiving 250 mg of gefitinib daily, and in 9% of patients receiving 500 mg daily (P = 0.51). Survival and symptom improvement did not differ between the two groups. Overall, survival at 1 year was 25%. A similar schema was utilized in the IDEAL-1 study, conducted through Europe and Japan (88). In this study, randomizing 210 patients with advanced NSCLC who had failed one or two prior chemotherapy regimens, objective RRs were slightly higher (18.4% and 19.0% for 250 mg and 500 mg dosing, respectively). Both IDEAL-1 and IDEAL-2 suggested limited toxicity with gefitinib therapy with appreciable

RR, thus providing impetus for more extensive assessment of the agent.

Phase III trials were subsequently designed to assess the efficacy of gefitinib monotherapy in advanced lung cancer. The Iressa Survival Evaluation in Lung Cancer (ISEL) study enrolled patients with chemotherapy-refractory NSCLC, and randomized 1,692 participants to gefitinib (at 250 mg/d) or placebo (both in combination with best supportive care) (89). With a median follow-up of 7.2 months, median OS did not differ in the gefitinib- or placebo-treated arms (5.6 vs. 5.1 months, $P = 0.087$). Similarly, no difference in median OS was observed in a prespecified analysis of patients with adenocarcinoma. Separately reported subset analyses of 235 Asian patients enrolled in ISEL did suggest a statistical improvement in time to treatment failure (TTF; 4.4 vs. 2.2 months, $P = 0.0084$), objective RR (12% vs. 2%), and OS (9.5 vs. 5.5 months, $P = 0.01$) with gefitinib therapy as compared with placebo (90). Furthermore, molecular correlates suggested that patients with EGFR mutation had substantially higher RR as compared with patients without this finding (37.5% vs. 2.6%).

These unplanned subset analyses are thought provoking, but certainly require further prospective validation. To this end, preliminary data from a phase II trial including patients with EGFR-mutated advanced NSCLC has yielded RR of 76% with gefitinib therapy (91). The multicenter iTARGET trial carried a similar premise, enrolling patients with advanced NSCLC and mutations in EGFR exons 18 to 21 (92). In 31 patients treated with gefitinib, an RR of 55% was achieved with a median PFS of 9.2 months. A third similar phase II trial was conducted by the West Japan Thoracic Oncology Group, yielding comparable results in this enriched population (93). The phase II ONCOBELL trial used even more extensive selection criteria; advanced NSCLC patients enrolled in this study had either EGFR amplification, were never-smokers, or had phospho-Akt positive tumors (94). The latter inclusion criterion was derived from retrospective analyses of phase II studies of gefitinib monotherapy in an unselected population—phospho-Akt, an activated mediator along the PI3K-Akt signaling cascade, was found to predict tumor response, disease control, and TTP (95). Data from the ONCOBELL trial (reflecting 42 patients enrolled) showed an overall RR of 47.6%, with a median TTP of 6.4 months. Median OS was not reached at the time of the most recent update.

Perhaps the most compelling dataset suggesting the utility of appropriate patient selection is derived from the iPASS study (96). This phase III trial is being conducted in Asia and includes chemotherapy-naïve, never-smokers with NSCLC, adenocarcinoma subtype. Patients are randomized to either gefitinib or carboplatin/paclitaxel (1:1). With 1,217 patients randomized to date, at an interim analysis, gefitinib demonstrated superior PFS (HR 0.741, $P < 0.0001$). EGFR mutational analysis was performed in this study. A more recent update of biomarker analyses accompanying the trial suggests that EGFR mutational status can be an effective means of predicting benefit from gefitinib therapy; those patients that were mutation (+) had superior PFS and RRs with gefitinib, while those that were mutation (–) had superior PFS and RRs with carboplatin and paclitaxel (97).

Whereas the ISEL experience compares gefitinib with placebo, the INTEREST trial provides a comparison of gefitinib to an approved second-line chemotherapy regimen, docetaxel (98). Designed as a noninferiority study, this phase III experience randomized patients who had been treated with ≥1 platinum-based chemotherapy regimen for advanced NSCLC to either gefitinib (250 mg/d) or docetaxel. With 1,433 assessable patients, the primary endpoint of noninferiority with respect to OS was met. A subsequent analysis of EGFR amplification showed no statistical difference in survival among those patients with high EGFR gene copy number treated with erlotinib as compared with docetaxel (8.4 vs. 7.5 months, $P = 0.62$).

Two studies have evaluated the role of chemotherapy in combination with gefitinib. In INTACT-1, chemotherapy-naïve patients with advanced NSCLC were randomized to cisplatin/gemcitabine with either placebo, gefitinib at 250 mg/d, or gefitinib at 500 mg/d (99). Gefitinib or placebo were continued until the time of disease progression, whereas chemotherapy was limited to six cycles. With 1,093 patients enrolled, no differences in OS were observed among the three arms (9.9 vs. 9.9 vs. 10.9 months, respectively; $P = 0.46$). RR on the three arms were 49.7%, 50.3%, and 44.8%, respectively. Similar results were observed in INTACT-2, a trial employing an identical randomization with a total of 1,037 patients enrolled. Median OS in arms receiving carboplatin/paclitaxel in combination with placebo, gefitinib at 250 mg/d, and gefitinib at 500 mg/d was 8.7, 9.8, and 9.9 months, respectively ($P = 0.64$) (100). Thus, similar to the experience with erlotinib, gefitinib therapy does not seem to augment the effect of chemotherapy in advanced lung cancer.

■ PAN-HER INHIBITORS

The activity of EGFR antagonists in lung cancer suggests a theoretic role for inhibition of other ErbB family members in the same malignancy. The compound HKI-272 has demonstrated activity against both EGFR and HER2 in xenograft models (101). Phase I experiences with the agent in advanced solid malignancies have shown that the agent is well tolerated, with diarrhea representing the most common adverse effect (102). Nine of the 73 patients included in this trial had NSCLC; no responses in this subgroup were noted.

Similar to HKI-272, the small molecule BIBW2992 inhibits activity of EGFR and HER2, thus leading to antitumor effects in preclinical models (103). Preliminary results from a phase I trial of the agent showed no clinical responses in patients with advanced solid tumors (104). However, 4 of 38 patients enrolled did experience stable disease for over 4 months. The LUX-Lung 2 trial represents a phase II experience with BIBW2992 enrolling patients who have failed first-line chemotherapy and harbor EGFR mutations (105). Reflecting a two-stage design, the trial has now proceeded to the second stage after 21 responses were observed among the first 38 patients enrolled. In 55 evaluable patients to date, 29 (53%) experienced a PR, and 23 (42%) had SD. The most common adverse events were diarrhea and skin rash—these were largely manageable, with only one patient discontinuing therapy on trial due to attributable side effects.

Extending the spectrum of activity of HKI-272 and BIBW2992, PF-00299804 inhibits EGFR, HER2, and HER4 activity. This agent is currently under investigation in a two-arm (adenocarcinoma and nonadenocarcinoma) phase II trial in patients with advanced NSCLC that has progressed on at least one prior chemotherapy regimen as well as erlotinib (106). At the time of a preliminary analysis, 34 patients had been enrolled. Of 20 evaluable patients, two unconfirmed PRs were reported, with SD in 10 patients.

■ INSULIN-LIKE GROWTH FACTOR 1 RECEPTOR–TARGETING THERAPIES

Insulin-like growth factor I receptor (IGF-1R) is frequently expressed in NSCLC, and activation of this moiety represents a potential bypass mechanism to circumvent ErbB-targeting agents in malignancies such as breast cancer (107). In the setting of lung cancer, the role of IGF-1R still remains somewhat unclear. Pathologic assessment of tissue specimens from 83 advanced NSCLC patients receiving gefitinib therapy through an expanded access trial demonstrated expression of IGF-1R in greater than 70% of tumors (108). Furthermore, it appeared that there was a correlation of IGF-1R expression with EGFR expression and EGFR gene amplification. The study, however, did not demonstrate a correlation between IGF-1R scoring and clinical outcome (i.e., PFS or OS). A contrasting result was obtained from a similarly sized cohort including 77 patients treated with gefitinib therapy—in this experience, IGF-1R positivity by IHC seemed to correlated with an improved OS (17.8 vs. 7.3 months, $P = 0.013$) (109). As the understanding of IGF-1R biology evolves, it may be that the moiety plays a more substantial role in the

progression of early stage NSCLC. Supporting this is a study of 184 patients with operable NSCLC (110). IGF-1R score in this setting was associated with worsened survival in both completely and incompletely resected patients. The amalgam of data implicating the role of IGF-1R in NSCLC pathogenesis (although admittedly not consistent) has led to the development of therapeutics targeting the receptor.

Several monoclonal antibodies targeting IGF-1R exist in various stages of development. CP-751,871 is one such agent that has been examined in a randomized phase II non-comparative study (111). In this trial, patients with treatment-naïve advanced NSCLC were assigned in a 2:1 ratio to receive either carboplatin/paclitaxel with CP-751,871 or carboplatin/paclitaxel alone (112). Chemotherapy was administered for up to six cycles, while the study agent was administered until the time of progression. At the time of most recent analysis, 156 patients were randomized, with safety and efficacy information available for 151 patients. Numerically, a greater percentage of patients receiving CP-751,871 demonstrated an objective response. Grade 3/4 hyperglycemia was more frequent with CP-751,871 therapy, but was generally controlled with insulin or oral hypoglycemic agents.

IMC-A12 represents a second monoclonal antibody with affinity for IGF-1R. The antibody appears to be well tolerated in the setting of a phase I clinical trial enrolling patients with advanced solid tumors (113). Other monoclonal antibodies currently under study include AMG 479, R1507, 19D12, and EM164 (114). The list of small molecule tyrosine kinase inhibitors targeting IGF-1R is similarly extensive, and includes (but is not limited to) AEW541, OSI906, INSM-18, and BMS536924 (114). All of these agents remain in early stages of clinical implementation.

■ MAMMALIAN TARGET OF RAPAMYCIN (mTOR) INHIBITORS

mTOR is a 289-kDA serine/threonine kinase in the PI3K family, playing a critical role in the regulation of cell cycle (Figure 20.3) (115). Activation of PI3K (frequently via ErbB or other transmembrane receptors) leads to phosphorylation of Akt. Akt subsequently leads to inhibition of the tuberous sclerosis 1/2 protein, which enhances activity of mTOR. Downstream of mTOR, moieties such as S6K1 and 4E-BP1 are thereby activated, leading to increased gene transcription, cell growth, and cell proliferation. Given the role of mTOR as an intermediary in these complex signaling cascades, it has been investigated extensively as a therapeutic target.

Everolimus represents an orally administered mTOR inhibitor that has demonstrated substantial clinical activity

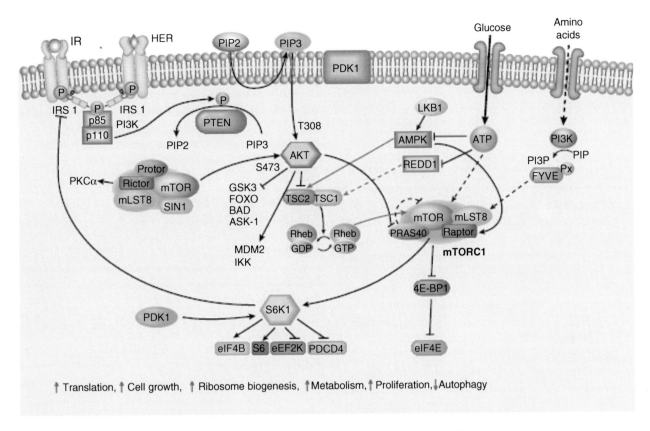

FIGURE 20.3 The mTOR pathway as it relates to cellular proliferation. (Adapted from Ref. 116, with permission.)

in advanced mRCC; the agent was recently approved in this setting on the basis of an improvement in PFS in patients refractory to VEGF-tyrosine kinase inhibitors (117). A phase I trial preceding this dataset suggested potential activity in NSCLC, as well (118). Among 12 patients enrolled with advanced NSCLC, 2 patients experienced PFS ≥6 months, and 2 patients experienced PFS between 4 and 6 months. In contrast to this data, a phase II trial of everolimus monotherapy for NSCLC produced rather discouraging results. In this two-arm trial, patients with advanced NSCLC who had failed ≤2 lines of chemotherapy (arm 1) or ≤2 lines of chemotherapy and an EGFR inhibitor (arm 2) were treated with everolimus at a dose of 10 mg oral daily until disease progression (119). The study employed a Simon 2-stage design, but did not proceed to the second stage in light of poor overall RR (5.3% for arm 1 and 2.8% for arm 2). Median PFS on the two study arms were 11.3 and 9.7 weeks, respectively. Data for everolimus in the setting of small cell lung cancer (SCLC) similarly showed low activity. Preliminary analyses from a phase II trial enrolling 17 patients with SCLC that had failed one to two prior chemotherapy regimens now yielded no objective responses with everolimus monotherapy. Only three patients (19%) experienced stable disease; the remainder (81%) experienced PD on therapy.

Like everolimus, temsirolimus has been approved for use in mRCC. Data from a phase III trial comparing temsirolimus to interferon and the combination of agents in poor-prognosis mRCC suggested improved survival with temsirolimus monotherapy (120). Temsirolimus has also been investigated in the setting of SCLC. In the ECOG 1500 trial, patients with stable or responding disease after four to six cycles of platinum chemotherapy with either etoposide or irinotecan were randomized between 4 (arm A) and 8 (arm B) weeks of maintenance therapy with temsirolimus (121). With a total of 87 patients enrolled, PFS on arm A was 1.9 months as compared with 2.5 months for arm B. Median OS from randomization was 8 months. These dismal outcomes do not seem to support implementation of temsirolimus maintenance therapy at this time.

Presently, the experience with mTOR inhibitors in both NSCLC and SCLC to date appears to be largely disappointing. However, it should be noted that the available datasets primarily examine monotherapy with mTOR inhibitors, and as such, the potential role of chemotherapy with mTOR inhibitors should not be dismissed. Furthermore, other novel mTOR inhibitors remain on the horizon. Deforolimus represents one such agent. A phase I trial has indicated responses to this agent in patients with NSCLC, and the agent is now being assessed in disease-specific trials (122).

■ CYCLOOXYGENASE-2 INHIBITORS

Cyclooxygenase (COX)-2 possesses a multitude of physiologic roles. In the setting of malignancy, COX-2 promotes growth and proliferation of cancer cells and stimulates tumor angiogenesis. Inhibition of COX-2 results in enhancement of IFN-γ dependent antitumor response, thereby making the moiety an attractive therapeutic target (123). Several large trials have evaluated the role of the COX-2 inhibitor celecoxib in NSCLC. A randomized phase II experience assigned patients with advanced NSCLC to either irinotecan and docetaxel or irinotecan and gemcitabine, with or without high-dose celecoxib (400 mg oral twice daily) (124). With 133 assessable patients, median OS was 6.31 months for celecoxib-treated patients, as compared with 8.99 months for patients treated with chemotherapy alone. Though these phase II results may be viewed as somewhat discouraging, it is difficult to ascertain whether therapeutic comparisons should be made in this small study with a 2 × 2 randomization.

A more straightforward assessment of celecoxib was reported in a separate phase II experience assessing the combination of celecoxib with paclitaxel. In this study, patients with platinum-refractory NSCLC received up to six cycles of weekly paclitaxel with twice daily celecoxib (400 mg) until the time of progression (125). With 58 patients enrolled, 14 patients (24.1%) experienced an objective response and 24 patients (41.3%) experienced stable disease. Interestingly, correlative studies suggested that decreases in serum VEGF was associated with clinical response.

In the largest experience to date with celecoxib, the phase III NVALT-4 study randomized 540 patients with advanced NSCLC to either carboplatin/docetaxel chemotherapy with celecoxib or with placebo (126). A total of 561 were randomized, with a median follow-up of 36 months. Hematologic toxicity was similar in the treatment arms, and there were no cardiovascular events observed with celecoxib therapy. A statistically significant improvement in RR was observed with the addition of celecoxib (32% vs. 27%; P = 0.05). No differences in PFS and OS were seen in this study. Importantly, no interaction was seen between survival endpoints and tumor histology. Several trials are ongoing to further clarify the benefit of combining celecoxib with chemotherapy for lung cancer. Notably, more selective and potent COX-2 inhibitors such as apricoxib show promise in early clinical trials; further clinical data related to these agents is eagerly anticipated (127).

Obtaining benefit from therapy with COX-2 inhibitors may be contingent upon COX-2 expression, as one randomized phase II study suggests (128). In this trial, the combination of carboplatin/gemcitabine was assessed with celecoxib or the 5-lipoxygenase inhibitor, zileuton, in patients with advanced NSCLC and no prior therapy. With 140 patients randomized in this study, no difference in OS was seen between the two treatment arms. Interestingly, COX-2 expression correlated with poorer OS among those patients not receiving celecoxib therapy (using a threshold COX-2 expression level ≥4, HR = 2.51, P = 0.019). Using the same metrics for COX-2 expression, patients receiving celecoxib actually had better survival with increased expression. Thus, future studies may assess the role of COX-2 as a biomarker to predict response to celecoxib therapy.

■ HISTONE DEACETYLASE (HDAC) INHIBITORS

Preclinical studies suggest that inhibitors of HDAC may augment the effect of platinating agents and taxanes via tubulin acetylation and DNA fragmentation (129). Data from a randomized phase II trial supports these observations (130). In this placebo-controlled, double-blinded effort, 94 patients with advanced NSCLC were enrolled and randomized in a 2:1 fashion to receive carboplatin and paclitaxel either with vorinostat (a novel HDAC inhibitor) or placebo. Overall RR was superior in the experimental arm (34% vs. 12%, P = 0.02), as was median TTP (5.75 vs. 4.1 months).

Recently, attention has been focused on patients with *EML-ALK* fusion, which may serve as a driver in 3% to 8% of patients with NSCLC (131). Although a relatively small subset, this population can potentially be enriched by selecting individuals with male gender, younger age, never-smoker status, or lack of EGFR or KRAS mutation (131–136). The agent PF-02341066 dually targets MET and ALK, and recent clinical data has shown substantial activity in patients with the EML-ALK fusion (137). Specifically, in a phase I study including 76 NSCLC patients harboring this fusion, an overall response rate of 57% was observed, with a disease control rate of 87% at 8 weeks (138). Common toxicities with the agent included nausea (54%) and vomiting (44%), although the agent was generally well tolerated. These impressive clinical data have prompted subsequent trials examining PF-02341066 in combination with other agents—for example, a phase I is exploring the use of the agent in combination with PF-00299804, a novel pan-HER inhibitor (139). Furthermore, a phase III trial is underway comparing the agent to standard second-line chemotherapy in patients with *EML-ALK* fusion (140).

■ RATIONAL COMBINATIONS OF TARGETED THERAPEUTICS

With a burgeoning repertoire of targeted agents under investigation in lung cancer, researchers have simultaneously turned their attention to developing effective combinations of these agents in hopes of harnessing synergistic or additive effects. These efforts can be subdivided into various mechanistic categories.

Combining Antiangiogenic and EGFR-Targeting Therapy

Promising activity has been observed for the combination of chemotherapy, bevacizumab and cetuximab in Southwest Oncology Group trial 0536 (141). In this phase II study, patients with advanced nonsquamous NSCLC were treated with the combination of carboplatin, paclitaxel cetuximab, and bevacizumab. With a total of 95 evaluable patients at the time of most recent analysis, 51 patients (54%) experienced a PR and 22 patients (23%) had SD, reflecting an overall clinical benefit rate of 77%. Notably, analysis of a limited sample set suggested no association of clinical benefit from cetuximab therapy and KRAS status (142). This encouraging data has led to the implementation of a phase III trial assessing carboplatin/paclitaxel chemotherapy with bevacizumab (in eligible patients), with or without cetuximab.

Following encouraging data in a phase I/II study, the combination of erlotinib and bevacizumab has been assessed in larger randomized phase II trial (143). In this unique design, patients with nonsquamous NSCLC that had progressed on platinum chemotherapy were randomized to receive either bevacizumab with chemotherapy (docetaxel or pemetrexed), bevacizumab with erlotinib, or chemotherapy alone. A total of 120 patients were enrolled; fewer patients in the bevacizumab-erlotinib arm discontinued therapy (13%) as compared with bevacizumab-chemotherapy (28%) or chemotherapy alone (24%). Though not achieving statistical significance, it did appear that the risk of disease progression or death with bevacizumab-erlotinib compared favorably with that of chemotherapy alone (HR 0.72, 95% CI 0.42–1.23). Notably, MALDI-TOF proteomic analyses paired with studies of bevacizumab and erlotinib have identified a signature that may ultimately identify appropriate candidates for this regimen (144,145).

The ATLAS trial compared three distinct chemotherapy regimens (carboplatin/paclitaxel, carboplatin/docetaxel, or carboplatin/gemcitabine) with bevacizumab (146). In this study, bevacizumab was either administered alone or in combination with erlotinib as maintenance treatment until the time of progression (after receipt of four cycles of chemotherapy with bevacizumab). With a total of 768 patients randomized, median PFS was prolonged with the combination of bevacizumab and erlotinib (4.8 months vs. 3.7 months, $P = 0.0012$) (147). In subset analysis, none of the platinum doublets assessed in this trial used in combination with targeted therapy appeared to result in superior survival. Until further data is available, several current and ongoing trials independently assess other platinum doublets with bevacizumab. As one such example,

bevacizumab with erlotinib is now being tested as first-line therapy in a phase II study of sequential targeted therapy and chemotherapy (148). In this trial, therapy is divided into three discrete modules. Module A consists of bevacizumab with erlotinib for a total of four cycles, and is followed by module B. Module B consists of four cycles of carboplatin/paclitaxel chemotherapy with bevacizumab. Patients who mount a response or experience stable disease with treatment on module A proceed to module C, bevacizumab and erlotinib, until the time of progression. With 48 patients enrolled, median survival for all patients was 12.9 months. In the subset of patients who experienced an objective response or stable disease during module A, survival was an impressive 23.2 months. Side effects associated with therapy were varied among the treatment modules; notable toxicities include bowel perforation (4% on module A) and thrombosis (10% on module C).

While the combination of EGFR-targeting small molecule inhibitors with bevacizumab remains promising, current studies have also focused on the combination of the former with small molecule VEGF-tyrosine kinase inhibitors. A phase I trial combining gefitinib with sorafenib (200–400 mg twice daily) has currently enrolled 31 patients (149). One patient experienced a PR, while 20 patients (38%) experienced stable disease. The combination of sorafenib with gefitinib appears to be well tolerated. Phase II data is available for the combination of sorafenib with erlotinib, as well (150). In a series of 50 patients with unresectable advanced NSCLC, a median PFS of 4.6 months was achieved, and median OS had not been reached at the time of a preliminary report. Paired radiographic studies suggested a median standardized uptake value decrease of 35% on [18]fluorodeoxyglucose–positron emission tomography, with a more substantial decrease occurring in responders as compared with non-responders (51% vs. 18.5%, $P = 0.031$). A randomized phase II trial comparing the combination of erlotinib with either placebo, low-dose sorafenib, or high-dose sorafenib is ongoing (151). With clinical data pending, this trial has already been applauded for use of tumor size (measured on a continuous scale) as the primary outcome variable. This novel trial design may allow for the selection of optimal regimens for testing in phase III studies.

Dual Inhibition of EGFR

Targeting EGFR from both the intracellular and extracellular domain has theoretic rationale. In a phase I trial in patients with advanced NSCLC previously treated with platinum-based chemotherapy, a regimen of weekly cetuximab with gefitinib was examined (152). A total of 13 patients were enrolled at the time of a preliminary report, with two episodes of grade 3 hypomagnesemia and one episode of grade 3 skin rash in the highest of three dosing cohorts. Though no responses were observed with this regimen, stable disease was observed in four patients. Screening for EGFR mutation or amplification was negative in all patients enrolled in this trial—presumably, this may have contributed to the absence of responses to therapy.

Investigators have also examined a distinct ErbB family inhibitor, pertuzumab, in combination with erlotinib. Pertuzumab has shown activity in the setting of breast cancer, and functions via inhibition of HER2 dimerization (153). In a phase I trial including patients with advanced NSCLC, patients received weekly intravenous pertuzumab with erlotinib. For dosing of the latter, patients were divided into two cohorts, with the first cohort receiving erlotinib at 100 mg oral daily, and the second receiving erlotinib at 150 mg oral daily. In the six patients enrolled in the first cohort, rash (100%) and diarrhea (50%) represented the most common adverse events. In the second cohort of patients, no dose-limiting toxicities have been observed, leading to the recommendation of pertuzumab with full-dose erlotinib (150 mg oral daily) for evaluation in phase II clinical trials.

Combining EGFR and COX-2 Inhibitors

Clinical trials are underway to see if the antitumor activity of EGFR inhibitors can be optimized through combination with COX-2-inhibitors. A phase I study of patients with advanced NSCLC examined celecoxib (with doses ranging from 200 to 800 mg oral twice daily) with erlotinib at a fixed dose (154). With 21 evaluable subjects, seven PRs (33%) were observed. Furthermore, five patients experienced stable disease. Molecular analyses confirmed that responses occurred in patients both with and without EGFR-activating mutations. Dermatologic toxicities represented the most frequent adverse effects, occurring in 86% of patients enrolled. Other biologic correlates examined in this trial pointed to the potential utility of baseline matrix metalloproteinase-9 in predicting responders to this combination of agents (155). This study demonstrated that the optimal dose of celecoxib combined with erlotinib at 150 mg daily was 600 mg twice daily based on the percentage decline in the major urinary metabolite of prostaglandin E2 (PGE2), PGE-M. In studies combining COX-2 inhibition with chemotherapy in lung cancer, it has been shown that patients who experience a significant decline in PGE-M have improved survival (156). The regimen is currently being examined in a randomized phase II trial comparing erlotinib with placebo to erlotinib with celecoxib (19).

Other combinations of erlotinib and gefitinib with COX-2 inhibitors do not appear to be as promising in unselected populations. Gefitinib and celecoxib were evaluated in a phase II study in platinum-refractory advanced NSCLC patients (157). With 27 patients enrolled, two PRs were observed with no CRs. Median TTP and OS were

2.2 and 4.6 months, respectively. A separate phase I/II study evaluated rofecoxib with gefitinib in patients with advanced NSCLC (158). With 42 assessable patients, only one CR and two PRs were observed. Median TTP and OS were 55 and 144 days, respectively. The authors of both studies suggested that the clinical activity observed with combination therapy was similar to that anticipated for gefitinib monotherapy. However, in the latter trial, use of matrix-assisted laser desorption/ionization (MALDI) proteomic analysis of baseline tumor specimens allowed for differentiation of responders and nonresponders. Though warranting prospective validation, MALDI proteomics may thus be a manner in which patients suitable for gefitinib and COX-2-inhibitor combination therapy could be identified.

A phase II trial evaluating erlotinib plus celecoxib in patients with advanced NSCLC who had failed one prior chemotherapy regimen identified disease control in 10 of 26 patients (159). They found that COX-2 tumor expression could be a marker for response to this combination. It will be important to understand how to select patients for this combined therapy for maximal benefit. COX-2 has been shown to be a prognostic marker in NSCLC (160). Recent efforts have been made to identify a predictive marker for selecting patients with NSCLC who might benefit from COX-2 inhibitor therapy. Several phase I and II trials have recently investigated tumor expression of COX-2 in a retrospective manner to help define a selected patient population with improved outcomes to therapy with COX-2 inhibitors (128,159,161).

Combining EGFR and mTOR Inhibitors

Similar to the aforementioned trials evaluating combinations with COX-2 inhibitors, ongoing clinical efforts seek to determine whether the activity of EGFR inhibitors can be augmented with mTOR inhibition. Phase I data suggested that gefitinib and everolimus could be safely coadministered, with responses observed in patients with NSCLC (162). A subsequent phase II trial included patients with advanced NSCLC that was either previously untreated or previously treated with carboplatin or cisplatin and docetaxel. With data from 23 evaluable patients, four PRs have been observed (17%). Notably, one responding patient was found to harbor the *KRAS* mutation and another possessed an EGFR mutation. A second trial using a similar molecular strategy has assessed the combination of everolimus with erlotinib. Phase I data is available from this phase I/II effort. With 61 patients treated in this portion of the trial, one CR and three PRs were observed. Furthermore, 17 cases of stable disease were noted. Several feasible regimens combining erlotinib and everolimus were identified, and the efficacy of these regimens will be assessed in the phase II component of this trial.

FUTURE DIRECTIONS

A number of agents are currently under investigation in both NSCLC and SCLC outside of those described herein. A challenge for future investigators will be to define appropriate combinations of novel therapies for the treatment of NSCLC. Furthermore, in the interest of identifying appropriate patients for these treatments, it will be critical to incorporate the growing body of knowledge related to lung cancer biomarkers into clinical trial design. A current example of this process is the Biomarker-Integrated Approaches of Targeted Therapy for Lung Cancer Elimination clinical trial program (163). In this randomized phase II effort, patients receive two fresh core-needle biopsies. Specimens are then tested for several biomarkers (EGR, *Braf* gene mutation, KRAS, EGFR mutation, cyclin D1 copy number, etc.) that more globally pertain to four molecular pathways. Based on these biomarker analyses, eligible patients are then randomized to one of four treatments: (a) sorafenib; (b) erlotinib; (c) vandetanib; or (d) erlotinib with bexarotene. Forward thinking designs such as these that utilize the results of ongoing translational efforts will surely serve as a paradigm for clinical trials in the future.

Further research efforts must also be directed at understanding mechanisms of resistance to targeted agents. In an ongoing study at the Memorial Sloan-Kettering Cancer Center, patients who have advanced NSCLC with progression on an EGFR tyrosine kinase inhibitor receive a rebiopsy of their tumor. EGFR mutational status and *MET* amplification status are then assessed, and compared with baseline characteristics (164). In this manner, molecular changes that accompany erlotinib resistance can be deciphered. Results of this trial and similar efforts are eagerly awaited. With multiple targeted therapies now at the disposal of the oncologist, studies such as these will inform the appropriate sequential use of agents.

KEY POINTS

- A randomized, phase III trial (ECOG 4599) demonstrated improved overall survival with the addition of bevacizumab to carboplatin and paclitaxel in the setting of advanced, nonsquamous NSCLC.
- TKIs with affinity for the VEGF receptor family (i.e., sunitinib, vandetanib, etc.) have an emerging role in the treatment of advanced NSCLC.
- Phase III trials examining platinum-based chemotherapy in combination with the EGFR-directed monoclonal antibody cetuximab have demonstrated a modest survival benefit in patients with advanced NSCLC.
- Erlotinib, a TKI with specifity for EGFR, is approved for second- or third-line therapy of advanced NSCLC

on the basis of a phase III study (NCIC-CTG BR.21) showing improved survival with this agent as compared to placebo.

- Gefitinib, mechanistically similar to erlotinib, has been compared with platinum-based chemotherapy in a phase III trial (iPASS) including advanced adenocarcinoma-type NSCLC patients with a limited smoking history. PFS was improved in gefitinib-treated patients, and EGFR mutation was a strong predictor of clinical outcome.
- A rapidly enlarging pipeline of agents is being assessed in the setting of advanced NSCLC, including pan-HER inhibitors, IGF-IR targeting antibodies, mTOR inhibitors, and COX-2 inhibitors.
- A current focus of clinical research is the development of rational combinations of targeted therapies. For instance, several studies have assessed the combination of antiangiogenic and EGFR-targeting strategies.

REFERENCES

1. Schiller JH, Harrington D, Belani CP, et al.; Eastern Cooperative Oncology Group. Comparison of four chemotherapy regimens for advanced non-small-cell lung cancer. *N Engl J Med.* 2002;346(2):92–98.
2. Folkman J. Tumor angiogenesis: therapeutic implications. *N Engl J Med.* 1971;285(21):1182–1186.
3. Hicklin DJ, Ellis LM. Role of the vascular endothelial growth factor pathway in tumor growth and angiogenesis. *J Clin Oncol.* 2005;23(5):1011–1027.
4. Kerbel R, Folkman J. Clinical translation of angiogenesis inhibitors. *Nat Rev Cancer.* 2002;2(10):727–739.
5. Kerbel RS. Tumor angiogenesis. *N Engl J Med.* 2008;358:2039–2049.
6. Frederick PJ, Straughn JM Jr, Alvarez RD, Buchsbaum DJ. Preclinical studies and clinical utilization of monoclonal antibodies in epithelial ovarian cancer. *Gynecol Oncol.* 2009;113(3):384–390.
7. Hurwitz H, Fehrenbacher L, Novotny W, et al. Bevacizumab plus irinotecan, fluorouracil, and leucovorin for metastatic colorectal cancer. *N Engl J Med.* 2004;350(23):2335–2342.
8. Miller K, Wang M, Gralow J, et al. Paclitaxel plus bevacizumab versus paclitaxel alone for metastatic breast cancer. *N Engl J Med.* 2007;357(26):2666–2676.
9. Zuniga RM, Torcuator R, Jain R, et al. Efficacy, safety and patterns of response and recurrence in patients with recurrent high-grade gliomas treated with bevacizumab plus irinotecan. *J Neurooncol.* 2009;91(3):329–336.
10. Johnson DH, Fehrenbacher L, Novotny WF, et al. Randomized phase II trial comparing bevacizumab plus carboplatin and paclitaxel with carboplatin and paclitaxel alone in previously untreated locally advanced or metastatic non-small-cell lung cancer. *J Clin Oncol.* 2004;22(11):2184–2191.
11. Sandler A, Gray R, Perry MC, et al. Paclitaxel-carboplatin alone or with bevacizumab for non-small-cell lung cancer. *N Engl J Med.* 2006;355(24):2542–2550.
12. Zhang W, Dahlberg SE, Yang D, et al. Genetic variants in angiogenesis pathway associated with clinical outcome in NSCLC patients (pts) treated with bevacizumab in combination with carboplatin and paclitaxel: subset pharmacogenetic analysis of ECOG 4599 [suppl; abstract 8032]. *J Clin Oncol.* 2009;27:15s.

13. Dahlberg SE, Sandler AB, Brahmer JR, et al. Clinical course of advanced non-small cell lung cancer (NSCLC) patients (pts) experiencing hypertension (HTN) during treatment (TX) with bevacizumab (B) in combination with carboplatin (C) and paclitaxel (P) on E4599 [suppl; abstract 8042]. *J Clin Oncol.* 2009;27:15s.

14. Reck M, von Pawel J, Zatloukal P, et al. Phase III trial of cisplatin plus gemcitabine with either placebo or bevacizumab as first-line therapy for nonsquamous non-small-cell lung cancer: AVAiL. *J Clin Oncol.* 2009;27(8):1227–1234.

15. Manegold C, Pawel Jv, Zatloukal P, et al. Randomised, double-blind multicentre phase III study of bevacizumab in combination with cisplatin and gemcitabine in chemotherapy-naïve patients with advanced or recurrent non-squamous non-small cell lung cancer (NSCLC): BO17704. ASCO Annual Meeting Proceedings Part I. *J Clin Oncol.* 2007;25(18S, June 20 suppl):LBA7514

16. Ferrer N, Paredes A, Muñoz-Langa JM, et al: Bevacizumab in combination with cisplatin and docetaxel as first line treatment of patients (pts) with advanced or metastatic, non squamous, non-small-cell lung cancer (NSCLC) [abstract 19109]. *J Clin Oncol.* 2008;26(May 20 suppl).

17. Scagliotti GV, Parikh P, von Pawel J, et al. Phase III study comparing cisplatin plus gemcitabine with cisplatin plus pemetrexed in chemotherapy-naive patients with advanced-stage non-small-cell lung cancer. *J Clin Oncol.* 2008;26(21):3543–3551.

18. Patel JD, Hensing TA, Rademaker A, et al. Phase II study of pemetrexed and carboplatin plus bevacizumab with maintenance pemetrexed and bevacizumab as first-line therapy for nonsquamous non-small-cell lung cancer. *J Clin Oncol.* 2009;27:3284–3289.

19. Morey MC, Snyder DC, Sloane R, et al. Effects of home-based diet and exercise on functional outcomes among older, overweight long-term cancer survivors: RENEW: a randomized controlled trial. *JAMA.* 2009;301(18):1883–1891.

20. Ramalingam SS, Dahlberg SE, Langer CJ, et al.; Eastern Cooperative Oncology Group. Outcomes for elderly, advanced-stage non small-cell lung cancer patients treated with bevacizumab in combination with carboplatin and paclitaxel: analysis of Eastern Cooperative Oncology Group Trial 4599. *J Clin Oncol.* 2008;26(1):60–65.

21. Ramies DA, Sandler A, Gray R, et al. Bevacizumab: analysis of clinical benefit in females across trials in colorectal cancer and non-small cell lung cancer. ASCO Annual Meeting Proceedings Part I. *J Clin Oncol.* 2007;25(18S,suppl):7634.

22. Akerley WL, Langer CJ, Oh Y, et al. Acceptable safety of bevacizumab therapy in patients with brain metastases due to non-small cell lung cancer [abstract 8043]. *J Clin Oncol.* 2008;26(May 20 suppl).

23. Mendel DB, Laird AD, Xin X, et al. *In vivo* antitumor activity of SU11248, a novel tyrosine kinase inhibitor targeting vascular endothelial growth factor and platelet-derived growth factor receptors: determination of a pharmacokinetic/pharmacodynamic relationship. *Clin Cancer Res.* 2003;9(1):327–337.

24. Abrams TJ, Lee LB, Murray LJ, et al. SU11248 inhibits KIT and platelet-derived growth factor receptor β in preclinical models of human small cell lung cancer. *Mol Cancer Ther.* 2003;2:471–478.

25. Faivre S, Delbaldo C, Vera K, et al. Safety, pharmacokinetic, and antitumor activity of SU11248, a novel oral multitarget tyrosine kinase inhibitor, in patients with cancer. *J Clin Oncol.* 2006;24(1):25–35.

26. Figlin RA, Hutson TE, Tomczak P, et al. Overall survival with sunitinib versus interferon (IFN)-alfa as first-line treatment of metastatic renal cell carcinoma (mRCC) [abstract 5024]. *J Clin Oncol.* 2008;26(May 20 suppl).

27. Socinski MA, Novello S, Brahmer JR, et al. Multicenter, phase II trial of sunitinib in previously treated, advanced non-small-cell lung cancer. *J Clin Oncol.* 2008;26:650–656.

28. Shepherd FA, Dancey J, Ramlau R, et al. Prospective randomized trial of docetaxel versus best supportive care in patients with non-small-cell lung cancer previously treated with platinum-based chemotherapy. *J Clin Oncol.* 2000;18:2095–2103.

29. Shepherd FA, Rodrigues Pereira J, Ciuleanu T, et al.; National Cancer Institute of Canada Clinical Trials Group. Erlotinib in previously treated non-small-cell lung cancer. *N Engl J Med.* 2005;353(2):123–132.

30. Hanna N, Shepherd FA, Fossella FV, et al. Randomized phase III trial of pemetrexed versus docetaxel in patients with non-small-cell lung cancer previously treated with chemotherapy. *J Clin Oncol.* 2004;22(9):1589–1597.

31. Reck M, Frickhofen N, Gatzemeier U, et al. A phase I dose escalation study of sunitinib in combination with gemcitabine + cisplatin for advanced non-small cell lung cancer (NSCLC). ASCO Annual Meeting Proceedings Part I. *J Clin Oncol.* 2007;25(18S, June 20 suppl):18057

32. Carter CA, Chen C, Brink C, et al. Sorafenib is efficacious and tolerated in combination with cytotoxic or cytostatic agents in preclinical models of human non-small cell lung carcinoma. *Cancer Chemother Pharmacol.* 2007;59(2):183–195.

33. Adjei AA, Molina JR, Hillman SL, et al. A front-line window of opportunity phase II study of sorafenib in patients with advanced non-small cell lung cancer: A North Central Cancer Treatment Group study. ASCO Annual Meeting Proceedings Part I. *J Clin Oncol.* 2007;25(18S, June 20 suppl):7547.

34. Schiller JH, Lee JW, Hanna NH, et al. A randomized discontinuation phase II study of sorafenib versus placebo in patients with non-small cell lung cancer who have failed at least two prior chemotherapy regimens: E2501 [abstract 8014]. *J Clin Oncol.* 2008;26(May 20 suppl).

35. Xin H, Zhang C, Herrmann A, Du Y, Figlin R, Yu H. Sunitinib inhibition of Stat3 induces renal cell carcinoma tumor cell apoptosis and reduces immunosuppressive cells. *Cancer Res.* 2009;69(6):2506–2513.

36. Matsumori Y, Yano S, Goto H, et al. ZD6474, an inhibitor of vascular endothelial growth factor receptor tyrosine kinase, inhibits growth of experimental lung metastasis and production of malignant pleural effusions in a non-small cell lung cancer model. *Oncol Res.* 2006;16(1):15–26.

37. Wedge SR, Ogilvie DJ, Dukes M, et al. ZD6474 inhibits vascular endothelial growth factor signaling, angiogenesis, and tumor growth following oral administration. *Cancer Res.* 2002;62(16):4645–4655.

38. Kiura K, Nakagawa K, Shinkai T, et al. A randomized, double-blind, phase IIa dose-finding study of Vandetanib (ZD6474) in Japanese patients with non-small cell lung cancer. *J Thorac Oncol.* 2008;3(4):386–393.

39. Heymach JV, Paz-Ares L, De Braud F, et al. Randomized phase II study of vandetanib alone or with paclitaxel and carboplatin as first-line treatment for advanced non-small-cell lung cancer. *J Clin Oncol.* 2008;26(33):5407–5415.

40. Hanrahan EO, Lin HY, Du DZ, et al. Correlative analyses of plasma cytokine/angiogenic factor (C/AF) profile, gender and outcome in a randomized, three-arm, phase II trial of first-line vandetanib (VAN) and/or carboplatin plus paclitaxel (CP) for advanced non-small cell lung cancer (NSCLC). ASCO Annual Meeting Proceedings Part I. *J Clin Oncol.* 2007;25(18S, June 20 suppl):7593.

41. Heymach JV, Johnson BE, Prager D, et al. Randomized, placebo-controlled phase II study of vandetanib plus docetaxel in previously treated non small-cell lung cancer. *J Clin Oncol.* 2007;25(27):4270–4277.

42. Herbst RS, Sun Y, Korfee S, et al. Vandetanib plus docetaxel versus docetaxel as second-line treatment for patients with advanced non-small cell lung cancer (NSCLC): a randomized, double-blind phase III trial (ZODIAC) [abstract CRA8003]. *J Clin Oncol.* 2009;27:18s(suppl).

43. De Boer R, Arrieta Ó, Gottfried M, et al. Vandetanib plus pemetrexed versus pemetrexed as second-line therapy in patients with advanced non small cell lung cancer (NSCLC): a randomized,

double-blind phase III trial (ZEAL) [abstract 8010]. *J Clin Oncol.* 2009;27:15s(suppl).

44. Natale RB, Thongprasert S, Greco FA, et al. Vandetanib versus erlotinib in patients with advanced non-small cell lung cancer (NSCLC) after failure of at least one prior cytotoxic chemotherapy: a randomized, double-blind phase III trial (ZEST) [abstract 8009]. *J Clin Oncol.* 2009;27:15s(suppl).

45. Natale RB, Bodkin D, Govindan R, et al. Vandetanib versus gefitinib in patients with advanced non-small-cell lung cancer: results from a two-part, double-blind, randomized phase ii study. *J Clin Oncol.* 2009;27:2523–2529.

46. Sonpavde G, Hutson TE. Pazopanib: a novel multitargeted tyrosine kinase inhibitor. *Curr Oncol Rep.* 2007;9(2):115–119.

47. Altorki N, Guarino M, Lee P, et al. Preoperative treatment with pazopanib (GW786034), a multikinase angiogenesis inhibitor in early-stage non-small cell lung cancer (NSCLC): a proof-of-concept phase II study [abstract 7557]. *J Clin Oncol.* 2008;26(May 20 suppl).

48. Nikolinakos P, Altorki N, Guarino M, et al. Analyses of plasma cytokine/angiogenic factors (C/AFs) profile during preoperative treatment with pazopanib (GW786034) in early-stage non-small cell lung cancer [abstract 7568]. *J Clin Oncol.* 2008;26(May 20 suppl).

49. Yarden Y, Sliwkowski MX. Untangling the ErbB signaling network. *Nat Rev Mol Cell Biol.* 2001;2:127–137.

50. Rusch V, Klimstra D, Venkatraman E, Pisters PW, Langenfeld J, Dmitrovsky E. Overexpression of the epidermal growth factor receptor and its ligand transforming growth factor alpha is frequent in resectable non-small cell lung cancer but does not predict tumor progression. *Clin Cancer Res.* 1997;3(4):515–522.

51. Brabender J, Danenberg KD, Metzger R, et al. Epidermal growth factor receptor and HER2-neu mRNA expression in non-small cell lung cancer Is correlated with survival. *Clin Cancer Res.* 2001;7(7):1850–1855.

52. Baselga J, Pfister D, Cooper MR, et al. Phase I studies of anti-epidermal growth factor receptor chimeric antibody C225 alone and in combination with cisplatin. *J Clin Oncol.* 2000;18:904–914.

53. Borghaei H, Langer CJ, Millenson M, et al. Phase II study of paclitaxel, carboplatin, and cetuximab as first line treatment, for patients with advanced non-small cell lung cancer (NSCLC): results of OPN-017. *J Thorac Oncol.* 2008;3(11):1286–1292.

54. Thienelt CD, Bunn PA Jr, Hanna N, et al. Multicenter phase I/II study of cetuximab with paclitaxel and carboplatin in untreated patients with stage IV non-small-cell lung cancer. *J Clin Oncol.* 2005;23(34):8786–8793.

55. Herbst RS, Chansky K, Kelly K, et al. A phase II randomized selection trial evaluating concurrent chemotherapy plus cetuximab or chemotherapy followed by cetuximab in patients with advanced non-small cell lung cancer (NSCLC): final report of SWOG 0342. ASCO Annual Meeting Proceedings Part I [abstract 7545]. *J Clin Oncol.* 2007;25:18S(June 20 suppl).

56. Saleh MN, Socinski MA, Trent D, et al. Randomized phase II trial of two dose schedules of carboplatin/paclitaxel/cetuximab in stage IIIB/IV non-small cell lung cancer (NSCLC). ASCO Annual Meeting Proceedings Part I. *J Clin Oncol.* 2007;25(18S, June 20 suppl):7586.

57. Rosell R, Robinet G, Szczesna A, et al. Randomized phase II study of cetuximab plus cisplatin/vinorelbine compared with cisplatin/vinorelbine alone as first-line therapy in EGFR-expressing advanced non-small-cell lung cancer. *Ann Oncol.* 2008;19(2):362–369.

58. Pirker R, Szczesna A, Pawel Jv, et al. FLEX: a randomized, multicenter, phase III study of cetuximab in combination with cisplatin/vinorelbine (CV) versus CV alone in the first-line treatment of patients with advanced non-small cell lung cancer (NSCLC) [abstr 3]. *J Clin Oncol.* 2008;26(May 20 suppl).

59. Robert F, Blumenschein G, Herbst RS, et al. Phase I/IIa study of cetuximab with gemcitabine plus carboplatin in patients with chemotherapy-naive advanced non-small cell lung cancer. *J Clin Oncol.* 2005;23(36):9089–9096.

60. Pilz LR, Cicenas S, Eschbach C, et al. Feasibility of cetuximab in combination with gemcitabine or docetaxel or carboplatin/gemcitabine for chemonaïve patients with advanced non-small cell lung cancer (NSCLC): observations from an ongoing randomized phase II/III trial (GemTax IV) [abstract 19005]. *J Clin Oncol.* 2008;26(May 20 suppl).

61. Jonker DJ, O'Callaghan CJ, Karapetis CS, et al. Cetuximab for the treatment of colorectal cancer. *N Engl J Med.* 2007;357:2040–2048.

62. Hirsch FR, Herbst RS, Olsen C, et al. Increased EGFR gene copy number detected by fluorescent in situ hybridization predicts outcome in non-small-cell lung cancer patients treated with cetuximab and chemotherapy. *J Clin Oncol.* 2008;26(20):3351–3357.

63. Van Cutsem E, Köhne CH, Hitre E, et al. Cetuximab and chemotherapy as initial treatment for metastatic colorectal cancer. *N Engl J Med.* 2009;360(14):1408–1417.

64. O'Byrne KJ, Bondarenko I, Barrios C, et al. Molecular and clinical predictors of outcome for cetuximab in non-small cell lung cancer (NSCLC): data from the FLEX study [abstract 8007]. *J Clin Oncol.* 2009;27:15s(suppl).

65. Khambata-Ford S, Harbison CT, Hart LL, et al. *K-RAS* mutations (MT) and EGFR-related markers as potential predictors of cetuximab benefit in 1st line advanced NSCLC: results from the BMS099 study. *J Thor Oncol.* 2008;3:S304.

66. Maitland ML, Kasza KE, Lacouture ME, et al. Refining epidermal growth factor receptor (EGFR) -inhibition-related rash (EIRR) phenotypes with a cetuximab (C) monotherapy stage of a phase II trial for non-small cell lung cancer (C) [abstract 8089]. *J Clin Oncol.* 2008;26(May 20 suppl).

67. Bonner JA, Harari PM, Giralt J, et al. Radiotherapy plus cetuximab for squamous-cell carcinoma of the head and neck. *N Engl J Med.* 2006;354(6):567–578.

68. Hughes S, Liong J, Miah A, et al. A brief report on the safety study of induction chemotherapy followed by synchronous radiotherapy and cetuximab in stage III non-small cell lung cancer (NSCLC): SCRATCH study. *J Thorac Oncol.* 2008;3(6):648–651.

69. Jensen AD, Münter MW, Bischoff H, et al. Treatment of non-small cell lung cancer with intensity-modulated radiation therapy in combination with cetuximab: the NEAR protocol (NCT00115518). *BMC Cancer.* 2006;6:122.

70. Govindan R, Bogart J, Wang X, et al. A phase II study of pemetrexed, carboplatin and thoracic radiation with or without cetuximab in patients with locally advanced unresectable non-small cell lung cancer: CALGB 30407—Early evaluation of feasibility and toxicity [abstract 7518]. *J Clin Oncol.* 2008;26(May 20 suppl).

71. Coate LE, Gately K, Barr M, et al. Phase II pilot study of neoadjuvant cetuximab in combination with cisplatin and gemcitabine in patients with resectable IB-IIIA non small cell lung cancer. ASCO Annual Meeting Proceedings Part I. *J Clin Oncol.* 2006;24(18S, June 20 suppl):17107.

72. Pérez-Soler R, Chachoua A, Hammond LA, et al. Determinants of tumor response and survival with erlotinib in patients with non–small-cell lung cancer. *J Clin Oncol.* 2004;22(16):3238–3247.

73. Massarelli E, Andre F, Liu DD, et al. A retrospective analysis of the outcome of patients who have received two prior chemotherapy regimens including platinum and docetaxel for recurrent non-small-cell lung cancer. *Lung Cancer.* 2003;39(1):55–61.

74. Tsao MS, Sakurada A, Cutz JC, et al. Erlotinib in lung cancer – molecular and clinical predictors of outcome. *N Engl J Med.* 2005;353(2):133–144.

75. Florescu M, Hasan B, Seymour L, Ding K, Shepherd FA; National Cancer Institute of Canada Clinical Trials Group. A clinical prognostic index for patients treated with erlotinib in National Cancer Institute of Canada Clinical Trials Group study BR.21. *J Thorac Oncol.* 2008;3(6):590–598.

76. Wheatley-Price P, Ding K, Seymour L, Clark GM, Shepherd FA. Erlotinib for advanced non-small-cell lung cancer in the elderly: an analysis of the National Cancer Institute of Canada Clinical Trials Group Study BR.21. *J Clin Oncol.* 2008;26(14):2350–2357.

77. Jackman DM, Yeap BY, Lindeman NI, et al. Phase II clinical trial of chemotherapy-naive patients > or = 70 years of age treated with erlotinib for advanced non-small-cell lung cancer. *J Clin Oncol.* 2007;25(7):760–766.

78. Lilenbaum R, Axelrod R, Thomas S, et al. Randomized phase II trial of erlotinib or standard chemotherapy in patients with advanced non-small-cell lung cancer and a performance status of 2. *J Clin Oncol.* 2008;26(6):863–869.

79. Cappuzzo F, Ciuleanu T, Stelmakh L, et al. SATURN: a double-blind, randomized, phase III study of maintenance erlotinib versus placebo following nonprogression with first-line platinum-based chemotherapy in patients with advanced NSCLC [abstract 8001]. *J Clin Oncol.* 2009;27:15s(suppl).

80. Brugger W, Triller N, Blasinska-Morawiec M, et al. Biomarker analyses from the phase III placebo-controlled SATURN study of maintenance erlotinib following first-line chemotherapy for advanced NSCLC [abstract 8020]. *J Clin Oncol.* 2009;27:15s(suppl).

81. Gatzemeier U, Pluzanska A, Szczesna A, et al. Phase III study of erlotinib in combination with cisplatin and gemcitabine in advanced non-small-cell lung cancer: the Tarceva Lung Cancer Investigation Trial. *J Clin Oncol.* 2007;25(12):1545–1552.

82. Herbst RS, Prager D, Hermann R, et al.; TRIBUTE Investigator Group. TRIBUTE: a phase III trial of erlotinib hydrochloride (OSI-774) combined with carboplatin and paclitaxel chemotherapy in advanced non-small-cell lung cancer. *J Clin Oncol.* 2005;23(25):5892–5899.

83. Choong NW, Mauer AM, Haraf DJ, et al. Phase I trial of erlotinib-based multimodality therapy for inoperable stage III non-small cell lung cancer. *J Thorac Oncol.* 2008;3:1003–1011.

84. Casal J, Vázquez S, Barón FJ, et al. An open label non-randomized phase II trial of erlotinib following concurrent chemo-radiotherapy as maintenance therapy in patients (p) with stage III non-small cell lung cancer (NSCLC): A Galician Lung Cancer Group study [abstract 18501]. *J Clin Oncol.* 2008;26(May 20 suppl).

85. Lind JS, Lagerwaard FJ, Smit EF, et al. Whole brain radiotherapy with concurrent erlotinib for brain metastases from non-small cell lung cancer: a phase I study [abstract 19122]. *J Clin Oncol.* 2008;26(May 20 suppl).

86. Wakeling AE, Guy SP, Woodburn JR, et al. ZD1839 (Iressa): an orally active inhibitor of epidermal growth factor signaling with potential for cancer therapy. *Cancer Res.* 2002;62(20):5749–5754.

87. Kris MG, Natale RB, Herbst RS, et al. Efficacy of gefitinib, an inhibitor of the epidermal growth factor receptor tyrosine kinase, in symptomatic patients with non-small cell lung cancer: a randomized trial. *JAMA.* 2003;290(16):2149–2158.

88. Fukuoka M, Yano S, Giaccone G, et al. Multi-institutional randomized phase II trial of gefitinib for previously treated patients with advanced non-small-cell lung cancer (The IDEAL 1 Trial) [corrected]. *J Clin Oncol.* 2003;21(12):2237–2246.

89. Thatcher N, Chang A, Parikh P, et al. Gefitinib plus best supportive care in previously treated patients with refractory advanced non-small-cell lung cancer: results from a randomised, placebo-controlled, multicentre study (Iressa Survival Evaluation in Lung Cancer). *Lancet.* 2005;366(9496):1527–1537.

90. Chang A, Parikh P, Thongprasert S, et al. Gefitinib (IRESSA) in patients of Asian origin with refractory advanced non-small cell lung cancer: subset analysis from the ISEL study. *J Thorac Oncol.* 2006;1(8):847–855.

91. Sunaga N, Tomizawa Y, Yanagitani N, et al. Phase II prospective study of the efficacy of gefitinib for the treatment of stage III/IV non-small cell lung cancer with EGFR mutations, irrespective of previous chemotherapy. *Lung Cancer.* 2007;56(3):383–389.

92. Sequist LV, Martins RG, Spigel D, et al. First-line gefitinib in patients with advanced non-small-cell lung cancer harboring somatic EGFR mutations. *J Clin Oncol.* 2008;26(15):2442–2449.

93. Tamura K, Okamoto I, Kashii T, et al.; West Japan Thoracic Oncology Group. Multicentre prospective phase II trial of gefitinib for advanced non-small cell lung cancer with epidermal growth factor receptor mutations: results of the West Japan Thoracic Oncology Group trial (WJTOG0403). *Br J Cancer.* 2008;98(5):907–914.

94. Cappuzzo F, Ligorio C, Jänne PA, et al. Prospective study of gefitinib in epidermal growth factor receptor fluorescence in situ hybridization-positive/phospho-Akt-positive or never smoker patients with advanced non-small-cell lung cancer: the ONCOBELL trial. *J Clin Oncol.* 2007;25(16):2248–2255.

95. Cappuzzo F, Magrini E, Ceresoli GL, et al. Akt phosphorylation and gefitinib efficacy in patients with advanced non-small-cell lung cancer. *J Natl Cancer Inst.* 2004;96(15):1133–1141.

96. Mok T, Wu YL, Thongprasert S, et al. Phase III, randomised, open-label, first-line study of gefitinib vs. carboplatin/paclitaxel in clinically selected patients with advanced non-small cell lung cancer (IPASS). Presented at the 2008 European Society of Medical Oncology Congress meeting; 2008; Stockholm, Sweden.

97. Fukuoka M, Wu Y, Thongprasert S, et al. Biomarker analyses from a phase III, randomized, open-label, first-line study of gefitinib (G) versus carboplatin/paclitaxel (C/P) in clinically selected patients (pts) with advanced non-small cell lung cancer (NSCLC) in Asia (IPASS) [abstract 8006]. *J Clin Oncol.* 2009;27:15s(suppl).

98. Kim ES, Hirsh V, Mok T, et al. Gefitinib versus docetaxel in previously treated non-small-cell lung cancer (INTEREST): a randomised phase III trial. *Lancet.* 2008;372(9652):1809–1818.

99. Giaccone G, Herbst RS, Manegold C, et al. Gefitinib in combination with gemcitabine and cisplatin in advanced non-small-cell lung cancer: a phase III trial–INTACT 1. *J Clin Oncol.* 2004;22(5):777–784.

100. Herbst RS, Giaccone G, Schiller JH, et al. Gefitinib in combination with paclitaxel and carboplatin in advanced non-small-cell lung cancer: a phase III trial–INTACT 2. *J Clin Oncol.* 2004;22(5):785–794.

101. Rabindran SK, Discafani CM, Rosfjord EC, et al. Antitumor activity of HKI-272, an orally active, irreversible inhibitor of the HER-2 tyrosine kinase. *Cancer Res.* 2004;64(11):3958–3965.

102. Wong KK, Fracasso PM, Bukowski RM, et al. HKI-272, an irreversible pan erbB receptor tyrosine kinase inhibitor: preliminary phase 1 results in patients with solid tumors. ASCO Annual Meeting Proceedings Part I. *J Clin Oncol.* 2006;24(18S, June 20 suppl):3018.

103. Li D, Ambrogio L, Shimamura T, et al. BIBW2992, an irreversible EGFR/HER2 inhibitor highly effective in preclinical lung cancer models. *Oncogene.* 2008;27(34):4702–4711.

104. Eskens FA, Mom CH, Planting AS, et al. A phase I dose escalation study of BIBW 2992, an irreversible dual inhibitor of epidermal growth factor receptor 1 (EGFR) and 2 (HER2) tyrosine kinase in a 2-week on, 2-week off schedule in patients with advanced solid tumours. *Br J Cancer.* 2008;98(1):80–85.

105. Shih J, Yang C, Su W, et al. A phase II study of BIBW 2992, a novel irreversible dual EGFR and HER2 tyrosine kinase inhibitor (TKI), in patients with adenocarcinoma of the lung and activating EGFR mutations after failure of one line of chemotherapy (LUX-Lung 2) [abstract 8013]. *J Clin Oncol.* 2009;27:15s(suppl).

106. Janne PA, Reckamp K, Koczywas M, et al. Efficacy and safety of PF-00299804 (PF299) in patients (pt) with advanced NSCLC after failure of at least one prior chemotherapy regimen and prior treatment with erlotinib (E): a two-arm, phase II trial [abstract 8063]. *J Clin Oncol.* 2009;27:15s(suppl).

107. Nahta R, Yu D, Hung MC, Hortobagyi GN, Esteva FJ. Mechanisms of disease: understanding resistance to HER2-targeted therapy in human breast cancer. *Nat Clin Pract Oncol.* 2006;3(5):269–280.

108. Batus M, Fidler MJ, Basu S, et al. Frequency of insulin-like growth factor 1 (IGFR-1) expression and correlation with clinical and selected molecular parameters in advanced non-small cell lung cancer (NSCLC) patients (pts) [abstract 22080]. *J Clin Oncol.* 2008;26(May 20 suppl).

109. Cappuzzo F, Toschi L, Tallini G, et al. Insulin-like growth factor receptor 1 (IGFR-1) is significantly associated with longer survival

in non-small-cell lung cancer patients treated with gefitinib. *Ann Oncol.* 2006;17(7):1120–1127.

110. Merrick DT, Dziadziuszko R, Szostakiewicz B, et al. High insulin-like growth factor 1 receptor (IGF1R) expression is associated with poor survival in surgically treated non-small cell lung cancer (NSCLC) patients (pts). ASCO Annual Meeting Proceedings Part I. *J Clin Oncol.* 2007;25(18S, June 20 suppl):7550.

111. Karp DD, Paz-Ares LG, Blakely LJ, et al. Efficacy of the anti-insulin like growth factor I receptor (IGF-IR) antibody CP-751871 in combination with paclitaxel and carboplatin as first-line treatment for advanced non-small cell lung cancer (NSCLC). ASCO Annual Meeting Proceedings Part I. *J Clin Oncol.* 2007;25(18S, June 20 suppl):7506.

112. Karp DD, Paz-Ares LG, Novello S, et al. Phase II study of the anti-insulin-like growth factor type 1 receptor antibody CP-751,871 in combination with paclitaxel and carboplatin in previously untreated, locally advanced, or metastatic non-small-cell lung cancer. *J Clin Oncol.* 2009;27(15):2516–2522.

113. Higano CS, Yu EY, Whiting SH, et al. A phase I, first in man study of weekly IMC-A12, a fully human insulin like growth factor-I receptor IgG1 monoclonal antibody, in patients with advanced solid tumors. ASCO Annual Meeting Proceedings Part I. *J Clin Oncol.* 2007;25(18S, June 20 suppl):3505.

114. Giaccone G. New opportunities in systemic therapy. Presented at the 2008 European Society of Medical Oncology Congress meeting; September 13, 2008; Stockholm, Sweden.

115. Pal SK, Figlin RA, Reckamp KL. The role of targeting mammalian target of rapamycin in lung cancer. *Clin Lung Cancer.* 2008;9(6):340–345.

116. Meric-Bernstam F, Gonzalez-Angulo AM. Targeting the mTOR signaling network for cancer therapy. *J Clin Oncol.* 2009;27: 2278–2287.

117. Motzer RJ, Escudier B, Oudard S, et al.; RECORD-1 Study Group. Efficacy of everolimus in advanced renal cell carcinoma: a double-blind, randomised, placebo-controlled phase III trial. *Lancet.* 2008;372(9637):449–456.

118. O'Donnell A, Faivre S, Burris HA 3rd, et al. Phase I pharmacokinetic and pharmacodynamic study of the oral mammalian target of rapamycin inhibitor everolimus in patients with advanced solid tumors. *J Clin Oncol.* 2008;26(10):1588–1595.

119. Papadimitrakopoulou V, Soria JC, Douillard JY, et al. A phase II study of RAD001 (R) (everolimus) monotherapy in patients (pts) with advanced non small cell lung cancer (NSCLC) failing prior platinum-based chemotherapy (C) or prior C and EGFR inhibitors (EGFR-I). ASCO Annual Meeting Proceedings Part I. *J Clin Oncol.* 2007;25(18S, June 20 suppl):7589.

120. Hudes G, Carducci M, Tomczak P, et al.; Global ARCC Trial. Temsirolimus, interferon alfa, or both for advanced renal-cell carcinoma. *N Engl J Med.* 2007;356(22):2271–2281.

121. Pandya KJ, Dahlberg S, Hidalgo M, et al.; Eastern Cooperative Oncology Group (E1500). A randomized, phase II trial of two dose levels of temsirolimus (CCI-779) in patients with extensive-stage small-cell lung cancer who have responding or stable disease after induction chemotherapy: a trial of the Eastern Cooperative Oncology Group (E1500). *J Thorac Oncol.* 2007;2(11):1036–1041.

122. Mita MM, Mita AC, Chu QS, et al. Phase I trial of the novel mammalian target of rapamycin inhibitor deforolimus (AP23573; MK-8669) administered intravenously daily for 5 days every 2 weeks to patients with advanced malignancies. *J Clin Oncol.* 2008;26(3):361–367.

123. Sharma S, Zhu L, Yang SC, et al. Cyclooxygenase 2 inhibition promotes IFN-gamma-dependent enhancement of antitumor responses. *J Immunol.* 2005;175(2):813–819.

124. Lilenbaum R, Socinski MA, Altorki NK, et al. Randomized phase II trial of docetaxel/irinotecan and gemcitabine/irinotecan with or without celecoxib in the second-line treatment of non-small-cell lung cancer. *J Clin Oncol.* 2006;24(30):4825–4832.

125. Gasparini G, Meo S, Comella G, et al. The combination of the selective cyclooxygenase-2 inhibitor celecoxib with weekly paclitaxel is a safe and active second-line therapy for non-small cell lung cancer: a phase II study with biological correlates. *Cancer J.* 2005;11(3):209–216.

126. Groen H, Hochstenbag MM, Putten JWv, et al. A randomized placebo-controlled phase III study of docetaxel/carboplatin with celecoxib in patients (pts) with advanced non-small cell lung cancer (NSCLC): the NVALT-4 study [abstract 8005]. *J Clin Oncol.* 2009;27:15s(suppl).

127. Reckamp KL, Patel R, Gitlitz B, et al. Biomarker based phase I study of Apricoxib, a potent COX-2 inhibitor in combination with erlotinib in non-small cell lung cancer (NSCLC) patients [abstract 5621]. Presented at the 100th Annual Meeting of the American Association of Cancer Research; April 22, 2009; Denver, CO.

128. Edelman MJ, Watson D, Wang X, et al. Eicosanoid modulation in advanced lung cancer: cyclooxygenase-2 expression is a positive predictive factor for celecoxib + chemotherapy—Cancer and Leukemia Group B Trial 30203. *J Clin Oncol.* 2008;26(6):848–855.

129. Catalano MG, Poli R, Pugliese M, Fortunati N, Boccuzzi G. Valproic acid enhances tubulin acetylation and apoptotic activity of paclitaxel on anaplastic thyroid cancer cell lines. *Endocr Relat Cancer.* 2007;14(3):839–845.

130. Ramalingam SS, Maitland M, Frankel P, et al. Randomized, double-blind, placebo-controlled phase II study of carboplatin and paclitaxel with or without vorinostat, a histone deacetylase inhibitor (HDAC), for first-line therapy of advanced non-small cell lung cancer (NCI 7863) [abstract 8004]. *J Clin Oncol.* 2009;27:15s(suppl).

131. Horn L, Pao W. EML4-ALK: Honing in on a new target in non-small-cell lung cancer. J Clin Oncol. 2009;27:4232–4235.

132. Inamura K, Takeuchi K, Togashi Y, et al. EML4-ALK lung cancers are characterized by rare other mutations, a TTF-1 cell lineage, an acinar histology, and young onset. Mod Pathol. 2009;22:508–515.

133. Inamura KMDP, Takeuchi KMDP, Togashi YM, et al. EML4-ALK fusion is linked to histological characteristics in a subset of lung cancers. J Thorac Oncol. 2008;3:13–17.

134. Koivunen JP, Mermel C, Zejnullahu K, et al. EML4-ALK fusion gene and efficacy of an ALK kinase inhibitor in lung cancer. Clin Cancer Res. 2008;14:4275–4283.

135. Martelli MP, Sozzi G, Hernandez L, et al. EML4-ALK rearrangement in non-small cell lung cancer and non-tumor lung tissues. Am J Pathol. 2009;174:661–670.

136. Wong DW-S, Leung EL-H, So KK-T, et al. The *EML4-ALK* fusion gene is involved in various histologic types of lung cancers from nonsmokers with wild-type *EGFR* and *KRAS*. Cancer. 2009;115:1723–1733.

137. Timofeevski SL, McTigue MA, Ryan K, et al. Enzymatic characterization of c-Met receptor tyrosine kinase oncogenic mutants and kinetic studies with aminopyridine and triazolopyrazine inhibitors. Biochemistry. 2009;48:5339–5349.

138. Bang Y, Kwak EL, Shaw AT, et al. Clinical activity of the oral ALK inhibitor PF-02341066 in ALK-positive patients with non-small cell lung cancer (NSCLC) [meeting abstracts]. J Clin Oncol. 2010;28:3.

139. NCT01121575: A Phase 1, Open Label, Dose Escalation Study To Evaluate Safety, Pharmacokinetics And Pharmacodynamics Of Combined Oral C- MET/ALK Inhibitor (PF- 02341066) And PAN-HER Inhibitor (PF- 00299804) In Patients With Advanced Non-Small Cell Lung Cancer http://www.clinicaltrials.gov. Accessed August 3, 2010.

140. NCT01154140: Phase 3, Randomized, Open-Label Study Of The Efficacy And Safety Of Crizotinib Versus Pemetrexed/Cisplatin Or Pemetrexed/Carboplatin In Previously Untreated Patients With Non-squamous Carcinoma Of The Lung Harboring A Translocation Or Inversion Event Involving The Anaplastic Lymphoma Kinase (ALK) Gene Locus. http://www.clinicaltrials.gov. Accessed August 3, 2010.

141. Gandara D, Kim ES, Herbst RS, et al. S0536: carboplatin, paclitaxel, cetuximab, and bevacizumab followed by cetuximab and bevacizumab maintenance in advanced non-small cell lung cancer (NSCLC): a SWOG phase II study [abstract 8015]. *J Clin Oncol.* 2009;27:15s(suppl).

142. Mack PC, Holland WS, Redman M, et al. KRAS mutation analysis in cetuximab-treated advanced stage non-small cell lung cancer (NSCLC): SWOG experience with S0342 and S0536 [abstract 8022]. *J Clin Oncol.* 2009;27:15s(suppl).

143. Herbst RS, O'Neill VJ, Fehrenbacher L, et al. Phase II study of efficacy and safety of bevacizumab in combination with chemotherapy or erlotinib compared with chemotherapy alone for treatment of recurrent or refractory non small-cell lung cancer. *J Clin Oncol.* 2007;25(30):4743–4750.

144. Dang TP, Salmon JS, Chen H, et al. Predictive value of serum MALDI-TOF proteomic profiling from patients treated with erlotinib and bevacizumab for survival in patients with non-small cell lung cancer (NSCLC) treated with erlotinib alone [abstract 11014]. *J Clin Oncol.* 2008;26(May 20 suppl).

145. Salmon JS, Dang TP, Billheimer D, et al. VeriStrat predicts survival in patients with non-small cell lung cancer (NSCLC) treated with erlotinib and bevacizumab [abstract 8008]. *J Clin Oncol.* 2008;26(May 20 suppl).

146. Polikoff J, Hainsworth JD, Fehrenbacher L, et al. Safety of bevacizumab (Bv) therapy in combination with chemotherapy in subjects with non-small cell lung cancer (NSCLC) treated on ATLAS [abstract 8079]. *J Clin Oncol.* 2008;26(May 20 suppl).

147. Miller VA, O'Connor P, Soh C, et al. A randomized, double-blind, placebo-controlled, phase IIIb trial (ATLAS) comparing bevacizumab (B) therapy with or without erlotinib (E) after completion of chemotherapy with B for first-line treatment of locally advanced, recurrent, or metastatic non-small cell lung cancer (NSCLC) [abstract LBA8002]. *J Clin Oncol.* 2009;27: 18s(suppl).

148. Faoro L, Cohen EE, Govindan R, et al.Phase II trial of sequential bevacizumab (B), erlotinib (E) and chemotherapy for first line treatment of clinical stage IIIB or IV non-small cell lung cancer (NSCLC) [abstract 19130]. *J Clin Oncol.* 2008;26(May 20 suppl).

149. Adjei AA, Molina JR, Mandrekar SJ, et al. Phase I trial of sorafenib in combination with gefitinib in patients with refractory or recurrent non-small cell lung cancer. *Clin Cancer Res.* 2007;13(9):2684–2691.

150. Lind JS, Dingemans AC, Groen HJ, et al. A phase II study of erlotinib and sorafenib in chemotherapy-naive patients with locally advanced/metastatic non-small cell lung cancer (NSCLC) [abstract 8018]. *J Clin Oncol.* 2009;27:15s(suppl).

151. Karrison TG, Maitland ML, Stadler WM, Ratain MJ. Design of phase II cancer trials using a continuous endpoint of change in tumor size: application to a study of sorafenib and erlotinib in non small-cell lung cancer. *J Natl Cancer Inst.* 2007;99(19):1455–1461.

152. Ramalingam S, Forster J, Naret C, et al. Dual inhibition of the epidermal growth factor receptor with cetuximab, an IgG1 monoclonal antibody, and gefitinib, a tyrosine kinase inhibitor, in patients with refractory non-small cell lung cancer (NSCLC): a phase I study. *J Thorac Oncol.* 2008;3(3):258–264.

153. Pal SK, Pegram M. HER2 targeted therapy in breast cancer.beyond Herceptin. *Rev Endocr Metab Disord.* 2007;8(3):269–277.

154. Reckamp KL, Krysan K, Morrow JD, et al. A phase I trial to determine the optimal biological dose of celecoxib when combined with erlotinib in advanced non-small cell lung cancer. *Clin Cancer Res.* 2006;12(11 Pt 1):3381–3388.

155. Reckamp KL, Gardner BK, Figlin RA, et al. Tumor response to combination celecoxib and erlotinib therapy in non-small cell lung cancer is associated with a low baseline matrix metalloproteinase-9 and a decline in serum-soluble E-cadherin. *J Thorac Oncol.* 2008;3(2):117–124.

156. Csiki I, Morrow JD, Sandler A, et al. Targeting cyclooxygenase-2 in recurrent non-small cell lung cancer: a phase II trial of celecoxib and docetaxel. *Clin Cancer Res.* 2005;11(18):6634–6640.

157. Gadgeel SM, Ruckdeschel JC, Heath EI, Heilbrun LK, Venkatramanamoorthy R, Wozniak A. Phase II study of gefitinib, an epidermal growth factor receptor tyrosine kinase inhibitor (EGFR-TKI), and celecoxib, a cyclooxygenase-2 (COX-2) inhibitor, in patients with platinum refractory non-small cell lung cancer (NSCLC). *J Thorac Oncol.* 2007;2(4):299–305.

158. O'Byrne KJ, Danson S, Dunlop D, et al. Combination therapy with gefitinib and rofecoxib in patients with platinum-pretreated relapsed non small-cell lung cancer. *J Clin Oncol.* 2007;25(22):3266–3273.

159. Fidler MJ, Argiris A, Patel JD, et al. The potential predictive value of cyclooxygenase-2 expression and increased risk of gastrointestinal hemorrhage in advanced non-small cell lung cancer patients treated with erlotinib and celecoxib. *Clin Cancer Res.* 2008;14:2088–2094.

160. Khuri FR, Wu H, Lee JJ, et al. Cyclooxygenase-2 overexpression is a marker of poor prognosis in stage I non-small cell lung cancer. *Clin Cancer Res.* 2001;7(4):861–867.

161. Sekine S, Oshima K, Ishida T. Phase II study of S-1 in non-small cell lung cancer (NSCLC) patients previously treated with a platinum-based regimen. *J Thorac Oncol.* 2007;2:S687.

162. Milton DT, Kris MG, Azzoli CG, et al. Phase I/II trial of gefitinib and RAD001 (everolimus) in patients (pts) with advanced non-small cell lung cancer (NSCLC). ASCO Annual Meeting Proceedings. *J Clin Oncol.* 2005;23(16S, Part I of II, June 1 suppl):7104.

163. Kim ES, Herbst RS, Lee JJ, et al. Phase II randomized study of biomarker-directed treatment for non-small cell lung cancer (NSCLC): the BATTLE (biomarker-integrated approaches of targeted therapy for lung cancer elimination) clinical trial program [abstract 8024]. *J Clin Oncol.* 2009;27:15s(suppl).

164. Arcila ME, Riely GJ, Zakowski MF, et al. Rebiopsy of patients (pts) with acquired resistance to epidermal growth factor tyrosine kinase inhibitors (EGFR-TKIs) in non-small cell lung cancer (NSCLC) [abstract 8025]. *J Clin Oncol.* 2009;27:15s(suppl).

21 Role of Personalized Medicine: Now and the Future

NIR PELED

CELINE MASCAUX

MURRY W. WYNES

FRED R. HIRSCH

■ INTRODUCTION

The International Association for the Study of Lung Cancer recently published a proposal for a new staging classification of lung cancer (1). Data on which this staging system was based showed that the 5-year survival rates for stage IA, IB, IIA, and IIB lung cancer were 73%, 58%, 46%, and 36%, respectively. In other words, disease will recur in 27% of stage IA and 42% of stage IB patients (1). How do we identify those patients who are most likely to suffer disease recurrence and how do we choose the most effective therapy? While adjuvant therapy is established for stage II disease, there is no consensus regarding adjuvant therapy for stages IA and IB despite the relatively low survival rates. Thus, there is a need for biomarker selection of patients in these stages in order to better select those who would benefit from adjuvant therapy.

Biomarkers in lung cancer can be applied for different purposes: prognosis and/or for prediction of outcome to specific therapies. It is important to distinguish between prognosis and prediction. Prediction represents the power of a measure to predict tumor response and outcome to a certain therapy, whereas prognosis represents the association between a measure and outcome, independent of therapy. Those measures are not always similar, as tumor response does not necessarily affect survival. In this chapter, we will explore mainly predictive biomarkers for response and outcome and focus on tailoring therapy for lung cancer.

■ PROGNOSTIC ASSOCIATION OF BIOMARKERS IN NON–SMALL CELL LUNG CANCER

Over the past few decades, many biomarkers have been published with claims of a prognostic association in lung cancer. The biomarker analyses are based on different assay platforms; that is, protein expression by immunohistochemistry (IHC), messenger (m)RNA level by polymerase chain reaction (PCR), gene copy number by fluorescence in situ hybridization (FISH) or comparative genomic hybridization, and proteomic profiling.

Many candidate biomarkers are proposed to predict the prognosis for patients with non–small cell lung cancer (NSCLC) in earlier stages of disease. However, it should be emphasized that even if a biomarker or prognostic classifier identifies a subgroup with poor prognosis, it does not necessarily mean that this group will benefit from any adjuvant chemotherapy. For that purpose, a predictive classifier is needed. For example, at Duke University (Durham, NC) the "metagene array model," which includes 133 genes, has been proposed to separate stage I patients into good and bad prognostic groups (2). In addition, the National Cancer Institute of Canada presented a 15-gene model that was derived from the adjuvant BR.10 study (observation vs. cisplatin plus vinorelbine) (3,4). The data were encouraging for different groups: those who benefited from adjuvant therapy and those without any benefit (4). A three-gene classifier (STX1A, HIF1A, and CCR7) for overall survival (OS) (hazard ratio [HR] 3.8, 95% confidence interval [CI] 1.7–8.2, $P < 0.001$) has also been identified. The classifier was able to stratify stage I and II early-stage NSCLC patients with significantly different prognoses, and further improved the predictive ability of clinical factors such as histology and tumor stage (5).

Focusing on the epidermal growth factor receptor (EGFR), there are conflicting data about the prognostic importance of EGFR protein levels in NSCLC. A meta-analysis failed to show a consistent correlation between EGFR expression levels and survival (6). Most studies have shown no prognostic effect of EGFR expression or a slight negative effect. Studies of EGFR gene copy numbers assessed by FISH have also failed to show a consistent association between EGFR gene copy number and prognosis, although few studies have reported a worse survival with EGFR gene amplification (7,8). The results for activating EGFR gene mutations are strikingly different. Nearly all studies have reported that patients with these mutations have a superior outcome compared with those without these mutations (9–16).

Several other studies have been published describing prognostic markers identified through PCR (17) and proteomics (18). However, rigorous prospective validation studies are needed for all of these biomarkers before they can be used in routine clinical practice.

■ TAILORING CHEMOTHERAPY BY BIOMARKERS

ERCC1 as a Predictor of Clinical Benefit from Platinum-Based Therapy

Platinum doublets remain the backbone of treatment for patients with NSCLC. Large randomized studies have demonstrated the equivalence of several platinum doublets, including gemcitabine, docetaxel, vinorelbine, paclitaxel, and pemetrexed (19). However, it should be noted that response and outcome varies significantly between patients, highlighting the need for molecular predictive markers for these therapeutic combinations.

Nucleotide excision repair is a highly versatile pathway for DNA damage removal and is often dysfunctional in NSCLC. Excision repair cross-complementation group 1 (ERCC1) performs an essential late step in the nucleotide excision repair process, where it nicks the damaged DNA strand at the 5′ site of the helix-distorting cisplatin lesion. ERCC1 might also play several other important roles in the DNA repair process (20).

A joint Spanish-U.S. study has observed longer survival and a trend toward improved response in NSCLC patients with stage IV disease and low ERCC1 mRNA levels who were treated with gemcitabine plus cisplatin (Figure 21.1) (21). In another study from the Spanish Lung Cancer Group, 444 patients with NSCLC (stage IV disease) were prospectively randomized based on ERCC1 mRNA level (22). In the genotyped treatment arm, the response rate was 50.7% compared with 39.3% in the control arm (P = 0.02). The study demonstrated that assessment of ERCC1 mRNA expression is feasible in the clinical setting, and predicts a response to docetaxel and cisplatin in combination. Ceppi et al. (23) have also shown, in a retrospective study of 70 patients, that a low level of ERCC1 predicts longer survival on cisplatin-based chemotherapy.

In another large randomized study, IALT (International Adjuvant Lung Cancer Trial), 766 NSCLC patients were assessed for ERCC1 protein expression by IHC (24). The ERCC1 was found to be positive in 44% of patients and negative in 56% of patients. The ERCC1-negative was associated with a benefit from cisplatin-based adjuvant chemotherapy. The ERCC1-negative tumors had an adjusted HR of 0.65 (95% CI 0.50–0.86,

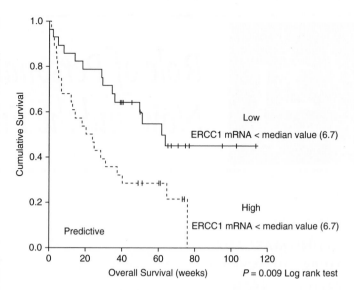

FIGURE 21.1 Excision repair cross-complementation group 1 (ERCC1) as a predictive marker for platinum-based therapy in non–small cell lung cancer. Adapted from Ref. 21.

P = 0.002) compared with an HR of 1.14 (95% CI 0.84–1.55, P = 0.40) for ERCC1-positive patients (24). Among patients who did not receive adjuvant chemotherapy, those with ERCC1-positive tumors survived longer than those with ERCC1-negative tumors (adjusted HR for death 0.66; 95% CI, 0.49–0.90; P = 0.009). It was concluded that NSCLC patients with completely resected ERCC1-negative tumors were stronger candidates for adjuvant cisplatin-based chemotherapy than those who had resected ERCC1-positive tumors (24). In the same cohort, the human MutS homolog 2 (MSH2) protein showed the same trend as with ERCC1, low expression predicted a higher benefit from platinum-based therapy. Chemotherapy compared to observation prolonged survival in the MSH2 negative group (HR for death 0.76; P = 0.03), but not in the MSH2 positive group (HR for death 1.12; P = 0.48) (25).

Based on these results, there is a high probability that in the near future platinum-based chemotherapy could be selected according to ERCC1 and MSH2 expression in tumor tissue. Nevertheless, additional studies are warranted to standardize and optimize methodologies for ERCC1 and MSH2 analysis in tumor tissue in order to define a biomarker profile for predicting outcome.

RRM1 as a Predictor of Clinical Benefit from Gemcitabine-Based Therapy

The gene *RRM1* (ribonucleotide reductase subunit M1) encodes the large regulatory subunit of ribonucleotide reductase and is located on the short arm of chromosome 11 in segment 15.5. Because RRM1 regulates ribonucleotide reductase function and thus deoxynucleotide production, it is likely that the RRM1 protein has a substantial effect on drugs that directly or indirectly influence nucleotide metabolism, namely antimetabolites and, in particular, nucleoside analogs. Among nucleoside analogs, gemcitabine (2′,2′-difluorodeoxycytidine) has been extensively studied. RRM1 is the major cellular determinant of the efficacy of gemcitabine.

Many preclinical studies have documented the relationship between RRM1 expression and gemcitabine cytotoxicity. In a clinical trial by Bepler et al. (26,27), a prospective assessment of tumoral RRM1 expression was performed (Figure 21.2). In 35 patients, disease response was inversely correlated with the level of RRM1 expression, indicating that low-level RRM1 expression is associated with tumor response to gemcitabine-based chemotherapy, and high-level RRM1 expression is associated with tumor resistance (28). Zheng et al. (29) have published an analysis of *RRM1* and *ERCC1* gene expression in relation to tumor response in patients with advanced NSCLC treated with gemcitabine plus platinum chemotherapy. Through the use of a PCR technique, both markers were found to be predictive. Therefore, a combination of ERCC1 and RRM1 is likely to predict an outcome based on gemcitabine plus platinum chemotherapy, and ongoing prospective multi-institutional studies are exploring the potential of this combination. Further studies are warranted for RRM1 to standardize methodology.

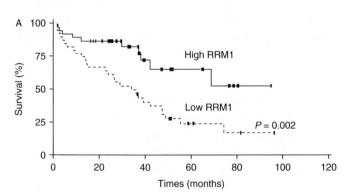

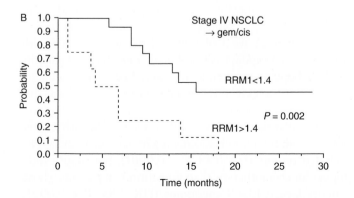

FIGURE 21.2 Ribonucleotide reductase subunit M1 (RRM1) as a (A) prognostic measure and (B) predictive marker in non–small cell lung cancer. Adapted with permission from Refs. 27 and 28.

Thymidylate Synthase as a Predictor of Clinical Benefit from Pemetrexed-Based Therapy

Pemetrexed, a multitargeted folic acid antagonist (antimetabolite), has recently been approved for the first-line treatment and for maintenance therapy of advanced NSCLC (combined with platinum) and is the standard of care for treatment of mesothelioma. In a noninferiority, phase III, randomized study, Scagliotti et al. (30) looked at OS in 1,725 chemotherapy-naïve patients with advanced NSCLC. Patients received cisplatin plus gemcitabine or cisplatin plus pemetrexed every 3 weeks for up to six cycles. OS for the cisplatin plus pemetrexed combination was noninferior to cisplatin plus gemcitabine (median survival 10.3 vs. 10.3 months, respectively; HR 0.94, 95% CI 0.84–1.05). OS was significantly superior for the cisplatin plus pemetrexed combination versus that of cisplatin plus gemcitabine in patients with adenocarcinoma (n = 847; 12.6 vs. 10.9 months, respectively) or large-cell carcinoma histology (n = 153; 10.4 vs. 6.7 months, respectively).

The mechanisms of action for pemetrexed are related to the inhibition of important enzymes for RNA and DNA synthesis in folate receptor downstream signaling, including thymidylate synthase (TS), glycinamide ribonucleotide formyltransferase, and dihydrofolate reductase. In several preclinical studies, pemetrexed resistance has been shown to be associated with increased TS expression, both at the mRNA and protein level (31–33). Basal TS levels were found to be higher in lung cancer tissue than in normal lung tissue and, more importantly, higher in chemonaïve squamous cell carcinomas than in chemonaïve adenocarcinomas (34). Thus, TS expression may be associated with the differential sensitivity to pemetrexed in various histologic groups.

In a nonsquamous population—that is, patients with a low TS level—pemetrexed has demonstrated superiority for median OS in both second-line therapy compared with docetaxel (9.3 vs. 8.0 months, HR 0.78, 95% CI 0.61–1.00, P = 0.047) and first-line therapy in combination with cisplatin compared with gemcitabine plus cisplatin (11.8 vs. 10.4, HR 0.81, 95% CI 0.70–0.94), as shown in the JMEI (35) and JMDB (30) trials, respectively. Among patients with adenocarcinomas in the JMDB trial, OS was 12.6 versus 10.9 months (HR 0.84, P = 0.033) for pemetrexed plus cisplatin versus gemcitabine plus cisplatin, respectively (30). Recent data from the JMEN trial, presented at the American Society of Clinical Oncology 2008 congress, confirmed the superior efficacy of pemetrexed in a nonsquamous patient population (36).

Based on data from the JMEI, JMDB, and JMEN trials, the European Medicines Agency has changed the label for pemetrexed usage. Because of its superior efficacy (and tolerability) in the treatment of adenocarcinoma and large cell carcinoma, pemetrexed is now indicated for the first line, second line, and for maintenance therapy of patients with NSCLC without predominantly squamous carcinoma.

Levels of TS have also been shown to correlate with pemetrexed efficacy in other tumor types. Preliminary data from breast cancer studies with pemetrexed have shown that low TS mRNA values correspond to long survival, while high TS mRNA values correspond to shorter survival (37). Likewise, in gastroenteropancreatic patients treated with 5-fluorouracil (5-FU) (which is in the same class of agents as pemetrexed), high TS mRNA values have been associated with a shorter time to progression (TTP) and OS (38). Together with the data mentioned earlier on NSCLC, these findings strongly indicate that TS is a possible predictive marker of treatment efficacy with agents in the same group as pemetrexed. This hypothesis is currently being tested in a prospective large adjuvant therapy study in patients with NSCLC. The most optimal methodology to TS determination has yet to be defined.

Tailoring EGFR-Related Therapies

EGFR inhibitors have proven to be effective in some patients with advanced NSCLC who were previously treated with chemotherapy (39) and most recently also proven effective in first-line treatment particularly in patients with EGFR mutation (40). Most of the data published exist for the EGFR tyrosine kinase inhibitors (TKIs) gefitinib and erlotinib as second-line therapy. Objective response rates with gefitinib and erlotinib are 10% to 18% in Western populations and up to 27% in Asian populations (41–43). In addition, a substantial fraction of NSCLC patients who failed previous chemotherapy regimens have achieved long-term stable disease on EGFR inhibitors (leading to a disease control in >50% of patients) that is often associated with symptomatic improvement and prolonged survival (44). Thus, developing a biomarker capable of predicting the disease control rate is equally important as to know who will have an objective response.

Several clinical and pathologic factors are known to predict the tumor response or OS benefit of EGFR-TKI therapy. Better response is related to East Asian ethnicity, female sex, never-smoking status, and/or adenocarcinoma histology. In addition, there are several molecular biomarkers that, retrospectively, have been shown to discriminate the clinical benefit of EGFR TKIs and EGFR-targeting monoclonal antibodies in the therapy of NSCLC (45). The recent IPASS (40,46) (Iressa Pan Asia Study) and OSI-774–203 (47) studies suggest that molecular biomarkers are more important than clinical features in selecting NSCLC patients for first-line therapy with EGFR TKIs. The observation was that in clinically selected patients, survival rate was superior with EGFR-TKI therapy versus chemotherapy only in patients with EGFR mutations, whereas survival was inferior with EGFR-TKI therapy in patients without EGFR mutations.

Tailoring by EGFR Gene Mutation

Somatic mutations in the kinase domain of EGFR in lung carcinoma exist in approximately 10% of specimens in the United States and 25% to 50% in Asia (9). About 90% of EGFR-activating mutations are clustered in exons 19 and 21 (48). A recent survey by Rosell R (49) et al in Europe (N = 2,105) showed that 16.6% of the patients had EGFR mutation. The mutations were more frequent in women (69.7%), never smokers (66.6%) and adenocarcinomas (80.9%). The mutations were deletions in exon 19 (62.2%) and a point mutation (L858R) in exon 21 (37.8%). Patients with these mutations have greater response rates to EGFR TKIs (approximately 60–80%) than patients without these mutations (approximately 10–20%) (10). Clinically, there seem to be differences in outcome based on the type of EGFR mutation. Patients with del19 mutations demonstrate a higher response rate and longer survival with EGFR-TKI therapy than patients with point mutations in exon 21 (10–12,50,51) (Figure 21.3). Deletions in exon 19, substitution mutations in exon 21 (L858R), or less common mutations (e.g., G719X, L861Q) cluster in the kinase domain around the adenosine 5′-triphosphate (ATP)-binding site. These mutations lead to preferential phosphorylation of protein kinase B (AKT) and signal transducers and activators of transcription 3 and 5 as opposed to extracellular signal-regulated kinases 1 and 2, and cell lines harboring these mutations show increased sensitivity to gefitinib (52–54). The T790M mutation (exon 20) was identified in patients with existing activating mutations of EGFR who developed (acquired) resistance to gefitinib or erlotinib (55). Unrelated to T790M mutation (56), MET gene amplification was also reported in 7% to 22% of lung cancer specimens that developed resistant to EGFR TKIs (57,58).

Several prospective phase II and III studies have studied EGFR TKIs as first-line therapy in NSCLC patients with EGFR mutations (11,59–63). These studies reported high response rates and longer progression-free survival (PFS) and OS than would be expected from chemotherapy alone, based upon historical controls. In the recent IPASS trial (40,46), 1,217 chemotherapy-naïve patients with advanced NSCLC were clinically selected. These patients had Asian ethnicity, adenocarcinoma histology, and were never- or light-smokers. A total of 609 patients were treated with gefitinib (250 mg/day) as first-line therapy and 608 patients with carboplatin (area under the curve 5 or 6) and paclitaxel (200 mg/m^2) weekly. Overall, PFS but not survival was different between the two arms (HR 0.69, $P < 0.0191$) (46). Of particular interest was that PFS was significantly higher for gefitinib than for chemotherapy in patients with EGFR-mutated tumors (HR 0.48, $P < 0.0001$), but significantly higher for chemotherapy than for gefitinib in patients whose tumors lacked EGFR mutations (HR 2.85, $P < 0.0001$; Figure 21.4) (40,64). Toxicity and quality of life analysis favored gefitinib over chemotherapy. The superiority of EGFR TKI alone as first line therapy over chemotherapy in

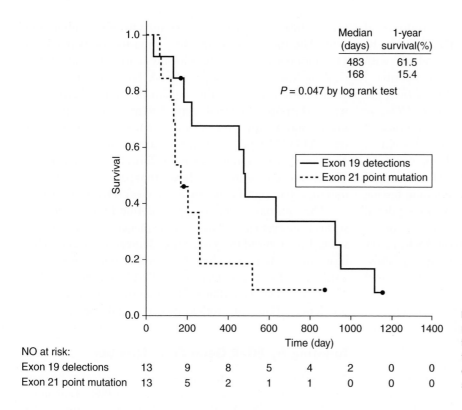

Median (days)	1-year survival(%)
483	61.5
168	15.4

$P = 0.047$ by log rank test

— Exon 19 detections
---- Exon 21 point mutation

NO at risk:

Exon 19 deletions	13	9	8	5	4	2	0	0
Exon 21 point mutation	13	5	2	1	1	0	0	0

FIGURE 21.3 Overall survival plot on EGFR mutation type. Patients with EGFR exon 19 deletion had a significantly longer median survival than those with exon 21 point mutation (483 vs. 168 days; log-rank $P = 0.047$). Adapted with permission from Ref. 51.

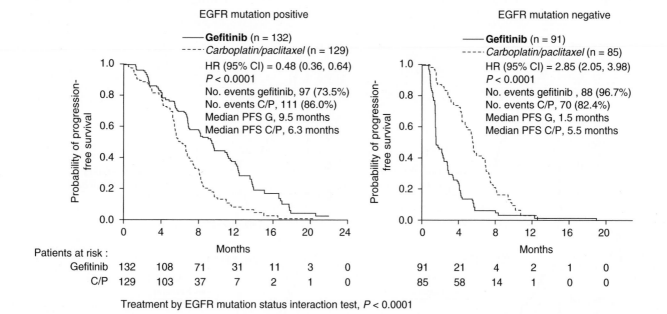

EGFR mutation positive

— **Gefitinib** (n = 132)
---- *Carboplatin/paclitaxel* (n = 129)
HR (95% CI) = 0.48 (0.36, 0.64)
$P < 0.0001$
No. events gefitinib, 97 (73.5%)
No. events C/P, 111 (86.0%)
Median PFS G, 9.5 months
Median PFS C/P, 6.3 months

EGFR mutation negative

— **Gefitinib** (n = 91)
---- *Carboplatin/paclitaxel* (n = 85)
HR (95% CI) = 2.85 (2.05, 3.98)
$P < 0.0001$
No. events gefitinib , 88 (96.7%)
No. events C/P, 70 (82.4%)
Median PFS G, 1.5 months
Median PFS C/P, 5.5 months

Patients at risk :

Gefitinib	132	108	71	31	11	3	0
C/P	129	103	37	7	2	1	0

91	21	4	2	1	0
85	58	14	1	0	0

Treatment by EGFR mutation status interaction test, $P < 0.0001$

Cox analysis with covariates; HR < 1 implies a lower risk of progression on gefitinib; ITT population

FIGURE 21.4 Progression-free survival in EGFR-mutation–positive and –negative patients. IPASS Trial. Adapted with permission from Ref. 40.

patients with advanced NSCLC and with tumors harboring mutations was also clearly demonstrated in two other large Asian studies (Mitsudomi T, Morita S, Yatabe Y et al. Gefitinib versus cisplatin plus docetaxel in patients with non-small-cell lung cancer harbouring mutations of the epidermal growth factor receptor (WJTOG3405): an open label, randomized phase 3 trial. Lancet Oncol 2010; 11: 121–128. Maemondo M, Inoue A, Kobayashi K et al. Gefitinib or chemotherapy for non-small-cell lung cancer with mutated EGFR. *N Engl J Med* 2010; 362: 2380–2388.). Furthermore, the significant role of EGFR mutations for first line therapy was also demonstrated in Western NSCLC population (Rosell R, Moran T, Queralt C et al. Screening for Epidermal Growth Factor Receptor Mutations in

Lung Cancer. *N Engl J Med* 2009.). Also a randomized phase II study by Hirsch et al (Hirsch FR, Dziadziuszko R, Camidge DR et al. Biomarker Status Correlates with Clinical Benefit: Phase 2 Study of Single-agent Erlotinib (E) or E Intercalated with Carboplatin and Paclitaxel (ECP) in an EGFR Biomarkerselected NSCLC Population. *J Thorac Oncol* 2008; 3: S267.) showed the clinical importance of EGFR mutations for first line therapy of advanced NSCLC. Thus, an EGFR TKI may be preferential to chemotherapy in chemonaïve patients with EGFR mutations. The most optimal and cost effective method for EGFR mutation testing has to be determined. While DNA sequencing is considered the "gold-standard", more sensitive PCR-based methods are currently used (e.g. DxS Scorpion). Immunohistochemistry with EGFR mutation specific antibody seems also promising (Kato Y, Peled N, Wynes MW et al. Novel Epidermal Growth Factor Receptor Mutation-Specific Antibodies for Non-Small Cell Lung Cancer: Immunohistochemistry as a Possible Screening Method for Epidermal Growth Factor Receptor Mutations. *J Thorac Oncol* 2010 in press).

In the OSI-774–203 protocol, patients expressing EGFR by IHC or FISH were randomized to receive chemotherapy (carboplatin and paclitaxel) intercalated with erlotinib or erlotinib alone in cycles of 21 days (65). Preliminary results showed a median PFS of 2.7 months

for the erlotinib arm and 4.6 months for the combination arm. The median OS was 16.7 months compared with 11.9 months favoring the erlotinib arm, although statistical significance was not achieved. However, in patients with EGFR mutations, the median PFS was 18.2 months with erlotinib compared with 4.9 months on alternating chemotherapy and erlotinib. Moreover, analysis of the SATURN trial (Sequential Tarceva in Unresectable Non-Small Cell Lung Cancer, Erlotinib Versus Placebo Maintenance Therapy) has shown that patients with EGFR mutation had significant better survival (HR of 0.1) (66).

The optimal methodology to define EGFR mutation status is not yet clear. The DNA sequencing has been considered as a standard procedure. However, newer PCR-based methods are developed, as well as mutation-specific antibodies for the detection of EGFR mutations (67). There is no evidence that EGFR mutations play a role in prediction of outcome following cetuximab therapy.

Tailoring by EGFR Gene Copy Number

The EGFR gene is located at the p14–12 region of human chromosome 7 and can be detected by FISH. True gene amplification or high polysomy is defined according to the Colorado EGFR scoring system (68). We have evaluated

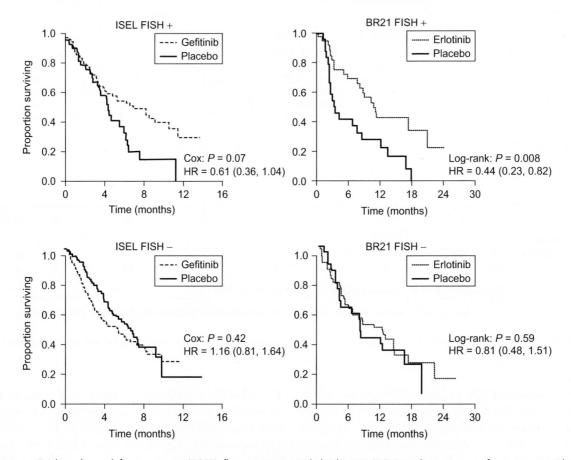

FIGURE 21.5 Epidermal growth factor receptor (EGFR)–fluorescence in situ hybridization (FISH) predicts outcome after treatment with EGFR tyrosine kinase inhibitors in advanced non-small cell lung cancer. BR.21, National Cancer Institute of Canada Clinical Trials Group Study; CI, confidence interval; HR, hazard ratio; ISEL, Iressa Survival Evaluation in Lung Cancer. Adapted with permission from Refs. 71 and 73.

the predictive value of FISH status in several phase II studies of EGFR TKIs in the second- and third-line settings. FISH-positive patients had superior response rates and longer survival times than FISH-negative patients in these studies (50,68–70).

FISH Positivity in the Second- or Third-Line Setting

The predictive value of FISH positivity has now been assessed in prospective randomized studies of erlotinib and gefitinib in the second- and third-line settings. In the BR.21 study, FISH-positive patients who were randomized to erlotinib had a significantly superior OS versus FISH-positive patients randomized to placebo (HR 0.44, $P = 0.01$). In the FISH-negative patients, there were no significant differences in survival between those receiving erlotinib and placebo (HR 0.80; Figure 21.5) (71,72). In the Iressa Survival Evaluation in Lung Cancer (ISEL) study, FISH-positive patients receiving gefitinib also had a superior survival compared with FISH-positive patients receiving placebo (HR 0.61, $P = 0.06$; Figure 21.5) (73).

Contradictory findings have been reported in randomized studies comparing EGFR TKIs with chemotherapy in second- and third-line settings. In the INTEREST (Iressa Non-small Cell Lung Cancer Trial Evaluating Response and Survival Against Taxotere) trial, which compared gefitinib with docetaxel, EGFR FISH did not predict a superior outcome with gefitinib (74). There was a trend for better PFS in patients treated with gefitinib who had both EGFR mutations and FISH-positive status. Thus, while there are consistent data regarding the predictive value of EGFR mutations in the first-line setting, data obtained in the second-line setting are less certain.

FISH Positivity in the First-Line Setting

There are fewer data about the predictive value of FISH positivity in the first-line setting. FISH positivity predicted a superior outcome following gefitinib therapy in patients with bronchioloalveolar carcinoma in a Southwest Oncology Group (SWOG) study (69). Patients with FISH-positive tumors had a superior outcome in the first-line IPASS study, but nearly all FISH-positive patients also had EGFR mutations, as EGFR gene copy number is higher when mutation exists. In the TRIBUTE (Tarceva Responses in Conjunction with Taxol and Carboplatin) phase III trial, in which carboplatin and paclitaxel, with or without erlotinib, were assessed in the first-line setting, subanalysis by EGFR FISH showed that there was no difference in OS between FISH-positive and FISH-negative patients in either the chemotherapy plus erlotinib or chemotherapy plus placebo arms (75). In FISH-positive patients, median TTP was 6.3 months in the erlotinib arm versus 5.8 months with placebo (HR 0.59, 95% CI 0.35–0.99, $P = 0.0430$); in FISH-negative patients, median TTP was 4.6 months versus 6.0 months, respectively (HR 1.42, 95%

CI 0.95–2.14, $P = 0.0895$; treatment interaction test, $P = 0.007$) (75). After 6 months of treatment, a notable separation of the TTP curves in favor of erlotinib emerged, indicating a role for erlotinib as maintenance therapy. This has been verified in the SATURN (Sequential Tarceva in Unresectable Non-Small Cell Lung Cancer, Erlotinib Versus Placebo Maintenance Therapy) trial (66,76).

FISH Status as a Predictive Biomarker of Response and Outcome to Cetuximab

Since EGFR-activating mutations do not appear to predict response to cetuximab (77), it is important to develop biomarkers in order to select patients who are more likely to benefit from this targeted agent. In a study from SWOG comparing sequential and concurrent cetuximab treatment in addition to carboplatin and paclitaxel chemotherapy (S0342), FISH-positive patients demonstrated improved median survival (15 vs. 7 months, $P = 0.04$), median PFS (6 vs. 3 months, $P = 0.0008$), and objective response rate (45% vs. 26%, $P = 0.14$) versus FISH-negative patients (45). These results suggest that FISH status might be a predictive biomarker for response to cetuximab therapy. However, similar results were not observed in the Bristol-Myers Squibb (BMS)-099 study (78) or the FLEX study (O'Byrne KJ, Bondarenko I, Barrios C et al. Molecular and clinical predictors of outcome for cetuximab in non-small cell lung cancer (NSCLC): Data from the FLEX study. *J Clin Oncol* (Meeting Abstracts) 2009; 27: 8007), where there was no association observed between FISH status and outcome with cetuximab. Therefore, the SWOG group has initiated a validation of EGFR FISH in a large prospective phase III trial (0819), which is also assessing chemotherapy, with or without cetuximab, as first-line therapy.

Tailoring by EGFR Protein Expression

Based on EGFR expression, IHC-positive patients (score >200) (68) had significantly higher response and disease control rates, and significantly longer TTP and survival than patients with lower scores (<200) when treated with gefitinib. In the randomized phase III BR.21 trial comparing erlotinib and placebo, IHC-positive patients treated with erlotinib had a significantly superior survival compared with placebo-treated patients (HR 0.68, $P = 0.02$) (71). In the ISEL trial, gefitinib produced a reduction in the HR for survival in IHC-positive patients (HR 0.77), but this was not significant when compared with placebo in IHC-positive patients ($P = 0.13$). However, the interaction coefficient (comparison of HR values for IHC-positive and IHC-negative groups) was statistically significant (73).

There are fewer studies evaluating the relationship between EGFR protein expression and efficacy of cetuximab. The FLEX (First line Erbitux in Lung Cancer) study, which compared chemotherapy alone (cisplatin and vinorelbine) with chemotherapy plus cetuximab, included only patients whose tumor expressed EGFR by IHC (approximately 85%) (79). The study showed a statistically significant survival advantage for the chemotherapy plus cetuximab group (HR 0.871, 95% CI 0.762–0.996, $P = 0.044$). However, there was no association between the degree of EGFR expression and improved outcome. The BMS-099 (Bristol-Myers Squibb-099) study compared a different chemotherapy regimen, carboplatin plus a taxane, with chemotherapy plus cetuximab (80). In this study all patients were included, irrespective of EGFR expression. There was no significant effect of cetuximab on median OS, although patients receiving cetuximab had a slightly greater PFS (HR 0.89, P = not significant). It is not clear if the differences in outcome between the FLEX and BMS-099 studies could be related to selection by IHC. The inability of EGFR protein expression to serve as a predictive biomarker in NSCLC is similar to observations with the use of cetuximab in metastatic colon cancer, and thus invites the exploration of other biomarkers for EGFR-targeted antibodies (81).

KRAS Gene Mutation as a Predictor of Clinical Benefit

KRAS is an important downstream mediator of EGFR signaling and harbors an activating mutation in codon 12 or 13 (exon 2). EGFR- and KRAS-activating mutations are nearly always mutually exclusive. Activating mutations in KRAS are associated with lower response rates to EGFR TKIs and worse survival periods (7,15,16,55,72,82,83). Based on that knowledge, it has been hypothesized that KRAS mutation is a negative predictive marker for treatment of NSCLC with EGFR inhibitors. In contrast to colorectal cancer, in which KRAS mutations occur in 40% to 50% of patients and have been shown to be associated with a lack of response and shortened survival, the situation for NSCLC is different, where KRAS mutations occur less frequently (in approximately 15–26% of unselected patients). Moreover, in NSCLC, KRAS mutations occur more frequently in adenocarcinomas, and are found significantly less frequently in tumors with squamous histology (84). Thus, based on the lower frequency compared to colorectal cancer patients, the KRAS marker might be of less clinical importance as a single marker in NSCLC. In NSCLC, KRAS mutation is associated with a poor prognosis and is thus a negative prognostic factor. This needs consideration when the predictive performance is assessed.

Recent analysis by Massarelli et al. (85) of 59 patients with NSCLC who were treated with EGFR TKIs showed that KRAS gene mutation is associated with a poor response to TKIs and overcomes the potential favorable role of increased EGFR gene copy number in NSCLC tumors.

In relation to the EGFR monoclonal antibody (cetuximab), the Flex study trial has shown a survival benefit with the addition of cetuximab to chemotherapy in the first-line treatment of NSCLC, unrelated to KRAS status in 379 patients (86). Likewise, in the BS099 study, which compared carboplatin plus paclitaxel with carboplatin plus paclitaxel and cetuximab in 676 patients with advanced NSCLC, the presence of KRAS mutations was not associated with a decreased benefit from cetuximab (78).

■ NOVEL DIRECTIONS

Serum Proteomics as a Predictor of Clinical Benefit

Serum proteomics is an emerging science in which the serum is analyzed by mass spectrometry for specific proteins. Numerous studies have provided evidence that this technology can be used to uncover proteomic expression patterns linked to a disease state. Taguchi et al. (87) have tested the serum from 139 patients with NSCLC in order to classify a proteomic profile that may predict a clinical benefit from EGFR-TKI therapy. Based on their classification, they identified patients who showed improved outcomes after EGFR-TKI treatment. In the validation cohort treated with gefitinib, the median survival of patients in the good and poor predictive groups was 207 and 92 days, respectively (HR of death in the good vs. poor groups 0.50, 95% CI 0.24–0.78). In the other cohort treated with erlotinib, median survival was 306 versus 107 days, respectively (HR 0.41, 95% CI 0.17–0.63). The classifier did not predict outcomes in patients who did not receive EGFR-TKI treatment. This proteomic classifier has been commercialized under the name VeriStrat® (Biodesix, Broomfield, CO). In a recent retrospective analysis of patients treated in the placebo-controlled BR-21 study, the proteomic classifier also showed to have a prognostic association (Carbone DP, Seymour L, Ding K et al. Serum proteomic prediction of outcomes in advanced NSCLC patients treated with erlotinib/placebo in the NCIC clinical trials group BR.21 trial. *J Thorac Oncol* (Meeting Abstracts) 2010; 5: S80.). Further validation studies with the VerisStrat® classifier are ongoing and will benefit the field. Salmons et al. has just published (88) another proteomic profile to predict PFS and OS in patients treated by erlotinib alone in the Eastern Cooperative Oncology Group (ECOG) 3503 cohort.

Class III β-Tubulin as a Predictor of Clinical Benefit from Taxane- and Vinorelbine-Based Therapy

Data from preclinical and some clinical studies (89–92) show that overexpression of class III β-tubulin is associated with resistance to tubulin-binding agents. Therefore, this overexpression could be used to predict outcome to such therapies, which are commonly used as the standard of care for patients with NSCLC.

High expression of class III β-tubulin is correlated with low response rates and shorter survival following treatment with regimens containing taxanes (and vinorelbine) in NSCLC and other tumors. Seve et al. (93) have shown that those patients with advanced NSCLC who received paclitaxel or vinorelbine and whose tumors expressed high levels of class III β-tubulin had a lower response rate and shorter survival time. However, this variable was not found to be prognostic in patients who received regimens without tubulin-binding agents (90). Conversely, analysis from the BR.10 study, which compared adjuvant chemotherapy with no further therapy in operable NSCLC, showed that chemotherapy seemed to overcome the negative prognostic effect of a high level of expression of class III β-tubulin. The greatest benefit from the cisplatin plus vinorelbine combination was observed in patients who had a high expression level of class III β-tubulin (94). Furthermore, while tubulin and microtubules are the main targets of the vinca alkaloids (e.g., vinorelbine, vinblastine, vincristine), the role of class III β-tubulin as a predictive marker is still controversial and additional preclinical and clinical studies are required. While more of these studies are conclusive, they suggest that class III β-tubulin could be both a prognostic and predictive marker. Thus, future prospective validation studies are warranted.

Insulin-Like Growth Factor Receptor Inhibition

Many new agents targeting the insulin-like growth factor pathway, both monoclonal antibodies and small molecules, are in clinical trials (95). Encouraging phase II data have already been presented with response rates exceeding 50% and long PFS (96). Histology seems to play a role in sensitivity to these agents, as the response rates were significantly better for patients with a squamous histology than those with a nonsquamous histology. Large phase III trials were launched, but prematurely stopped due to toxicity and futility (Jassem J, Langer CJ, Karp DD et al. Randomized, open label, phase III trial of figitumumab in combination with paclitaxel and carboplatin versus paclitaxel and carboplatin in patients with non-small cell lung cancer (NSCLC). *J Clin Oncol* (Meeting Abstracts) 2010; 28: 7500–). Unfortunately, the large phase III-studies were performed without a biomarker-driven selection approach. While there are many potential candidates for predictive markers beyond histology, so far, no predictive marker is in clinical use. However, IGF-1R is highly expressed both in NSCLC and SCLC tumors (Dziadziuszko R, Merrick DT, Witta SE et al. Insulin-like growth factor receptor 1 (IGF1R) gene copy number is associated with survival in operable non-small-cell lung cancer: a comparison between IGF1R fluorescent in situ hybridization, protein expression, and mRNA expression. *J Clin Oncol* 2010; 28: 2174–2180., Badzio A*, Wynes MW*, Dziadziuszko R, et al. *Co-First Authors. Increased Insulin-Like Growth Factor 1 Receptor Protein Expression and Gene Copy Number in Small Cell Lung Cancer. *J Thorac Oncol*. 2010. Accepted, In Press.) and may be a potential predictive biomarker, i.e. gene copy number and protein expression should be further explored.

Antiangiogenic Agents

Several agents targeting the vascular endothelial growth factor receptor (VEGFR) system, either alone or combined with EGFR-targeting, have been developed and entered into clinical studies. Based on the positive ECOG 5499 study comparing chemotherapy with or without bevacizumab, bevacizumab (Avastin) has been approved for the first-line treatment of NSCLC in the United States and Europe (97). Detailed survival data from a similar large European trial—the AVAiL (Avastin in Lung) study—showed significantly improved survival with bevacizumab in combination with chemotherapy, but failed to show improved OS (98). In respect to predictive biomarkers, studies to date have been challenging and no predictive biomarker has yet emerged for the clinical use of antiangiogenic agents. Candidate markers have included tissue expression of VEGFRs (as a potential marker for adjuvant therapy) and platelet-derived growth factor receptor among many others; studies evaluating different VEGFRs in the peripheral blood are ongoing (99).

Gene Expression

Based on cell line assays, the Duke University group indentified gene signatures predicting response to different chemotherapy agents, for example, docetaxel, topotecan, adriamycin, etoposide, 5-FU, placlitaxel, and cyclophosphamide (100). The predicted sensitivities to etoposide, docetaxel, and paclitaxel approached those observed for response to these agents in lung cancer patients. They also highlighted that, in lung cancer, docetaxel-sensitive patients seem to be resistant to etoposide. Such signatures could thus provide a tool to better select first-line chemotherapy for lung cancer patients (100). By the same genomic approach, the same team identified molecular pathways associated with chemotherapy resistance and open the perspective that we could create a map of molecular pathways for each tumor and thereby determine the best sequence to prescribe chemotherapy and/or targeted therapy in first-, second-, and third-line setting for each patient. These promising data require further development and validation (101,102). In parallel, the Duke University team (103) generated a gene expression model, also based on *in vitro* assays, for a priori prediction of response to

EGFR TKIs. Using their predictor, they were able to capture the majority of lung adenocarcinoma with high levels of EGFR activation or with activating mutations. These results are preliminary and should be compared with the other individual biomarkers like gene copy number or mutation assessment or even their combination.

BRCA1 in Lung Cancer

A growing body of evidence indicates that *BRCA1* (breast cancer susceptibility gene 1) confers sensitivity to apoptosis induced by antimicrotubule drugs (e.g., paclitaxel, vincristine), but induces resistance to DNA-damaging agents (e.g., cisplatin, etoposide) and radiotherapy (104). This differential modulating effect of BRCA1 mRNA expression has also been observed in tumor cells isolated from malignant effusions of NSCLC patients, where BRCA1 mRNA levels correlated negatively with cisplatin sensitivity and positively with docetaxel sensitivity (105). One retrospective study in NSCLC showed that low or intermediate BRCA1 mRNA levels correlated with significantly longer survival following platinum-based chemotherapy (106).

In a phase II trial with 123 advanced NSCLC patients (107), patients received chemotherapy, with or without cisplatin, based on their BRCA1 mRNA levels: low (cisplatin plus gemcitabine), intermediate (cisplatin plus docetaxel), and high (docetaxel alone). In addition, the tumors were analyzed for RAP80 (receptor-associated protein 80) and Abraxas protein, both of which are interacting proteins that form complexes with BRCA1 and could modulate the effect of BRCA1. The study showed high rates of 2-year survival in the group with low BRCA1 and RAP80 expression. However, this field needs to be studied further.

ELM4-ALK Fusion

Chromosome translocation may lead to the generation of novel fusion genes at the ligation points of chromosomes, or may juxtapose growth-promoting genes to aberrant promoter or enhancer fragments, resulting in dysregulated expression of the genes. A fusion-type protein tyrosine kinase, echinoderm microtubule-associated protein like-4 (EML4)–anaplastic lymphoma kinase (ALK), was recently associated with 5% to 13% of lung cancer patients (108–110). The EML4-ALK fusion results from a small inversion within chromosome 2p, which leads to expression of a chimeric tyrosine kinase, in which the N-terminal half of echinoderm microtubule-associated protein-like 4 (EML4) is fused to the intracellular kinase domain of ALK (111) and possesses potent oncogenic activity both in vitro and in vivo (112). This activity can be effectively blocked by small molecule inhibitors that target ALK (112), which supports a role for EML4-ALK as a key driver of lung tumorigenesis.

Epidemiologically, patients with EML4-ALK fusion tend to be younger, never/light smoking men with adenocarcinoma, particularly signet ring subtype (109). Patients with demonstrated EML4-ALK fusion genes were found to have an unprecedented high response rate (OR: 64%, DCR 90%) in a phase II study despite progression on previous chemotherapy (Bang Y, Kwak EL, Shaw AT et al. Clinical activity of the oral ALK inhibitor PF-02341066 in ALK-positive patients with non-small cell lung cancer (NSCLC). *J Clin Oncol* (Meeting Abstracts) 2010; 28: 3–). Clinical phase III studies are currently ongoing in patients with tumors harboring EML4-ALK fusion genes. There are several ALK-fusion partners identified and the clinical role of other fusion partners in NSCLC are not known. Furthermore, ALK-amplification and gene copy number gain are frequent and the clinical role of these findings are also unknown (Salido M, Pijuan L, Martínez-Avilés L, Galván AB, Rovira A, Zanui M, Cañadas I, Martínez A, Longarón R, Sole F, Serrano S, Bellosillo B, Wynes MW, Albanell J, Hirsch FR, Arriola E. Increased ALK Gene Copy Number and Amplification are Frequent in Non-Small Cell Lung Cancer. *J Thorac Oncol.* 2010. Accepted, In Press). While FISH is the assay method used in the current crizotinib studies, the most optimal assay method for screening for ALK-fusion genes are not yet determined, but immunohistochemistry may be a possibility (Salido M, Pijuan L, Martínez-Avilés L, Galván AB, Rovira A, Zanui M, Cañadas I, Martínez A, Longarón R, Sole F, Serrano S, Bellosillo B, Wynes MW, Albanell J, Hirsch FR, Arriola E. Increased ALK Gene Copy Number and Amplification are Frequent in Non-Small Cell Lung Cancer. *J Thorac Oncol.* 2010. Accepted, In Press).

■ THE FUTURE

Personalized medicine has finally come to NSCLC. We are currently focusing on a few already "established" biomarkers but in the future multiple biomarkers will most likely be needed in order to determine the best choice of therapy. Encouraging steps towards personalized medicine was recently demonstrated by the BATTLE study (Kim ES, Herbst RS, Lee JJ et al. The BATTLE trial (Biomarker-integrated Approaches of Targeted Therapy for Lung Cancer Elimination): personalizing therapy for lung cancer. AACR Annual Meeting (Meeting Abstracts) 2010; LB-1), in which pathway biomarkers were applied to determine therapy. An important requirement for personalized medicine will be robust validation of the biomarkers assays and very carefully designed prospective clinical trials. To summarize, the main predictive biomarkers are as follows:

- A high ERCC1 level predicts a lower benefit from platinum-based therapy.
- A high RRM1 level predicts a lower benefit from gemcitabine therapy.

- A high TS level might suggest a lower benefit from pemetrexed therapy.
- EGFR mutations predict a better outcome to EGFR TKIs.
- A high EGFR gene copy number might predict a better outcome to EGFR TKIs, but prospective validation is awaited.
- KRAS mutations do not seem to predict poor outcome for EGFT TKIs therapy in NSCLC.
- EML4-ALK fusion translocations indicate good response to ALK fusion specific targeted therapies.

Further studies should be conducted in order to be able to use these biomarkers in the routine clinical algorithms.

■ REFERENCES

1. Goldstraw P, Crowley J, Chansky K, et al.; International Association for the Study of Lung Cancer International Staging Committee; Participating Institutions. The IASLC Lung Cancer Staging Project: proposals for the revision of the TNM stage groupings in the forthcoming (seventh) edition of the TNM Classification of malignant tumours. *J Thorac Oncol.* 2007;2(8):706–714.
2. Potti A, Mukherjee S, Petersen R, et al. A genomic strategy to refine prognosis in early-stage non-small-cell lung cancer. *N Engl J Med.* 2006;355(6):570–580.
3. Tsao MS, Zhu C, Ding K, et al. Shepherd A 15-gene expression signature prognostic for survival and predictive for adjuvant chemotherapy benefit in JBR-10 patietns [abstract 7510]. *J Clin Oncol.* 2008;26(15S).
4. Shedden K, Taylor JM, Enkemann SA, et al.; Director's Challenge Consortium for the Molecular Classification of Lung Adenocarcinoma. Gene expression-based survival prediction in lung adenocarcinoma: a multi-site, blinded validation study. *Nat Med.* 2008;14(8):822–827.
5. Lau SK, Boutros PC, Pintilie M, et al. Three-gene prognostic classifier for early-stage non small-cell lung cancer. *J Clin Oncol.* 2007;25(35):5562–5569.
6. Meert AP, Martin B, Delmotte P, et al. The role of EGF-R expression on patient survival in lung cancer: a systematic review with meta-analysis. *Eur Respir J.* 2002;20(4):975–981.
7. Sasaki H, Shimizu S, Okuda K, et al. Epidermal growth factor receptor gene amplification in surgical resected Japanese lung cancer. *Lung Cancer.* 2009;64(3):295–300.
8. Hirsch FR, Varella-Garcia M, Bunn PA Jr, et al. Epidermal growth factor receptor in non-small-cell lung carcinomas: correlation between gene copy number and protein expression and impact on prognosis. *J Clin Oncol.* 2003;21(20):3798–3807.
9. Sequist LV, Bell DW, Lynch TJ, Haber DA. Molecular predictors of response to epidermal growth factor receptor antagonists in non-small-cell lung cancer. *J Clin Oncol.* 2007;25(5):587–595.
10. Riely GJ, Pao W, Pham D, et al. Clinical course of patients with non-small cell lung cancer and epidermal growth factor receptor exon 19 and exon 21 mutations treated with gefitinib or erlotinib. *Clin Cancer Res.* 2006;12(3 Pt 1):839–844.
11. Jackman DM, Yeap BY, Sequist LV, et al. Exon 19 deletion mutations of epidermal growth factor receptor are associated with prolonged survival in non-small cell lung cancer patients treated with gefitinib or erlotinib. *Clin Cancer Res.* 2006;12(13):3908–3914.
12. Mitsudomi T, Kosaka T, Endoh H, et al. Mutations of the epidermal growth factor receptor gene predict prolonged survival after gefitinib treatment in patients with non-small-cell lung cancer with postoperative recurrence. *J Clin Oncol.* 2005;23(11):2513–2520.
13. Marks JL, Broderick S, Zhou Q, et al. Prognostic and therapeutic implications of EGFR and KRAS mutations in resected lung adenocarcinoma. *J Thorac Oncol.* 2008;3(2):111–116.
14. Sasaki H, Endo K, Mizuno K, et al. EGFR mutation status and prognosis for gefitinib treatment in Japanese lung cancer. *Lung Cancer.* 2006;51(1):135–136.
15. Eberhard DA, Johnson BE, Amler LC, et al. Mutations in the epidermal growth factor receptor and in KRAS are predictive and prognostic indicators in patients with non-small-cell lung cancer treated with chemotherapy alone and in combination with erlotinib. *J Clin Oncol.* 2005;23(25):5900–5909.
16. Kosaka T, Yatabe Y, Onozato R, Kuwano H, Mitsudomi T. Prognostic implication of EGFR, KRAS, and TP53 gene mutations in a large cohort of Japanese patients with surgically treated lung adenocarcinoma. *J Thorac Oncol.* 2009;4(1):22–29.
17. Chen HY, Yu SL, Chen CH, et al. A five-gene signature and clinical outcome in non-small-cell lung cancer. *N Engl J Med.* 2007;356(1):11–20.
18. Yanagisawa K, Tomida S, Shimada Y, Yatabe Y, Mitsudomi T, Takahashi T. A 25-signal proteomic signature and outcome for patients with resected non-small-cell lung cancer. *J Natl Cancer Inst.* 2007;99(11):858–867.
19. Schiller JH, Harrington D, Belani CP, et al.; Eastern Cooperative Oncology Group. Comparison of four chemotherapy regimens for advanced non-small-cell lung cancer. *N Engl J Med.* 2002;346(2):92–98.
20. Altaha R, Liang X, Yu JJ, Reed E. Excision repair cross complementing-group 1: gene expression and platinum resistance. *Int J Mol Med.* 2004;14(6):959–970.
21. Lord RV, Brabender J, Gandara D, et al. Low ERCC1 expression correlates with prolonged survival after cisplatin plus gemcitabine chemotherapy in non-small cell lung cancer. *Clin Cancer Res.* 2002;8(7):2286–2291.
22. Cobo M, Isla D, Massuti B, et al. Customizing cisplatin based on quantitative excision repair cross-complementing 1 mRNA expression: a phase III trial in non-small-cell lung cancer. *J Clin Oncol.* 2007;25(19):2747–2754.
23. Ceppi P, Volante M, Novello S, et al. ERCC1 and RRM1 gene expressions but not EGFR are predictive of shorter survival in advanced non-small-cell lung cancer treated with cisplatin and gemcitabine. *Ann Oncol.* 2006;17(12):1818–1825.
24. Olaussen KA, Dunant A, Fouret P, et al.; IALT Bio Investigators. DNA repair by ERCC1 in non-small-cell lung cancer and cisplatin-based adjuvant chemotherapy. *N Engl J Med.* 2006;355(10):983–991.
25. Kamal NS, Soria JC, Mendiboure J, et al.; International Adjuvant Lung Trial-Bio investigators. MutS homologue 2 and the long-term benefit of adjuvant chemotherapy in lung cancer. *Clin Cancer Res.* 2010;16(4):1206–1215.
26. Bepler G, Kusmartseva I, Sharma S, et al. RRM1 modulated *in vitro* and *in vivo* efficacy of gemcitabine and platinum in non-small-cell lung cancer. *J Clin Oncol.* 2006;24(29):4731–4737.
27. Bepler G, Sharma S, Cantor A, et al. RRM1 and PTEN as prognostic parameters for overall and disease-free survival in patients with non-small-cell lung cancer. *J Clin Oncol.* 2004;22(10):1878–1885.
28. Rosell R, Scagliotti G, Danenberg KD, et al. Transcripts in pretreatment biopsies from a three-arm randomized trial in metastatic non-small-cell lung cancer. *Oncogene.* 2003;22(23):3548–3553.
29. Zheng Z, Chen T, Li X, Haura E, Sharma A, Bepler G. DNA synthesis and repair genes RRM1 and ERCC1 in lung cancer. *N Engl J Med.* 2007;356(8):800–808.
30. Scagliotti GV, Parikh P, von Pawel J, et al. Phase III study comparing cisplatin plus gemcitabine with cisplatin plus pemetrexed in chemotherapy-naive patients with advanced-stage non-small-cell lung cancer. *J Clin Oncol.* 2008;26(21):3543–3551.

31. Hanauske AR, Eismann U, Oberschmidt O, et al. *In vitro* chemosensitivity of freshly explanted tumor cells to pemetrexed is correlated with target gene expression. *Invest New Drugs.* 2007;25(5):417–423.

32. Sigmond J, Backus HH, Wouters D, Temmink OH, Jansen G, Peters GJ. Induction of resistance to the multitargeted antifolate Pemetrexed (ALIMTA) in WiDr human colon cancer cells is associated with thymidylate synthase overexpression. *Biochem Pharmacol.* 2003;66(3):431–438.

33. Giovannetti E, Mey V, Nannizzi S, et al. Cellular and pharmacogenetics foundation of synergistic interaction of pemetrexed and gemcitabine in human non-small-cell lung cancer cells. *Mol Pharmacol.* 2005;68(1):110–118.

34. Ceppi P, Volante M, Saviozzi S, et al. Squamous cell carcinoma of the lung compared with other histotypes shows higher messenger RNA and protein levels for thymidylate synthase. *Cancer.* 2006;107(7):1589–1596.

35. Peterson P, Park K, Fossella F, et al. Is pemetrexed more effective in adenocarcinoma and large cell lung cancer than in squamous cell carcinoma? A retrospective analysis of a phase III trial of pemetrexed vs docetaxel in previously treated patients with advanced non-small cell lung cancer (NSCLC) [abstract]. *J Thorac Oncol.* 2008;2(suppl 4):S851.

36. Ciuleanu T, Brodowicz T, Zielinski C, et al. Maintenance pemetrexed plus best supportive care versus placebo plus best supportive care for non-small-cell lung cancer: a randomised, double-blind, phase 3 study. *Lancet.* 2009;374(9699):1432–1440.

37. Gomez HL, Santillana SL, Vallejos CS, et al. A phase II trial of pemetrexed in advanced breast cancer: clinical response and association with molecular target expression. *Clin Cancer Res.* 2006;12(3 Pt 1):832–838.

38. Shirota Y, Stoehlmacher J, Brabender J, et al. ERCC1 and thymidylate synthase mRNA levels predict survival for colorectal cancer patients receiving combination oxaliplatin and fluorouracil chemotherapy. *J Clin Oncol.* 2001;19(23):4298–4304.

39. Shepherd FA, Rodrigues Pereira J, Ciuleanu T, et al.; National Cancer Institute of Canada Clinical Trials Group. Erlotinib in previously treated non-small-cell lung cancer. *N Engl J Med.* 2005;353(2):123–132.

40. Mok TS, Wu YL, Thongprasert S, et al. Gefitinib or carboplatin-paclitaxel in pulmonary adenocarcinoma. *N Engl J Med.* 2009;361(10):947–957.

41. Fukuoka M, Yano S, Giaccone G, et al. Multi-institutional randomized phase II trial of gefitinib for previously treated patients with advanced non-small-cell lung cancer (The IDEAL 1 Trial) [corrected]. *J Clin Oncol.* 2003;21(12):2237–2246.

42. Kris MG, Natale RB, Herbst RS, et al. Efficacy of gefitinib, an inhibitor of the epidermal growth factor receptor tyrosine kinase, in symptomatic patients with non-small cell lung cancer: a randomized trial. *JAMA.* 2003;290(16):2149–2158.

43. Perez-Soler R. Phase II clinical trial data with the epidermal growth factor receptor tyrosine kinase inhibitor erlotinib (OSI-774) in non-small-cell lung cancer. *Clin Lung Cancer.* 2004;6(suppl 1):S20–S23.

44. Bezjak A, Tu D, Seymour L, et al.; National Cancer Institute of Canada Clinical Trials Group Study BR.21. Symptom improvement in lung cancer patients treated with erlotinib: quality of life analysis of the National Cancer Institute of Canada Clinical Trials Group Study BR.21. *J Clin Oncol.* 2006;24(24):3831–3837.

45. Hirsch FR, Herbst RS, Olsen C, et al. Increased EGFR gene copy number detected by fluorescent in situ hybridization predicts outcome in non-small-cell lung cancer patients treated with cetuximab and chemotherapy. *J Clin Oncol.* 2008;26(20):3351–3357.

46. Yukito I, Yutaka N, Yuichiro O, et al. Analyses of Japanese patients recruited in IPASS, a phase III, randomized, open-label, first-line study of gefitinib vs carboplatin/paclitaxel in selected pts with advanced non-small-cell lung cancer. IASLC Meeting abstracts [abstract PD3.1.3]. 13th World Conference on Lung Cancer. *J Thorac Oncol.* 2009(suppl).

47. Hirsch FR, Camidge DR, Kabbinavar F, et al. Biomarker status correlates with clinical benefit: phase 2 study of single-agent erlotinib (E) or E intercalated with carboplatin and paclitaxel (ECP) in an EGFR biomarkerselected NSCLC population. *J Thorac Oncol.* 2008;3(11):S267.

48. Sharma SV, Bell DW, Settleman J, Haber DA. Epidermal growth factor receptor mutations in lung cancer. *Nat Rev Cancer.* 2007;7(3):169–181.

49. Rosell R, Moran T, Queralt C, et al.; Spanish Lung Cancer Group. Screening for epidermal growth factor receptor mutations in lung cancer. *N Engl J Med.* 2009;361(10):958–967.

50. Hirsch FR, Varella-Garcia M, Cappuzzo F, et al. Combination of EGFR gene copy number and protein expression predicts outcome for advanced non-small-cell lung cancer patients treated with gefitinib. *Ann Oncol.* 2007;18(4):752–760.

51. Zhu JQ, Zhong WZ, Zhang GC, et al. Better survival with EGFR exon 19 than exon 21 mutations in gefitinib-treated non-small cell lung cancer patients is due to differential inhibition of downstream signals. *Cancer Lett.* 2008;265(2):307–317.

52. Sordella R, Bell DW, Haber DA, Settleman J. Gefitinib-sensitizing EGFR mutations in lung cancer activate anti-apoptotic pathways. *Science.* 2004;305(5687):1163–1167.

53. Lynch TJ, Bell DW, Sordella R, et al. Activating mutations in the epidermal growth factor receptor underlying responsiveness of non-small-cell lung cancer to gefitinib. *N Engl J Med.* 2004;350(21):2129–2139.

54. Paez JG, Jänne PA, Lee JC, et al. EGFR mutations in lung cancer: correlation with clinical response to gefitinib therapy. *Science.* 2004;304(5676):1497–1500.

55. Pao W, Miller VA, Politi KA, et al. Acquired resistance of lung adenocarcinomas to gefitinib or erlotinib is associated with a second mutation in the EGFR kinase domain. *PLoS Med.* 2005;2(3):e73.

56. Bean J, Brennan C, Shih JY, et al. MET amplification occurs with or without T790M mutations in EGFR mutant lung tumors with acquired resistance to gefitinib or erlotinib. *Proc Natl Acad Sci USA.* 2007;104(52):20932–20937.

57. Engelman JA, Zejnullahu K, Mitsudomi T, et al. MET amplification leads to gefitinib resistance in lung cancer by activating ERBB3 signaling. *Science.* 2007;316(5827):1039–1043.

58. Cappuzzo F, Jänne PA, Skokan M, et al. MET increased gene number and primary resistance to gefitinib therapy in non-small-cell lung cancer patients. *Ann Oncol.* 2009;20(2):298–304.

59. Sugio K, Uramoto H, Onitsuka T, et al. Prospective phase II study of gefitinib in non-small cell lung cancer with epidermal growth factor receptor gene mutations. *Lung Cancer.* 2009;64(3): 314–318.

60. Cappuzzo F, Ligorio C, Ligorio C, et al. EGFR and HER2 gene copy number and response to first-line chemotherapy in patients with advanced non-small cell lung cancer (NSCLC). *J Thorac Oncol.* 2007;2(5):423–429.

61. Okamoto I, Kashii T., Urata Y, et al. EGFR mutation-based phase II multicenter trial of gefitinib in advanced non-small cell lung cancer (NSCLC) patients (pts): results of West Japan Thoracic Oncology Group trial (WJTOG0403). *Proc Am Soc Clin Oncol.* 2006;24(suppl):382s.

62. West H, Chansky K, Franklin WA, et al. Long-term survival with gefitinib (ZD 1839) therapy for advanced bronchioloalveolar lung cancer (BAC): Southwest Oncology Group (SWOG) study S0126 [abstract]. *J Clin Oncol.* 2008;26(suppl):8047.

63. Paz-Ares L, Sanchez JM, Garcia-Velasco A, et al. A prospective phase II study of erlotinib in advanced non-small cell lung cancer (NSCLC) patients (p) with mutations in the tyrosine kinase (TK) domain of the epidermal growth factor receptor (EGFR) [abstract]. *Proc Am Soc Clin Oncol.* 2006;24(suppl):7020.

64. Mok TST, Kai Fai T, Vichien S, et al. Clinical outcomes of patients with epidermal growth factor receptor (EGFR) mutations (Mut) in

IPASS (IRESSATM Pan ASia Study) [abstract B9.5]. 13th World Conference on Lung Cancer. *J Thorac Oncol.* 2009(suppl).

65. Camidge DR, Kabbinavar F, Martins R, et al. EGFR biomarker-selected randomized phase II study of erlotinib (E) or intercalated E with carboplatin/paclitaxel (C/P) in chemo-naive advanced NSCLC. *J Thorac Oncol.* 2008;3:S268.

66. Cappuzzo F, Ciuleanu T, Stelmakh L et al. Erlotinib as maintenance treatment in advanced non-small-cell lung cancer: a multicentre, randomised, placebo-controlled phase 3 study. *Lancet Oncol.* 2010; 11: 521–529.

67. Yu J, Kane S, Wu J, et al. Mutation-specific antibodies for the detection of EGFR mutations in non-small-cell lung cancer. *Clin Cancer Res.* 2009;15(9):3023–3028.

68. Cappuzzo F, Hirsch FR, Rossi E, et al. Epidermal growth factor receptor gene and protein and gefitinib sensitivity in non-small-cell lung cancer. *J Natl Cancer Inst.* 2005;97(9):643–655.

69. Hirsch FR, Varella-Garcia M, McCoy J, et al.; Southwest Oncology Group. Increased epidermal growth factor receptor gene copy number detected by fluorescence in situ hybridization associates with increased sensitivity to gefitinib in patients with bronchioloalveolar carcinoma subtypes: a Southwest Oncology Group Study. *J Clin Oncol.* 2005;23(28):6838–6845.

70. Goss G, Ferry D, Wierzbicki R, et al. Randomized phase II study of gefitinib compared with placebo in chemotherapy-naive patients with advanced non-small-cell lung cancer and poor performance status. *J Clin Oncol.* 2009;27(13):2253–2260.

71. Tsao MS, Sakurada A, Cutz JC, et al. Erlotinib in lung cancer - molecular and clinical predictors of outcome. *N Engl J Med.* 2005;353(2):133–144.

72. Zhu CQ, da Cunha Santos G, Ding K, et al.; National Cancer Institute of Canada Clinical Trials Group Study BR.21. Role of KRAS and EGFR as biomarkers of response to erlotinib in National Cancer Institute of Canada Clinical Trials Group Study BR.21. *J Clin Oncol.* 2008;26(26):4268–4275.

73. Hirsch FR, Varella-Garcia M, Bunn PA Jr, et al. Molecular predictors of outcome with gefitinib in a phase III placebo-controlled study in advanced non-small-cell lung cancer. *J Clin Oncol.* 2006;24(31):5034–5042.

74. Kim ES, Hirsh V, Mok T, et al. Gefitinib versus docetaxel in previously treated non-small-cell lung cancer (INTEREST): a randomised phase III trial. *Lancet.* 2008;372(9652):1809–1818.

75. Hirsch FR, Varella-Garcia M, Dziadziuszko R, et al. Fluorescence in situ hybridization subgroup analysis of TRIBUTE, a phase III trial of erlotinib plus carboplatin and paclitaxel in non-small cell lung cancer. *Clin Cancer Res.* 2008;14(19):6317–6323.

76. Cappuzzo F, Ciuleanu T, Stelmakh L, et al.; on behalf of the SATURN Investigators. SATURN: a double-blind, randomized, phase III study of maintenance erlotinib versus placebo following nonprogression with first-line platinum-based chemotherapy in patients with advanced NSCLC [abstract 8001]. *ASCO.* 2009.

77. Tsuchihashi Z, Khambata-Ford S, Hanna N, Jänne PA. Responsiveness to cetuximab without mutations in EGFR. *N Engl J Med.* 2005;353(2):208–209.

78. Khambata-Ford S, Harbison CT, Hart LL, et al. Analysis of potential predictive markers of cetuximab benefit in BMS099, a phase III study of cetuximab and first-line taxane/carboplatin in advanced non-small-cell lung cancer. *J Clin Oncol.* 2010;28(6):918–927.

79. Pirker R, Pereira JR, Szczesna A, et al.; FLEX Study Team. Cetuximab plus chemotherapy in patients with advanced non-small-cell lung cancer (FLEX): an open-label randomised phase III trial. *Lancet.* 2009;373(9674):1525–1531.

80. Lynch TJ, Patel T, Dreisbach L, et al. Cetuximab and first-line taxane/carboplatin chemotherapy in advanced non-small-cell lung cancer: results of the randomized multicenter phase III trial BMS099. *J Clin Oncol.* 2010;28(6):911–917.

81. Cunningham D, Humblet Y, Siena S, et al. Cetuximab monotherapy and cetuximab plus irinotecan in irinotecan-refractory metastatic colorectal cancer. *N Engl J Med.* 2004;351(4):337–345.

82. Miller VA, Riely GJ, Zakowski MF, et al. Molecular characteristics of bronchioloalveolar carcinoma and adenocarcinoma, bronchioloalveolar carcinoma subtype, predict response to erlotinib. *J Clin Oncol.* 2008;26(9):1472–1478.

83. Huncharek M, Muscat J, Geschwind JF. K-ras oncogene mutation as a prognostic marker in non-small cell lung cancer: a combined analysis of 881 cases. *Carcinogenesis.* 1999;20(8):1507–1510.

84. Shigematsu H, Gazdar AF. Somatic mutations of epidermal growth factor receptor signaling pathway in lung cancers. *Int J Cancer.* 2006;118(2):257–262.

85. Massarelli E, Varella-Garcia M, Tang X, et al. KRAS mutation is an important predictor of resistance to therapy with epidermal growth factor receptor tyrosine kinase inhibitors in non-small-cell lung cancer. *Clin Cancer Res.* 2007;13(10):2890–2896.

86. O'Byrne KJ, Bondarenko I, Barrios C, et al. Molecular and clinical predictors of outcome for cetuximab in non-small cell lung cancer (NSCLC): data from the FLEX study. *J Clin Oncol.* 2009;18S:8007.

87. Taguchi F, Solomon B, Gregorc V, et al. Mass spectrometry to classify non-small-cell lung cancer patients for clinical outcome after treatment with epidermal growth factor receptor tyrosine kinase inhibitors: a multicohort cross-institutional study. *J Natl Cancer Inst.* 2007;99(11):838–846.

88. Salmon S, Chen H, Chen S, et al. Classification by mass spectrometry can accurately and reliably predict outcome in patients with non-small cell lung cancer treated with erlotinib-containing regimen. *J Thorac Oncol.* 2009;4(6):689–696.

89. Hayashi Y, Kuriyama H, Umezu H, et al. Class III beta-tubulin expression in tumor cells is correlated with resistance to docetaxel in patients with completely resected non-small-cell lung cancer. *Intern Med.* 2009;48(4):203–208.

90. Sève P, Mackey J, Isaac S, et al. Class III beta-tubulin expression in tumor cells predicts response and outcome in patients with non-small cell lung cancer receiving paclitaxel. *Mol Cancer Ther.* 2005;4(12):2001–2007.

91. Burkhart CA, Kavallaris M, Band Horwitz S. The role of beta-tubulin isotypes in resistance to antimitotic drugs. *Biochim Biophys Acta.* 2001;1471(2):O1–O9.

92. Ranganathan S, Benetatos CA, Colarusso PJ, Dexter DW, Hudes GR. Altered beta-tubulin isotype expression in paclitaxel-resistant human prostate carcinoma cells. *Br J Cancer.* 1998;77(4):562–566.

93. Sève P, Isaac S, Trédan O, et al. Expression of class III {beta}-tubulin is predictive of patient outcome in patients with non-small cell lung cancer receiving vinorelbine-based chemotherapy. *Clin Cancer Res.* 2005;11(15):5481–5486.

94. Sève P, Lai R, Ding K, et al. Class III beta-tubulin expression and benefit from adjuvant cisplatin/vinorelbine chemotherapy in operable non-small cell lung cancer: analysis of NCIC JBR.10. *Clin Cancer Res.* 2007;13(3):994–999.

95. Gualberto A, Pollak M. Emerging role of insulin-like growth factor receptor inhibitors in oncology: early clinical trial results and future directions. *Oncogene.* 2009;28(34):3009–3021.

96. Karp DD, Paz-Ares LG, Novello S, et al. Phase II study of the anti-insulin-like growth factor type 1 receptor antibody CP-751,871 in combination with paclitaxel and carboplatin in previously untreated, locally advanced, or metastatic non-small-cell lung cancer. *J Clin Oncol.* 2009;27(15):2516–2522.

97. Sandler A, Gray R, Perry MC, et al. Paclitaxel-carboplatin alone or with bevacizumab for non-small-cell lung cancer. *N Engl J Med.* 2006;355(24):2542–2550.

98. Di Costanzo F, Mazzoni F, Micol Mela M, et al. Bevacizumab in non-small cell lung cancer. *Drugs.* 2008;68(6):737–746.

99. Dowlati A, Gray R, Sandler AB, Schiller JH, Johnson DH. Cell adhesion molecules, vascular endothelial growth factor, and basic fibroblast growth factor in patients with non-small cell lung cancer treated with chemotherapy with or without bevacizumab–an Eastern Cooperative Oncology Group Study. *Clin Cancer Res.* 2008;14(5):1407–1412.

100. Potti A, Dressman HK, Bild A, et al. Genomic signatures to guide the use of chemotherapeutics. *Nat Med.* 2006;12(11): 1294–1300.

101. Chang JT, Carvalho C, Mori S, et al. A genomic strategy to elucidate modules of oncogenic pathway signaling networks. *Mol Cell.* 2009;34(1):104–114.

102. Riedel RF, Porrello A, Pontzer E, et al. A genomic approach to identify molecular pathways associated with chemotherapy resistance. *Mol Cancer Ther.* 2008;7(10):3141–3149.

103. Balko JM, Potti A, Saunders C, Stromberg A, Haura EB, Black EP. Gene expression patterns that predict sensitivity to epidermal growth factor receptor tyrosine kinase inhibitors in lung cancer cell lines and human lung tumors. *BMC Genomics.* 2006;7:289.

104. Lafarge S, Sylvain V, Ferrara M, Bignon YJ. Inhibition of BRCA1 leads to increased chemoresistance to microtubule-interfering agents, an effect that involves the JNK pathway. *Oncogene.* 2001;20(45):6597–6606.

105. Wang L, Wei J, Qian X, et al. ERCC1 and BRCA1 mRNA expression levels in metastatic malignant effusions is associated with chemosensitivity to cisplatin and/or docetaxel. *BMC Cancer.* 2008;8:97.

106. Taron M, Rosell R, Felip E, et al. BRCA1 mRNA expression levels as an indicator of chemoresistance in lung cancer. *Hum Mol Genet.* 2004;13(20):2443–2449.

107. Rosell R, Perez-Roca L, Sanchez JJ, et al. Customized treatment in non-small-cell lung cancer based on EGFR mutations and BRCA1 mRNA expression. *PLoS ONE.* 2009;4(5):e5133.

108. Mano H. Non-solid oncogenes in solid tumors: EML4-ALK fusion genes in lung cancer. *Cancer Sci.* 2008;99(12):2349–2355.

109. Shaw AT, Yeap BY, Mino-Kenudson M, et al. Clinical features and outcome of patients with non-small-cell lung cancer who harbor EML4-ALK. *J Clin Oncol.* 2009;27(26):4247–4253.

110. Wong DW, Leung EL, So KK, et al.; University of Hong Kong Lung Cancer Study Group. The EML4-ALK fusion gene is involved in various histologic types of lung cancers from nonsmokers with wild-type EGFR and KRAS. *Cancer.* 2009;115(8):1723–1733.

111. Chiarle R, Voena C, Ambrogio C, Piva R, Inghirami G. The anaplastic lymphoma kinase in the pathogenesis of cancer. *Nat Rev Cancer.* 2008;8(1):11–23.

112. Soda M, Takada S, Takeuchi K, et al. A mouse model for EML4-ALK-positive lung cancer. *Proc Natl Acad Sci USA.* 2008;105(50):19893–19897.

22 Lung Cancer in Older Adults

SUMANTA KUMAR PAL

ARTI HURRIA

■ INTRODUCTION

Lung cancer represents the most common cause of cancer death among both men and women in the United States (1). Older adults constitute a substantial proportion of the lung cancer population—it is estimated that 47% of patients are over the age of 70, and 14% of patients are over the age of 80 (2). Although lung cancer is a disease of older adults, patients at the extremes of age or those in poor overall health are under-represented on clinical trials which set the standard of care (3–5). Therefore, there is less evidence-based data regarding the risks and benefits of treatment in this population. This lack of evidence-based data likely contributes to variations in treatment patterns (6) and poorer clinical outcomes (2). This chapter provides an overview of general considerations in the care of older adults with lung cancer, as well as the specific studies of surgery, radiation, and systemic therapy for non–small cell lung cancer (NSCLC) and small cell lung cancer (SCLC).

■ GENERAL CONSIDERATIONS IN TREATING THE OLDER ADULT

There are many unique considerations when treating the older adult with cancer. With increasing age, there is a decrease in physiologic reserve, which affects virtually every organ system. This decrease in reserve can affect an older adult's ability to tolerate cancer therapy. Aging is associated with a decrease in both renal mass and blood flow and a decrease in glomerular filtration rate. After age 40, there is an estimated loss in glomerular filtration rate of 0.75 ml/min/year (7). In addition, both hepatic mass and blood flow decrease with age; however, these changes are not reflected in liver function tests. Neurological changes with aging include a decrease in cerebral blood flow, decrease in brain weight, and slowed reaction time (8,9).

Both vision and hearing decline, with the development of presbyopia (impaired ability to focus on near objects) and presbycusis (sensorineural hearing loss with a loss of high-frequency hearing) (10). Cardiovascular changes with aging include increase in arterial stiffening, increase in systolic blood pressure, and decrease in maximum heart rate (11,12). Pulmonary changes include a decrease in vital capacity, diffusion capacity, and forced expiratory volume in 1 second (13). These and other age-related changes in physiology can affect an older adult's ability to tolerate cancer therapy.

Bone marrow reserve decreases with increasing age, placing older adults at increased risk for myelosuppressive complications (14). Strategies to curtail the risk of infectious complications associated with chemotherapy are of prime importance in older adults. A prospective randomized study of older adults with either solid tumor or non-Hodgkin's lymphoma demonstrated that the receipt of white blood cell growth factor beginning with the first cycle of chemotherapy decreased the risk of fever and neutropenia (15). The APRONTA trial evaluated the utility of antibiotic prophylaxis to decrease the risk of infectious complications associated with chemotherapy (16). In this study, 192 patients with advanced NSCLC age 65 or older were randomized to receive carboplatin and docetaxel every 3 weeks with either placebo or levofloxacin (a fluoroquinolone antibiotic) on days 5 to 11 of each cycle. The rate of grade 3 or 4 infection (the primary endpoint of the study) was reduced with levofloxacin prophylaxis as compared with placebo (27.5% vs. 36.7%).

In the theme of personalized medicine, metrics to appropriately assess and risk stratify older adults may ultimately aid in determining the optimal therapy for individual patients. These metrics, captured in a geriatric assessment, evaluate factors other than chronological age, which predict the risk of morbidity and mortality in older adults, including evaluation of an individual's functional status, comorbid medical conditions, cognitive function, psychological state, social support, and nutritional status (17). Examples of the utility of a geriatric assessment are emerging in the lung cancer literature. For example, in the phase III MILES-01 study of patients with advanced NSCLC, baseline functional status as measured by ability to complete instrumental activities of daily living ($P = 0.04$) and quality of life (QOL) ($P = 0.0003$) were associated with better prognosis (18). In another phase III study, patients with a higher comorbidity score were more likely to discontinue treatment (19). Integrating a geriatric assessment into oncology care may help to identify older individuals at risk for morbidity, mortality, or potential drug interactions. Studies are underway to develop a cancer-specific geriatric assessment and to identify how the elements in this assessment predict risk of cancer treatment toxicity, in order to identify rationale interventions to optimize outcomes for older adults with cancer (20,21).

■ NON–SMALL CELL LUNG CANCER

Surgery for NSCLC

Several studies have identified age as an important predictor of clinical outcome in patients receiving surgery for NSCLC. A prospective study of patients enrolled in the Nova Scotia Cancer Registry included all individuals (N = 130) who were undergoing resection of NSCLC in 1994, with 10 years of subsequent clinical follow-up (22). The mean age of this group at the time of surgery was 67.7 years (SD 8.2 years). In multivariate analysis, age of 70 or older was found to be a predictor of survival (hazard ratio [HR] 1.79, 95% confidence interval [CI] 1.20–2.68); other factors identified as independent predictors of survival included stage III disease at the time of diagnosis, large cell carcinoma, and extent of lymph node sampling. A larger Surveillance, Epidemiology and End Result (SEER) registry review produced corroborating results, though limited to individuals with stage IA disease (23). In a cohort of 10,761 patients, age (more than the median of 67) was again found to be a significant predictor of poorer 5-year survival (52% vs. 65%, $P < 0.0001$), in addition to larger tumor size, male gender, and greater extent of surgical resection. As a result of these compelling data, a number of subsequent studies have sought to discern predictors of poorer outcome among older adults with NSCLC.

A report from the Norway Cancer Registry aimed to determine whether surgical methodology in older adults resulted in disparate outcomes (24). A total of 763 patients aged 70 or older were assessed. Postoperative mortality was 9% and was highest in those patients that had received more extensive procedures, such as bilobectomy and pneumonectomy. The most common cause of postoperative mortality was pneumonia. Survival was improved in patients with lower stage tumors, as anticipated. Women had significantly better 5-year survival as compared with men (62.8% vs. 35.7%).

In addition to surgical technique, the use of neoadjuvant chemotherapy may affect surgical outcomes in older adults. A nested case-control study of 6,450 patients with

NSCLC who underwent surgical resection for NSCLC included 363 patients aged 70 or older (25). Analysis of these patients was paired with a younger cohort of patients (age < 65) matched for stage, pulmonary function, performance status, and type of resection. Ultimately, there was no difference in major morbidity or postoperative mortality between the older adults assessed and the paired younger controls. Receipt of neoadjuvant therapy, however, was associated with a significantly higher rate of major postoperative morbidity (OR 2.8, 95%CI 1.14–7.41).

Several studies have assessed the effect of functional status and comorbidity on surgical outcome for localized NSCLC. In an institutional series of 126 patients aged 70 or older who underwent lung resection for NSCLC, each patient was assessed with the Charlson Comorbidity Index (CCI) prior to surgery (26). Postoperative events were characterized as either major or minor complications. Minor complications were observed in 71 patients (57%), and major complications were observed in 16 patients (13%). A poor CCI score (i.e., grade 3–4) was found to be predictive of major complications (odds ratio [OR] 12.6, 95%CI 1.5–108.6). A second study assessed the longitudinal association of surgery on performance status (27). In a review of the Minneapolis Veterans Affairs Medical Center database, a total of 143 patients received lobectomies for NSCLC, with Karnofsky performance status (KPS) measured in all patients preoperatively. At 1-year follow-up, KPS score had declined in only 8% of patients aged 70 or older, as compared with 24% of patients aged 70 or younger. Thus, surgical intervention in older adults with limited stage NSCLC is not necessarily accompanied by a more pronounced change in global functioning as compared with younger patients.

Surgery for NSCLC in Octogenarians

The largest experience to date describing surgical outcomes in octogenarians with NSCLC is derived from an institutional analysis at the Mayo Clinic extending over 17 years (28). Between 1985 and 2002, 294 patients between age 80 and 94 underwent pulmonary resection for NSCLC. This study cited a high rate of complications in this cohort (48.0%), including atrial fibrillation, retained secretions requiring bronchoscopy, and pneumonia. Furthermore, several predictors of complications were identified, including male gender, previous history of stroke, and previous history of hemoptysis. In spite of the frequent adverse events, the 1- and 5-year survival were 80% and 34%, respectively. In subset analysis, female gender was associated with improved survival (36.2% vs. 32.7% at 5 years; $P = 0.04$). In contrast, dyspnea at the time of initial presentation was noted to be a negative predictor of survival.

Other studies have evaluated the morbidity and mortality of surgery in octogenarians with early NSCLC. As an example, a prospective database of patients aged 75 or older undergoing pulmonary resection for NSCLC was assessed and results stratified into two groups based on age (group 1: 75–79 years, and group 2: >80 years) (29). With data available from 110 and 47 patients in groups 1 and 2, respectively, there were no substantial differences in morbidity or mortality between the two groups. In another study of 40 octogenarians receiving surgery for localized disease (primarily IA and IB disease), survival at 1 year was 92.4% (30). A slightly smaller series of 20 octogenarians with higher baseline stage (only 50% had stage I disease) reported a median OS of 21.1 months.

The utility of varying surgical approaches in octogenarians has been examined. In a review of the Nigata University experience between 1985 and 2001, 49 patients aged 80 or older received surgical resection for stage I NSCLC (31). Of these, 22 were treated with lobectomy and systematic lymphadenectomy. The remaining 27 were treated with lobectomy alone. A trend toward improvement in 5-year survival was seen among patients receiving the lymphadenectomy, although this was not statistically significant (55.5% vs. 44.8%; $P = 0.88$). However, this observation was tempered by a trend toward increasing postoperative pulmonary complications with lymphadenectomy (32% vs. 11%; $P = 0.07$). Thus, the use of lymphadenectomy as an adjunct to lobectomy may lead to modest survival gains, but comes with an increased risk of postoperative complications. The role of video-assisted thoracic surgery (VATS) for stage I disease has also been examined in octogenarians. In a retrospective analysis including 55 consecutive patients aged 80 or older treated with VATS, actuarial survival was 76.4% at 3 years and 65.9% at 5 years. VATS was used for lobectomy in most of these cases (67%), though it was also applied to perform bilobectomy (2%), segmentectomy (13%), and wedge resection (18%). Postoperative complications were observed in a total of 14 patients (25%), with the most frequent complications being bacterial pneumonia, arrythmia, and air leak. Two operative deaths occurred, both secondary to pneumonia. The authors of the study concluded that VATS could be considered in appropriately selected octogenarians after a balanced consideration of the associated risks.

Adjuvant Therapy for NSCLC

Support for adjuvant therapy in early-stage NSCLC is derived from the intergroup JBR.10 trial, randomizing patients with surgically resected stage IB or II NSCLC to either observation or four cycles of cisplatin and vinorelbine chemotherapy (32). Median OS was prolonged with use of chemotherapy as compared to observation (94 months vs. 73 months, HR 0.69; $P = 0.04$). In an age-based subset analysis of this trial, pretreatment characteristics and survival were compared for patients age > 65 (N = 155) or ≤ 65 (N = 327) (33). Chemotherapy was noted

to prolong OS in the older cohort in a manner similar to that in the generalized trial population (HR 0.61; $P = 0.04$) (Figure 22.1), despite receipt of fewer doses of vinorelbine ($P = 0.014$) and cisplatin ($P = 0.006$) in comparison to younger patients. No substantial differences in toxicity or treatment-related death occurred in the two groups.

The Lung Adjuvant Cisplatin Analysis (LACE) pooled results from five major trials of adjuvant cisplatin-based chemotherapy (34). Of the 4,585 patients included in this analysis, 414 patients (95%) were aged 70 or older. Overall, an improvement in OS was observed with the use of adjuvant cisplatin-based chemotherapy (HR 0.89, 95% CI 0.82–0.96; $P = 0.005$). When considering variation in age in relation to treatment effect, no significant interaction ($P = 0.26$) or trend ($P = 0.29$) was observed.

Although data from JBR.10 and the LACE pooled analysis suggest that older adults derive similar benefit from adjuvant therapy. Limitations of these studies include the low representation of older adults, the lack of inclusion of a geriatric assessment in order to provide insight into the functional age of older adults enrolled on these clinical trials, and the limited information about the longitudinal

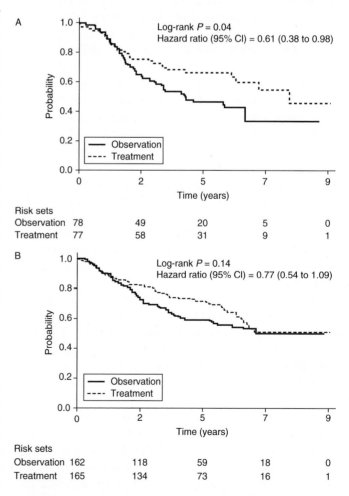

FIGURE 22.1 OS in patients age ≥65 (A) or age <65 (B) enrolled on intergroup trial JBR.10, comparing adjuvant cisplatin and vinorelbine to placebo in fully resected NSCLC.

effect of adjuvant therapy on functional status and QOL. In addition, evolving genetic tests may be able to better identify patients at a higher risk for developing recurrence (35) or patients that are sensitive to platinum-based chemotherapy (36). Though ultimately these strategies may refine the approach to selecting those older adults who derive the greatest benefit from adjuvant therapy (37).

Locally Advanced NSCLC

An ongoing debate in lung cancer therapy centers on the management of stage III NSCLC. At present, various permutations of surgical resection, chemotherapy, and radiation are employed. It appears that in patients with unresectable stage IIIA or IIIB disease, combined modality therapy (chemoradiation) may be superior to radiation alone (38,39). As a result, National Comprehensive Cancer Network (NCCN) guidelines recommend consideration of chemoradiation for unresectable stage III disease (40).

Several studies have assessed subsets of older adults enrolled on large trials of chemoradiation or sequential therapy for NSCLC. In Radiation Therapy Oncology Group trial 94–10, chemoradiation with cisplatin and vinblastine was compared to chemotherapy followed by thoracic radiation (41). Concurrent radiotherapy was administered either once daily or twice daily. Of 610 patients enrolled, 104 patients (17%) were aged 70 or older. Grade 3 or 4 neutropenia was higher in this older cohort with both sequential and concurrent radiotherapy. With concurrent radiotherapy specifically, a higher rate of esophagitis was observed in patients aged 70 or older as compared to those younger than 70. With respect to efficacy, median OS favored concurrent radiotherapy as compared to sequential therapy (22.4 months with once daily concurrent radiotherapy vs. 16.4 months with twice daily concurrent radiotherapy vs. 10.8 months with sequential therapy; $P = 0.069$). In contrast, little difference in median OS was observed among subsets aged 70 or younger (15.5 months vs. 16.0 months vs. 15.7 months for the same comparison).

An analysis of older adults enrolled in Cancer and Leukemia Group B (CALGB) trial 9130 provides further insight into the benefit of chemoradiation (42). CALGB 9130 examined a regimen of cisplatin and vinblastine for stage IIIA or IIIB NSCLC, followed by thoracic radiation with or without concomitant carboplatin. Stratifying patients by age, 98 patients (39%) enrolled in CALGB 9130 were between age 60 and 69, and 54 patients (22%) were between age 70 and 79. Notably, the trial did not enroll any octogenarians, despite the absence of an upper age limit in the eligibility criteria. An assessment of toxicity in the cohort of patients aged 70 to 79 suggested an increased rate of nephrotoxicity during induction chemotherapy with cisplatin and vinblastine (11% in this group vs. 0% in patients aged < 60). Grade 3/4 leucopenia during

induction therapy was also found to be more severe in this age group ($P = 0.04$); however, there was no increase in the rate of febrile neutropenia in older adults. No significant differences in median OS were observed in any age-based cohorts (age 50–59, 12.7 months vs. age 60–69, 15.4 months vs. age 70–79, 13.4 months; $P = 0.84$).

A third subset analysis provides similar data supporting the efficacy of chemoradiation in older adults, albeit with moderately increased toxicity. In North Central Cancer Treatment Group (NCCTG) trial 94–24–52, patients with stage IIIA or IIIB NSCLC were treated with cisplatin and etoposide with concomitant radiotherapy, split into either once daily or twice daily fractions (43). In patients older than 70 years, there were no differences in survival by the radiation fractionation strategy. Furthermore, there were no differences in 2- or 5-year survival between patients in this older cohort and patients younger than age 70 ($P = 0.4$). With respect to adverse effects, there were no differences in grade 3 toxicities among older and younger patients; however, there were substantially more grade 4 to 5 toxicities in patients older than 70 as compared with patients younger than 70 (81% vs. 62%, $P = 0.007$). Specifically, the incidence of grade 4 to 5 leucopenia ($P = 0.0005$), thrombocytopenia ($P = 0.05$), and pneumonitis ($P = 0.02$) were higher in this cohort.

The aforementioned cooperative group efforts indicating a similar benefit from chemoradiation in older and younger cohorts has prompted prospective evaluation of this modality in older adults. In a phase II trial, patients aged 70 or older with locally advanced NSCLC received two cycles of carboplatin and paclitaxel (both administered every 3 weeks), followed by thoracic radiation with concomitant chemotherapy (composed of weekly paclitaxel, followed by weekly carboplatin) (44). With 30 patients enrolled, median progression-free survival (PFS) was 8.7 months (95%CI 3.4–37.8 months) and median OS was 15 months (95%CI 4.2–52.1 months). A total of 12 patients (40%) experienced grade 3 or 4 neutropenia, while 6 patients (20%) experienced grade 3 esophagitis (primarily during concomitant radiotherapy). No treatment-related mortality was observed with this regimen. This prospective experience with chemoradiation in older adults seems to support what has been observed in retrospective analyses—specifically, that the strategy appears to be efficacious, albeit with slightly increased toxicity as compared with younger adults.

Despite the existence of recommendations for chemoradiation, a patient's health status (i.e., comorbidity, functional status, etc.) influences the decision to recommend this modality in older adults. For example, a study at the H. Lee Moffitt Cancer Center of older adults with stage III lung cancer, ECOG performance status demonstrated that the existence of severe medical comorbidity significantly influenced treatment recommendations and survival (45). Ideally, chemoradiation will be evaluated in prospective, randomized trials including older adults, with use of metrics to account for variations in health status.

Chemotherapy for Advanced Disease

Phase III Clinical Trials

Chemotherapy versus Best Supportive Care. The Elderly Lung Cancer Study Group reported a randomized trial comparing vinorelbine to best supportive care (BSC) in patients aged 70 or older with stage IIIB or IV NSCLC (46). QOL represented the primary endpoint of the study, assessed via several lung cancer-specific metrics. Ultimately, the study was closed to accrual due to poor enrollment. QOL assessments from 151 assessable patients suggested that patients treated with vinorelbine (as compared with patients receiving BSC) had decreased pain (*P* = 0.02) and dyspnea (*P* = 0.05). More broadly, patients receiving BSC had worse lung-cancer related symptoms, while patients receiving chemotherapy had worse toxicity-related symptoms. Furthermore, as compared to BSC, treatment with vinorelbine was associated with an improvement in median OS (28 vs. 21 weeks, *P* = 0.03) (Figure 22.2).

Single-Agent Chemotherapy. A phase III effort evaluated the efficacy of single-agent vinorelbine versus single-agent docetaxel in older adults. In the West Japan Thoracic Oncology Group (WJTOG) trial 9904, 182 advanced NSCLC patients aged 70 or older with an Eastern Cooperative Oncology Group (ECOG) performance status (PS) ≤ 2 were randomized to receive four cycles of docetaxel or vinorelbine (47). Though the study failed to meet its primary endpoint of improving OS, docetaxel was associated with an improvement in PFS(5.5 vs. 3.1 months, *P* < 0.001; Figure 22.3) and overall response rate (RR; 22.7% vs. 9.9%, *P* = 0.019) as compared with

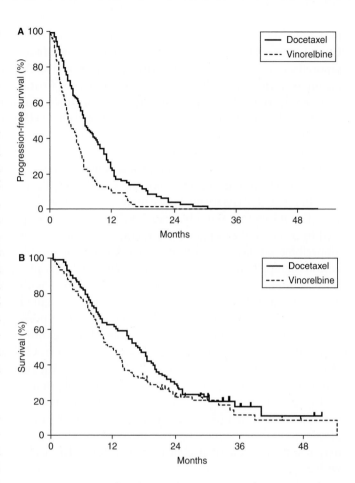

FIGURE 22.3 In the phase III West Japanese Thoracic Oncology Group trial 9904, docetaxel improved PFS as compared to vinorelbine in patients aged 70 or older with advanced NSCLC (A). However, there was no difference in OS (B).

vinorelbine. Grade 3 and 4 neutropenia was more common among patients receiving docetaxel (82.9% vs. 62.9%, *P* = 0.031); however, other toxicities were mild.

Combination versus Single-Agent Chemotherapy. Three phase III trials have focused on comparisons of single- to multiagent chemotherapy. The MILES phase III trial compared vinorelbine alone, gemcitabine alone, or the combination of both (administered for a maximum of 6 cycles) in patients with advanced NSCLC aged 70 or older (48). With 698 patients assessed in an intention-to-treat (ITT) analysis, combination therapy did not improve OS (the primary endpoint) as compared to either vinorelbine alone (HR 1.17, 95%CI 0.95–1.44; *P* = 0.93) or gemcitabine alone (HR 1.06, 95%CI 0.86–1.29; *P* = 0.65). Combination therapy also appeared to be more toxic than single-agent therapy. As compared to vinorelbine alone, combination therapy resulted in greater thrombocytopenia and hepatic toxicity (all grades). Furthermore, as compared with gemcitabine alone, combination therapy resulted in increased cardiac toxicity, neutropenia, extravasation sequelae, vomiting, fatigue, and constipation (all grades). Contrasting results were obtained

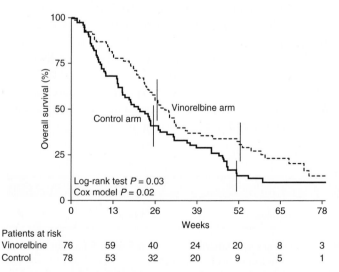

FIGURE 22.2 The Elderly Lung Cancer Study Group reported improved OS with vinorelbine as compared to BSC in chemotherapy-naïve NSCLC patients aged 70 or older.

in a separate (albeit smaller) trial by the Southern Italy Cooperative Oncology Group (SICOG) comparing vinorelbine alone to vinorelbine with gemcitabine (19). At an interim analysis including 120 patients (with a total planned accrual of 240 patients), the risk of death was significantly lower with combination chemotherapy (HR 0.48, 95%CI 0.28–0.79; $P < 0.01$).

The most recent phase III trial to address the use of combination chemotherapy in older adults was conducted by the French Intergroup for Thoracic Oncology (IFCT) (49). In IFCT-0501, patients between the ages of 70 and 89 with ECOG PS 0-2 and advanced NSCLC were randomized to receive either single-agent therapy (gemcitabine or vinorelbine on days 1 and 8 of a 3-week cycle) or combination therapy with carboplatin with paclitaxel (carboplatin was administered every 4 weeks in combination with weekly paclitaxel on days 1, 8, and 15). Accrual was halted after inclusion of 451 of a planned 522 patients given positive interim efficacy data. PFS was prolonged with combination therapy (6.3 vs. 3.2 months, $P < 0.0001$), as was OS (10.4 vs. 6.2 months, $P = 0.0001$). Though no significant difference was observed in early deaths, the rate of grade 3 to 4 hematologic toxicities was greater with combination therapy (54.1% vs. 17.9%). Juxtaposing a commonly used platinum doublet regimen against single agents, these data may result in a new treatment paradigm for older adults with advanced lung cancer.

Randomized Phase II Trials

Several age-specific randomized phase II trials have been designed to address older adults with lung cancer. In one such effort, patients with a poor PS (defined as ECOG PS 2 or 3) aged 70 or greater with chemotherapy-naïve advanced NSCLC were assigned to receive single-agent therapy with gemcitabine, vinorelbine, or docetaxel (50). With 134 evaluable patients, RRs of 16%, 20%, and 22% were observed for gemcitabine, vinorelbine, and docetaxel, respectively (P = NS). All groups experienced improvements in QOL indicators through the course of therapy.

As noted previously, the phase III WJTOG 9904 trial demonstrated improved PFS and overall RR with docetaxel as compared with vinorelbine in patients aged 70 or older

(47). In this trial, docetaxel was dosed at 60 mg/m^2 every 3 weeks. A randomized, multicenter phase II trial directly compared two distinct schedules of docetaxel in patients aged 70 or older—specifically, docetaxel at 75 mg/m^2 every 21 days, and docetaxel at 30 mg/m^2 weekly for 3 out of 4 weeks per cycle (Table 22.1) (51). With 111 patients enrolled, a nonsignificant trend toward improved OS was observed in the weekly docetaxel group (6.7 vs. 3.5 months). Notably, in this study, outcomes for octogenarians were similar to those of patients between the ages of 70 and 79. No differences in QOL were observed between the two arms.

Similar to the previously noted MILES and SICOG trials comparing single- to multiagent chemotherapy, a randomized phase II trial has been reported that compared vinorelbine alone to the combination of vinorelbine with cisplatin (52). In this study, a total of 65 patients aged 70 or older were randomized. Patients were treated with up to six cycles of chemotherapy if a complete response (CR) or partial response (PR) was observed and four cycles if stable disease (SD) was observed with initial therapy. As in the MILES study, no improvement in OS was noted with combination chemotherapy. Furthermore, toxicities such as neutropenia and anemia were significantly higher with cisplatin and vinorelbine. However, median time to progression (TTP) was improved with combination therapy (5.2 vs. 3.1 months, $P = 0.03$), and disease control rates were higher (defined as the sum of CR, PR, and SD; 32.4% vs. 16.1%, $P = 0.009$).

Two distinct multiagent chemotherapy regimens were compared in yet another randomized phase II experience. In this study, patients aged 70 or older with chemotherapy-naïve NSCLC were assigned to receive paclitaxel with either carboplatin or cisplatin (53). A median of four cycles of therapy was delivered to 81 patients enrolled on the trial. No difference in median OS was observed with carboplatin or cisplatin therapy (10.3 vs. 10.5 months, respectively), nor was there a difference observed in PFS (6.6 vs. 6.9 months, respectively). It was noted that the combination of paclitaxel plus carboplatin had less alopecia ($P < 0.001$), peripheral neuropathy ($P = 0.017$) and fatigue ($P < 0.001$) as compared to paclitaxel plus cisplatin; however, there were no differences in hematologic toxicity (including all grades in both comparisons).

■ **Table 22.1**	Randomized phase II trials assessing standard regimens for NSCLC in older adults					
Author/Study Title	**Entry Criteria**	**N**	**Regimen 1**	**Regimen 2**	**OS**	**P**
Lilenbaum et al. (50)	Age ≥ 70	111	Docetaxel, 75 mg/m^2 every 21 days	Docetaxel, 30 mg/m^2, 3 out of 4 weeks per cycle	6.7 vs. 3.5 months	NS
Chen et al. (51)	Age ≥ 70	81	Carboplatin/paclitaxel	Cisplatin/paclitaxel	10.3 vs. 10.5 months	NS

NS, not specified; OS, overall survival.

Nonrandomized Phase II Trials

Several nonrandomized phase II trials in older adults provide important insights into unique patient populations and/or utilize unique and promising therapeutic regimens. As an example of both, Southwest Oncology Group (SWOG) trial 0027 treated a combined group of advanced NSCLC patients either aged 70 or older (stratum 1) or with an ECOG PS of 2 (stratum 2) with sequential vinorelbine followed by docetaxel (54). Median survival was 9.1 months and 5.5 months in strata 1 and 2, respectively. The most common grade 3 or 4 toxicity was neutropenia, seen in 32% and 31% of each stratum, respectively. These results compared favorably to historical benchmarks cited by the authors of this trial. Sequential therapy may thus warrant further evaluation in the setting of a phase III trial.

A separate phase II trial investigated the combination of gemcitabine and vinorelbine in advanced NSCLC patients who either possessed a contraindication to cisplatin therapy or were aged 70 or older (55). A total of 49 patients (38 of age 70 or older and 11 with a contraindication to cisplatin) were ultimately treated with this combined regimen. The overall RR was 26%, with 2 patients (4%) achieving a CR and 11 patients (22%) achieving a PR. Albeit with a relatively small sample size, it was noted that patients experiencing grade 3 or 4 neutropenia were older (median age 75 vs. 72, $P = 0.047$). On this basis, it was recommended that growth factor support be administered to older adults receiving this regimen.

Use of standard NSCLC chemotherapy regimens in older adults has been assessed in the setting of several age-specific phase II trials. The regimens assessed include carboplatin and paclitaxel, cisplatin and docetaxel, and cisplatin and gemcitabine (56–59). Data from these efforts are listed in Table 22.2.

Retrospective Analyses

Given inherent challenges in designing age-specific trials for older adults, much information regarding this subgroup has been derived from retrospective analyses of large phase III efforts including patients of all ages. As an example of this, the Lineberger Comprehensive Cancer Center (LCCC) trial 9719 compared administration of four cycles of carboplatin and paclitaxel chemotherapy to the same therapy administered until the time of disease progression in patients with advanced NSCLC (60). With 239 patients randomized, this trial demonstrated no difference in OS or overall RR between the two therapeutic strategies. A separately reported subset analysis provided data related to 67 patients (29%) enrolled in LCCC 9719 that were aged 70 or older (61). This analysis yielded no statistically significant difference in toxicities associated with carboplatin and paclitaxel chemotherapy in this older cohort as compared with younger patients enrolled on the trial. Furthermore, survival rates were not different between the two subgroups, suggesting the feasibility of carboplatin and paclitaxel in older adults. The most suitable dosing of this regimen in patients older than 70 years can be interpreted from subset analysis of a phase II randomized trial comparing three distinct regimens of carboplatin and paclitaxel (62). In patients older than 70 years, it appeared that weekly paclitaxel (at 100 mg m²) in combination with carboplatin every 4 weeks (area under the curve [AUC] = 6 mg/ml/min) resulted in superior survival and lesser toxicity.

Useful data in an older cohort was also derived from subset analysis of ECOG trial 5592, a comparison of cisplatin in combination with either etoposide or paclitaxel in chemotherapy-naïve patients with advanced NSCLC. The study demonstrated superior survival with paclitaxel treatment as compared with etoposide (9.9 vs. 7.6 months, $P = 0.048$) (63). In a separate analysis of patients aged 70 or older, outcomes for 86 patients (representing 15% of the evaluable population) were assessed (64). Survival distributions were similar in patients older than and younger than 70 years, as were most toxicities attributable to therapy. It was observed, however, that older adults did more frequently experience leucopenia and

■ **Table 22.2** Nonrandomized phase II trials assessing standard regimens for NSCLC in older adults

Author	Entry Criteria	N	Regimen	Overall RR (%)	Median OS (wks)
Choi et al. (55)	Age ≥ 65 or PS 2	35	Carboplatin (AUC = 5) IV q3wks + paclitaxel 135 mg/m² IV q3wks	40	37
Feliu et al. (56)	Age ≥ 70	46	Cisplatin 50 mg/m² IV q3wks + gemcitabine 1,000 mg/m² d1,8 IV q3wks	35	44
Giorgio et al. (57)	Age > 70	40	Carboplatin (AUC = 5) IV q3wks + P paclitaxel 175 mg/m² IV q3wks	25	31
Ohe et al. (58)	Age ≥ 75	33	Cisplatin 25 mg/m² IV d1,8,15 q4wks + docetaxel 20 mg/m² IV d1,8,15 q4wks	52	63

AUC, area under the curve; RR, response rate; OS, overall survival.

neuropsychiatric symptoms from these platinum-based therapies.

With a favorable toxicity profile and comparable (if not superior) efficacy to other platinum-based doublets, the combination of cisplatin with pemetrexed has emerged as an attractive regimen in patients with advanced NSCLC (65). Furthermore, single-agent pemetrexed has demonstrated efficacy similar to that of other approved second-line agents (66). A combined analysis of older patients enrolled in three randomized trials of pemetrexed (for first- and second-line therapy of NSCLC and for treatment of advanced pancreatic cancer) suggested similar median OS and TTP in cohorts older than and younger than 70 years (67). Grade 3 or 4 myelosuppression did occur more frequently in older adults; however, the rate of febrile neutropenia was similar in both groups.

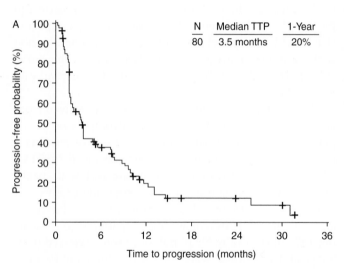

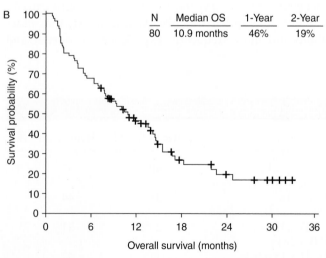

FIGURE 22.4 PFS (A) and OS (B) in a phase II trial of erlotinib in patients aged 70 or older with advanced NSCLC.

Biologic Therapy for Advanced Disease

Small Molecule Inhibitors

The most prevalent class of small molecule inhibitors in clinical use for NSCLC targets the epidermal growth factor receptor (EGFR). This class includes erlotinib and gefitinib, and there is emerging data for each in the setting of older adults. Erlotinib was approved as second-line therapy for NSCLC on the basis of a randomized phase III trial showing an OS benefit with this agent relative to placebo (68). Of the 731 patients enrolled in this trial in total, 57% and 49% of patients treated with erlotinib and placebo, respectively, were aged 60 or older. Response rates and survival benefit with erlotinib were similar in patients older than and younger than 60 years. Data related to erlotinib therapy in an older cohort is derived from a separate phase II effort enrolling patients aged 70 or older with chemotherapy-naïve advanced NSCLC to receive erlotinib therapy (Figure 22.4) (69). In 88 eligible patients, 8 PRs (10%) were observed and 33 patients (41%) had SD for 2 months or greater. In this cohort of older adults, it was found that EGFR mutation strongly correlated with disease control, prolonged TTP, and prolonged OS. Interestingly, these correlative data contrasted with those from the aforementioned phase III experience with erlotinib, where EGFR expression, copy number, and mutation had no correlation with survival on multivariate analysis (70).

In a study conducted by the National Health Research Institute of Taiwan, erlotinib has been compared with cytotoxic chemotherapy (71). In this randomized phase II effort, patients aged 70 or older with advanced NSCLC were treated with either erlotinib or oral vinorelbine until the time of progression. With data available in 77 patients, a greater percentage of objective responses were observed in patients treated with erlotinib (21.6% vs. 12.8%). At the time of preliminary analysis, no difference in median TTP was observed (4.4 months with erlotinib vs. 3.9 months with vinorelbine; *P* = 0.60). Both treatments were well tolerated, with erlotinib resulting in a greater frequency of dermatologic toxicity, and vinorelbine resulting in a greater frequency of gastrointestinal toxicity.

Results to date from phase III studies of gefitinib in unselected populations have failed to show an improvement in OS with the agent either alone or in combination with chemotherapy (72–74). However, there are encouraging signals for activity of gefitinib in older adults. In a multicenter, phase II trial, chemotherapy-naïve patients aged 75 or older with advanced NSCLC were assigned to receive gefitinib monotherapy (75). A total of 49 patients were enrolled; 32 patients (65%) were women and 40 patients (82%) had adenocarcinoma. An objective RR of 25% was observed, with a median OS of 10 months (95%CI 7–20 months). The most common adverse toxicities were dermatologic, and 15 patients (30%) experienced grade ≥ 3 toxicity. PCR analysis of tumor samples from 17 patients demonstrated EGFR mutation in 7 patients. Of these, 5 patients (71%) obtained a PR with gefitinib monotherapy.

Similar outcomes were derived from a study assessing the combination of chemotherapy with gefitinib in older adults. In this phase II study, patients aged 70 or older with chemotherapy-naïve NSCLC were treated with docetaxel and gefitinib in combination for two cycles beyond maximal response (gefitinib alone was subsequently continued until disease progression) (76). A total of 44 patients were enrolled, and 17 patients (40%) achieved a PR with this regimen. A further 21 patients (48%) experienced SD. Median PFS and OS in this trial were 6.9 and 9.6 months, respectively. Interestingly, markedly different outcomes were observed by gender. Median OS in women was 22.8 months, as compared to 4.8 months in men. Female gender was found to be a predictor of survival on multivariate analysis in this study.

More modest response rates were observed in a trial examining older adults (age ≥ 70) with chemotherapy-refractory advanced NSCLC (77). In this study, gefitinib monotherapy in 40 eligible patients resulted in 1 CR (2.5%) and 1 PR (2.5%). Importantly, 18 patients (45%) had SD lasting over 2 months (with 6 patients, 15%, experiencing SD lasting over 6 months) for an overall disease control rate of 50%. Adverse effects associated with gefitinib were generally mild, with grade 1 or 2 dermatologic toxicity occurring in 20 patients (52.6%). Given these results in combination with data for gefitinib in chemotherapy-naïve patients, it appears that the agent may have clinical utility in older adults.

Monoclonal Antibodies

More limited data in older adults is available regarding the two monoclonal antibodies approved for clinical use in NSCLC (namely, cetuximab and bevacizumab). Similar to gefitinib and erlotinib, cetuximab targets EGFR, albeit in the extracellular domain. A phase III trial randomized patients with previously untreated, EGFR-detectable advanced NSCLC to cisplatin and vinorelbine alone or with cetuximab (78). Median OS was prolonged with the addition of cetuximab. A substantial number of older adults were included in the trial, with roughly 31% of the trial population being age 65 or older. A recent update of this dataset indicated that age (older than and younger than 65) did not correlate with prognosis (78).

Bevacizumab is a monoclonal antibody with affinity for vascular endothelial growth factor (VEGF). In preclinical models, bevacizumab exerts an antitumor effect through abrogation of tumor-related angiogenesis (79). In the phase III ECOG trial 4599, patients with advanced NSCLC (nonsquamous histology) were randomized to receive carboplatin and paclitaxel alone or in combination with bevacizumab (80). Median OS was 12.3 months in patients receiving bevacizumab therapy, as compared to 10.3 months with chemotherapy alone ($P = 0.003$). Importantly, this marked the first occasion on which a phase III trial in NSCLC demonstrated a median OS in excess of 1 year. A formal analysis of the subset of older adults enrolled in this trial suggests that there was a trend toward higher RR (29% vs. 17%, $P = 0.067$) and PFS (5.9 vs. 4.9 months, $P = 0.063$) with the addition of bevacizumab therapy (81). However, grade 3 to 5 toxicities appeared to be more common with the addition of bevacizumab (87% vs. 61%, $P < 0.001$), with two treatment-related deaths occurring on the chemotherapy alone arm as compared with 7 on the bevacizumab-containing arm. As compared with younger patients, older adults had a higher rate of grades 3 to 5 neutropenia, bleeding, and proteinuria with bevacizumab therapy. Furthermore, in contrast to the overall study population, it did not appear that the addition of bevacizumab enhanced overall survival (OS) as compared with chemotherapy alone (11.3 vs. 12.1 months, respectively; $P = 0.4$).

The AVAiL trial assessed the combination of cisplatin and gemcitabine, either with placebo or with bevacizumab (administered at two distinct dose levels). With a total of 1,043 patients enrolled, the addition of bevacizumab at either dose level led to a prolongation in median PFS (82). A separate analysis of patients aged 65 or older (N = 304) suggested a similar benefit in PFS with bevacizumab therapy as compared with patients of age 65 or younger (83). Overall, the rates of grade ≥ 3 toxicity were similar among older adults enrolled on all three treatment arms. Though no specific safety concerns emerged from this analysis, separate studies have identified adverse events somewhat unique to bevacizumab. A pooled analysis of studies comparing chemotherapy with bevacizumab to chemotherapy alone in metastatic NSCLC, colorectal cancer, and breast cancer suggested an increased rate of arterial thromboembolism with bevacizumab (HR 2.0, 95%CI 1.05–3.75; $P = 0.031$) (84). Among all patient characteristics evaluated, only prior arterial thrombotic event ($P < 0.001$) and age of 65 or older ($P = 0.01$) were associated with arterial thrombosis with bevacizumab. Therefore, consideration should be given to counseling older adults regarding this potential adverse effect before embarking upon treatment with bevacizumab.

Radiation Therapy Alone for NSCLC

NCCN guidelines recommend potentially curative radiation for early-stage disease (clinical stage I or stage II) if the patient is deemed inoperable by a thoracic surgeon (40). Though this recommendation may only apply to a fraction of patients in an unselected population, single-modality therapy with radiation has more bearing among older adults who frequently possess comorbidities that preclude surgery. Supporting this approach in older adults is a retrospective review of 347 patients receiving 50 Gy of external beam radiotherapy for node-negative, pT1, or T2 NSCLC (85). The median age of the study population was 70 years. Interestingly, a trend toward improved survival was observed in patients aged 70 or older as compared with patients aged 70 or younger (26 vs. 22 months, P = NS). In fact, among cohorts divided into 5-year age groups, patients between the ages of 75 and 79 had superior 5-year survival relative to all other groups (53%).

A separate institutional review including patients with slightly more advanced disease suggested that the benefit of radiotherapy may be contingent upon histology. In a series of 112 patients aged 75 or older with stage IB or II NSCLC, either surgery or radiation was used for definitive therapy (86). Though a trend toward improved survival was seen in the group receiving surgery as compared to radiotherapy (53% vs. 35% at 2 years; P = NS), the outcome of patients with adenocarcinoma histology treated with radiotherapy compared favorably (2-year survival: 58%).

Radiation therapy alone may be considered at later stages for use as palliative therapy. A prospective study has assessed this strategy in older patients (age ≥ 75) with poor KPS score (≤60) with stage IIIA NSCLC who were deemed unfit for combined-modality therapy (87). All of the 40 patients enrolled in this study had one or more medical comorbidities, and 7 patients (18%) had a CCI score > 2. Patients were treated with 60 Gy of radiation therapy encompassing the primary tumor and associated lymph node regions. Median OS in this study was an appreciable 19 months. Furthermore, no treatment related mortality was observed.

■ SMALL CELL LUNG CANCER

Limited Disease

The benefit of adding thoracic radiotherapy to chemotherapy in SCLC-limited disease (LD) has been established through two comprehensive meta-analyses published in 1992, both citing a survival benefit with this strategy (88,89). Several studies have assessed the role of this strategy specifically in older adults. Intergroup Trial 0096 randomized patients with SCLC-LD to once daily or twice daily radiotherapy in conjunction with cisplatin and etoposide (90). At a median follow-up of 8 years, median OS was significantly improved with twice daily radiotherapy (23 vs. 19 months, P = 0.04). In a separately reported subset analysis of patients aged 70 or older enrolled on this trial, there were no differences in response rate or duration of response as compared to younger patients (91). However, survival was improved in patients younger than 70 (5-year survival: 22% vs. 16%; P = 0.05). Furthermore, severe hematologic toxicity and treatment-related mortality occurred more frequently among older adults.

Somewhat contrasting data is provided in a retrospective review of patients treated on two National Cancer Institute of Canada-Clinical Trials Group protocols, BR.3 and BR.6 (92). A combined analysis of these studies evaluated the role of age on efficacy and tolerance of thoracic radiotherapy in SCLC-LD. In both BR.3 and BR.6, chemotherapy with cyclophosphamide, doxorubicin, and vincristine was given sequentially or alternating with cisplatin and etoposide chemotherapy. In BR.3, thoracic radiotherapy was given following chemotherapy with a randomization to one of two dose levels. Alternatively, in BR.6, radiation was administered with cisplatin and etoposide either early or late in the course of treatment. With 608 patients eligible for analysis, 88 were aged 70 or older. No statistical difference in RR or OS was observed in this older age group. Furthermore, among patients who completed radiation therapy, no difference in toxicity was observed.

Outside of prospective clinical trials, there is a suggestion that reluctance to treat older adults with combined modality therapy for SCLC-LD may result in inferior outcomes. A retrospective analysis of the British Columbia Cancer Agency (BCCA) registry included 174 patients with SCLC-LD divided into age-based cohorts (<65, 65–74, and ≥75) (93). Notably, older adults were less likely to be treated with chemotherapy and radiation (P < 0.0001). In addition, use of less aggressive chemotherapy regimens, fewer cycles of chemotherapy and lower dose intensity was more frequent with increasing age (P < 0.05). Alongside these observations, it was noted that older adults did have inferior overall RRs (P = 0.014) and 2-year OS (P = 0.003); however, on multivariate analysis, age or CCI were not related to treatment response or survival. As such, the decrement in response and survival in older adults may be attributed to suboptimal treatment in this group.

The aforementioned BCCA registry analysis also suggested a decrease in the use of prophylactic cranial irradiation (PCI) among older adults (93). Notably, PCI has been shown in two large meta-analyses of improve OS in the setting of SCLC in complete remission and has more recently demonstrated an OS benefit in a prospective analysis including SCLC-extensive disease (ED) (94–96). Though no subset analysis by age is offered in the latter prospective analysis, data from the meta-analysis suggest that the benefit of PCI exists across all strata of age (89).

Extensive Disease

For more than 20 years, the combination of platinum chemotherapy with etoposide has remained a standard therapy for SCLC-ED (97). The regimen has stood the test of time, despite comparison to alternative three-drug regimens or high-dose therapy (98,99). There is available, though conflicting, data to guide use of this therapy in older adults. In one phase II experience, six cycles of carboplatin and etoposide were administered to patients with SCLC-ED aged 70 or older. Of 38 patients enrolled, 18 patients (47%) received the planned six cycles (100). In 30 evaluable patients, 2 CRs and 20 PRs were observed (overall RR, 73%), with a median OS of 237 days. These encouraging data were tempered by the toxicities encountered with therapy, including five episodes of febrile neutropenia with one associated death. Slightly disparate results (poorer efficacy and more severe toxicity) were noted in a separate phase II study of patients with both ED and LD SCLC (101). In 34 patients treated with a nearly identical regimen (with thoracic radiotherapy added to patients with LD SCLC), an overall RR of 59% was achieved. Notably, this response rate was inferior to that observed in the aforementioned trial, despite inclusion of patients with LD SCLC. Furthermore, toxic deaths due to febrile neutropenia were observed in 3 patients (9%).

A randomized phase II trial has examined two strategies to mitigate the excessive rates of febrile neutropenia with platinum/etoposide therapy in older adults: (a) reduction of chemotherapy dose and (b) use of growth factor support (102). In this study, patients aged 70 or older were randomized to receive either cisplatin at 25 mg/m^2 (on days 1 and 2) with etoposide at 60 mg/m^2 (on days 1, 2, and 3) every 3 weeks (Arm 1), or cisplatin at 40 mg/m^2 (on days 1 and 2) with etoposide at 100 mg/m^2 (on days 1, 2, and 3) every 3 weeks in addition to lenogastrim support at 5 mg/kg (days 5–12; Arm 2). Response rates for Arm 1 were substantially lower than those for Arm 2 (39% vs. 69%). Importantly, limited grade 3 or 4 myelotoxicity was observed on either arm (0% on Arm 1; 12% on Arm 2). Thus, attenuated doses of chemotherapy seem to severely compromise RR as compared to offering standard dose chemotherapy with growth factor support in older adults with SCLC-ED, with similar toxicity using either approach. Historically, efforts to curtail the dose intensity or number of drugs administered have failed in the setting of SCLC. As one example, initial phase II studies of single-agent etoposide in older adults produced moderate response rates with reasonable toxicity (103,104). However, two randomized studies thereafter comparing single-agent etoposide to intravenous combination chemotherapy in ECOG PS 2–4 patients demonstrated inferior RR and shorter OS with etoposide alone (105).

Treatment of SCLC-ED with platinum and irinotecan has produced mixed results in the literature. A randomized, phase III study by the Japan Clinical Oncology Group (JCOG) was terminated early when the combination of cisplatin and irinotecan showed superior survival to cisplatin and etoposide for patients with SCLC-ED (12.8 vs. 9.4 months, P = 0.002) (106). However, the study has been criticized for the relatively small sample size (N = 154). Furthermore, conflicting data has emerged from a larger,

U.S.-led trial (107). In this effort, patients with SCLC-ED were randomized in a 2:1 fashion to either cisplatin and irinotecan or cisplatin and etoposide. With a substantially larger sample size (N = 331), there was no difference in median OS between the two groups, respectively (9.3 vs. 10.2 months, P = 0.74).

The regimen of cisplatin and irinotecan has specifically been assessed in older adults with SCLC-ED. In a phase II study, previously untreated patients aged 65 or older received a maximum of six cycles of cisplatin and irinotecan chemotherapy (108). A total of 46 patients were enrolled, with an overall response rate of 76.1%. Nine patients (19.6%) obtained a CR, while 26 patients (56.5%) obtained a PR with this regimen. The most frequent grade 3 or 4 toxicities were neutropenia (58.7%), leucopenia (49.9%), and diarrhea (30.4%). Thus, in an older cohort, the regimen of cisplatin and irinotecan produces impressive response rates, albeit with considerable associated morbidity.

■ PALLIATIVE CARE

Despite recent advances in the treatment of advanced lung cancer, prognosis with this disease remains somewhat limited and end-of-life care is inevitable in most cases. An assessment of SEER-Medicare data between 1992 and 2002 identified a total of 45,627 patients aged 65 or older with stage IIIB or IV NSCLC who died within 1 year of their cancer diagnosis (109). During the study period, there was a 6.6% annual increase in the use of ICU care during the last 6 months of life (from 17.5% to 24.7%; P < 0.001). Use of hospice care also rose from 28.8% to 49.9% during the study period (P < 0.001); however, a limited number of patients (6.2%) used both hospice and ICU services. Overall costs were substantially lower with use of hospice care relative to ICU use ($27,160 vs. $40,929 for the last 6 months of life; P < 0.001), of increasing concern in a financially constrained health care system. These analyses demonstrate the importance of developing studies to not only improve treatment but also palliation and end-of-life care in older adults with lung cancer.

■ CONCLUSIONS

Most of the patients diagnosed with lung cancer are aged 65 or older (110). As such, it is critical that future research efforts focus on refining the treatment approach for older adults with this disease. While subset analyses from large, randomized trials do provide certain insights into this population, a pooled analysis of the NCCTG experience suggests that age-specific trials in lung cancer may offer older adults lower rates of severe adverse events with no statistically significant differences in survival (111). A more individualized approach to the older adult may also be warranted; as opposed to a focus on chronologic age, more comprehensive tools (such as the cancer-specific geriatric assessment) may help stratify patients according to functional status and medical comorbidity (20,112). To facilitate these efforts, the dismal accrual of older adults onto clinical trial will have to be improved (113). Until then, critical questions regarding the management of this unique group will remain unanswered.

■ KEY POINTS

- Multiple physiologic changes accompany the aging process; consequent changes in drug metabolism may affect the efficacy and tolerability of anticancer agents
- Subset analyses of pivotal trials assessing adjuvant chemotherapy for non–small cell lung cancer (NSCLC) in older adults suggest similar benefit as compared with younger adults
- Concurrent chemoradiation appears to yield benefit in older adults with unresectable, stage III NSCLC, although this approach may result in higher rates of hematologic toxicity as compared with younger adults
- The Elderly Lung Cancer Study Group randomized patients aged 70 or older with advanced NSCLC to receive either best supportive care or vinorelbine, showing a survival advantage with the latter strategy
- Data for the efficacy of targeted agents in older adults with NSCLC is emerging; pivotal studies of erlotinib and bevacizumab suggest that clinical benefit is largely maintained in this subset
- Treatment of both limited- and extensive-stage SCLC in older adults is accompanied by critical toxicity considerations.

■ REFERENCES

1. Lynn TT, Scott G. Treatment of lung cancer in older patients. *Clin Chest Med.* 2007;28:735–749.
2. Owonikoko TK, Ragin CC, Belani CP, et al. Lung cancer in elderly patients: an analysis of the surveillance, epidemiology, and end results database. *J Clin Oncol.* 2007;25(35):5570–5577.
3. Hutchins LF, Unger JM, Crowley JJ, Coltman CA Jr, Albain KS. Underrepresentation of patients 65 years of age or older in cancer-treatment trials. *N Engl J Med.* 1999;341(27):2061–2067.
4. Yee KW, Pater JL, Pho L, Zee B, Siu LL. Enrollment of older patients in cancer treatment trials in Canada: why is age a barrier? *J Clin Oncol.* 2003;21(8):1618–1623.
5. Talarico L, Chen G, Pazdur R. Enrollment of elderly patients in clinical trials for cancer drug registration: a 7-year experience by the US Food and Drug Administration. *J Clin Oncol.* 2004;22(22):4626–4631.
6. Reddy SK, Berdan M, Curti M, et al. Non-small cell lung cancer in patients aged 75 years and older: A community-based experience [abstract 20676]. *J Clin Oncol.* 2008;26:(May 20 suppl).
7. Lindeman RD, Tobin J, Shock NW. Longitudinal studies on the rate of decline in renal function with age. *J Am Geriatr Soc.* 1985;33(4):278–285.
8. Larsson A, Skoog I, Aevarsson, et al. Regional cerebral blood flow in normal individuals aged 40, 75 and 88 years studied by 99Tc(m)-d,l-HMPAO SPET. *Nucl Med Commun.* 2001;22(7):741–746.
9. Fozard JL, Vercryssen M, Reynolds SL, Hancock PA, Quilter RE. Age differences and changes in reaction time: the Baltimore Longitudinal Study of Aging. *J Gerontol.* 1994;49(4):P179–P189.
10. Helzner EP, Cauley JA, Pratt SR, et al. Race and sex differences in age-related hearing loss: the Health, Aging and Body Composition Study. *J Am Geriatr Soc.* 2005;53(12):2119–2127.
11. Tanaka H, Monahan KD, Seals DR. Age-predicted maximal heart rate revisited. *J Am Coll Cardiol.* 2001;37(1):153–156.
12. Ferrari AU, Radaelli A, Centola M. Invited review: aging and the cardiovascular system. *J Appl Physiol.* 2003;95(6):2591–2597.
13. Sawhney R, Sehl M, Naeim A. Physiologic aspects of aging: impact on cancer management and decision making, part I. *Cancer J.* 2005;11(6):449–460.
14. Repetto L, Carreca I, Maraninchi D, et al. Use of growth factors in the elderly patient with cancer: a report from the Second International Society for Geriatric Oncology (SIOG) 2001 meeting. *Crit Rev Oncol Hematol.* 2003;45:123–128.
15. Balducci L, Al-Halawani H, Charu V, et al. Elderly cancer patients receiving chemotherapy benefit from first-cycle pegfilgrastim. *Oncologist.* 2007;12(12):1416–1424.
16. Schuette W, Nagel S, Weikersthal LFv, et al. Docetaxel plus carboplatin with or without levofloxacin prophylaxis in elderly patients (pts) with advanced non-small cell lung cancer (NSCLC): The APRONTA trial [abstract 8047]. *J Clin Oncol.* 2009;27:15s(suppl).
17. Extermann M, Hurria A. Comprehensive geriatric assessment for older patients with cancer. *J Clin Oncol.* 2007;25(14):1824–1831.
18. Maione P, Perrone F, Gallo C, et al. Pretreatment quality of life and functional status assessment significantly predict survival of elderly patients with advanced non-small-cell lung cancer receiving chemotherapy: a prognostic analysis of the multicenter Italian lung cancer in the elderly study. *J Clin Oncol.* 2005;23(28):6865–6872.
19. Frasci G, Lorusso V, Panza N, et al. Gemcitabine plus vinorelbine versus vinorelbine alone in elderly patients with advanced non-small-cell lung cancer. *J Clin Oncol.* 2000;18(13):2529–2536.
20. Hurria A, Gupta S, Zauderer M, et al. Developing a cancer-specific geriatric assessment: a feasibility study. *Cancer.* 2005;104(9):1998–2005.
21. Hurria A, Mohile S, Lichtman S, et al. Geriatric assessment of older adults with cancer: baseline data from a 500 patient multicenter study. American Society of Clinical Oncology, Orlando, FL; 2009.
22. Wong DR, Henteleff HJ. Ten-year follow-up of a province-wide cohort of surgical lung cancer patients in Nova Scotia. *Can J Surg.* 2008;51(4):257–262.
23. Chang MY, Mentzer SJ, Colson YL, et al. Factors predicting poor survival after resection of stage IA non-small cell lung cancer. *J Thorac Cardiovasc Surg.* 2007;134(4):850–856.
24. Rostad H, Naalsund A, Strand TE, Jacobsen R, Talleraas O, Norstein J. Results of pulmonary resection for lung cancer in Norway, patients older than 70 years. *Eur J Cardiothorac Surg.* 2005;27(2):325–328.
25. Cerfolio RJ, Bryant AS. Survival and outcomes of pulmonary resection for non-small cell lung cancer in the elderly: a nested case-control study. *Ann Thorac Surg.* 2006;82:424–429.
26. Birim O, Zuydendorp HM, Maat AP, Kappetein AP, Eijkemans MJ, Bogers AJ. Lung resection for non-small-cell lung cancer in patients older than 70: mortality, morbidity, and late

survival compared with the general population. *Ann Thorac Surg.* 2003;76(6):1796–1801.

27. Sullivan V, Tran T, Holmstrom A, et al. Advanced age does not exclude lobectomy for non-small cell lung carcinoma. *Chest.* 2005;128(4):2671–2676.

28. Dominguez-Ventura A, Cassivi SD, Allen MS, et al. Lung cancer in octogenarians: factors affecting long-term survival following resection. *Eur J Cardiothorac Surg.* 2007;32(2):370–374.

29. Bölükbas S, Beqiri S, Bergmann T, Trainer S, Fisseler-Eckhoff A, Schirren J. Pulmonary resection of non-small cell lung cancer: is survival in the elderly not affected by tumor stage after complete resection? *Thorac Cardiovasc Surg.* 2008;56(8):476–481.

30. Matsuoka H, Okada M, Sakamoto T, Tsubota N. Complications and outcomes after pulmonary resection for cancer in patients 80 to 89 years of age. *Eur J Cardiothorac Surg.* 2005;28(3):380–383.

31. Aoki T, Tsuchida M, Watanabe T, et al. Surgical strategy for clinical stage I non-small cell lung cancer in octogenarians. *Eur J Cardiothorac Surg.* 2003;23(4):446–450.

32. Winton T, Livingston R, Johnson D, et al.; National Cancer Institute of Canada Clinical Trials Group; National Cancer Institute of the United States Intergroup JBR.10 Trial Investigators. Vinorelbine plus cisplatin vs. observation in resected non-small-cell lung cancer. *N Engl J Med.* 2005;352(25):2589–2597.

33. Pepe C, Hasan B, Winton TL, et al.; National Cancer Institute of Canada and Intergroup Study JBR.10. Adjuvant vinorelbine and cisplatin in elderly patients: National Cancer Institute of Canada and Intergroup Study JBR.10. *J Clin Oncol.* 2007;25(12):1553–1561.

34. Früh M, Rolland E, Pignon JP, et al. Pooled analysis of the effect of age on adjuvant cisplatin-based chemotherapy for completely resected non-small-cell lung cancer. *J Clin Oncol.* 2008;26(21):3573–3581.

35. Potti A, Mukherjee S, Petersen R, et al. A genomic strategy to refine prognosis in early-stage non-small-cell lung cancer. *N Engl J Med.* 2006;355(6):570–580.

36. Olaussen KA, Dunant A, Fouret P, et al.; IALT Bio Investigators. DNA repair by ERCC1 in non-small-cell lung cancer and cisplatin-based adjuvant chemotherapy. *N Engl J Med.* 2006;355(10):983–991.

37. Muss HB, Biganzoli L, Sargent DJ, et al. Adjuvant therapy in the elderly: making the right decision. *J Clin Oncol.* 2007;25:1870–1875.

38. Dillman RO, Herndon J, Seagren SL, Eaton WL Jr, Green MR. Improved survival in stage III non-small-cell lung cancer: seven-year follow-up of cancer and leukemia group B (CALGB) 8433 trial. *J Natl Cancer Inst.* 1996;88(17):1210–1215.

39. Le Chevalier T, Arriagada R, Quoix E, et al. Radiotherapy alone versus combined chemotherapy and radiotherapy in nonresectable non-small-cell lung cancer: first analysis of a randomized trial in 353 patients. *J Natl Cancer Inst.* 1991;83(6):417–423.

40. National Comprehensive Cancer Network (NCCN) Treatment Guidelines: Non-small cell lung cancer. http://www.nccn.org. Accessed May 25, 2009.

41. Langer CJ, Hsu C, Curran WJ, et al. Elderly patients (pts) with locally advanced non-small cell lung cancer (LA-NSCLC) benefit from combined modality therapy: secondary analysis of Radiation Therapy Oncology Group (RTOG) 94–10 [abstract 1193]. *Proc Am Soc Clin Oncol.* 2002;21.

42. Rocha Lima CMS, Herndon JE II, Kosty M, et al. Therapy choices among older patients with lung carcinoma. *Cancer.* 2002;94:181–187.

43. Schild SE, Stella PJ, Geyer SM, et al.; North Central Cancer Treatment Group. The outcome of combined-modality therapy for stage III non-small-cell lung cancer in the elderly. *J Clin Oncol.* 2003;21(17):3201–3206.

44. Giorgio CG, Pappalardo A, Russo A, et al. A phase II study of induction chemotherapy followed by concurrent chemoradiotherapy in elderly patients with locally advanced non-small-cell lung cancer. *Anticancer Drugs.* 2007;18(6):713–719.

45. Luong DD, Poon D, Gao G, et al. Predictors of outcome and treatment decisions of older patients with stage III non-small cell lung cancer. ASCO Annual Meeting Proceedings Part I. *J Clin Oncol.* 2007;25:18S(June 20 suppl):19574.

46. Elderly Lung Cancer Vinorelbine Italian Study Group T. Effects of vinorelbine on quality of life and survival of elderly patients with advanced non-small-cell lung cancer. *J Natl Cancer Inst.* 1999;91:66–72.

47. Kudoh S, Takeda K, Nakagawa K, et al. Phase III study of docetaxel compared with vinorelbine in elderly patients with advanced non-small-cell lung cancer: results of the West Japan Thoracic Oncology Group Trial (WJTOG 9904). *J Clin Oncol.* 2006;24(22):3657–3663.

48. Gridelli C, Perrone F, Gallo C, et al.; MILES Investigators. Chemotherapy for elderly patients with advanced non-small-cell lung cancer: the Multicenter Italian Lung Cancer in the Elderly Study (MILES) phase III randomized trial. *J Natl Cancer Inst.* 2003;95(5):362–372.

49. Quoix EA, Oster J, Westeel V, et al. Weekly paclitaxel combined with monthly carboplatin versus single-agent therapy in patients age 70 to 89: IFCT-0501 randomized phase III study in advanced non-small cell lung cancer (NSCLC) (meeting abstracts). *J clin Oncol.* 2010;28:2.

50. Leong SS, Toh CK, Lim WT, et al. A randomized phase II trial of single-agent gemcitabine, vinorelbine, or docetaxel in patients with advanced non-small cell lung cancer who have poor performance status and/or are elderly. *J Thorac Oncol.* 2007;2(3): 230–236.

51. Lilenbaum R, Rubin M, Samuel J, et al. A randomized phase II trial of two schedules of docetaxel in elderly or poor performance status patients with advanced non-small cell lung cancer. *J Thorac Oncol.* 2007;2(4):306–311.

52. Chen YM, Perng RP, Shih JF, Whang-Peng J. A phase II randomized study of vinorelbine alone or with cisplatin against chemo-naïve inoperable non-small cell lung cancer in the elderly. *Lung Cancer.* 2008;61(2):214–219.

53. Chen YM, Perng RP, Tsai CM, et al. A Phase II randomized study of paclitaxel plus carboplatin or cisplatin against chemo-naive inoperable non-small cell lung cancer in the elderly. *J Thorac Oncol.* 2006;1:141–145.

54. Hesketh PJ, Chansky K, Lau DH, et al. Sequential vinorelbine and docetaxel in advanced non-small cell lung cancer patients age 70 and older and/or with a performance status of 2: a phase II trial of the Southwest Oncology Group (S0027). *J Thorac Oncol.* 2006;1:537–44.

55. Feliu J, López Gómez L, Madroñal C, et al. Gemcitabine plus vinorelbine in nonsmall cell lung carcinoma patients age 70 years or older or patients who cannot receive cisplatin. Oncopaz Cooperative Group. *Cancer.* 1999;86(8):1463–1469.

56. Choi IS, Kim BS, Park SR, et al. Efficacy of modified regimen with attenuated doses of paclitaxel plus carboplatin combination chemotherapy in elderly and/or weak patients with advanced non-small cell lung cancer. *Lung Cancer.* 2003;39(1):99–101.

57. Feliu J, Martín G, Madroñal C, et al. Combination of low-dose cisplatin and gemcitabine for treatment of elderly patients with advanced non-small-cell lung cancer. *Cancer Chemother Pharmacol.* 2003;52(3):247–252.

58. Giorgio CG, Pappalardo A, Russo A, et al. A phase II study of carboplatin and paclitaxel as first line chemotherapy in elderly patients with advanced non-small cell lung cancer (NSCLC). *Lung Cancer.* 2006;51(3):357–362.

59. Ohe Y, Niho S, Kakinuma R, et al. A phase II study of cisplatin and docetaxel administered as three consecutive weekly infusions for advanced non-small-cell lung cancer in elderly patients. *Ann Oncol.* 2004;15(1):45–50.

60. Socinski MA, Schell MJ, Peterman A, et al. Phase III trial comparing a defined duration of therapy versus continuous therapy followed by second-line therapy in advanced-stage IIIB/IV non-small-cell lung cancer. *J Clin Oncol.* 2002;20(5):1335–1343.

61. Hensing TA, Peterman AH, Schell MJ, Lee JH, Socinski MA. The impact of age on toxicity, response rate, quality of life, and survival in patients with advanced, Stage IIIB or IV nonsmall cell lung carcinoma treated with carboplatin and paclitaxel. *Cancer.* 2003;98(4):779–788.

62. Ramalingam S, Barstis J, Perry MC, et al. Treatment of elderly non-small cell lung cancer patients with three different schedules of weekly paclitaxel in combination with carboplatin: subanalysis of a randomized trial. *J Thorac Oncol.* 2006;1(3):240–244.

63. Bonomi P, Kim K, Fairclough D, et al. Comparison of survival and quality of life in advanced non-small-cell lung cancer patients treated with two dose levels of paclitaxel combined with cisplatin versus etoposide with cisplatin: results of an Eastern Cooperative Oncology Group trial. *J Clin Oncol.* 2000;18(3):623–631.

64. Langer CJ, Manola J, Bernardo P, et al. Cisplatin-based therapy for elderly patients with advanced non-small-cell lung cancer: implications of Eastern Cooperative Oncology Group 5592, a randomized trial. *J Natl Cancer Inst.* 2002;94(3):173–181.

65. Scagliotti GV, Parikh P, von Pawel J, et al. Phase III study comparing cisplatin plus gemcitabine with cisplatin plus pemetrexed in chemotherapy-naive patients with advanced-stage non-small-cell lung cancer. *J Clin Oncol.* 2008;26(21):3543–3551.

66. Hanna N, Shepherd FA, Fossella FV, et al. Randomized phase III trial of pemetrexed versus docetaxel in patients with non-small-cell lung cancer previously treated with chemotherapy. *J Clin Oncol.* 2004;22(9):1589–1597.

67. Pandurang MK, Ruqin C, Taruna A, et al. Efficacy and safety of pemetrexed in elderly cancer patients: Results of an integrated analysis. *Crit Rev Oncol Hematol.* 2008;67:64–70.

68. Shepherd FA, Rodrigues Pereira J, Ciuleanu T, et al.; National Cancer Institute of Canada Clinical Trials Group. Erlotinib in previously treated non-small-cell lung cancer. *N Engl J Med.* 2005;353(2):123–132.

69. Jackman DM, Yeap BY, Lindeman NI, et al. Phase II clinical trial of chemotherapy-naive patients > or = 70 years of age treated with erlotinib for advanced non-small-cell lung cancer. *J Clin Oncol.* 2007;25(7):760–766.

70. Tsao MS, Sakurada A, Cutz JC, et al. Erlotinib in lung cancer - molecular and clinical predictors of outcome. *N Engl J Med.* 2005;353(2):133–144.

71. Chen Y, Tsai C, Shih J, et al. Phase II randomized trial of erlotinib versus vinorelbine in chemotherapy-naive patients with advanced non-small-cell lung cancer (NSCLC) aged ≥70 years in Taiwan [abstract 8051]. *J Clin Oncol.* 2009;27:15s(suppl).

72. Giaccone G, Herbst RS, Manegold C, et al. Gefitinib in combination with gemcitabine and cisplatin in advanced non-small-cell lung cancer: a phase III trial–INTACT 1. *J Clin Oncol.* 2004;22(5):777–784.

73. Herbst RS, Giaccone G, Schiller JH, et al. Gefitinib in combination with paclitaxel and carboplatin in advanced non-small-cell lung cancer: a phase III trial–INTACT 2. *J Clin Oncol.* 2004;22(5):785–794.

74. Thatcher N, Chang A, Parikh P, et al. Gefitinib plus best supportive care in previously treated patients with refractory advanced non-small-cell lung cancer: results from a randomised, placebo-controlled, multicentre study (Iressa Survival Evaluation in Lung Cancer). *Lancet.* 2005;366(9496):1527–1537.

75. Ebi N, Semba H, Tokunaga SJ, et al.; Lung Oncology Group in Kyushu, Japan. A phase II trial of gefitinib monotherapy in chemotherapy-naïve patients of 75 years or older with advanced non-small cell lung cancer. *J Thorac Oncol.* 2008;3(10):1166–1171.

76. Simon GR, Extermann M, Chiappori A, et al. Phase 2 trial of docetaxel and gefitinib in the first-line treatment of patients with advanced nonsmall-cell lung cancer (NSCLC) who are 70 years of age or older. *Cancer.* 2008;112:2021–2029.

77. Cappuzzo F, Bartolini S, Ceresoli GL, et al. Efficacy and tolerability of gefitinib in pretreated elderly patients with advanced non-small-cell lung cancer (NSCLC). *Br J Cancer.* 2004;90(1):82–86.

78. Pirker R, Szczesna A, Pawel Jv, et al. FLEX: a randomized, multicenter, phase III study of cetuximab in combination with cisplatin/vinorelbine (CV) versus CV alone in the first-line treatment of patients with advanced non-small cell lung cancer (NSCLC) [abstract 3]. *J Clin Oncol.* 2008;26(May 20 suppl).

79. Kerbel RS. Tumor angiogenesis. *N Engl J Med.* 2008;358:2039–2049.

80. Sandler A, Gray R, Perry MC, et al. Paclitaxel-carboplatin alone or with bevacizumab for non-small-cell lung cancer. *N Engl J Med.* 2006;355(24):2542–2550.

81. Ramalingam SS, Dahlberg SE, Langer CJ, et al.; Eastern Cooperative Oncology Group. Outcomes for elderly, advanced-stage non small-cell lung cancer patients treated with bevacizumab in combination with carboplatin and paclitaxel: analysis of Eastern Cooperative Oncology Group Trial 4599. *J Clin Oncol.* 2008;26(1):60–65.

82. Reck M, von Pawel J, Zatloukal P, et al. Phase III trial of cisplatin plus gemcitabine with either placebo or bevacizumab as first-line therapy for nonsquamous non-small-cell lung cancer: AVAiL. *J Clin Oncol.* 2009;27(8):1227–1234.

83. Leighl NB, Zatloukal P, Mezger J, et al. Efficacy and safety of first-line bevacizumab (Bv) and cisplatin/gemcitabine (CG) in elderly patients (pts) with advanced non-small cell lung cancer (NSCLC) in the BO17704 study (AVAiL) [abstract 8050]. *J Clin Oncol.* 2009;27:15s(suppl).

84. Scappaticci FA, Skillings JR, Holden SN, et al. Arterial thromboembolic events in patients with metastatic carcinoma treated with chemotherapy and bevacizumab. *J Natl Cancer Inst.* 2007;99(16):1232–1239.

85. Gauden SJ, Tripcony L. The curative treatment by radiation therapy alone of Stage I non-small cell lung cancer in a geriatric population. *Lung Cancer.* 2001;32(1):71–79.

86. Okamoto T, Maruyama R, Shoji F, et al. Clinical patterns and treatment outcome of elderly patients in clinical stage IB/II non-small cell lung cancer. *J Surg Oncol.* 2004;87(3):134–138.

87. Pergolizzi S, Santacaterina A, Renzis CD, et al. Older people with non small-cell lung cancer in clinical stage IIIA and co-morbid conditions. Is curative irradiation feasible? Final results of a prospective study. *Lung Cancer.* 2002;37(2):201–206.

88. Warde P, Payne D. Does thoracic irradiation improve survival and local control in limited-stage small-cell carcinoma of the lung? A meta-analysis. *J Clin Oncol.* 1992;10(6):890–895.

89. Pignon JP, Arriagada R, Ihde DC, et al. A meta-analysis of thoracic radiotherapy for small-cell lung cancer. *N Engl J Med.* 1992;327(23):1618–1624.

90. Turrisi AT 3rd, Kim K, Blum R, et al. Twice-daily compared with once-daily thoracic radiotherapy in limited small-cell lung cancer treated concurrently with cisplatin and etoposide. *N Engl J Med.* 1999;340(4):265–271.

91. Yuen AR, Zou G, Turrisi AT, et al. Similar outcome of elderly patients in Intergroup Trial 0096. *Cancer.* 2000;89:1953–1960.

92. Quon H, Shepherd FA, Payne DG, et al. The influence of age on the delivery, tolerance, and efficacy of thoracic irradiation in the combined modality treatment of limited stage small cell lung cancer. *Int J Radiat Oncol Biol Phys.* 1999;43(1):39–45.

93. Ludbrook JJ, Truong PT, MacNeil MV, et al. Do age and comorbidity impact treatment allocation and outcomes in limited stage small-cell lung cancer? a community-based population analysis. *Int J Radiat Oncol Biol Phys.* 2003;55(5):1321–1330.

94. Aupérin A, Arriagada R, Pignon JP, et al. Prophylactic cranial irradiation for patients with small-cell lung cancer in complete remission. Prophylactic Cranial Irradiation Overview Collaborative Group. *N Engl J Med.* 1999;341(7):476–484.

95. Meert AP, Paesmans M, Berghmans T, et al. Prophylactic cranial irradiation in small cell lung cancer: a systematic review of the literature with meta-analysis. *BMC Cancer.* 2001;1:5.

96. Slotman B, Faivre-Finn C, Kramer G, et al.; EORTC Radiation Oncology Group and Lung Cancer Group. Prophylactic cranial irradiation in extensive small-cell lung cancer. *N Engl J Med.* 2007;357(7):664–672.

97. Evans WK, Shepherd FA, Feld R, Osoba D, Dang P, Deboer G. VP-16 and cisplatin as first-line therapy for small-cell lung cancer. *J Clin Oncol.* 1985;3(11):1471–1477.

98. Sundstrøm S, Bremnes RM, Kaasa S, et al.; Norwegian Lung Cancer Study Group. Cisplatin and etoposide regimen is superior to cyclophosphamide, epirubicin, and vincristine regimen in small-cell lung cancer: results from a randomized phase III trial with 5 years' follow-up. *J Clin Oncol.* 2002;20(24):4665–4672.

99. Ihde D, Mulshine J, Kramer B, et al. Prospective randomized comparison of high-dose and standard-dose etoposide and cisplatin chemotherapy in patients with extensive-stage small-cell lung cancer. *J Clin Oncol.* 1994;12:2022–2034.

100. Quoix E, Breton JL, Daniel C, et al. Etoposide phosphate with carboplatin in the treatment of elderly patients with small-cell lung cancer: a phase II study. *Ann Oncol.* 2001;12(7):957–962.

101. Larive S, Bombaron P, Riou R, et al.; Groupe Lyon-Saint Etienne d'Oncologie Thoracique. Carboplatin-etoposide combination in small cell lung cancer patients older than 70 years: a phase II trial. *Lung Cancer.* 2002;35(1):1–7.

102. Ardizzoni A, Favaretto A, Boni L, et al. Platinum-etoposide chemotherapy in elderly patients with small-cell lung cancer: results of a randomized multicenter phase II study assessing attenuated-dose or full-dose with lenograstim prophylaxis–a Forza Operativa Nazionale Italiana Carcinoma Polmonare and Gruppo Studio Tumori Polmonari Veneto (FONICAP-GSTPV) study. *J Clin Oncol.* 2005;23(3):569–575.

103. Smit EF, Carney DN, Harford P, Sleijfer DT, Postmus PE. A phase II study of oral etoposide in elderly patients with small cell lung cancer. *Thorax.* 1989;44(8):631–633.

104. Carney DN, Grogan L, Smit EF, Harford P, Berendsen HH, Postmus PE. Single-agent oral etoposide for elderly small cell lung cancer patients. *Semin Oncol.* 1990;17(1 suppl 2):49–53.

105. Girling DJ. Comparison of oral etoposide and standard intravenous multidrug chemotherapy for small-cell lung cancer: a stopped multicentre randomised trial. *The Lancet.* 1996;348:563–566.

106. Noda K, Nishiwaki Y, Kawahara M, et al.; Japan Clinical Oncology Group. Irinotecan plus cisplatin compared with etoposide plus cisplatin for extensive small-cell lung cancer. *N Engl J Med.* 2002;346(2):85–91.

107. Hanna N, Bunn PA, Jr, Langer C, et al. Randomized phase III trial comparing irinotecan/cisplatin with etoposide/cisplatin in patients with previously untreated extensive-stage disease small-cell lung cancer. *J Clin Oncol.* 2006;24:2038–2043.

108. Kim HG, Lee GW, Kang JH, et al. Combination chemotherapy with irinotecan and cisplatin in elderly patients (>or= 65 years) with extensive-disease small-cell lung cancer. *Lung Cancer.* 2008;61(2):220–226.

109. Sharma G, Freeman J, Zhang D, Goodwin JS. Trends in end-of-life ICU use among older adults with advanced lung cancer. *Chest.* 2008;133(1):72–78.

110. Hurria A, Kris MG. Management of lung cancer in older adults. *CA Cancer J Clin.* 2003;53(6):325–341.

111. Jatoi A, Hillman S, Stella P, et al.; North Central Cancer Treatment Group. Should elderly non-small-cell lung cancer patients be offered elderly-specific trials? Results of a pooled analysis from the North Central Cancer Treatment Group. *J Clin Oncol.* 2005;23(36):9113–9119.

112. Goodwin JA, Coleman EA, Shaw J. Short Functional Dependence Scale: development and pilot test in older adults with cancer. *Cancer Nurs.* 2006;29(1):73–81.

113. Murthy VH, Krumholz HM, Gross CP. Participation in cancer clinical trials: race-, sex-, and age-based disparities. *JAMA.* 2004;291(22):2720–2726.

23 Racial Disparities in Lung Cancer

CHRISTOPHER LATHAN

■ INTRODUCTION

It is well known that lung cancer is the leading cause of cancer mortality for both men and women in the United States, accounting for 161,840 deaths in the year 2008 (1). Due to the low overall survival for lung cancer (1) the disparities by race and class can be easily overlooked. In fact, African American men have the highest incidence and mortality of lung cancer in the United States (2). While over the past 40 years there has been a decrease in lung cancer incidence and mortality in all races, the differential between African American men and white men in mortality and incidence remains (2). The National Cancer Institute sponsored cancer monitoring system in the United States, Surveillance Epidemiology and End Report (SEER) lists the 2001-to-2005 incidence rate of lung cancer for U.S. white men to be 79.3 per 100,000 versus 107.6 per 100,000 for African American men, and the mortality rate for white men with lung cancer is 71.3 per 100,000 versus 93.1 per 100,000 for African American men (3). The numbers for African American women versus white women for incidence and survival do not demonstrate such a disparate pattern, indicating the racial disparities in lung cancer more pronounced in African American men. The incidence for other ethnic groups (Asian Americans, Native Americans, and nonblack Hispanics) in the United States is lower than that of whites for lung cancer (3).

Lung cancer mortality for men peaked in the last decade, while the mortality for women has only started to plateau (1,4). The survival gap by race in lung cancer started in the early 1980s and has been sustained since (5). Smoking rates for both African American and white men have decreased dramatically, with rates now approximately 26% for black men, and 23.5% for white men. This difference is essentially negative once age and socioeconomic status (SES) is accounted for (6,7). Black women and white women continued to have similarly low smoking rates (8). Although African Americans have historically smoked at higher rates than white Americans, this alone is not enough to explain for the difference in mortality, and African American men are two to four times more likely to have lung cancer even when adjusting for smoking habits (2).

■ RACIAL DISPARITIES MODEL

This data has prompted research and clinical trials to examine the root causes of the differences in outcome. Studies of health care disparities have become an integral part of the medical research landscape over the past 2 decades. Lately, the field has combined the talents of social scientists and health service researchers with those of biomedical researchers and clinical trialists. Studies in numerous medical fields have depicted disparities in the utilization of health care (9–11). Research into disparities in cancer care has also become a priority for the National Cancer Institute, which has targeted task force resources and allocated grant funding to elucidate the factors behind the unequal burden of cancer borne by ethnic minorities, and those of low SES in the United States (12). There is marked disparity in incidence and mortality in colon cancer, head and neck cancer, prostate cancer, pancreatic cancer, esophageal cancer, as well as lung cancer (3).

The differences in mortality and incidence for lung cancer in African Americans are well documented (2,11,13–15). Likewise there is substantial evidence documenting differences in treatment for African Americans in the United States as compared with their white counterparts across disease areas, including lung cancer (10,16,17). However, the underlying reasons for these disparities are not well delineated. Access to care, patient factors, and provider factors have all been implicated in treatment disparities by race (18,19). Our conceptual model on disparities, adapted from the provider-based model presented in the Institute of Medicine's study of racial disparities in health, Unequal Treatment (20), is shown in Figure 23.1.

The role of access to care has always been very important in the discussion of the disparities evident in health care for African Americans (21–23). In our model, access to care includes income, insurance, segregation, and geographic factors. A study by McDavid et al. (24) evaluated

Racial Disparities in Cancer Treatment

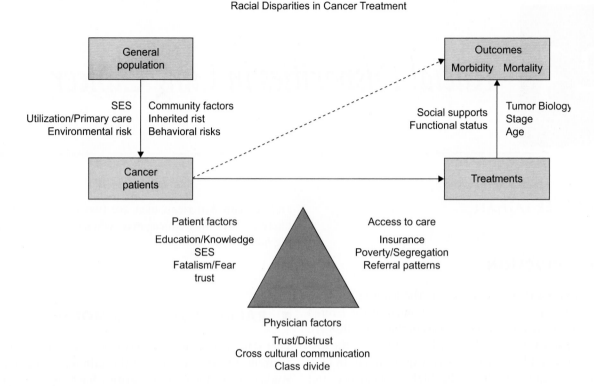

FIGURE 23.1 Racial disparities in cancer treatment.

the role of health insurance on cancer survival and found that patients without insurance had worse outcomes than cancer patients with insurance. African Americans are more likely not to have health insurance (21), and the effect of lack of access on obtaining specialized care has been well documented in systematic reviews and recent research on health disparities and recent studies (18,25). Both the Institute of Medicine Report Unequal Treatment and individual studies, show that disparities exist even in equal access systems like Medicare (10,11,16,17).

In truth, racial disparities often have multiple causes, access to care, cultural differences, and communication with providers leading to refusal of care, biological differences, as well as the systemic and structural effects of racial exclusion. With the dawn of targeted therapy and personalized medicine in lung cancer (26,27), the importance of obtaining appropriate treatment for all racial, ethnic, and socioeconomic groups takes on added importance.

■ SOCIOECONOMIC STATUS

Socioeconomic status takes on special importance separate from race in lung cancer, as examination of the role of SES in lung cancer reveals a double jeopardy phenomenon, with low income increasing the risk due to tobacco use, and also increasing the risk of dying from lung cancer presumably from lack of appropriate treatment (28,29).

Work by Schwartz et al. (30) has demonstrated that SES is often directly related to stage of disease at presentation, and this often adversely affects treatment choice and other processes of care. Similar research has shown that patients of lower SES obtain treatment of poor quality both in the United States and in the United Kingdom (23,31). Health care systems that provide universal access have been shown to attenuate racial and ethnic disparities in treatment (22,32), evidence that further supports the important role of income and access in explaining observed differences by race.

Lung cancer is unique among solid tumor cancers due to its relentless mortality rate, social stigma, and lack of a suitable screening tool for high-risk patients, and as such, the relationship between socioeconomic position and race might have a different pattern than that of other cancers (29). Qualitative studies demonstrated that patients with lung cancer often carry a stigma that separates them from other cancer patients (33). A study by Albano et al. (29) indicated that lung cancer mortality varied dramatically by years of education as well as race, whereas disparities in colon cancer varied more by sex and race as opposed to education. Lung cancer's SES effect has been documented in other places in the literature as well (28). Other studies have demonstrated a difference in stage distribution by SES (34,35), with lower SES resulting in later stage presentation of disease regardless of race. Clegg et al. discovered that socioeconomic patterns in incidence varied by specific cancers. Lung cancer and cervical cancer had an inverse relationship between SES gradient and incidence, while breast cancer and melanoma had incidence increase with increasing SES. Colon cancer did not appear to have an income gradient (34). In the United Kingdom, a significant regional socioeconomic gradient link to survival was seen, with the majority of the effect seen in the first year of diagnosis (36). Low SES was seen to be an independent poor prognostic finding for patients with stage I lung cancer in a SEER-based analysis (37). In a review of clinical trial data from the Southwest Oncology Group, Albain et al. (38) found that for patients on clinical trials, lung cancer did not show any difference in survival by race after adjusting for confounders. This is similar to work done by Blackstock et al. (32) in small cell lung cancer clinical trials. These studies suggest that equal treatment can lead to equal outcomes even when patients present with worsening stage and comorbid disease. The weight of the evidence suggests that even when SES is considered, it explains only part of observed differences in treatment and outcomes by race (14,15,39,40). The unique role of SES in lung cancer is only beginning to be examined.

■ LUNG CANCER DISPARITIES

Advanced Disease

Treatment disparities by race are well documented in advanced disease (10,16). Work by Earle et al. (10,17) demonstrated that black patients on Medicare were found to get chemotherapy at a significantly lower rate than their white counterparts, even when comorbid disease and SES were accounted for. The same is true for radiation in stage III disease (16). Given that treatment for late-stage lung cancer is palliative, this does not translate into a difference in long-term survival. There has been little data on lung cancer disparities in treatment with the targeted agents. At this time few papers have evaluated the frequency of the EGFR mutation in African Americans. Patients of Asian descent appear to have a higher frequency of the mutations than white patients with African Americans having very low frequency of the mutation (41). Unfortunately, there are only a handful of papers that examine this issue, and the question of the use of targeted agents with the underserved remains understudied. Even allowing for the advances made with targeted therapy, surgery for early-stage disease is the only treatment modality that can be potentially curative for lung cancer, and it is here that the disparities in treatment have maximum effect.

Early-Stage Disease

The majority of patients with lung cancer present with advanced disease, and early-stage lung cancer is usually discovered incidentally. There is no recommended screening for lung cancer at this time, and as such patients usually present with symptoms (42). African Americans tend to present with later stage disease and this could contribute to the treatment disparities. Although early-stage lung cancer only makes up 14% to 16% of the total cases of lung cancer (43), failure to use curative treatment in even a small subset of patients with this common disease represents a public health problem, and one that affects African Americans disproportionately (14). Surgery for early-stage disease is the only treatment modality that can be potentially curative. African Americans are nearly 50% less likely to receive surgery for early-stage non–small cell lung cancer when compared with white patients (11). The reasons for this difference in lung cancer treatment have not been fully elucidated, though it has been suggested that increased comorbid disease in African American men (32), differences in patient preferences due to mistrust and prevalent beliefs (44), poor physician and patient communication (45), and access to care (22,23,46,47) may all contribute.

Previous studies have documented that African American race was a negative predictor of obtaining surgery for early stage lung cancer (48). Bach et al. used the SEER-Medicare database to evaluate surgery patterns, and discovered treatment disparities in surgery for early-stage lung cancer by race. The data suggested that differences in survival between African Americans and whites could be explained by the difference in rates of surgery for early-stage disease. Some researchers have postulated that the difference in rates of surgery for African Americans was due to an increased rate of refusal by patients (49).

In a follow-up study by Earle et al. (15), investigators updated the seminal Bach study on the effect of race on surgery rates for Medicare but with a cohort of patients who had undergone invasive staging. The importance of invasive staging in lung cancer as a necessary part of the assessment of the primary tumor is well documented (49,50). Current recommendations advise the use of mediastinoscopy in addition to computed tomography scanning on every patient with possibly operable non–small cell lung cancer. In this study, even after controlling for potential confounding factors, African American patients were significantly less likely to undergo invasive staging in the workup of their lung cancer. Even when African American patients had invasive staging, they remained far less likely than their white counterparts to have potentially curative surgery. When they did have surgery, however, similar treatment resulted in similar outcomes, with no difference in survival between the races. Review of the reasons that surgery was not performed indicated that African American patients had surgery recommended less often than whites and also refused surgery slightly more than white patients (51). Data using SEER-Medicare revealed that while African American patients refused surgery for lung cancer more than white patients, they were also offered treatment less often than their white counterparts (52,53). This has been replicated in state cancer registries as well (54).

Due to the results of these studies, some have asked what role patient preference plays in exploring these patterns among ethnic minorities (55). This question was asked in respect to surgery for non–small cell lung cancer by Margolis et al. (44). In this study, the authors found that African American men at various hospitals believed that surgery for lung cancer caused the disease to spread. Some patients indicated that they would decline lung cancer surgery if offered for this very reason. The idea that African American patients refuse treatment more that white patients due to distrust of the medical system is prevalent, and is often attributed to the devastating effect of the Tuskegee experiments (21). While mistrust likely plays a role in health disparities, it is but one of the many factors that account for treatment choices.

Tobacco

The high incidence of lung cancer among African Americans, in addition to the aggressive targeting of African Americans by tobacco manufacturers, has prompted many in the public health community to focus on factors that enhance smoking cessation campaigns (56,57). Lower SES directly impacts smoking rates, with low SES resulting in higher smoking rates across all races (7,8,58).

These studies demonstrate that low income and education adversely affect cessation attempts, and that, often, African Americans underestimate the link between cancer and tobacco smoking when compared with white smokers. Investigators have examined cigarette additives such as menthol, as a potential explanation for the increased incidence in lung cancer and the evidence is as of yet, inconclusive (59). Epidemiologic studies have suggested that black patients might metabolize tobacco smoke in a different manner leaving them more vulnerable to the effects of smoking when compared with their white counterparts (7). Other studies have implicated Tp53 genetic variations found in African Americans (60). Further studies of tobacco carcinogenesis are needed to determine the role that tobacco metabolism plays in the increased incidence of lung cancer in African Americans.

■ SUMMARY

The fact that differential outcomes by race and SES exist in lung cancer is not in doubt (2,5,7,10,15,16,41,44,46, 54,58,61–63). Neither is the fact that these disparities by race and class have an effect on survival, particularly in early-stage disease, but will also likely have an effect in the advanced setting as lung cancer treatment makes advances in personalized medicine and treatments in adjuvant and

maintenance settings (27,64–66). Disparities in health care are multifactorial, and interventions to address these issues must take that into account. Access to care, patient/provider interaction, and biology all interact to create differences, and it is imperative to realize that scientific advances in the treatment of lung cancer should extend to all patients and not exclude those who are most adversely affected, low SES and ethnic minorities. Further research on the factors leading to disparities in cancer treatment and outcomes is urgently needed if we hope to relieve the unequal burden of cancer on vulnerable patient populations such as, ethnic minorities, immigrants and those of lower SES.

■ REFERENCES

1. American Cancer Society. *Cancer Facts and Figures 2008*. Atlanta: American Cancer Society; 2008
2. Stewart JH 4th. Lung carcinoma in African Americans: a review of the current literature. *Cancer*. 2001;91(12):2476–2482.
3. Ries LAG, Kosary CL, Hankey BF, et al. *SEER Cancer Statistics Review, 1973–2005*. Bethesda, MD: National Cancer Institute NIH publication, 2008. *SEER Cancer Statistics Review 1973–1996*. Bethesda, MD: National Cancer Institute NIH publication; 2008.
4. DeLancey JO, Thun MJ, Jemal A, Ward EM. Recent trends in Black-White disparities in cancer mortality. *Cancer Epidemiol Biomarkers Prev*. 2008;17(11):2908–2912.
5. Gadgeel SM, Kalemkerian GP. Racial differences in lung cancer. *Cancer Metastasis Rev*. 2003;22(1):39–46.
6. Alberg AJ, Brock MV, Samet JM. Epidemiology of lung cancer: looking to the future. *J Clin Oncol*. 2005;23(14):3175–3185.
7. Haiman CA, Stram DO, Wilkens LR, et al. Ethnic and racial differences in the smoking-related risk of lung cancer. *N Engl J Med*. 2006;354(4):333–342.
8. National Center for Health Statistics. *Chartbook on Trends in the Health of Americans*. Hyattsville, MD: National Center for Health Statistics; 2006.
9. Ayanian JZ, Udvarhelyi IS, Gatsonis CA, Pashos CL, Epstein AM. Racial differences in the use of revascularization procedures after coronary angiography. *JAMA*. 1993;269(20):2642–2646.
10. Earle CC, Venditti LN, Neumann PJ, et al. Who gets chemotherapy for metastatic lung cancer? *Chest*. 2000;117(5):1239–1246.
11. Bach PB, Cramer L, Warren JL, Begg CB. Racial differences in the treatment of early-stage lung cancer. *N Engl J Med*. 1999;34(16):1198–1205.
12. The Nation's Investment in Cancer Research: a plan and budget proposal for FY 2006. NCI, 2005. http://plan.cancer.gov/disparities.shtml. Accessed August 24, 2006.
13. Piffath TA, Whiteman MK, Flaws JA, Fix AD, Bush TL. Ethnic differences in cancer mortality trends in the US 1950–1992. *Ethn Health*. 2001;6(2):105–119.
14. Potosky AL, Saxman S, Wallace RB, Lynch CF. Population variations in the initial treatment of non-small-cell lung cancer. *J Clin Oncol*. 2004;22(16):3261–3268.
15. Lathan CS, Neville BA, Earle CC. The effect of race on invasive staging and surgery in non-small-cell lung cancer. *J Clin Oncol*. 2006;24(3):413–418.
16. Potosky AL, Saxman S, Wallace RB, Lynch CF. Population variations in the initial treatment of non-small-cell lung cancer. *J Clin Oncol*. 2004;22(16):3261–3268.
17. Earle CC, Neumann PJ, Gelber RD, Weinstein MC, Weeks JC. Impact of referral patterns on the use of chemotherapy for lung cancer. *J Clin Oncol*. 2002;20(7):1786–1792.
18. Medicine Io. Unequal Treatment: Institute of Medicine.

19. Laviest. Race, Ethnicity, and Health, a public health reader; 1999.
20. Institute of Medicine. Unequal Treatment: Institute of Medicine; 2002.
21. Clayton B. The African American Health Dilemma Volume I–II; 2002.
22. Mulligan CR, Meram AD, Proctor CD, Wu H, Zhu K, Marrogi AJ. Unlimited access to care: effect on racial disparity and prognostic factors in lung cancer. *Cancer Epidemiol Biomarkers Prev.* 2006;15(1):25–31.
23. Jack RH, Gulliford MC, Ferguson J, Møller H. Explaining inequalities in access to treatment in lung cancer. *J Eval Clin Pract.* 2006;12(5):573–582.
24. McDavid K, Tucker TC, Sloggett A, Coleman MP. Cancer survival in Kentucky and health insurance coverage. *Arch Intern Med.* 2003;163(18):2135–2144.
25. Bach PB, Pham HH, Schrag D, Tate RC, Hargraves JL. Primary care physicians who treat blacks and whites. *N Engl J Med.* 2004;351(6):575–584.
26. Paez JG, Jänne PA, Lee JC, et al. EGFR mutations in lung cancer: correlation with clinical response to gefitinib therapy. *Science.* 2004;304(5676):1497–1500.
27. Lynch TJ, Bell DW, Sordella R, et al. Activating mutations in the epidermal growth factor receptor underlying responsiveness of non-small-cell lung cancer to gefitinib. *N Engl J Med.* 2004;350(21):2129–2139.
28. Geyer S. Social inequalities in the incidence and case fatality of cancers of the lung, the stomach, the bowels, and the breast. *Cancer Causes Control.* 2008;19(9):965–974.
29. Albano JD, Ward E, Jemal A, et al. Cancer mortality in the United States by education level and race. *J Natl Cancer Inst.* 2007;99(18):1384–1394.
30. Schwartz KL, Crossley-May H, Vigneau FD, Brown K, Banerjee M. Race, socioeconomic status and stage at diagnosis for five common malignancies. *Cancer Causes Control.* 2003;14(8):761–766.
31. Weissman JS, Schneider EC. social disparities in cancer: lessons from a multidisciplinary workshop. *Cancer Causes and Control.* 2005;16:71–74.
32. Blackstock WB HJ, Paskett ED, Perry MC, et al. Outcomes among African-American/Non African American patients with advanced non small cell lung carcinoma: report from the Cancer and Leukemia Group B. *J Natl Cancer Inst.* 2002;94:284–290.
33. Chapple A, Ziebland S, McPherson A. Stigma, shame, and blame experienced by patients with lung cancer: qualitative study. *BMJ.* 2004;328(7454):1470.
34. Clegg LX, Reichman ME, Miller BA, et al. Impact of socioeconomic status on cancer incidence and stage at diagnosis: selected findings from the surveillance, epidemiology, and end results: National Longitudinal Mortality Study. *Cancer Causes Control.* 2009;20(4):417–435.
35. Herndon JE 2nd, Kornblith AB, Holland JC, Paskett ED. Patient education level as a predictor of survival in lung cancer clinical trials. *J Clin Oncol.* 2008;26(25):4116–4123.
36. Rachet B, Quinn MJ, Cooper N, Coleman MP. Survival from cancer of the lung in England and Wales up to 2001. *Br J Cancer.* 2008;99(suppl 1):S40–S42.
37. Ou SH, Zell JA, Ziogas A, Anton-Culver H. Low socioeconomic status is a poor prognostic factor for survival in stage I nonsmall cell lung cancer and is independent of surgical treatment, race, and marital status. *Cancer.* 2008;112(9):2011–2020.
38. Albain KS, Unger JM, Crowley JJ, Coltman CA Jr, Hershman DL. Racial disparities in cancer survival among randomized clinical trials patients of the Southwest Oncology Group. *J Natl Cancer Inst.* 2009;101(14):984–992.
39. Ward E, Jemal A, Cokkinides V, et al. Cancer disparities by race/ethnicity and socioeconomic status. *CA Cancer J Clin.* 2004;54(2):78–93.
40. Baldwin LM, Dobie SA, Billingsley K, et al. Explaining black-white differences in receipt of recommended colon cancer treatment. *J Natl Cancer Inst.* 2005;97(16):1211–1220.
41. Yang SH, Mechanic LE, Yang P, et al. Mutations in the tyrosine kinase domain of the epidermal growth factor receptor in non-small cell lung cancer. *Clin Cancer Res.* 2005;11(6):2106–2110.
42. Skarin AT LC. *Lung Cancer: Screening Staging and Treatment.* Edinburgh: Mosby Elsevier; 2007.
43. SEER Registry Statistics by Cancer Site. 2005. http://seer.cancer.gov/faststats/. Accessed August 24, 2005.
44. Margolis ML, Christie JD, Silvestri GA, Kaiser L, Santiago S, Hansen-Flaschen J. Racial differences pertaining to a belief about lung cancer surgery: results of a multicenter survey. *Ann Intern Med.* 2003;139(7):558–563.
45. Gordon HS, Street RL Jr, Sharf BF, Kelly PA, Souchek J. Racial differences in trust and lung cancer patients' perceptions of physician communication. *J Clin Oncol.* 2006;24(6):904–909.
46. Lathan CS, Neville BA, Earle CC. Racial composition of hospitals: effects on surgery for early-stage non-small-cell lung cancer. *J Clin Oncol.* 2008;26(26):4347–4352.
47. Greenwald HP, Polissar NL, Borgatta EF, McCorkle R, Goodman G. Social factors, treatment, and survival in early-stage non-small cell lung cancer. *Am J Public Health.* 1998;88(11):1681–1684.
48. Bach PB, Cramer LD, Warren JL, Begg CB. Racial differences in the treatment of early-stage lung cancer. *N Engl J Med.* 1999;341(16):1198–1205.
49. Mentzer SJ, Swanson SJ, DeCamp MM, Bueno R, Sugarbaker DJ. Mediastinoscopy, thoracoscopy, and video-assisted thoracic surgery in the diagnosis and staging of lung cancer. *Chest.* 1997;112(4 suppl):239S–241S.
50. NCCN. Clinical Practice Guidelines in Oncology v.1.2004 Non Small Cell lung Cancer. 2004.
51. Ayanian JZ, Cleary PD, Weissman JS, Epstein AM. The effect of patients' preferences on racial differences in access to renal transplantation. *N Engl J Med.* 1999;341(22):1661–1669.
52. Lathan CS, Neville BA, Earle CC. The effect of race on invasive staging and surgery in non-small-cell lung cancer. *J Clin Oncol.* 2006;24(3):413–418.
53. Detterbeck FC, Falen S, Rivera MP, Halle JS, Socinski MA. Seeking a home for a PET, part 2: Defining the appropriate place for positron emission tomography imaging in the staging of patients with suspected lung cancer. *Chest.* 2004;125(6):2300–2308.
54. Esnaola NF, Gebregziabher M, Knott K, et al. Underuse of surgical resection for localized, non-small cell lung cancer among whites and African Americans in South Carolina. *Ann Thorac Surg.* 2008;86(1):220–6; discussion 227.
55. Cykert S, Phifer N. Surgical decisions for early stage, non-small cell lung cancer: which racially sensitive perceptions of cancer are likely to explain racial variation in surgery? *Med Decis Making.* 2003;23(2):167–176.
56. Manfredi C, Lacey L, Warnecke R, Buis M. Smoking-related behavior, beliefs, and social environment of young black women in subsidized public housing in Chicago. *Am J Public Health.* 1992;82(2):267–272.
57. Klesges RC, Somes G, Pascale RW, et al. Knowledge and beliefs regarding the consequences of cigarette smoking and their relationships to smoking status in a biracial sample. *Health Psychol.* 1988;7(5):387–401.
58. Molina JR, Yang P, Cassivi SD, Schild SE, Adjei AA. Non-small cell lung cancer: epidemiology, risk factors, treatment, and survivorship. *Mayo Clin Proc.* 2008;83(5):584–594.
59. Carpenter CL, Jarvik ME, Morgenstern H, McCarthy WJ, London SJ. Mentholated cigarette smoking and lung cancer risk. *Ann Epidemiol.* 1999;9:114–20.
60. Mechanic LE, Bowman ED, Welsh JA, et al. Common genetic variation in TP53 is associated with lung cancer risk and prognosis in African Americans and somatic mutations in lung tumors. *Cancer Epidemiol Biomarkers Prev.* 2007;16(2):214–222.
61. Hardy D, Liu CC, Xia R, et al. Racial disparities and treatment trends in a large cohort of elderly black and white patients with nonsmall cell lung cancer. *Cancer.* 2009;115(10):2199–2211.

62. Menvielle G, Boshuizen H, Kunst AE, et al. The role of smoking and diet in explaining educational inequalities in lung cancer incidence. *J Natl Cancer Inst.* 2009;101(5):321–330.

63. Neighbors CJ, Rogers ML, Shenassa ED, Sciamanna CN, Clark MA, Novak SP. Ethnic/racial disparities in hospital procedure volume for lung resection for lung cancer. *Med Care.* 2007;45(7):655–663.

64. Arriagada R, Bergman B, Dunant A, Le Chevalier T, Pignon JP, Vansteenkiste J; International Adjuvant Lung Cancer Trial Collaborative Group. Cisplatin-based adjuvant chemotherapy in patients with completely resected non-small-cell lung cancer. *N Engl J Med.* 2004;350(4):351–360.

65. Pirker R, Pereira JR, Szczesna A, et al.; FLEX Study Team. Cetuximab plus chemotherapy in patients with advanced non-small-cell lung cancer (FLEX): an open-label randomised phase III trial. *Lancet.* 2009;373(9674):1525–1531.

66. Sandler A, Gray R, Perry MC, et al. Paclitaxel-carboplatin alone or with bevacizumab for non-small-cell lung cancer. *N Engl J Med.* 2006;355(24):2542–2550.

24 Immunological Approaches to the Treatment of Lung Cancer

NICK LEVONYAK

MITCHELL MAGEE

JOHN NEMUNAITIS

■ INTRODUCTION

Evidence of an endogenous immune-modulating effect in non–small cell lung cancer (NSCLC) is suggested based on heterogeneity of clinical progression observed in patients with the same histologic type of malignancy (1,2). There is also evidence for shared antigens in lung cancers (3–10) as seen in other tumor types (11,12). Dendritic cells (DCs), responsible for antigen presentation and induction of antitumor immunity in tumor-bearing hosts (13,14), have been shown to be activated in NSCLC, and biopsies of responsive disease have occasionally demonstrated tumor-infiltrating lymphocytes within the cancer, suggestive of endogenous immune effect (15). Lastly, improved survival of lung cancer patients who develop empyema has been rarely observed (16), further suggesting a potential positive role of the modulated host immune system against cancer.

Recent advances in molecular biology have identified antigens, cytokines, and mechanisms that have furthered our understanding of immunotherapeutic approaches.

The role of DCs in cell-mediated immunity has been extensively investigated (17–21). DCs play a central role in the induction of antitumor immunity through tumor antigen cross-presentation and the efficient display of these antigens in the context of major histocompatability complexes (MHC). This ultimately results in stimulation, proliferation, and activation of CD4+ and CD8+ T cells. CD4+ cells further augment the activity of natural killer (NK) cells and macrophages, in addition to amplifying antigen-specific immunity by local secretion of cytokines (22–26). These attributes make DCs a pivotal component in therapeutic strategies of many current immune-based therapies in NSCLC.

However, previous approaches to immunotherapy in lung cancer have failed to realize the potential of this promising strategy. There are several hypotheses to explain potential lack of activity, including ineffective priming of tumor-specific T cells, lack of high avidity of primed tumor-specific T cells, and physical or functional disabling of primed tumor-specific T cells by the primary host, and/or tumor-related mechanism. For example, in NSCLC a high proportion of the tumor-infiltrating lymphocytes are immunosuppressive T regulatory cells (CD4+ CD25+) that secrete transforming growth factor-β (TFG-β) and express a high level of cytotoxic T-lymphocyte (CTL) antigen-4 (27,28). These cells have been shown to impede immune activation by facilitating T-cell tolerance to tumor-associated antigens (TAAs) rather than cross-priming CD8+ T cells, resulting in the nonproliferation of killer T cells that recognize the tumor (27–33). Additionally, elevated levels of interleukin-10 (IL-10) and TFG-β found in patients with NSCLC have been shown in animal models to mediate immunosuppression, which may in turn alter host defense against malignant cells (34–43). These mechanisms are manipulated in different ways in the design of recent vaccine therapeutics described in this review.

■ NSCLC VACCINE DEVELOPMENT

Belagenpumatucel

Belagenpumatucel-L (Lucanix) (44) is a nonviral gene-based allogeneic vaccine that incorporates the TGF-β2 antisense gene into a cocktail of four different NSCLC cell lines. Elevated levels of TGF-β2 are linked to immunosuppression in cancer patients (45–50), and the level of TGF-β2 is inversely correlated with prognosis in patients with NSCLC (51). TGF-β2 has antagonistic effects on NK cells, lymphokine-activated killer cells, and DCs (34,39,40,52–54). Using an antisense gene to inhibit TGF-β2, several groups have demonstrated an inhibition of cellular TGF-β2 expression resulting in an increased immunogenicity of gene-modified cancer cells (10–14,55–58). In a recent phase II study involving 75 early- (n = 14) and late-stage (n = 61) NSCLC patients, a dose-related effect of belagenpumatucel was defined (44). Patients were randomized to one of the three dose cohorts. Grade 3 arm swelling existed in one patient with no other serious side effects. Of all 75 patients, the median survival was 441 days with a 1-year survival of 54%. In 41 advanced-stage (IIIB, IV) patients, the investigators found no adverse toxicity and an impressive survival advantage at dose levels $\geq 2.5 \times 10^7$ cells/injection, with an estimated 2-year survival of 47%. This compared favorably with the historical 2-year survival rate of <20% of stage IIIB/IV NSCLC patients (3–6,59,60). Furthermore, induction of an enhanced immune response to tumor antigen correlated with a more favorable outcome. Immune function was explored in the 61 advanced-stage (IIIB/IV) patients. Cytokine production (interferon [IFN]-γ, $P = 0.006$; IL-6, $P = 0.004$; and IL-4, $P = 0.007$) was induced, an antibody-mediated response to vaccine human leukocyte antigen (HLA) antigen was observed ($P = 0.014$), and there was a trend toward a correlation between a cell-mediated response and achievement of stable disease or better ($P = 0.086$).

In a recent open-label phase II trial of belagenpumatucel involving 21 confirmed stage IV NSCLC patients, safety and efficacy as well as the correlation between circulating tumor cells (CTCs) in blood and overall survival of advanced NSCLC patients were investigated. Patients were given intradermal (61) immunization of 2.5×10^7 TGF-β2 antisense gene–transfected allogeneic tumor cells (belagenpumatucel) one time per month for a 16-month period. The trial took place from September 2005 to January 2008.

There were no significant grade 3 or 4 toxicities related to therapy. There was grade 2 transient injection-site erythema in three patients and grade 1 and 2 injection-site induration in five patients.

Twenty of 21 patients enrolled were evaluable, with a median survival of 562 days; however, those patients whose baseline CTC levels were 0 to 1 had a significantly improved median survival of 660 days ($P = 0.025$). This adds further support to the hypothesis that lower CTC count may be correlated with better survival (61).

A phase III trial is ongoing to test the effect of belagenpumatucel in patients with stage IIIB, IV NSCLC who demonstrate initial responsiveness to platinum-based therapy.

There have been several investigations involving immune stimulation through TGF-β "blockade." One technique involves a TGF-β type 1 receptor kinase inhibitor, SM16. Inhibition of this particular receptor was shown to increase immunostimulatory cytokines and ICAM-1. In addition, there was an increase in number and function of antitumor CD8+ cells in mice containing lung cancer tumors (62).

Another study was done to explore the effectiveness of silencing TGF-β1. Tumor cultures of SW1 melanoma and Ag104 sarcoma cells were transfected with short hairpin RNA (shRNA) that inhibited the production of TGF-β1 utilizing a lentivirus vector. The concentration of TGF-β1 decreased by 98% in the SW1 culture and by 94% in the Ag104 culture. To explore the efficacy of using these TGF-β1 inhibited tumor cultures (SW1-TGF-β1 or Ag104-TGF-β1) as vaccines, in vivo studies were performed in mice. In one study, four SW1 mice treated with the SW1-TGF-β1 culture had a significant delay in tumor growth and two had a complete regression. All four of the control mice had consistent tumor growth. Similar results were found in studies with the Ag104-TGF-β1 cells (63).

GVAX

Vaccines transduced with granulocyte-macrophage colony-stimulating factor (GM-CSF) gene were potent inducers of tumor immunity in animal models (64). Secretion of GM-CSF by genetically modified tumor cells induced local tumor antigen expression and stimulated cytokine release at the vaccine site, which activated and attracted antigen-presenting cells, thereby inducing a tumor-specific cellular immune response (65). Preclinical studies conducted with GVAX showed no significant local and systemic toxicities at clinically relevant doses (64,66–68).

Several phase I/II human trials using GM-CSF–secreting autologous or allogeneic tumor cell vaccines have been performed (69–74). One multicenter phase I/II trial involving patients with early-stage and advanced-stage NSCLC evaluated an autologous GVAX vaccine (8). For vaccine preparation, tumor tissue was obtained surgically or by thoracentesis in the case of malignant effusions. Cells were exposed overnight to an adenoviral vector supernatant (Ad-GM). GVAX was administered intradermally. A total of 43 NSCLC patients (10 early-stage, 33 late-stage) were vaccinated. The most common vaccine-related adverse events were local vaccine injection-site reactions (93%), followed by fatigue (16%) and nausea (12%). Three advanced-stage patients achieved durable, complete tumor regression. Two remain without disease more than 5 years following vaccine. Both had failed prior frontline and second-line therapy prior to vaccination and had multisite disease. One complete responder showed an in vitro T-cell response to autologous tumor-pulsed DCs after vaccination. Survival at 1 year was 44% for all advanced-stage–treated patients and median survival was 12 months. Medial survival among patients receiving vaccines secreting GM-CSF at a rate of ≥ 40 ng/24 hours/10^6 cells was 17 months, compared with 7 months for those receiving vaccines secreting less GM-CSF.

A subsequent trial in advanced NSCLC using a vaccine composed of autologous tumor cells mixed with an allogeneic GM-CSF–secreting cell line (K562 cells) failed to demonstrate evidence of clinical efficacy (75). Evidence of vaccine-induced immune activation was demonstrated; however, objective tumor responses were not seen despite a 25-fold higher GM-CSF–secretion concentration with the bystander GVAX vaccine.

α-Galactosylceramide

αGalCer is a glycolipid-based vaccine that has demonstrated capacity to activate Vα24 NK T cells which have been shown to demonstrate antitumor activity via several mechanisms including the production of cytokines such as IFN-γ. Combination with peripheral blood mononuclear cells pulsed with low-dose IL-2 and GM-CSF appeared to enhance vaccine activity (76). A phase 1 study involving 11 patients with NSCLC demonstrated minimal toxicity (grade I or II toxicity) and predicted immune response. However, only two patients achieved stable disease.

In a more recent phase I–II trial of the same vaccine, 23 advanced-stage NSCLC patients received treatment and 17 patients completed the study which took place from February 2004 to August 2006 (77). In 10 of the 17 patients, there was a measurable increase in IFN-γ producing cells. More significantly, those 10 patients had a 2-year survival of 60% and also had an appreciably greater median survival of 31.9 months in comparison with the 9.7-month median survival of the unresponsive patients ($P = 0.0015$). The median survival of the unresponsive patients is consistent with historical survival of similar patients undergoing standard treatment.

L-BLP-25

Mucin (MUC)-1 is a high molecular-weight protein containing large amounts of o-linked sugars and is expressed on the apical borders of most normal secretory epithelial cells (78). It is expressed in many cancers, including NSCLC (79). Tumor-associated MUC1 is antigenically distinct from normal MUC1 (80). Recent studies have identified that MUC1 is associated with cellular transformation, as demonstrated by tumorigenicity (81), and can confer resistance to genotoxic agents (82). Both the oligosaccharide portion and the tandem repeat of the MUC extracellular domain have potential for immunotherapeutic activity.

L-BLP-25 vaccine has been tested in three NSCLC trials (83). Three doses and two regimens were tested, including one regimen using liposomal IL-2 as an adjuvant. Recently, results of a phase III study (84) of L-BLP-25 in 171 advanced-stage NSCLC patients were reported (75). Patients with stable or responding stage IIIB or IV NSCLC following standard first-line chemotherapy were randomized to either L-BLP-25 (88 patients) or best supportive care (83 patients). There was a 4.4-month longer median survival for patients on the L-BLP-25 arm (17.4 vs. 13 months), although this did not reach statistical significance. The median survival for a subset of 35 stage IIIB patients who received vaccine was 30 months versus 13.3 months for the 30 who received best supportive care ($P = 0.09$). There were no major toxicities.

The clinically meaningful survival advantages seen for stage IIIB patients are encouraging. A phase III randomized trial of L-BLP-25 for unresectable stage III NSCLC patients with response or stable disease after chemoradiation is now ongoing.

IDM-2101

IDM-2101 is a peptide-based vaccine designed to induce CTLs against five TAAs frequently overexpressed in NSCLC (i.e., carcinoembryonic antigen [CEA] (85), p53 (86,87), HER-2/neu (88,89), and melanoma antigens [MAGE] 2 and 3) (90). These TAAs have been used in previous vaccine studies involving patients with NSCLC (91–110) and have been extensively characterized in the literature. IDM-2101 is composed of 10 synthetic peptides from these TAAs. Nine of the peptides represent CTL epitopes and each CTL epitope is restricted by HLA-A2.1 and at least one other member of the HLA-A2 superfamily of MHC class I molecules, providing coverage of approximately 45% of the general population. The 10th synthetic peptide is the pan-DR epitope (PADRE), a rationally designed helper T-lymphocyte epitope included to augment the magnitude and duration of CTL responses (111).

IDM-2101 was tested in an open-label phase II study involving 63 HLA-A2–positive stage IIIB/IV NSCLC patients who had failed prior chemotherapy (112). No significant adverse events were noted. Low-grade erythema and pain at the injection site were the most common side effects. One-year survival in the treated patients was 60%, and median survival was 17.3 months. One complete and one partial response were identified. Survival was longer in patients demonstrating an immune response to epitope peptides ($P < 0.001$). Overall, treated patients appeared to do well when compared with historical controls.

Immune responses in 33 patients collectively showed induction of CTLs to all of the vaccine epitopes. Although patient-to-patient variability was observed with respect to the frequency and magnitude of the CTL responses, 85% of tested patients responded to at least two epitopes. These data are consistent with results from an earlier phase I trial (113). Moreover, longer survival was shown in patients achieving responses to two or more epitopes ($P < 0.001$).

B7.1 Vaccine

B7.1 (CD80⁺) is a costimulating molecule associated with induction of a T- and NK-cell response (96,114–116). Tumor cells transfected with B7.1 and HLA molecules have been shown to stimulate an avid immune response by direct antigen presentation and direct activation of T cells, in addition to allowing cross-presentation (117–120). In a Phase I trial, Raez et al. (121) used an allogeneic NSCLC tumor cell line (AD100) transfected with B7.1 (CD80) and HLA-A1 or -A2 to generate CD8 CTL responses. Patients who were HLA-A1 or -A2 allotype received the corresponding HLA-matched vaccine. A total of 19 patients with stage IIIB/IV NSCLC were treated, and most had received prior chemotherapy. Patients who were neither HLA-A1 nor -A2 received the HLA-A1–transfected vaccine.

A total of 18 patients received at least one full course of treatment. One patient was removed before the completion of the first course due to a serious adverse event not associated with the vaccine. Three more patients experienced serious adverse events, which were also not associated with the vaccine. Side effects included minimal skin erythema for four patients.

One patient showed a partial response for 13 months and five patients had stable disease ranging from 1.6 to >52 months (121,122). The Kaplan-Meyer estimate for the survival for the 19 patients was 18 months. One-year survival was estimated at 52%. The low toxicity and good survival in this study suggested benefit from clinical vaccination.

L523S Vaccine

L523S is a lung cancer antigen originally identified through screening of genes differentially expressed in cancer versus normal tissue (123,124). L523S is expressed in approximately 80% of NSCLC cells (123,124). The immunogenicity of L523S in humans was initially shown by detecting the presence of existent antibody and helper T-cell responses to L523S in patients with lung cancer. Subsequent studies further validated L532S immunogenicity by demonstrating that human CTLs could specifically recognize and kill cells that express L523S. In preclinical studies, the gene proved safe when injected intramuscularly as an expressive plasmid (pVAX/L523S) and when delivered following incorporation into an EIB-deleted adenovirus (Ad/L523S). In a phase I clinical trial in 13 stage IB, IIA, and IIB NSCLC patients, both delivery vehicles (pVAX/L523S and Ad/L523S) were used to administer the gene to three patients in each of three cohorts (125). No significant toxic effect was identified. All but one patient demonstrated at least twofold elevation in antiadenovirus antibodies; however, despite the positive preclinical studies, vaccination induced an immune response in only one patient in the phase I study. The reasons for a lack of significant detectable immune response are unknown. The use of alternative formulations and/or regimens and the assessment of other surrogate immune function parameters might be considered. Two patients developed disease recurrence and all remained alive after a median of 290 days follow-up.

Epidermal Growth Factor Vaccine

Overexpression of epidermal growth factor receptor (EGFR) and its ligand, epidermal growth factor (EGF), has been linked with the promotion of cell proliferation, survival, and motility. EGF transduces signaling through EGFR following binding to this cell surface receptor, ultimately resulting in the stimulation of cell proliferation. The immunotherapy developed by Ramos et al. (126) induces an immune response against self-produced EGF. This vaccine is a human recombinant EGF linked to a P64K recombinant carrier protein from *Neisseria meningitides*. Several pilot trials have been completed (126–128). Results from these studies have demonstrated that vaccination with EGF is immunogenic and appears to be well-tolerated.

In one study, 43 patients with stage IIIB/IV NSCLC randomly received either a single dosage or a double dose (126). Immune response against EGF was measured in 38 of the 43 patients, and 15 achieved a good antibody response (GAR) against EGF following vaccination. Kaplan-Meyer analysis separating patients by dose predicted a median estimated life expectancy of 6.4 months for patients who received the single dose, and 8.4 months for the patients who received the double dose. Based on immune response, however, patients classified as GARs had a life expectancy estimated at 12 months, whereas those who had a less favorable GAR had a life expectancy of 7 months.

Two other studies conducted by Gonzalez and colleagues compared the effect of different adjuvants on patients' antibody response (127,128). The patients were treated each time when antibody titers decreased to at least 50% of their induction-phase peak titer. The pooled data of the two trials suggested that higher antibody responses were obtained when the vaccine was emulsified in adjuvant montanide ISA 51 or when low-dose cyclophosphamide was administered before the vaccination; however, the difference was not statistically significant. Median survival of GAR patients was 9.1 months, whereas poor antibody responding patients had a survival of 4.5 months.

Previous results described justified a randomized phase II trial of 80 late-stage (IIIB/IV) NSCLC patients that was recently completed (129). Patients were randomized to either vaccine or standard therapy. Mild, grade 1 and 2 toxic events were associated with the vaccine. The investigators classified patients whose anti-EGF antibody titers were at least 1:4,000 or four times their preimmunization values to have GAR. Of the vaccinated patients, 51.4% of them achieved GAR while no patients achieved GAR in the control group. The vaccine did decrease EGF concentration in 64.3% of vaccinated patients and those who achieved GAR survived significantly longer, with an 11.7-month median survival as opposed to 3.6 months in those with poor antibody response. Overall, there was a slight advantage for vaccinated patients with a 6.47-month median survival versus the 5.33-month median survival for the patients on the control arm. One-year survival was nonsignificantly higher ($P = 0.096$) in vaccinated patients at 67% in comparison with 33% for the controls.

A subsequent study investigated the same EGF-based vaccine in combination with chemotherapy in 20 advanced NSCLC patients (130). No serious side effects related to the combination therapy were observed. Also, median survival and 1-year survival were both encouraging at 9.3 months and 70%, respectively, suggesting support of further testing in combination with chemotherapy.

Melanoma-Associated Antigen E-3 Vaccine

MAGE-3 is the most commonly expressed testicular cancer antigen and is expressed in testicular germ cells, but no other normal tissue (131). It is aberrantly expressed in a wide variety of tumors, including NSCLC (131). Several CD8+ T-cell epitopes of MAGE-3 have been identified in vitro (132–140), including HLA-A1–restricted epitope 168–176 (141), and HLA-A2–restricted epitope 271–279 (142). Based on these findings, synthetic peptides corresponding to these epitopes have been introduced into clinical vaccination studies in which they were associated with regression of melanoma in individual cases (143). Clinical vaccination studies using full-length recombinant proteins may offer potential advantages in that this antigen includes the full range of epitopes for CD4+ and CD8+ T cells. In addition, it is likely that protein vaccination leads to presentation of epitopes in the context of various HLA alleles, and therefore, this type of vaccine should be applicable to any patient regardless of HLA restriction (144).

Atanackovic et al. (144) used a MAGE-3 protein as a vaccine to induce CD4+ T cells in patients with stage I or II NSCLC. All patients had undergone surgical resection of the primary lung tumor and had no evidence of disease at the onset of the study. Of the nine patients who received the MAGE-3 protein alone, three developed an increase in antibodies against MAGE-3 protein and one had a CD8+ T-cell response. By comparison, of the eight patients who received MAGE-3 antigen combined with the adjuvant ASO2B, seven showed an increase in serum concentrations of anti-MAGE-3 and four had a CD4+ response to HLA-DP4–restricted peptide. Based on these results, further testing in a larger randomized phase II trial was completed and recently reported (145), involving 182 (122 vaccine and 60 placebo) early-stage (IB, II) NSCLC MAGE-A3 positive patients. No significant toxicity issues were identified, and preliminary analysis revealed a 33% disease-free survival improvement in the vaccinated arm compared with the placebo arm. Results trended toward significance in the stage II patients.

Currently, a randomized, double-blind, placebo-controlled phase III trial with a target accrual of over 2,200 stage IB, II, and IIIA NSCLC patients is ongoing. The trial began in June 2007 and explores the vaccine both following adjuvant chemotherapy and without chemotherapy. The primary end-point for the trial is disease-free survival (146).

Transcriptase Catalytic Subunit Antigen Vaccine

It is well established that T cells of the human immune system can recognize telomerase (147–155). Although telomerase is also expressed in some normal cells, such as bone marrow stem cells (156) and epithelial cells in gastrointestinal tract crypts (157), it is highly expressed in virtually all cancer cells. GV1001 is a unique peptide corresponding to a sequence derived from the active site of the catalytic subunit of human telomerase reverse transcriptase (hTERT). It contains the 611–626 sequence of hTERT and is capable of binding to molecules encoded by multiple alleles of all three loci of HLA class II (158). HR2822 is a second peptide corresponding to sequences 540–548 of hTERT. Brunsvig et al. (159) initiated a phase I/II trial involving 26 patients with late-stage NSCLC. No clinically significant toxic events related to the treatment were reported. Importantly, no bone marrow or severe gastrointestinal toxicities were observed. Side effects were mild and included flu-like symptoms, chills, and fever.

Eleven patients demonstrated an immune response against GV1001, and only two patients demonstrated a response to HR2822. After receiving booster shots, two patients were converted to immune responders. One patient with stage IIIA NSCLC showed a complete tumor response and developed GV1001-specific CTLs that could be cloned from peripheral blood. The median survival time for all 26 patients was 8.5 months.

Dexosome Vaccine

Exosomes are cell-derived lipid vesicles that express high levels of a narrow spectrum of cell proteins (160–162). Vesicles released from DCs (dexosomes) have been demonstrated to play a role in the activation of the immune response (163,164). In vitro, dexosomes have the capacity to present antigen to naïve CD8+ cytolytic T cells and CD4+ T cells (161,165). Purified dexosomes were shown to be effective in both suppressing tumor growth and eradicating an established tumor in murine models (160). Morse et al. developed a vaccine using DC–derived exosomes loaded with MAGE tumor antigens (166). The phase I trial enrolled 13 patients with stage IIIB or IV NSCLC demonstrating MAGE-A3 or -A4 expression. Autologous DCs were harvested to produce dexosomes. They were loaded with MAGE-A3, -A4, -A10, and -3DPG4 peptides. Dexosome therapy was administered to nine patients. Patients experienced grade 1 to 2 toxicities, including injection-site reactions, flu-like symptoms, edema, and pain. Three patients exhibited delayed-type hypersensitivity reactions against MAGE peptides. Survival ranged from 52 to 665 days.

α(1,3)-Galactosyltransferase

α(1,3)-Galactosyltransferase (agal) epitopes are present on the surface of most nonhuman mammalian cells and are the primary antigen source responsible for hyperacute xenograft rejection. Expression of agal epitopes after gene transfer (using a retroviral vector) in human A375 melanoma cells prevented tumor formation in nude mice (167).

Preliminary results by Morris et al. (168), using three irradiated lung cancer cell lines genetically altered to express xenotransplantation antigens by retroviral transfer of the murine *agal* gene, were recently described in seven patients with stage IV, recurrent or refractory NSCLC. Toxicity involved grade 1 to 2 pain at the injection site, local skin reaction, fatigue, and hypertension. Four patients had stable disease for >16 months.

NSCLC Dendritic Cell Vaccines

DCs are potent antigen-presenting cells. As part of a phase II study, Hirshowitz et al. (169, 17-21) recently generated DC vaccines from CD14+ precursors, which were pulsed with apoptotic bodies of an allogeneic NSCLC cell line that overexpressed Her2/neu, CEA, WT1, MAGE-2, and survivin. A total of 16 patients with stage IA–IIIB NSCLC were vaccinated. There were 10 patients who experienced skin erythema at the injection site and 4 patients experienced minor fatigue. No patients experienced a serious adverse event. Five patients showed a tumor antigen-independent response, and 6 patients showed an antigen-specific response. The study concluded that the vaccine was safe and demonstrated biological activity.

Another phase I trial utilizing peripheral blood mononuclear cells from 15 patients with several different metastatic tumor types (melanoma, lung, renal cell carcinoma, sarcoma, and breast cancer) was also recently described (170). The DCs were stimulated with autologous tumor lysates and infused intravenously every 21 days for four total treatments. Toxicity was mild and included fever on the day of injection as well as well as asthenia. Seven of the 15 patients experienced stable disease for at least 3 months and 7 progressed while on treatment. The median time to progression was 3 months indicating that this DC approach should be pursued in further clinical testing.

Others have looked at use of postsurgical chemotherapy in combination with immunotherapy utilizing DCs and activated T-killer cells in late-stage lung cancer patients (171). The T-killer cells and DCs were harvested from tumor-draining lymph nodes and supplemented with peripheral blood lymphocytes. Thirty-one patients received four courses of chemotherapy in combination with immunotherapy every 2 months over the course of 2 years. These 31 patients were divided into two groups—those with N2 disease (group A) and those with N0 or N1 (group B). Group A received chemotherapy (calboplatin and paclitaqxel) and then underwent surgery. Group B went straight to surgery, and then both groups received a combination of chemotherapy and DC therapy or chemotherapy only. Those eligible for combination therapy

received two to four courses and then continued DC therapy every 2 months for 2 more years. Group A was treated with docetaxel while group B received calboplatin and paclitaxel. In both cases, DC therapy was administered 5 to 7 days after chemotherapy. Twenty-eight patients in total received the DC therapy.

There were no significant toxicities other than low-grade fever, chills, fatigue, and nausea on the day of immunotherapy. Two- and 5-year survival of 88.9% and 52.9%, respectively, are encouraging and support an evaluation of efficacy in a phase III trial. There was also a correlation between the number of cells transferred and the rate of patient survival. Patients receiving more than 5×10^{10} cells had a 5-year survival rate of 80.8% compared with 38.5% in those who received less.

Cyclophilin B

Cyclophilin-B (CypB) is a ubiquitous protein playing an important role in protein folding (172,173), and is expressed in both normal and cancerous cells. CypB-derived peptides are recognized by HLA-A24 restricted cytotoxic lymphocytes (CTL) isolated from lung adenocarcinoma. CypB peptides induce CTLs from leukemic patients, but failed to induce an immune response in cells isolated from patients with epithelial cancer or normal donors. Modification of a single amino acid of the CypB gene increases its immunogenicity and results in CTL activation in both cancer patients and healthy donors (174).

Gohara et al. (175) investigated the immune response in advanced-stage lung cancer patients treated with CypB vaccine. Sixteen HLA-A24 positive patients, 15 with NSCLC and 1 with small cell lung cancer (SCLC), were treated with CypB or modified CypB peptide vaccine following completion of chemotherapy. All patients had stable disease at 5-week follow-up. Following vaccination, IFN-γ production by peripheral blood mononuclear cells isolated from patient sera was elevated in 3 of 12 patients. Overall survival for NSCLC patients receiving CypB or modified CypB vaccine was 67+ and 28+ weeks, respectively. One patient with SCLC was not evaluable for response.

1E10 Vaccine

The 1E10 vaccine is a murine anti-idiotypic antibody that was primarily created by the immunization of BALB/c mice containing P3, an idiotypic antibody which recognizes gangliosides containing NeuGc. Such gangliosides are reasonable targets for immunotherapeutic techniques as they have been detected in a number of different tumor types, including lung cancer. In fact, there has been recent data to suggest that NeuGcGM3 is correlated closely with tumor progression (176). It was hypothesized that the 1E10 idiotypic vaccination could produce an idiotypic cascade specific to the NeuGcGM3 antigen.

In a recent study aimed to investigate efficacy of the 1E10 vaccine, 20 advanced-stage NSCLC patients were administered 15 doses of the vaccine over an 18-month period (177). Those patients who received at least five doses of the vaccine were considered immunologically evaluable.

The study investigated via serum analysis whether antibodies against both the 1E10 vaccine itself and against the NeuGcGM3 ganglioside were produced in vaccinated patients. Of the 20 patients, 18 elicited an immune response against the vaccine and 16 produced an immune response against the ganglioside. The 1E10 antibodies, however, showed no success in inducing cell death and it was development of the anti-NeuGcGM2 antibodies that showed a distinct significance in patient survival. The median survival time of all patients on study was 10.6 months, but a dramatic improvement in survival was observed in patients who developed antibodies against NeuGcGM3 (median survival of 14.26 months) compared with those who did not (median survival 6.35 months). There were no significant advanced-grade side effects observed in the study.

■ SMALL CELL LUNG CANCER VACCINE DEVELOPMENT

Fucosyl GM1

The ganglioside fucosyl-GM1 is a carbohydrate molecule present in most cases of SCLC (178,179), but absent in normal lung tissue. Immunostaining has demonstrated the presence of fucosyl-GM1 in culture media from SCLC cell lines, in tumor extracts, and in serum of mouse xenografts (180). Fucosyl-GM1 was detected in the serum of 4 of 20 SCLC patients with extensive-stage disease, but was not present in the serum of 12 patients with non-SCLC or in 20 healthy volunteers (180). The specificity of fucosyl-GM1 to SCLC makes it a potential target for immunotherapy.

Dickler et al. (181) treated 13 patients with Fuc-GM1 isolated from bovine thyroid tissue; 10 patients completed the study and were evaluable. All 10 patients demonstrated high titers of IgM and IgG antibodies to Fuc-GM1. The most common toxicity was local skin reaction, lasting 2 to 5 days. Three of 6 patients who completed the entire course of vaccinations remained relapse free at 18, 24, and 30 months from diagnosis. Subsequently, Krug et al. (182) administered synthetic fucosyl-GM1 after conventional chemotherapy to 17 patients. Five of 6 patients at the high dose demonstrated increased levels of antifucosyl GM1 IgM. Three of 6 patients receiving the middle dose showed antifucosyl GM1 IgM production, and none of 5 patients at the low dose showed elevated IgM levels. Toxicities were minimal.

Recently, a new vaccine was synthesized which utilizes the fucosyl-GM1 molecule but has been altered to enhance immunogenicity. The investigators have incorporated an MHC-II binding site into the existing carbohydrate which should aid in its activation of T cells. In particular, the chosen sequence has the capacity to bind up to nine variants of the human HLA-DR. Clinical testing will be underway in the near future (183).

BEC2

Ganglioside GD3 is a cell surface glycosphingolipid with differential expression limited to cells of neuroectodermal origin and a subset of T lymphocytes (184–186). High levels of expression have been demonstrated in SCLC tumors and cell lines (187). Because GD3 is present at low levels in normal tissues, it is poorly immunogenic. BEC2, an anti-idiotypic IgG2b mouse antibody that is structurally similar to GD3, demonstrated strong immunogenic properties in patients with melanoma (188).

Grant et al. (189) treated 15 SCLC patients, 8 with extensive-stage and 7 with limited-stage disease, with BEC2 vaccination. Thirteen patients were evaluable for response; all developed IgM antibodies to BEC2, and 3 developed IgG antibodies. Duration of antibody production was variable, with at least 1 patient demonstrating measurable antibody production 1 year following treatment. Median survival was 20.5 months from diagnosis, and patients with measurable anti-GD3 antibodies showed the longest relapse-free intervals. When compared with SCLC patients treated with conventional therapy alone, the authors found patients treated with BEC2 vaccine to have longer than expected survival time, though not statistically significant. Significant toxicity was minimized to local skin irritation.

In a randomized, phase III study of BEC3 vaccine in combination with standard chemotherapy, 515 SCLC patients either received standard therapy plus vaccine or were randomized to standard treatment (190). Those randomized to the vaccination arm received five vaccinations of Bec2 (2.5 mg)/BCG cavvine over a 10-week period. The primary side effects were mild including transient skin ulcerations and mild flu-like symptoms.

The results did not show a clinical benefit, however. In fact, it was concluded that there was no improvement in survival, progression-free survival, or quality of life when receiving vaccine. Median survival was 14.3 months in vaccinated patients and 16.4 months in standard treatment patients.

PolySA

Polysialic acid (polySA) is found on the surface of Gram-negative bacteria (such as group B meningococcus), embryonic neural crest cells, and some malignancies of neural crest origin (191,192). The large size and negative charge of this molecule inhibit binding of cell adhesion molecules, and it is this property that is believed to contribute to its role in neural crest cell migration and early metastasis of malignant cells (193). PolySA has been shown to be expressed abundantly by SCLC tissues (194–197), making it a potentially viable target for SCLC vaccine therapy.

Krug et al. (198) investigated the immunogenicity of polySA vaccination in 11 SCLC patients following conventional therapy. Two forms of polySA were administered to patients. Five patients received vaccination with polySA, and 6 patients received polySA manipulated by N-propionylation (NP-polySA), which has been shown to boost the IgG response in mice (199). One of 5 patients treated with unmodified polySA demonstrated an IgM response. Of the 6 patients vaccinated with NP-polySA, all produced measurable IgM antibody responses. In five of the six cases these antibodies cross-reacted with unmodified polySA. Flow cytometry confirmed the presence of IgM antibodies reactive to SCLC cell lines. Despite the demonstrable production of IgM antibodies to polySA, complement-dependent lysis of polySA-positive tumor cells with human complement could not be demonstrated. The median survival of all patients receiving PolySA treatment was 22 months after the first vaccination. Common adverse effects were minimal and included injection-site reaction and flu-like symptoms lasting 2 to 4 days. Four patients reported sensory neuropathy.

Wilm's Tumor Gene

The Wilm's tumor gene (WT1) is responsible for Wilm's tumor, a pediatric renal cancer, and encodes a protein involved in cell proliferation and differentiation, apoptosis, and organ development (200–202). WT1 is overexpressed in several hematologic malignancies as well as various solid tumors, including lung, breast, thyroid, and colorectal cancers (203,204). WT1-specific cytotoxic lymphocytes (CTL) lyse WT1 expressing tumor cells in vitro without damaging normal tissues that express WT1 physiologically (205,206).

Oka et al. (207) treated 26 patients, including 10 lung cancer patients (histologic type not specified), with WT1 vaccine following completion of conventional therapy. Three NSCLC patients showed decreased serum levels of tumor markers (CEA or SLX) following vaccination; 1 patient also showed a radiographic decrease in tumor size. One NSCLC patient had stable disease at follow-up; 4 patients developed progressive disease, and 2 were unevaluable. Three patients demonstrated increased activity of WT1-specific CTL activity. A correlation ($P = 0.0397$) between immunological and clinical response was observed for all study patients.

CONCLUSION

In conclusion, several approaches to vaccine therapy in lung cancer demonstrate promise of clinical efficacy. All appear remarkably safe. Limitations include identification of sensitive subset patient populations and surrogate measures of relevant immune reactivity. Vaccines described in this review focus on different elements of immune reactivity (i.e., antigen exposure, dendritic activation, T-cell activation, inhibition of T regulatory cells, inhibition of TGF-β expression). Any one of these approaches has demonstrated evidence of activity in subsets of patients. However, phase III trials are required to determine conclusive relevance to lung cancer therapy. Data appear encouraging particularly in a setting of minimal disease early in the therapeutic course and at earlier stages of disease. It is also enticing to consider combinations of vaccines, particularly those with varied mechanisms of action. Future trials will undoubtedly explore combined vaccine approaches, or products with multiple immune-component modulation.

REFERENCES

1. Shankaran V, Ikeda H, Bruce AT, et al. IFNgamma and lymphocytes prevent primary tumour development and shape tumour immunogenicity. *Nature.* 2001;410(6832):1107–1111.
2. Bell JW. Possible immune factors in spontaneous regression of bronchogenic carcinoma. Ten year survival in a patient treated with minimal (1,200 r) radiation alone. *Am J Surg.* 1970;120(6):804–806.
3. Hanna N, Shepherd FA, Fossella FV, et al. Randomized phase III trial of pemetrexed versus docetaxel in patients with non-small-cell lung cancer previously treated with chemotherapy. *J Clin Oncol.* 2004;22(9):1589–1597.
4. Tsao MS, Sakurada A, Cutz JC, et al. Erlotinib in lung cancer - molecular and clinical predictors of outcome. *N Engl J Med.* 2005;353(2):133–144.
5. Shepherd FA, Rodrigues Pereira J, Ciuleanu T, et al.; National Cancer Institute of Canada Clinical Trials Group. Erlotinib in previously treated non-small-cell lung cancer. *N Engl J Med.* 2005;353(2):123–132.
6. Kris MG, Natale RB, Herbst RS, et al. Efficacy of gefitinib, an inhibitor of the epidermal growth factor receptor tyrosine kinase, in symptomatic patients with non-small cell lung cancer: a randomized trial. *JAMA.* 2003;290(16):2149–2158.
7. Nemunaitis J. Vaccines in cancer: GVAX, a GM-CSF gene vaccine. *Expert Rev Vaccines.* 2005;4(3):259–274.
8. Nemunaitis J, Sterman D, Jablons D, et al. Granulocyte-macrophage colony-stimulating factor gene-modified autologous tumor vaccines in non-small-cell lung cancer. *J Natl Cancer Inst.* 2004;96(4):326–331.
9. Fakhrai H, Gramatikova S, Safaei R. *Down-Regulation of TGF-beta 2 as a Therapeutic Approach In Brain Tumor Immunotherapy.* Totowa, NJ: Humana Press; 2001.
10. Dorigo O, Shawler DL, Royston I, Sobol RE, Berek JS, Fakhrai H. Combination of transforming growth factor beta antisense and interleukin-2 gene therapy in the murine ovarian teratoma model. *Gynecol Oncol.* 1998;71(2):204–210.
11. Tzai TS, Shiau AL, Liu LL, Wu CL. Immunization with TGF-beta antisense oligonucleotide-modified autologous tumor vaccine enhances the antitumor immunity of MBT-2 tumor-bearing

mice through upregulation of MHC class I and Fas expressions. *Anticancer Res.* 2000;20(3A):1557–1562.

12. Tzai TS, Lin CI, Shiau AL, Wu CL. Antisense oligonucleotide specific for transforming growth factor-beta 1 inhibit both *in vitro* and *in vivo* growth of MBT-2 murine bladder cancer. *Anticancer Res.* 1998;18(3A):1585–1589.

13. Marzo AL, Fitzpatrick DR, Robinson BW, Scott B. Antisense oligonucleotides specific for transforming growth factor beta2 inhibit the growth of malignant mesothelioma both *in vitro* and in vivo. *Cancer Res.* 1997;57(15):3200–3207.

14. Park JA, Wang E, Kurt RA, Schluter SF, Hersh EM, Akporiaye ET. Expression of an antisense transforming growth factor-beta1 transgene reduces tumorigenicity of EMT6 mammary tumor cells. *Cancer Gene Ther.* 1997;4(1):42–50.

15. Wei YQ, Hang ZB. In situ observation of lymphocyte-tumor cell interaction in human lung carcinoma. *Immunol Invest.* 1989;18(9–10):1095–1105.

16. Ruckdeschel JC, Codish SD, Stranahan A, McKneally MF. Postoperative empyema improves survival in lung cancer. Documentation and analysis of a natural experiment. *N Engl J Med.* 1972;287(20):1013–1017.

17. Gilboa E, Nair SK, Lyerly HK. Immunotherapy of cancer with dendritic-cell-based vaccines. *Cancer Immunol Immunother.* 1998;46(2):82–87.

18. Timmerman JM, Levy R. Dendritic cell vaccines for cancer immunotherapy. *Annu Rev Med.* 1999;50:507–529.

19. Conrad C, Nestle FO. Dendritic cell-based cancer therapy. *Curr Opin Mol Ther.* 2003;5(4):405–412.

20. Keilholz U, Weber J, Finke JH, et al. Immunologic monitoring of cancer vaccine therapy: results of a workshop sponsored by the Society for Biological Therapy. *J Immunother.* 2002;25(2):97–138.

21. Cranmer LD, Trevor KT, Hersh EM. Clinical applications of dendritic cell vaccination in the treatment of cancer. *Cancer Immunol Immunother.* 2004;53(4):275–306.

22. Banchereau J, Briere F, Caux C, et al. Immunobiology of dendritic cells. *Annu Rev Immunol.* 2000;18:767–811.

23. Germain RN. MHC-dependent antigen processing and peptide presentation: providing ligands for T lymphocyte activation. *Cell.* 1994;76(2):287–299.

24. McAdam AJ, Schweitzer AN, Sharpe AH. The role of B7 co-stimulation in activation and differentiation of CD4+ and CD8+ T cells. *Immunol Rev.* 1998;165:231–247.

25. Pulendran B, Smith JL, Caspary G, et al. Distinct dendritic cell subsets differentially regulate the class of immune response in vivo. *Proc Natl Acad Sci USA.* 1999;96(3):1036–1041.

26. Akbari O, DeKruyff RH, Umetsu DT. Pulmonary dendritic cells producing IL-10 mediate tolerance induced by respiratory exposure to antigen. *Nat Immunol.* 2001;2(8):725–731.

27. Woo EY, Yeh H, Chu CS, et al. Cutting edge: Regulatory T cells from lung cancer patients directly inhibit autologous T cell proliferation. *J Immunol.* 2002;168(9):4272–4276.

28. Woo EY, Chu CS, Goletz TJ, et al. Regulatory CD4(+)CD25(+) T cells in tumors from patients with early-stage non-small cell lung cancer and late-stage ovarian cancer. *Cancer Res.* 2001;61(12):4766–4772.

29. Neuner A, Schindel M, Wildenberg U, Muley T, Lahm H, Fischer JR. Prognostic significance of cytokine modulation in non-small cell lung cancer. *Int J Cancer.* 2002;101(3):287–292.

30. Neuner A, Schindel M, Wildenberg U, Muley T, Lahm H, Fischer JR. Cytokine secretion: clinical relevance of immunosuppression in non-small cell lung cancer. *Lung Cancer.* 2001;34(suppl 2):S79–S82.

31. Dohadwala M, Luo J, Zhu L, et al. Non-small cell lung cancer cyclooxygenase-2-dependent invasion is mediated by CD44. *J Biol Chem.* 2001;276(24):20809–20812.

32. Schwartz RH. Models of T cell anergy: is there a common molecular mechanism? *J Exp Med.* 1996;184(1):1–8.

33. Lombardi G, Sidhu S, Batchelor R, Lechler R. Anergic T cells as suppressor cells in vitro. *Science.* 1994;264(5165):1587–1589.

34. Ruffini PA, Rivoltini L, Silvani A, Boiardi A, Parmiani G. Factors, including transforming growth factor beta, released in the glioblastoma residual cavity, impair activity of adherent lymphokine-activated killer cells. *Cancer Immunol Immunother.* 1993;36(6):409–416.

35. Roszman T, Elliott L, Brooks W. Modulation of T-cell function by gliomas. *Immunol Today.* 1991;12(10):370–374.

36. Smith KA. Interleukin-2: inception, impact, and implications. *Science.* 1988;240(4856):1169–1176.

37. Smith KA. Lowest dose interleukin-2 immunotherapy. *Blood.* 1993;81(6):1414–1423.

38. Tigges MA, Casey LS, Koshland ME. Mechanism of interleukin-2 signaling: mediation of different outcomes by a single receptor and transduction pathway. *Science.* 1989;243(4892):781–786.

39. Rook AH, Kehrl JH, Wakefield LM, et al. Effects of transforming growth factor beta on the functions of natural killer cells: depressed cytolytic activity and blunting of interferon responsiveness. *J Immunol.* 1986;136(10):3916–3920.

40. Tsunawaki S, Sporn M, Ding A, Nathan C. Deactivation of macrophages by transforming growth factor-beta. *Nature.* 1988;334(6179):260–262.

41. Fontana A, Frei K, Bodmer S, et al. Transforming growth factor-beta inhibits the generation of cytotoxic T cells in virus-infected mice. *J Immunol.* 1989;143(10):3230–3234.

42. Hirte HW, Clark DA, O'Connell G, Rusthoven J, Mazurka J. Reversal of suppression of lymphokine-activated killer cells by transforming growth factor-beta in ovarian carcinoma ascitic fluid requires interleukin-2 combined with anti-CD3 antibody. *Cell Immunol.* 1992;142(1):207–216.

43. Ranges GE, Figari IS, Espevik T, Palladino MA Jr. Inhibition of cytotoxic T cell development by transforming growth factor beta and reversal by recombinant tumor necrosis factor alpha. *J Exp Med.* 1987;166(4):991–998.

44. Nemunaitis J, Dillman RO, Schwarzenberger PO, et al. Phase II study of belagenpumatucel-L, a transforming growth factor beta-2 antisense gene-modified allogeneic tumor cell vaccine in non-small-cell lung cancer. *J Clin Oncol.* 2006;24(29):4721–4730.

45. Sporn MB, Roberts AB, Wakefield LM, Assoian RK. Transforming growth factor-beta: biological function and chemical structure. *Science.* 1986;233(4763):532–534.

46. Massagué J. The TGF-beta family of growth and differentiation factors. *Cell.* 1987;49(4):437–438.

47. Border WA, Ruoslahti E. Transforming growth factor-beta in disease: the dark side of tissue repair. *J Clin Invest.* 1992;90(1):1–7.

48. Bodmer S, Strommer K, Frei K, et al. Immunosuppression and transforming growth factor-beta in glioblastoma. Preferential production of transforming growth factor-beta 2. *J Immunol.* 1989;143(10):3222–3229.

49. Jakowlew SB, Mathias A, Chung P, Moody TW. Expression of transforming growth factor beta ligand and receptor messenger RNAs in lung cancer cell lines. *Cell Growth Differ.* 1995;6(4):465–476.

50. Constam DB, Philipp J, Malipiero UV, ten Dijke P, Schachner M, Fontana A. Differential expression of transforming growth factor-beta 1, -beta 2, and -beta 3 by glioblastoma cells, astrocytes, and microglia. *J Immunol.* 1992;148(5):1404–1410.

51. Kong F, Jirtle RL, Huang DH, Clough RW, Anscher MS. Plasma transforming growth factor-beta1 level before radiotherapy correlates with long term outcome of patients with lung carcinoma. *Cancer.* 1999;86(9):1712–1719.

52. Kasid A, Bell GI, Director EP. Effects of transforming growth factor-beta on human lymphokine-activated killer cell precursors. Autocrine inhibition of cellular proliferation and differentiation to immune killer cells. *J Immunol.* 1988;141(2):690–698.

53. Hirte H, Clark DA. Generation of lymphokine-activated killer cells in human ovarian carcinoma ascitic fluid: identification of transforming growth factor-beta as a suppressive factor. *Cancer Immunol Immunother.* 1991;32(5):296–302.

54. Naganuma H, Sasaki A, Satoh E, et al. Transforming growth factor-beta inhibits interferon-gamma secretion by lymphokine-activated killer cells stimulated with tumor cells. *Neurol Med Chir (Tokyo)*. 1996;36(11):789–795.

55. Fakhrai H, Mantil JC, Liu L, et al. Phase I clinical trial of a TGF-beta antisense-modified tumor cell vaccine in patients with advanced glioma. *Cancer Gene Ther*. 2006;13(12):1052–1060.

56. Liau LM, Fakhrai H, Black KL. Prolonged survival of rats with intracranial C6 gliomas by treatment with TGF-beta antisense gene. *Neurol Res*. 1998;20(8):742–747.

57. Kettering JD, Mohamedali AM, Green LM, Gridley DS. IL-2 gene and antisense TGF-beta1 strategies counteract HSV-2 transformed tumor progression. *Technol Cancer Res Treat*. 2003;2(3):211–221.

58. Fakhrai H, Dorigo O, Shawler DL, et al. Eradication of established intracranial rat gliomas by transforming growth factor beta antisense gene therapy. *Proc Natl Acad Sci USA*. 1996;93(7):2909–2914.

59. Shepherd FA, Dancey J, Ramlau R, et al. Prospective randomized trial of docetaxel versus best supportive care in patients with non-small-cell lung cancer previously treated with platinum-based chemotherapy. *J Clin Oncol*. 2000;18(10):2095–2103.

60. Fossella FV, DeVore R, Kerr RN, et al. Randomized phase III trial of docetaxel versus vinorelbine or ifosfamide in patients with advanced non-small-cell lung cancer previously treated with platinum-containing chemotherapy regimens. The TAX 320 Non-Small Cell Lung Cancer Study Group. *J Clin Oncol*. 2000;18(12):2354–2362.

61. Nemunaitis J, Nemunaitis M, Senzer N, et al. Phase II trial of Belagenpumatucel-L, a TGF-beta2 antisense gene modified allogeneic tumor vaccine in advanced non small cell lung cancer (NSCLC) patients. *Cancer Gene Ther*. 2009;16(8):620–624.

62. Kim S, Buchlis G, Fridlender ZG, et al. Systemic blockade of transforming growth factor-beta signaling augments the efficacy of immunogene therapy. *Cancer Res*. 2008;68(24):10247–10256.

63. Liu P, Jaffar J, Zhou Y, Yang Y, Hellström I, Hellström KE. Inhibition of TGFbeta1 makes nonimmunogenic tumor cells effective for therapeutic vaccination. *J Immunother*. 2009;32(3):232–239.

64. Dranoff G, Jaffee E, Lazenby A, et al. Vaccination with irradiated tumor cells engineered to secrete murine granulocyte-macrophage colony-stimulating factor stimulates potent, specific, and long-lasting anti-tumor immunity. *Proc Natl Acad Sci USA*. 1993;90(8):3539–3543.

65. Scheffer SR, Nave H, Korangy F, et al. Apoptotic, but not necrotic, tumor cell vaccines induce a potent immune response in vivo. *Int J Cancer*. 2003;103(2):205–211.

66. Borrello I, Pardoll D. GM-CSF-based cellular vaccines: a review of the clinical experience. *Cytokine Growth Factor Rev*. 2002;13(2):185–193.

67. Jaffee EM, Thomas MC, Huang AY, Hauda KM, Levitsky HI, Pardoll DM. Enhanced immune priming with spatial distribution of paracrine cytokine vaccines. *J Immunother Emphasis Tumor Immunol*. 1996;19(3):176–183.

68. Couch M, Saunders JK, O'Malley BW Jr, Pardoll D, Jaffee E. Genetically engineered tumor cell vaccine in a head and neck cancer model. *Laryngoscope*. 2003;113(3):552–556.

69. Simons JW, Mikhak B, Chang JF, et al. Induction of immunity to prostate cancer antigens: results of a clinical trial of vaccination with irradiated autologous prostate tumor cells engineered to secrete granulocyte-macrophage colony-stimulating factor using ex vivo gene transfer. *Cancer Res*. 1999;59(20):5160–5168.

70. Soiffer R, Lynch T, Mihm M, et al. Vaccination with irradiated autologous melanoma cells engineered to secrete human granulocyte-macrophage colony-stimulating factor generates potent antitumor immunity in patients with metastatic melanoma. *Proc Natl Acad Sci USA*. 1998;95(22):13141–13146.

71. Simons JW, Jaffee EM, Weber CE, et al. Bioactivity of autologous irradiated renal cell carcinoma vaccines generated by ex vivo granulocyte-macrophage colony-stimulating factor gene transfer. *Cancer Res*. 1997;57(8):1537–1546.

72. Jaffee EM, Hruban RH, Biedrzycki B, et al. Novel allogeneic granulocyte-macrophage colony-stimulating factor-secreting tumor vaccine for pancreatic cancer: a phase I trial of safety and immune activation. *J Clin Oncol*. 2001;19(1):145–156.

73. Salgia R, Lynch T, Skarin A, et al. Vaccination with irradiated autologous tumor cells engineered to secrete granulocyte-macrophage colony-stimulating factor augments antitumor immunity in some patients with metastatic non-small-cell lung carcinoma. *J Clin Oncol*. 2003;21(4):624–630.

74. Soiffer R, Hodi FS, Haluska F, et al. Vaccination with irradiated, autologous melanoma cells engineered to secrete granulocyte-macrophage colony-stimulating factor by adenoviral-mediated gene transfer augments antitumor immunity in patients with metastatic melanoma. *J Clin Oncol*. 2003;21(17):3343–3350.

75. Nemunaitis J, Jahan T, Ross H, et al. Phase ½ trial of autologous tumor mixed with an allogeneic GVAX vaccine in advanced-stage non-small-cell lung cancer. *Cancer Gene Ther*. 2006;13(6):555–562.

76. Ishikawa E, Motohashi S, Ishikawa A, et al. Dendritic cell maturation by CD11c- T cells and Valpha24+ natural killer T-cell activation by alpha-galactosylceramide. *Int J Cancer*. 2005;117(2):265–273.

77. Motohashi S, Nagato K, Kunii N, et al. A phase I-II study of alpha-galactosylceramide-pulsed IL-2/GM-CSF-cultured peripheral blood mononuclear cells in patients with advanced and recurrent non-small cell lung cancer. *J Immunol*. 2009;182(4):2492–2501.

78. Kufe D, Inghirami G, Abe M, Hayes D, Justi-Wheeler H, Schlom J. Differential reactivity of a novel monoclonal antibody (DF3) with human malignant versus benign breast tumors. *Hybridoma*. 1984;3(3):223–232.

79. Burchell J, Gendler S, Taylor-Papadimitriou J, et al. Development and characterization of breast cancer reactive monoclonal antibodies directed to the core protein of the human milk mucin. *Cancer Res*. 1987;47(20):5476–5482.

80. Gendler SJ, Lancaster CA, Taylor-Papadimitriou J, et al. Molecular cloning and expression of human tumor-associated polymorphic epithelial mucin. *J Biol Chem*. 1990;265(25):15286–15293.

81. Li Y, Liu D, Chen D, Kharbanda S, Kufe D. Human DF3/MUC1 carcinoma-associated protein functions as an oncogene. *Oncogene*. 2003;22(38):6107–6110.

82. Ren J, Agata N, Chen D, et al. Human MUC1 carcinoma-associated protein confers resistance to genotoxic anticancer agents. *Cancer Cell*. 2004;5(2):163–175.

83. MacLean GD, Reddish MA, Koganty RR, Longenecker BM. Antibodies against mucin-associated sialyl-Tn epitopes correlate with survival of metastatic adenocarcinoma patients undergoing active specific immunotherapy with synthetic STn vaccine. *J Immunother Emphasis Tumor Immunol*. 1996;19(1):59–68.

84. Butts C, Murray N, Maksymiuk A, et al. Randomized phase IIB trial of BLP25 liposome vaccine in stage IIIB and IV non-small-cell lung cancer. *J Clin Oncol*. 2005;23(27):6674–6681.

85. Slodkowska J, Szturmowicz M, Rudzinski P, et al. Expression of CEA and trophoblastic cell markers by lung carcinoma in association with histological characteristics and serum marker levels. *Eur J Cancer Prev*. 1998;7(1):51–60.

86. Fijolek J, Wiatr E, Rowinska-Zakrzewska E, et al. p53 and HER2/neu expression in relation to chemotherapy response in patients with non-small cell lung cancer. *Int J Biol Markers*. 2006;21(2):81–87.

87. Tsao MS, Aviel-Ronen S, Ding K, et al. Prognostic and predictive importance of p53 and RAS for adjuvant chemotherapy in non small-cell lung cancer. *J Clin Oncol*. 2007;25(33):5240–5247.

88. Brabender J, Danenberg KD, Metzger R, et al. Epidermal growth factor receptor and HER2-neu mRNA expression in non-small cell lung cancer Is correlated with survival. *Clin Cancer Res*. 2001;7(7):1850–1855.

89. Vallböhmer D, Brabender J, Yang DY, et al. Sex differences in the predictive power of the molecular prognostic factor HER2/neu in patients with non-small-cell lung cancer. *Clin Lung Cancer.* 2006;7(5):332–337.

90. Sienel W, Varwerk C, Linder A, et al. Melanoma associated antigen (MAGE)-A3 expression in Stages I and II non-small cell lung cancer: results of a multi-center study. *Eur J Cardiothorac Surg.* 2004;25(1):131–134.

91. Marshall JL, Hoyer RJ, Toomey MA, et al. Phase I study in advanced cancer patients of a diversified prime-and-boost vaccination protocol using recombinant vaccinia virus and recombinant nonreplicating avipox virus to elicit anti-carcinoembryonic antigen immune responses. *J Clin Oncol.* 2000;18(23):3964–3973.

92. Fong L, Hou Y, Rivas A, et al. Altered peptide ligand vaccination with Flt3 ligand expanded dendritic cells for tumor immunotherapy. *Proc Natl Acad Sci USA.* 2001;98(15):8809–8814.

93. Knutson KL, Schiffman K, Disis ML. Immunization with a HER-2/neu helper peptide vaccine generates HER-2/neu CD8 T-cell immunity in cancer patients. *J Clin Invest.* 2001;107(4):477–484.

94. Rosenberg SA, Yang JC, Schwartzentruber DJ, et al. Immunologic and therapeutic evaluation of a synthetic peptide vaccine for the treatment of patients with metastatic melanoma. *Nat Med.* 1998;4(3):321–327.

95. Arlen P, Tsang KY, Marshall JL, et al. The use of a rapid ELISPOT assay to analyze peptide-specific immune responses in carcinoma patients to peptide vs. recombinant poxvirus vaccines. *Cancer Immunol Immunother.* 2000;49(10):517–529.

96. Hörig H, Lee DS, Conkright W, et al. Phase I clinical trial of a recombinant canarypoxvirus (ALVAC) vaccine expressing human carcinoembryonic antigen and the B7.1 co-stimulatory molecule. *Cancer Immunol Immunother.* 2000;49(9):504–514.

97. Vierboom MP, Nijman HW, Offringa R, et al. Tumor eradication by wild-type p53-specific cytotoxic T lymphocytes. *J Exp Med.* 1997;186(5):695–704.

98. Vierboom MP, Bos GM, Ooms M, Offringa R, Melief CJ. Cyclophosphamide enhances anti-tumor effect of wild-type p53-specific CTL. *Int J Cancer.* 2000;87(2):253–260.

99. Rosenwirth B, Kuhn EM, Heeney JL, et al. Safety and immunogenicity of ALVAC wild-type human p53 (vCP207) by the intravenous route in rhesus macaques. *Vaccine.* 2001;19(13–14):1661–1670.

100. van der Burg SH, de Cock K, Menon AG, et al. Long lasting p53-specific T cell memory responses in the absence of anti-p53 antibodies in patients with resected primary colorectal cancer. *Eur J Immunol.* 2001;31(1):146–155.

101. Ferriès E, Connan F, Pagès F, et al. Identification of p53 peptides recognized by CD8(+) T lymphocytes from patients with bladder cancer. *Hum Immunol.* 2001;62(8):791–798.

102. Tartaglia J, Bonnet MC, Berinstein N, Barber B, Klein M, Moingeon P. Therapeutic vaccines against melanoma and colorectal cancer. *Vaccine.* 2001;19(17–19):2571–2575.

103. An open label study of a peptide vaccine in patients with Stage IIB or IIIA non-small cell lung cancer, www.clinicaltrials.gov, July 2010.

104. van der Bruggen P, Traversari C, Chomez P, et al. A gene encoding an antigen recognized by cytolytic T lymphocytes on a human melanoma. *Science.* 1991;254(5038):1643–1647.

105. Thurner B, Haendle I, Röder C, et al. Vaccination with mage-3A1 peptide-pulsed mature, monocyte-derived dendritic cells expands specific cytotoxic T cells and induces regression of some metastases in advanced stage IV melanoma. *J Exp Med.* 1999;190(11):1669–1678.

106. Weber JS, Hua FL, Spears L, Marty V, Kuniyoshi C, Celis E. A phase I trial of an HLA-A1 restricted MAGE-3 epitope peptide with incomplete Freund's adjuvant in patients with resected high-risk melanoma. *J Immunother.* 1999;22(5):431–440.

107. Coulie PG, Karanikas V, Colau D, et al. A monoclonal cytolytic T-lymphocyte response observed in a melanoma patient vaccinated with a tumor-specific antigenic peptide encoded by gene MAGE-3. *Proc Natl Acad Sci USA.* 2001;98(18):10290–10295.

108. Banchereau J, Palucka AK, Dhodapkar M, et al. Immune and clinical responses in patients with metastatic melanoma to CD34(+) progenitor-derived dendritic cell vaccine. *Cancer Res.* 2001;61(17):6451–6458.

109. Slamon DJ, Godolphin W, Jones LA, et al. Studies of the HER-2/neu proto-oncogene in human breast and ovarian cancer. *Science.* 1989;244(4905):707–712.

110. Disis ML, Calenoff E, McLaughlin G, et al. Existent T-cell and antibody immunity to HER-2/neu protein in patients with breast cancer. *Cancer Res.* 1994;54(1):16–20.

111. Alexander J, Sidney J, Southwood S, et al. Development of high potency universal DR-restricted helper epitopes by modification of high affinity DR-blocking peptides. *Immunity.* 1994;1(9):751–761.

112. Barve M, Bender J, Senzer N, et al. Induction of immune responses and clinical efficacy in a phase II trial of IDM-2101, a 10-epitope cytotoxic T-lymphocyte vaccine, in metastatic non-small-cell lung cancer. *J Clin Oncol.* 2008;26(27):4418–4425.

113. Ishioka GY, Disis ML, Morse MA, et al. Multi-epitope CTL responses induced by a peptide vaccine (EP-2101) in colon and non-small cell lung cancer patients [abstract]. *J Immunother* 2004;27(6):S23–S4.

114. Antonia SJ, Seigne J, Diaz J, et al. Phase I trial of a B7-1 (CD80) gene modified autologous tumor cell vaccine in combination with systemic interleukin-2 in patients with metastatic renal cell carcinoma. *J Urol.* 2002;167(5):1995–2000.

115. Hull GW, Mccurdy MA, Nasu Y, et al. Prostate cancer gene therapy: comparison of adenovirus-mediated expression of interleukin 12 with interleukin 12 plus B7-1 for in situ gene therapy and gene-modified, cell-based vaccines. *Clin Cancer Res.* 2000;6(10):4101–4109.

116. von Mehren M, Arlen P, Tsang KY, et al. Pilot study of a dual gene recombinant avipox vaccine containing both carcinoembryonic antigen (CEA) and B7.1 transgenes in patients with recurrent CEA-expressing adenocarcinomas. *Clin Cancer Res.* 2000;6(6):2219–2228.

117. Johnston JV, Malacko AR, Mizuno MT, et al. B7-CD28 costimulation unveils the hierarchy of tumor epitopes recognized by major histocompatibility complex class I-restricted CD8+ cytolytic T lymphocytes. *J Exp Med.* 1996;183(3):791–800.

118. Liu B, Podack ER, Allison JP, Malek TR. Generation of primary tumor-specific CTL *in vitro* to immunogenic and poorly immunogenic mouse tumors. *J Immunol.* 1996;156(3):1117–1125.

119. Nabel GJ, Gordon D, Bishop DK, et al. Immune response in human melanoma after transfer of an allogeneic class I major histocompatibility complex gene with DNA-liposome complexes. *Proc Natl Acad Sci USA.* 1996;93(26):15388–15393.

120. Yamazaki K, Spruill G, Rhoderick J, Spielman J, Savaraj N, Podack ER. Small cell lung carcinomas express shared and private tumor antigens presented by HLA-A1 or HLA-A2. *Cancer Res.* 1999;59(18):4642–4650.

121. Raez LE, Cassileth PA, Schlesselman JJ, et al. Allogeneic vaccination with a B7.1 HLA-A gene-modified adenocarcinoma cell line in patients with advanced non-small-cell lung cancer. *J Clin Oncol.* 2004;22(14):2800–2807.

122. Raez LE, Santos ES, Mudad R, Podack ER. Clinical trials targeting lung cancer with active immunotherapy: the scope of vaccines. *Expert Rev Anticancer Ther.* 2005;5(4):635–644.

123. Mueller-Pillasch F, Pohl B, Wilda M, et al. Expression of the highly conserved RNA binding protein KOC in embryogenesis. *Mech Dev.* 1999;88(1):95–99.

124. Aguiar JC, Hedstrom RC, Rogers WO, et al. Enhancement of the immune response in rabbits to a malaria DNA vaccine by immunization with a needle-free jet device. *Vaccine.* 2001;20(1–2):275–280.

125. Nemunaitis J, Meyers T, Senzer N, et al. Phase I Trial of sequential administration of recombinant DNA and adenovirus expressing L523S protein in early stage non-small-cell lung cancer. *Mol Ther.* 2006;13(6):1185–1191.

126. Ramos TC, Vinageras EN, Ferrer MC, et al. Treatment of NSCLC patients with an EGF-based cancer vaccine: report of a Phase I trial. *Cancer Biol Ther*. 2006;5(2):145–149.

127. González G, Crombet T, Catalá M, et al. A novel cancer vaccine composed of human-recombinant epidermal growth factor linked to a carrier protein: report of a pilot clinical trial. *Ann Oncol*. 1998;9(4):431–435.

128. Gonzalez G, Crombet T, Torres F, et al. Epidermal growth factor-based cancer vaccine for non-small-cell lung cancer therapy. *Ann Oncol*. 2003;14(3):461–466.

129. Neninger Vinageras E, de la Torre A, Osorio Rodríguez M, et al. Phase II randomized controlled trial of an epidermal growth factor vaccine in advanced non-small-cell lung cancer. *J Clin Oncol*. 2008;26(9):1452–1458.

130. Neninger E, Verdecia BG, Crombet T, et al. Combining an EGF-based cancer vaccine with chemotherapy in advanced nonsmall cell lung cancer. *J Immunother*. 2009;32(1):92–99.

131. Van den Eynde BJ, van der Bruggen P. T cell defined tumor antigens. *Curr Opin Immunol*. 1997;9(5):684–693.

132. Herman J, van der Bruggen P, Luescher IF, et al. A peptide encoded by the human MAGE3 gene and presented by HLA-B44 induces cytolytic T lymphocytes that recognize tumor cells expressing MAGE3. *Immunogenetics*. 1996;43(6):377–383.

133. Fleischhauer K, Fruci D, Van Endert P, et al. Characterization of antigenic peptides presented by HLA-B44 molecules on tumor cells expressing the gene MAGE-3. *Int J Cancer*. 1996;68(5):622–628.

134. Tanaka F, Fujie T, Tahara K, et al. Induction of antitumor cytotoxic T lymphocytes with a MAGE-3-encoded synthetic peptide presented by human leukocytes antigen-A24. *Cancer Res*. 1997;57(20):4465–4468.

135. Kawashima I, Hudson SJ, Tsai V, et al. The multi-epitope approach for immunotherapy for cancer: identification of several CTL epitopes from various tumor-associated antigens expressed on solid epithelial tumors. *Hum Immunol*. 1998;59(1):1–14.

136. Oiso M, Eura M, Katsura F, et al. A newly identified MAGE-3-derived epitope recognized by HLA-A24-restricted cytotoxic T lymphocytes. *Int J Cancer*. 1999;81(3):387–394.

137. Tanzarella S, Russo V, Lionello I, et al. Identification of a promiscuous T-cell epitope encoded by multiple members of the MAGE family. *Cancer Res*. 1999;59(11):2668–2674.

138. Russo V, Tanzarella S, Dalerba P, et al. Dendritic cells acquire the MAGE-3 human tumor antigen from apoptotic cells and induce a class I-restricted T cell response. *Proc Natl Acad Sci USA*. 2000;97(5):2185–2190.

139. Keogh E, Fikes J, Southwood S, Celis E, Chesnut R, Sette A. Identification of new epitopes from four different tumor-associated antigens: recognition of naturally processed epitopes correlates with HLA-A*0201-binding affinity. *J Immunol*. 2001;167(2):787–796.

140. Schultz ES, Chapiro J, Lurquin C, et al. The production of a new MAGE-3 peptide presented to cytolytic T lymphocytes by HLA-B40 requires the immunoproteasome. *J Exp Med*. 2002;195(4):391–399.

141. Gaugler B, Van den Eynde B, van der Bruggen P, et al. Human gene MAGE-3 codes for an antigen recognized on a melanoma by autologous cytolytic T lymphocytes. *J Exp Med*. 1994;179(3):921–930.

142. van der Bruggen P, Bastin J, Gajewski T, et al. A peptide encoded by human gene MAGE-3 and presented by HLA-A2 induces cytolytic T lymphocytes that recognize tumor cells expressing MAGE-3. *Eur J Immunol*. 1994;24(12):3038–3043.

143. Marchand M, van Baren N, Weynants P, et al. Tumor regressions observed in patients with metastatic melanoma treated with an antigenic peptide encoded by gene MAGE-3 and presented by HLA-A1. *Int J Cancer*. 1999;80(2):219–230.

144. Atanackovic D, Altorki NK, Stockert E, et al. Vaccine-induced CD4+ T cell responses to MAGE-3 protein in lung cancer patients. *J Immunol*. 2004;172(5):3289–3296.

145. Halmos BH. Lung cancer II. ASCO Annual Meeting Summaries 2006:156–60.

146. GSK1572932A Antigen-specific cancer immunotherapeutic as adjuvant therapy in patients with non-small cell lung cancer. www.clinicaltrials.gov, July 2010.

147. Vonderheide RH, Hahn WC, Schultze JL, Nadler LM. The telomerase catalytic subunit is a widely expressed tumor-associated antigen recognized by cytotoxic T lymphocytes. *Immunity*. 1999;10(6):673–679.

148. Minev B, Hipp J, Firat H, Schmidt JD, Langlade-Demoyen P, Zanetti M. Cytotoxic T cell immunity against telomerase reverse transcriptase in humans. *Proc Natl Acad Sci USA*. 2000;97(9):4796–4801.

149. Vonderheide RH, Anderson KS, Hahn WC, Butler MO, Schultze JL, Nadler LM. Characterization of HLA-A3-restricted cytotoxic T lymphocytes reactive against the widely expressed tumor antigen telomerase. *Clin Cancer Res*. 2001;7(11):3343–3348.

150. Arai J, Yasukawa M, Ohminami H, Kakimoto M, Hasegawa A, Fujita S. Identification of human telomerase reverse transcriptase-derived peptides that induce HLA-A24-restricted antileukemia cytotoxic T lymphocytes. *Blood*. 2001;97(9):2903–2907.

151. Hernandez J, Garcia-Pons F, Lone YC, et al. Identification of a human telomerase reverse transcriptase peptide of low affinity for HLA A2.1 that induces cytotoxic T lymphocytes and mediates lysis of tumor cells. *Proc Natl Acad Sci USA*. 2002;99(19):12275–12280.

152. Scardino A, Gross DA, Alves P, et al. HER-2/neu and hTERT cryptic epitopes as novel targets for broad spectrum tumor immunotherapy. *J Immunol*. 2002;168(11):5900–5906.

153. Gross DA, Graff-Dubois S, Opolon P, et al. High vaccination efficiency of low-affinity epitopes in antitumor immunotherapy. *J Clin Invest*. 2004;113(3):425–433.

154. Schroers R, Huang XF, Hammer J, Zhang J, Chen SY. Identification of HLA DR7-restricted epitopes from human telomerase reverse transcriptase recognized by CD4+ T-helper cells. *Cancer Res*. 2002;62(9):2600–2605.

155. Schroers R, Shen L, Rollins L, et al. Human telomerase reverse transcriptase-specific T-helper responses induced by promiscuous major histocompatibility complex class II-restricted epitopes. *Clin Cancer Res*. 2003;9(13):4743–4755.

156. Uchida N, Otsuka T, Shigematsu H, et al. Differential gene expression of human telomerase-associated protein hTERT and TEP1 in human hematopoietic cells. *Leuk Res*. 1999;23(12):1127–1132.

157. Tahara H, Yasui W, Tahara E, et al. Immuno-histochemical detection of human telomerase catalytic component, hTERT, in human colorectal tumor and non-tumor tissue sections. *Oncogene*. 1999;18(8):1561–1567.

158. Shepherd F, Carney D. *Textbook of Lung Cancer*, London, Martin Dunitz Ltd. for International Association for the Study of Lung Cancer, Hansen HH (Ed.), 2000.

159. Brunsvig PF, Aamdal S, Gjertsen MK, et al. Telomerase peptide vaccination: a phase I/II study in patients with non-small cell lung cancer. *Cancer Immunol Immunother*. 2006;55(12):1553–1564.

160. Zitvogel L, Regnault A, Lozier A, et al. Eradication of established murine tumors using a novel cell-free vaccine: dendritic cell-derived exosomes. *Nat Med*. 1998;4(5):594–600.

161. Théry C, Duban L, Segura E, Véron P, Lantz O, Amigorena S. Indirect activation of naïve CD4+ T cells by dendritic cell-derived exosomes. *Nat Immunol*. 2002;3(12):1156–1162.

162. Théry C, Regnault A, Garin J, et al. Molecular characterization of dendritic cell-derived exosomes. Selective accumulation of the heat shock protein hsc73. *J Cell Biol*. 1999;147(3):599–610.

163. Raposo G, Nijman HW, Stoorvogel W, et al. B lymphocytes secrete antigen-presenting vesicles. *J Exp Med*. 1996;183(3):1161–1172.

164. Denzer K, van Eijk M, Kleijmeer MJ, Jakobson E, de Groot C, Geuze HJ. Follicular dendritic cells carry MHC class II-expressing microvesicles at their surface. *J Immunol*. 2000;165(3):1259–1265.

165. Hsu DH, Paz P, Villaflor G, et al. Exosomes as a tumor vaccine: enhancing potency through direct loading of antigenic peptides. *J Immunother*. 2003;26(5):440–450.

166. Morse MA, Garst J, Osada T, et al. A phase I study of dexosome immunotherapy in patients with advanced non-small cell lung cancer. *J Transl Med.* 2005;3(1):9.

167. Link CJ Jr, Seregina T, Atchison R, Hall A, Muldoon R, Levy JP. Eliciting hyperacute xenograft response to treat human cancer: alpha(1,3) galactosyltransferase gene therapy. *Anticancer Res.* 1998;18(4A):2301–2308.

168. Morris JC, Vahanian, N, Janik, JE. Phase I study of an anti-tumor vaccination using α(1,3)galactosyltransferase expressing allogeneic tumor cells in patients (Pts) with refractory or recurrent non-small cell lung cancer (NSCLC). ASCO Annual Meeting Proceedings. *J Clin Oncol.* 2005;23(No. 16S, Part I of II, June 1 suppl):2586.

169. Hirschowitz EA, Foody T, Kryscio R, Dickson L, Sturgill J, Yannelli J. Autologous dendritic cell vaccines for non-small-cell lung cancer. *J Clin Oncol.* 2004;22(14):2808–2815.

170. Mayordomo JI, Andres R, Isla MD, et al. Results of a pilot trial of immunotherapy with dendritic cells pulsed with autologous tumor lysates in patients with advanced cancer. *Tumori.* 2007;93(1):26–30.

171. Kimura H, Iizasa T, Ishikawa A, et al. Prospective phase II study of post-surgical adjuvant chemo-immunotherapy using autologous dendritic cells and activated killer cells from tissue culture of tumor-draining lymph nodes in primary lung cancer patients. *Anticancer Res.* 2008;28(2B):1229–1238.

172. Price ER, Zydowsky LD, Jin MJ, Baker CH, McKeon FD, Walsh CT. Human cyclophilin B: a second cyclophilin gene encodes a peptidyl-prolyl isomerase with a signal sequence. *Proc Natl Acad Sci USA.* 1991;88(5):1903–1907.

173. Bergsma DJ, Eder C, Gross M, et al. The cyclophilin multigene family of peptidyl-prolyl isomerases. Characterization of three separate human isoforms. *J Biol Chem.* 1991;266(34):23204–23214.

174. Gomi S, Nakao M, Niiya F, et al. A cyclophilin B gene encodes antigenic epitopes recognized by HLA-A24-restricted and tumor-specific CTLs. *J Immunol.* 1999;163(9):4994–5004.

175. Gohara R, Imai N, Rikimaru T, et al. Phase 1 clinical study of cyclophilin B peptide vaccine for patients with lung cancer. *J Immunother.* 2002;25(5):439–444.

176. de Leòn J, Fernández A, Mesa C, Clavel M, Fernández LE. Role of tumour-associated N-glycolylated variant of GM3 ganglioside in cancer progression: effect over CD4 expression on T cells. *Cancer Immunol Immunother.* 2006;55(4):443–450.

177. Hernández AM, Toledo D, Martínez D, et al. Characterization of the antibody response against NeuGcGM3 ganglioside elicited in non-small cell lung cancer patients immunized with an anti-idiotype antibody. *J Immunol.* 2008;181(9):6625–6634.

178. Brezicka FT, Olling S, Nilsson O, et al. Immunohistological detection of fucosyl-GM1 ganglioside in human lung cancer and normal tissues with monoclonal antibodies. *Cancer Res.* 1989;49(5):1300–1305.

179. Brezicka T, Bergman B, Olling S, Fredman P. Reactivity of monoclonal antibodies with ganglioside antigens in human small cell lung cancer tissues. *Lung Cancer.* 2000;28(1):29–36.

180. Vangsted AJ, Clausen H, Kjeldsen TB, et al. Immunochemical detection of a small cell lung cancer-associated ganglioside (FucGM1) antigen in serum. *Cancer Res.* 1991;51(11):2879–2884.

181. Dickler MN, Ragupathi G, Liu NX, et al. Immunogenicity of a fucosyl-GM1-keyhole limpet hemocyanin conjugate vaccine in patients with small cell lung cancer. *Clin Cancer Res.* 1999;5(10):2773–2779.

182. Krug LM, Ragupathi G, Hood C, et al. Vaccination of patients with small-cell lung cancer with synthetic fucosyl GM-1 conjugated to keyhole limpet hemocyanin. *Clin Cancer Res.* 2004;10(18 Pt 1):6094–6100.

183. Nagorny P, Kim WH, Wan Q, Lee D, Danishefsky SJ. On the emerging role of chemistry in the fashioning of biologics: synthesis of a bidomainal fucosyl GM1-based vaccine for the treatment of small cell lung cancer. *J Org Chem.* 2009;74(15):5157–5162.

184. Graus F, Cordon-Cardo C, Houghton AN, Melamed MR, Old LJ. Distribution of the ganglioside GD3 in the human nervous system detected by R24 mouse monoclonal antibody. *Brain Res.* 1984;324(1):190–194.

185. Dippold WG, Dienes HP, Knuth A, Meyer zum Büschenfelde KH. Immunohistochemical localization of ganglioside GD3 in human malignant melanoma, epithelial tumors, and normal tissues. *Cancer Res.* 1985;45(8):3699–3705.

186. Welte K, Miller G, Chapman PB, et al. Stimulation of T lymphocyte proliferation by monoclonal antibodies against GD3 ganglioside. *J Immunol.* 1987;139(6):1763–1771.

187. Fuentes R, Allman R, Mason MD. Ganglioside expression in lung cancer cell lines. *Lung Cancer.* 1997;18(1):21–33.

188. McCaffery M, Yao TJ, Williams L, Livingston PO, Houghton AN, Chapman PB. Immunization of melanoma patients with BEC2 anti-idiotypic monoclonal antibody that mimics GD3 ganglioside: enhanced immunogenicity when combined with adjuvant. *Clin Cancer Res.* 1996;2(4):679–686.

189. Grant SC, Kris MG, Houghton AN, Chapman PB. Long survival of patients with small cell lung cancer after adjuvant treatment with the anti-idiotypic antibody BEC2 plus Bacillus Calmette-Guérin. *Clin Cancer Res.* 1999;5(6):1319–1323.

190. Giaccone G, Debruyne C, Felip E, et al. Phase III study of adjuvant vaccination with Bec2/bacille Calmette-Guerin in responding patients with limited-disease small-cell lung cancer (European Organisation for Research and Treatment of Cancer 08971–08971B; Silva Study). *J Clin Oncol.* 2005;23(28):6854–6864.

191. Rutishauser U. Polysialic acid at the cell surface: biophysics in service of cell interactions and tissue plasticity. *J Cell Biochem.* 1998;70(3):304–312.

192. Finne J, Finne U, Deagostini-Bazin H, Goridis C. Occurrence of alpha 2–8 linked polysialosyl units in a neural cell adhesion molecule. *Biochem Biophys Res Commun.* 1983;112(2):482–487.

193. Rutishauser U, Landmesser L. Polysialic acid in the vertebrate nervous system: a promoter of plasticity in cell-cell interactions. *Trends Neurosci.* 1996;19(10):422–427.

194. Daniel L, Trouillas J, Renaud W, et al. Polysialylated-neural cell adhesion molecule expression in rat pituitary transplantable tumors (spontaneous mammotropic transplantable tumor in Wistar-Furth rats) is related to growth rate and malignancy. *Cancer Res.* 2000;60(1):80–85.

195. Komminoth P, Roth J, Lackie PM, Bitter-Suermann D, Heitz PU. Polysialic acid of the neural cell adhesion molecule distinguishes small cell lung carcinoma from carcinoids. *Am J Pathol.* 1991;139(2):297–304.

196. Lantuejoul S, Moro D, Michalides RJ, Brambilla C, Brambilla E. Neural cell adhesion molecules (NCAM) and NCAM-PSA expression in neuroendocrine lung tumors. *Am J Surg Pathol.* 1998;22(10):1267–1276.

197. Zhang S, Cordon-Cardo C, Zhang HS, et al. Selection of tumor antigens as targets for immune attack using immunohistochemistry: I. Focus on gangliosides. *Int J Cancer.* 1997;73(1):42–49.

198. Krug LM, Ragupathi G, Ng KK, et al. Vaccination of small cell lung cancer patients with polysialic acid or N-propionylated polysialic acid conjugated to keyhole limpet hemocyanin. *Clin Cancer Res.* 2004;10(3):916–923.

199. Jennings HJ, Roy R, Gamian A. Induction of meningococcal group B polysaccharide-specific IgG antibodies in mice by using an N-propionylated B polysaccharide-tetanus toxoid conjugate vaccine. *J Immunol.* 1986;137(5):1708–1713.

200. Drummond IA, Madden SL, Rohwer-Nutter P, Bell GI, Sukhatme VP, Rauscher FJ 3rd. Repression of the insulin-like growth factor II gene by the Wilms tumor suppressor WT1. *Science.* 1992;257(5070):674–678.

201. Goodyer P, Dehbi M, Torban E, Bruening W, Pelletier J. Repression of the retinoic acid receptor-alpha gene by the Wilms' tumor suppressor gene product, wt1. *Oncogene.* 1995;10(6):1125–1129.

202. Hewitt SM, Hamada S, McDonnell TJ, Rauscher FJ 3rd, Saunders GF. Regulation of the proto-oncogenes bcl-2 and c-myc by the Wilms' tumor suppressor gene WT1. *Cancer Res.* 1995;55(22):5386–5389.

203. Oji Y, Miyoshi S, Maeda H, et al. Overexpression of the Wilms' tumor gene WT1 in de novo lung cancers. *Int J Cancer.* 2002;100(3):297–303.

204. Miyoshi Y, Ando A, Egawa C, et al. High expression of Wilms' tumor suppressor gene predicts poor prognosis in breast cancer patients. *Clin Cancer Res.* 2002;8(5):1167–1171.

205. Oka Y, Elisseeva OA, Tsuboi A, et al. Human cytotoxic T-lymphocyte responses specific for peptides of the wild-type Wilms' tumor gene (WT1) product. *Immunogenetics.* 2000;51(2):99–107.

206. Ohminami H, Yasukawa M, Fujita S. HLA class I-restricted lysis of leukemia cells by a CD8(+) cytotoxic T-lymphocyte clone specific for WT1 peptide. *Blood.* 2000;95(1):286–293.

207. Oka Y, Tsuboi A, Taguchi T, et al. Induction of WT1 (Wilms' tumor gene)-specific cytotoxic T lymphocytes by WT1 peptide vaccine and the resultant cancer regression. *Proc Natl Acad Sci USA.* 2004;101(38):13885–13890.

25 Multidisciplinary Approach to Palliative and Symptom Management of Disease

BETTY FERRELL

MARIANNA KOCZYWAS

Cancer and its treatments cause considerable symptom burden for individuals diagnosed with lung cancer. Throughout the disease trajectory, patients frequently suffer from complex disease- and treatment-related symptoms. These often debilitating symptoms negatively affect the quality of life (QOL) of patients. Despite the recognition of the symptom burden and impaired QOL in cancer patients, optimal symptom management and palliative care is often lacking. Furthermore, use of patient-reported outcomes (PROs) through assessment of symptoms and QOL is inconsistent both in the clinical setting as well as in research. In recent years, the Institute of Medicine report on palliative care and various national guidelines have increased emphasis on the provision of quality palliative care (1). Improving the quality of palliative care will allow patients to maximize disease treatment benefit by reducing debilitating symptoms and enhancing QOL (2). The purpose of this chapter is to review the current evidence on multidisciplinary symptom management and QOL in lung cancer, to discuss the importance of integrating PROs into clinical settings and clinical trials, and to review the current guidelines and national initiatives to improve the quality of palliative oncology care for lung cancer patients.

■ DEFINING PALLIATIVE CARE

Palliative care is a concept in medical care that has expanded within the last decade to address the supportive care needs that accompany the occurrence of life-threatening disease. The concept addresses different aspects in the trajectory of cancer. In its recent 2009 update, the National Consensus Project of Clinical Practice Guidelines for Quality Palliative Care defines palliative care as "medical care provided by an interdisciplinary team, including the professions of medicine, nursing, social work, chaplaincy, counseling, nursing assistant, and other health care professions focused on the relief of suffering and support for the best possible QOL for patients facing serious life-threatening illness and their families. It aims to identify and address the physical, psychologic, spiritual, and practical burdens of illness" (3). Figure 25.1 illustrates how palliative care fits with the treatment of lung cancer. Palliative care begins at the time of diagnosis of a serious disease, and continues throughout treatment and cure, or until death, and involves the family during the bereavement period.

■ SYMPTOMS AND QUALITY OF LIFE IN EARLY-STAGE LUNG CANCER

Several studies have described QOL in early-stage non–small cell lung cancer (NSCLC) postoperatively. Balduyck et al. (4) followed 100 NSCLC patients for 12 months postoperatively and found that the QOL evolution in patients who received a lobectomy or wedge resection was comparable with a 1-month transient decrease in functioning and increase in pain. Other studies have found similar transient QOL decreases postoperatively, with general recovery seen between 3 and 9 months postoperatively (5–8). Patients who underwent a pneumonectomy had the worst outcome, with poor physical functioning, role functioning, pain, dyspnea, emotional problems, and decreased pulmonary functions that did not recover to baseline (5,9,10). Pneumonectomy was also found to be predictive for hospital readmissions and mortality postoperatively (11).

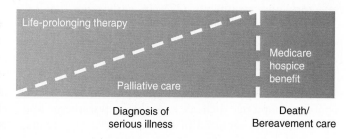

FIGURE 25.1 Palliative Care's Place in the Course of Illness.

In a longitudinal study exploring QOL in patients with resected NSCLC 2 years postoperatively, surgery substantially reduced QOL across all dimensions except emotional functioning (12). Approximately half of the patients continued to experience symptoms and diminished functioning after 2 years (12). In a study with long-term survivors of lung cancer (>5 years), Sarna et al. (13) found that 22% of survivors had distressed mood, and 50% experienced moderate to severe pulmonary distress.

Studies have also identified determinants of QOL following pulmonary resections. Preoperative QOL has been found to predict postoperative QOL, with continued declines in physical, social, and psychologic states and slower recovery (5,14–20). Patients who continued to smoke postoperatively reported higher rates of complications, mortality, and impaired QOL postoperatively (9,21–23). Preoperative dyspnea and fatigue have also been reported to predict QOL postoperatively (7,24). Finally, factors that provoke the most fear in resectable NSCLC patients are not surgical risks of perioperative morbidity or mortality, but the physical and mental handicaps that hinder recovery of physical and functional status postoperatively (25,26).

Physical and functional well-being are considered essential dimensions of overall QOL. It is well documented that disease- and treatment-related symptoms in NSCLC impact pulmonary function, strength, and functional status of patients (27). It has been reported that NSCLC patients experience the highest number of symptoms when compared with patients with other solid tumors. Common disease- and treatment-related symptoms include dyspnea, cough, fatigue, pain, lack of appetite, and insomnia (27,28). The average number of symptoms per patient in NSCLC has been reported to be around 14 with 2.3 symptoms rated as severe (28,29). The most distressing and prevalent symptoms in newly diagnosed adults with NSCLC are pain, cough, and fatigue (30,31). Fox and Lyon (32) studied symptom clusters and QOL in a cohort of 51 lung cancer survivors, and findings identified depression and fatigue as a common cluster, which explained 29% of variance in QOL in this cohort. Pain was significantly correlated with fatigue but not with depression or QOL (32).

In a systematic review of symptoms in lung cancer, Cooley concluded that patients with lung cancer experienced multiple symptoms that differed across illness trajectory and treatments (27). In early-stage NSCLC where surgical interventions are the primary treatment, postoperative symptoms include pain and dyspnea (33). Post-thoracotomy pain syndrome is defined as an aching or burning sensation that persists or recurs along the thoracotomy scar at least 2 months postoperatively, and neuropathic symptoms such as paresthesia-dysesthesia and hypoesthesia are reported in 69% and 40% of patients, respectively (34–36). Immediately following a thoracotomy, 90% of patients report varying degrees of pain (37).

The incidence of chronic post-thoracotomy pain (CPTP) is estimated to be around 26% to 67% in the current literature (36,38–40). Dajczman et al. (38) followed patients post-thoracotomy for up to 5 years and found that pain persisted in 50% of patients at 1 year, 73% at 2 years, 54% at 3 years, 50% at 4 years, and 30% at 5 years. Predictors of CPTP includes severe acute postoperative pain (36), high consumption of analgesics postoperatively (37,41), female gender (35,42), the extent of surgery (40), and psychologic distress (43,44). The long-term pain 1.5 years after thoracotomy was predicted by the intensity of pain experienced as early as 6 hours and up to 2 days postoperatively (36). The majority of patients do not seek pain management, even though approximately 50% of patients report functional limitations by CPTP at 1 year post-thoracotomy (37,45). Studies exploring post-thoracotomy pain in minimally invasive surgery versus open thoracotomy found a difference in favor of minimally invasive techniques for acute postoperative pain but no difference in CPTP occurrence 1 year after surgery (44–47). Studies have also revealed that the predominant symptoms in NSCLC patients receiving chemotherapy were nausea, vomiting, fatigue, hair loss, and peripheral neuropathy (48,49). The predominant symptoms in patients receiving radiation therapy were dysphagia, cough, heartburn, dyspnea, fatigue, and loss of appetite (50,51).

Respiratory symptoms such as cough, dyspnea, wheeze, and hemoptysis are common in NSCLC, occurring in 40% to 85% of patients (52). These symptoms may be present at diagnosis or as a direct result of treatment, and prevalence is dependent on tumor type, disease stage, gender, age, and living situations (53). Dyspnea occurs in 29% to 74% of cancer patients, and is most prevalent in lung cancer patients (53,54). It has been associated with physical, emotional, and cognitive changes, which includes poor concentration, fatigue, depression, anxiety, panic, and memory loss (54,55). Dales et al. (56) followed NSCLC patients after thoracic surgery and found that dyspnea and QOL deteriorated up to 3 months postoperatively, but returned to baseline at 9 months. In a study exploring dyspnea and QOL in both early- and late-stage NSCLC patients (n = 120), Smith et al. found that advanced disease was not correlated with dyspnea. This finding suggests that early-stage NSCLC patients who are most likely to be cured may also be faced with debilitating breathlessness that results in poor QOL during survivorship (54). Perceptions of respiratory symptoms among NSCLC survivors may be affected by age, tobacco use, and comorbid conditions that impact pulmonary functions (57). Likewise, the degree of pulmonary and functional compromise has been associated with the extent of thoracic resection (56,58–61). In a study with long-term lung cancer survivors (>5 years.), Sarna et al. (57) found that two thirds of subjects reported at least one respiratory symptom, and 11% reported that they are so breathless that they cannot leave their homes. Despite the symptoms, only 18% reported the use of prescribed bronchodilators. The presence of dyspnea was associated with reduced physical functioning, physical role activities, and decreased social functioning (57).

The trajectory and treatment of early-stage lung cancer may also affect the nature of the patient's social well-being and relationships with others. Alterations in work, family roles, and social activities for patients are associated with the illness (62–65). Research has shown that social support is associated with distress among cancer patients and is positively related to QOL (66–70). Walker et al. (67) found that the type of social support available to NSCLC patients predicted more adaptive coping in early-stage disease (n = 119). A more assisting and cooperative support that leaves responsibilities and choices to the patient was associated with adaptive coping, while support that entails others taking responsibility for tasks and telling the patient what to do was associated with less adaptive coping (67,71).

Diagnosis of a life-threatening disease such as NSCLC can cause enormous spiritual distress. Finding meaning in illness has shown to positively affect QOL. In a cross-sectional study conducted by Downe-Wamboldt et al. (72), results showed that overall QOL in NSCLC patients is predicted most by meaning of illness, specifically, the illness being perceived as manageable. In a study conducted among 60 NSCLC patients, Meraviglia found that people who reported more meaning in life had better psychologic well-being. Furthermore, as the level of meaning in life increased, symptom distress decreased among the study participants (73). Finally, Sarna et al. examined the relationship between meaning of illness and QOL in women with NSCLC (n = 217). Findings suggest that depressed mood, negative conceptualizations of meaning of illness, and younger age explained 37% of the variance of global QOL and were correlated with poorer QOL (74). In this study, more than a third of patients associated lung cancer with negative meaning (74).

■ SYMPTOMS AND QOL IN LATE-STAGE LUNG CANCER

In late-stage lung cancer where the disease is incurable, the approaches to palliative care are focused on maximizing QOL through aggressive symptom management. Studies suggest that palliative chemotherapy in advanced disease has the additional benefit of improving pain and other symptoms, although treatments should be given within the confounds of symptom palliation only (75–80). Results have shown that in late-stage disease, the goal of treatment is not survival but rather the improvement of QOL (17). QOL has also been identified as an independent prognostic

factor for survival, even after controlling for factors such as age or extent of disease (18,81–84). Ganz et al. (83) reported that median survival was 24 weeks for lung cancer patients reporting high QOL, as compared with 11.9 weeks for those who reported lower QOL. Predictors of QOL in late-stage lung cancer include type of treatment, age, psychologic distress, and pretreatment QOL (85–91). The importance of pretreatment QOL was tested in a phase II study of an integrative palliative care intervention that was administered early in the ambulatory setting for late-stage patients, and results show that early palliative care was feasible with a trend toward QOL improvements (92). In a study exploring the impact of QOL on women with lung cancer, Sarna found that younger subjects (<65 years.) had more serious disruptions in overall QOL (91). Bozcuk et al. (85) found that lung cancer patients who started chemotherapy with good baseline QOL benefited more on survival, and those with poorer QOL gained more benefits from symptom palliation.

The physical well-being of lung cancer patients with advanced disease is related to factors such as treatment and site of metastasis. Several studies have found that advanced disease patients experience more symptom severity and intensity than other solid tumor types (27,31,93,94). According to the literature, the most common symptoms in advanced disease are pain, dyspnea, cough, weight loss, insomnia, and fatigue, and these symptoms are also found in the terminally ill (95). Kreech et al. (96) found that late-stage patients reported an average of 9 symptoms. These findings suggest that patients with late-stage disease suffer from multiple, dynamic symptoms that require ongoing assessment and aggressive management.

Numerous descriptive studies have explored symptom prevalence, intensity, and distress in NSCLC patients with advanced diseases. The majority of these studies found that fatigue, pain, and dyspnea were the most prevalent and distressing for patients, and that symptom prevalence and distress increased during the terminal phases of illness (97–101). Gift et al. (29) studied 112 lung cancer patients and reported a symptom cluster that consisted of fatigue, weakness, weight loss, appetite loss, nausea, vomiting, and altered taste. This cluster had internal consistency that remained at 3 and 6 months. Stage of disease was the most significant predictor of the cluster, and death 6 to 9 months after diagnosis was predicted by age, stage of cancer at diagnosis, and symptom severity at 6 months (29). Sarna and Brecht found that symptom experience of lung cancer patients cluster together to form distinct congregations of distress. They revealed links between frequent, severe pain with poor bowel function, nausea with appetite loss, and respiratory symptoms with insomnia (102). Finally, Cooley et al. described symptom prevalence, distress, and progression during treatment for lung cancer (n = 117). Fatigue and pain were the most distressing symptoms, and significant differences were found among treatment groups (97). Overall, a decrease in symptom distress was found from 0 to 3 months, but this level increased from 3 to 6 months. Symptom distress at baseline was a strong predictor of nine distressing symptoms at 3 months and seven distressing symptoms at 6 months (97). These high levels of distress are also reported by other investigators (103,104).

Approximately 75% of patients with advanced cancers have pain (105). Potential causes in late-stage disease include tumor progression, metastatic disease (i.e., bone), nerve damage, and toxicities from chemotherapy and radiation (105). In a study on symptom prevalence and predictors in late-stage NSCLC, Skaug et al. (106) reported that 85% of patients experienced pain 8 weeks prior to death, even after controlling for factors such as gender, age, PS, stage, and histology. In another study, Hoffman et al. (98) reported that pain occurred in 69% of a cohort of 80 NSCLC patients, and that pain clustered with fatigue and insomnia.

Respiratory symptoms such as dyspnea are common in advanced lung cancer, with reported prevalence of 32% (107). As death approaches, 90% of patients have severe dyspnea (107). Incidence of dyspnea is higher when pain and anxiety levels are high (108–110). Other factors correlated with dyspnea include psychologic distress and cough (111). Edmonds et al. (112) found that the prevalence of dyspnea was high in the last week life (55%), and spiritual distress, weakness, and low family well-being were associated with dyspnea in a cohort of cancer patients receiving inpatient palliative care. Patients who reported severe dyspnea were also more likely to die in a hospital versus hospice or nursing homes (112). Tanaka et al. (113) found that dyspnea interfered with daily life and physical activities such as walking, as well as psychologic activities such as insomnia and social relationships.

In addition to dyspnea, advanced stage patients also suffer from severe fatigue. The prevalence of fatigue in lung cancer patients is high (78%), and data suggest that it is not correlated with either disease or treatment variables (114). Okuyama et al. (115) found that dyspnea on walking, appetite loss, and depression were significantly correlated with clinical fatigue in a cohort of ambulatory patients with late-stage NSCLC. In a separate study, Tanaka et al. (116) found that fatigue and dyspnea interfered with at least one daily life activity, and these include walking and work. Finally, studies with lung cancer patients receiving chemoradiation found that by the end of treatment, approximately 63% of patients experienced moderate to severe levels of symptom clusters, which included fatigue (117). In this cohort (n = 64), fatigue was the most severe symptom at baseline and over the course of treatment, and severity remained 5 to 6 weeks post-treatment (117). Fatigue was also the highest predictive factor for interference in daily living (117). Finally, sleep disturbances have been reported in late-stage disease, and findings suggest that this problem leads to excessive daytime sleepiness and impaired QOL (118,119).

Weight loss is a common feature of advanced cancer, and figures for weight loss are highest among lung cancer patients, with prevalence rates of 50% to 83% in late-stage disease (120). Weight loss is a significant, independent predictor of decreased survival and has been associated with impaired QOL, low physical functioning, and increased psychologic distress (121). Treatment effectiveness is also impaired, and studies have found that weight loss is associated with less chemotherapy and radiation, fewer objective responses, and more frequency and severity of side effects (122). Studies have found that patients who reported 5% or more weight loss and reduced food intake had more symptoms, and this correlation was significant (120,123). This finding suggests that symptom severity and the number of symptoms may play a part in the reduction of food intake and weight loss in late-stage disease.

Lung cancer patients have been identified as a group with increased needs yet those receiving less support as compared with other cancer groups. Li and Girgis explored supportive care needs in 1,492 lung cancer patients. The mean number of unmet needs (out of a maximum of 59) reported by patients was 15.6, compared with 10.9 in other cancer patients (124). Lung cancer patients reported more unmet psychologic and daily living needs (124). The spiritual challenges associated with late-stage NSCLC precipitate a need to search for meaning and can lead to spiritual distress (125). Murray et al. (126) found that spiritual issues were important and often the source of unmet needs for patients and their carers. Patients expressed fear, deep hurt, and desperation as they struggled with impending death. Feelings of loss of control were found to contribute greatly to the spiritual distress experienced by this sample. Furthermore, the study reported that patients perceived that health care professionals sometimes did provide spiritual care, but that they could inadvertently cause spiritual distress by undermining people's sense of identity and self-worth (126). Balboni et al. examined religiousness and spiritual support in advanced cancer patients, with 57 of the total subjects diagnosed with lung cancer. Findings demonstrate that religion is important to advanced cancer patients, but they are less able to participate in religious communities due to the progressive nature of the disease (127). Support of patient's spiritual needs was strongly associated with improved QOL (127). Patients reported that spiritual needs were not met through the medical systems. Surprisingly, the investigators also found an association between religiousness and desires for more aggressive treatments to extend survival. This finding may be related to the fact that religiousness may preserve meaning and the desire of remaining connected to others in the face of impending death and terminal illness (127).

■ ASSESSING SYMPTOMS AND QOL: PATIENT-REPORTED OUTCOMES

QOL is a concept that has been studied for many years both in clinical research as well as in practice settings. The application of QOL assessments in oncology research has been an ongoing process, and in recent years a steady increase and interest has been observed. At the City of Hope (COH), 20 years of collaborative, prospective research by Ferrell and Grant has resulted in the development of a QOL model (128). The COH-QOL model incorporates four domains of QOL: physical, psychologic, social, and spiritual well-being (see Figure 25.2). Physical well-being issues are focused on common disease or treatment-related symptoms such as pain, fatigue, and sleep disturbance. Psychologic well-being issues include anxiety, depression, fear of recurrence, and coping. Social well-being domain issues include family distress, financial burden, sexual function, and employment. Finally, spiritual well-being concerns include hope, finding meaning, and religiosity (128). A QOL assessment tool was developed based on this model, and measurements incorporate all aspects of the four domains. The measure is validated in several different cancer populations, and various versions are available, including a version for family caregivers (129).

The incorporation of QOL assessments into clinical trials is rapidly becoming a standard of practice. More recently, the term "patient-reported outcomes" has been used to describe all aspects of symptoms and QOL assessments that are patient-focused. In the United States, the emergence of this newer term was a result of the recommendations by the Food and Drug Administration of the inclusion of PROs as basis for new drug and medical device approvals (130). The FDA defines PROs as "measurement of any aspect of a patient's health status that comes directly from the patient (i.e., without the interpretation of the patient's response by a physician or anyone else), including disease symptoms, patient functioning, and QOL." (130). Thus, PROs focus for data gathering is patients rather than clinical views on the content covered by the questionnaire. Only through direct patient input in the assessment of QOL and symptoms can a more complete appreciation of the value and impact of treatment be obtained (131).

In late-stage lung cancer, where treatment intent is palliative in most cases, the impact of treatment on QOL is an important factor on treatment decisions. There is some evidence in the current literature that suggests that QOL might be significantly related to survival in NSCLC (132–135). A recent systematic review of cancer clinical trials that incorporated PROs into study design indicated that PROs provide unique prognostic information that are beyond the standard clinical measures used in traditional cancer clinical trials (136). Recommendations from this review suggest that PROs may be used for stratification purposes in future trials because they were often better predictors of survival than PS (136). Common symptom measures that frequently predicted survival include appetite/appetite loss, fatigue, pain, mood/emotion functioning, and role functioning (136).

Several issues need to be considered when integrating PROs into clinical research. A vital first step includes outlining the various types of measures that are currently available for the target population of interest. In late-stage lung cancer, several measures have been used and validated in clinical trials. These include tools for overall QOL assessments (EORTC QLQ-C30, EORTC QLQ-LC13, FACT-L) and more symptom-specific measures such as the *Lung Cancer Symptom Scale* (137–146). A second step involves reviewing the content of relevant measurements to assess the appropriateness of use. Focus

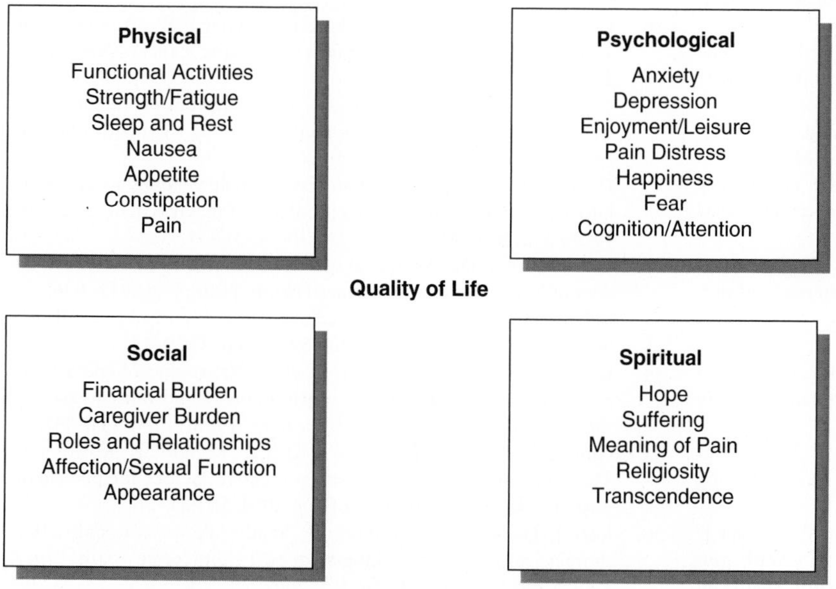

Physical

Functional Activities
Strength/Fatigue
Sleep and Rest
Nausea
Appetite
Constipation
Pain

Psychological

Anxiety
Depression
Enjoyment/Leisure
Pain Distress
Happiness
Fear
Cognition/Attention

Quality of Life

Social

Financial Burden
Caregiver Burden
Roles and Relationships
Affection/Sexual Function
Appearance

Spiritual

Hope
Suffering
Meaning of Pain
Religiosity
Transcendence

FIGURE 25.2 City of Hope quality of life model.

should be placed on the length of the measure, potential subject burdens, timing and frequency of measure, and scoring. This critical assessment will aid in determining how responses are organized and reported in order to ensure interpretable results (147). This in turn will aid in interpretation of clinically meaningful changes in trial results that can be used in treatment decision-making. The final step involves addressing the problem of missing data, which is the single biggest threat to validity of PRO data. Although controversial, many new statistical methods are being developed to address the issue, and the problem can be diminished with increased vigilance, commitment, and attention to data quality in clinical trials (147,148). The critical assessment of current available measures in combination with the incorporation of clear QOL and symptom-related hypotheses will ultimately lead to clinically meaningful interventions.

■ REFERENCES

1. Foley K, Gelband H. *Improving Palliative Care for Cancer.* Washington, DC: National Academy Press; 2009.
2. Ferrell B, Paice J, Koczywas M. New standards and implications for improving the quality of supportive oncology practice. *J Clin Oncol.* 2008;26(23):3824–3831.
3. National Consensus Project for Quality Palliative Care. *Clinical Practice Guidelines for Quality Palliative Care, Second Edition,* 2009. http://www.nationalconsensusproject.org. Accessed April 14, 2010.
4. Balduyck B, Hendriks J, Lauwers P, Van Schil P. Quality of life evolution after lung cancer surgery: a prospective study in 100 patients. *Lung Cancer.* 2007;56(3):423–431.
5. Brunelli A, Socci L, Refai M, Salati M, Xiumé F, Sabbatini A. Quality of life before and after major lung resection for lung cancer: a prospective follow-up analysis. *Ann Thorac Surg.* 2007;84(2):410–416.
6. Li WW, Lee TW, Lam SS, et al. Quality of life following lung cancer resection: video-assisted thoracic surgery vs thoracotomy. *Chest.* 2002;122(2):584–589.
7. Paull DE, Thomas ML, Meade GE, et al. Determinants of quality of life in patients following pulmonary resection for lung cancer. *Am J Surg.* 2006;192(5):565–571.
8. Win T, Sharples L, Wells FC, Ritchie AJ, Munday H, Laroche CM. Effect of lung cancer surgery on quality of life. *Thorax.* 2005;60(3):234–238.
9. Myrdal G, Valtysdottir S, Lambe M, Ståhle E. Quality of life following lung cancer surgery. *Thorax.* 2003;58(3):194–197.
10. Zieren HU, Müller JM, Hamberger U, Pichlmaier H. Quality of life after surgical therapy of bronchogenic carcinoma. *Eur J Cardiothorac Surg.* 1996;10(4):233–237.
11. Handy JR Jr, Child AI, Grunkemeier GL, et al. Hospital readmission after pulmonary resection: prevalence, patterns, and predisposing characteristics. *Ann Thorac Surg.* 2001;72(6):1855–9; discussion 1859.
12. Kenny PM, King MT, Viney RC, et al. Quality of life and survival in the 2 years after surgery for non small-cell lung cancer. *J Clin Oncol.* 2008;26(2):233–241.
13. Sarna L, Padilla G, Holmes C, Tashkin D, Brecht ML, Evangelista L. Quality of life of long-term survivors of non-small-cell lung cancer. *J Clin Oncol.* 2002;20(13):2920–2929.
14. Barlési F, Doddoli C, Loundou A, Pillet E, Thomas P, Auquier P. Preoperative psychological global well being index (PGWBI) predicts postoperative quality of life for patients with non-small cell
15. Buccheri GF, Ferrigno D, Tamburini M, Brunelli C. The patient's perception of his own quality of life might have an adjunctive prognostic significance in lung cancer. *Lung Cancer.* 1995;12(1–2):45–58.
16. Handy JR Jr, Asaph JW, Skokan L, et al. What happens to patients undergoing lung cancer surgery? Outcomes and quality of life before and after surgery. *Chest.* 2002;122(1):21–30.
17. Montazeri A, Gillis CR, McEwen J. Quality of life in patients with lung cancer: a review of literature from 1970 to 1995. *Chest.* 1998;113(2):467–481.
18. Montazeri A, Milroy R, Hole D, McEwen J, Gillis CR. Quality of life in lung cancer patients: as an important prognostic factor. *Lung Cancer.* 2001;31(2–3):233–240.
19. Parsons JA, Johnston MR, Slutsky AS. Predicting length of stay out of hospital following lung resection using preoperative health status measures. *Qual Life Res.* 2003;12(6):645–654.
20. Svobodník A, Yang P, Novotny PJ, et al. Quality of life in 650 lung cancer survivors 6 months to 4 years after diagnosis. *Mayo Clin Proc.* 2004;79(8):1024–1030.
21. Evangelista LS, Sarna L, Brecht ML, Padilla G, Chen J. Health perceptions and risk behaviors of lung cancer survivors. *Heart Lung.* 2003;32(2):131–139.
22. Harpole DH Jr, DeCamp MM Jr, Daley J, et al. Prognostic models of thirty-day mortality and morbidity after major pulmonary resection. *J Thorac Cardiovasc Surg.* 1999;117(5):969–979.
23. Myrdal G, Gustafsson G, Lambe M, Hörte LG, Ståhle E. Outcome after lung cancer surgery. Factors predicting early mortality and major morbidity. *Eur J Cardiothorac Surg.* 2001;20(4):694–699.
24. Ostlund U, Wennman-Larsen A, Gustavsson P, Wengström Y. What symptom and functional dimensions can be predictors for global ratings of overall quality of life in lung cancer patients? *Support Care Cancer.* 2007;15(10):1199–1205.
25. Cykert S, Kissling G, Hansen CJ. Patient preferences regarding possible outcomes of lung resection: what outcomes should preoperative evaluations target? *Chest.* 2000;117(6):1551–1559.
26. Rocco G, Vaughan R. Outcome of lung surgery: what patients don't like. *Chest.* 2000;117(6):1531–1532.
27. Cooley ME. Symptoms in adults with lung cancer. A systematic research review. *J Pain Symptom Manage.* 2000;19(2):137–153.
28. Hopwood P, Stephens RJ. Symptoms at presentation for treatment in patients with lung cancer: implications for the evaluation of palliative treatment. The Medical Research Council (MRC) Lung Cancer Working Party. *Br J Cancer.* 1995;71(3):633–636.
29. Gift AG, Stommel M, Jablonski A, Given W. A cluster of symptoms over time in patients with lung cancer. *Nurs Res.* 2003;52(6):393–400.
30. Cooley ME, Short TH, Moriarty HJ. Symptom prevalence, distress, and change over time in adults receiving treatment for lung cancer. *Psychooncology.* 2003;12(7):694–708.
31. Degner LF, Sloan JA. Symptom distress in newly diagnosed ambulatory cancer patients and as a predictor of survival in lung cancer. *J Pain Symptom Manage.* 1995;10(6):423–431.
32. Fox SW, Lyon DE. Symptom clusters and quality of life in survivors of lung cancer. *Oncol Nurs Forum.* 2006;33(5):931–936.
33. Belani CP. Adjuvant and neoadjuvant therapy in non-small cell lung cancer. *Semin Oncol.* 2005;32(2 suppl 2):S9–15.
34. Benedetti F, Vighetti S, Ricco C, et al. Neurophysiologic assessment of nerve impairment in posterolateral and muscle-sparing thoracotomy. *J Thorac Cardiovasc Surg.* 1998;115(4):841–847.
35. Gotoda Y, Kambara N, Sakai T, Kishi Y, Kodama K, Koyama T. The morbidity, time course and predictive factors for persistent post-thoracotomy pain. *Eur J Pain.* 2001;5(1):89–96.
36. Katz J, Jackson M, Kavanagh BP, Sandler AN. Acute pain after thoracic surgery predicts long-term post-thoracotomy pain. *Clin J Pain.* 1996;12(1):50–55.

37. Perttunen K, Tasmuth T, Kalso E. Chronic pain after thoracic surgery: a follow-up study. *Acta Anaesthesiol Scand.* 1999;43(5):563–567.

38. Dajczman E, Gordon A, Kreisman H, Wolkove N. Long-term postthoracotomy pain. *Chest.* 1991;99(2):270–274.

39. Kalso E, Perttunen K, Kaasinen S. Pain after thoracic surgery. *Acta Anaesthesiol Scand.* 1992;36(1):96–100.

40. Pluijms WA, Steegers MA, Verhagen AF, Scheffer GJ, Wilder-Smith OH. Chronic post-thoracotomy pain: a retrospective study. *Acta Anaesthesiol Scand.* 2006;50(7):804–808.

41. Tiippana E, Nilsson E, Kalso E. Post-thoracotomy pain after thoracic epidural analgesia: a prospective follow-up study. *Acta Anaesthesiol Scand.* 2003;47(4):433–438.

42. Ochroch EA, Gottschalk A, Augostides J, et al. Long-term pain and activity during recovery from major thoracotomy using thoracic epidural analgesia. *Anesthesiology.* 2002;97(5):1234–1244.

43. Perkins FM, Kehlet H. Chronic pain as an outcome of surgery. A review of predictive factors. *Anesthesiology.* 2000;93(4):1123–1133.

44. Rogers ML, Duffy JP. Surgical aspects of chronic post-thoracotomy pain. *Eur J Cardiothorac Surg.* 2000;18(6):711–716.

45. Landreneau RJ, Mack MJ, Hazelrigg SR, et al. Prevalence of chronic pain after pulmonary resection by thoracotomy or video-assisted thoracic surgery. *J Thorac Cardiovasc Surg.* 1994;107(4):1079–85; discussion 1085.

46. Furrer M, Rechsteiner R, Eigenmann V, Signer C, Althaus U, Ris HB. Thoracotomy and thoracoscopy: postoperative pulmonary function, pain and chest wall complaints. *Eur J Cardiothorac Surg.* 1997;12(1):82–87.

47. Kirby TJ, Mack MJ, Landreneau RJ, Rice TW. Lobectomy–video-assisted thoracic surgery versus muscle-sparing thoracotomy. A randomized trial. *J Thorac Cardiovasc Surg.* 1995;109(5):997–1001; discussion 1001.

48. Lyne ME, Coyne PJ, Watson AC. Pain management issues for cancer survivors. *Cancer Pract.* 2002;10(suppl 1):S27–S32.

49. Polomano RC, Farrar JT. Pain and neuropathy in cancer survivors. Surgery, radiation, and chemotherapy can cause pain; research could improve its detection and treatment. *Am J Nurs.* 2006;106(3 suppl):39–47.

50. Borthwick D, Knowles G, McNamara S, Dea RO, Stroner P. Assessing fatigue and self-care strategies in patients receiving radiotherapy for non-small cell lung cancer. *Eur J Oncol Nurs.* 2003;7(4):231–241.

51. Dagnelie PC, Pijls-Johannesma MC, Lambin P, Beijer S, De Ruysscher D, Kempen GI. Impact of fatigue on overall quality of life in lung and breast cancer patients selected for high-dose radiotherapy. *Ann Oncol.* 2007;18(5):940–944.

52. Hollen PJ, Gralla RJ, Kris MG, Eberly SW, Cox C. Normative data and trends in quality of life from the Lung Cancer Symptom Scale (LCSS). *Support Care Cancer.* 1999;7(3):140–148.

53. Chernecky C, Sarna L, Waller JL, Brecht ML. Assessing coughing and wheezing in lung cancer: a pilot study. *Oncol Nurs Forum.* 2004;31(6):1095–1101.

54. Smith EL, Hann DM, Ahles TA, et al. Dyspnea, anxiety, body consciousness, and quality of life in patients with lung cancer. *J Pain Symptom Manage.* 2001;21(4):323–329.

55. Brown ML, Carrieri V, Janson-Bjerklie, Dodd MJ. Lung cancer and dyspnea: the patient's perception. *Oncol Nurs Forum.* 1986;13(5):19–24.

56. Dales RE, Bélanger R, Shamji FM, Leech J, Crépeau A, Sachs HJ. Quality-of-life following thoracotomy for lung cancer. *J Clin Epidemiol.* 1994;47(12):1443–1449.

57. Sarna L, Evangelista L, Tashkin D, et al. Impact of respiratory symptoms and pulmonary function on quality of life of long-term survivors of non-small cell lung cancer. *Chest.* 2004;125(2):439–445.

58. Bolliger CT, Jordan P, Solèr M, et al. Pulmonary function and exercise capacity after lung resection. *Eur Respir J.* 1996;9(3):415–421.

59. Larsen KR, Svendsen UG, Milman N, Brenøe J, Petersen BN. Cardiopulmonary function at rest and during exercise after resection for bronchial carcinoma. *Ann Thorac Surg.* 1997;64(4):960–964.

60. Nugent AM, Steele IC, Carragher AM, et al. Effect of thoracotomy and lung resection on exercise capacity in patients with lung cancer. *Thorax.* 1999;54(4):334–338.

61. Pelletier C, Lapointe L, LeBlanc P. Effects of lung resection on pulmonary function and exercise capacity. *Thorax.* 1990;45(7):497–502.

62. De Valck C, Vinck J. Health locus of control and quality of life in lung cancer patients. *Patient Educ Couns.* 1996;28(2):179–186.

63. Klemm PR. Variables influencing psychosocial adjustment in lung cancer: a preliminary study. *Oncol Nurs Forum.* 1994;21(6):1059–1062.

64. Kuo TT, Ma FC. Symptom distresses and coping strategies in patients with non-small cell lung cancer. *Cancer Nurs.* 2002;25(4):309–317.

65. Stavraky KM, Donner AP, Kincade JE, Stewart MA. The effect of psychosocial factors on lung cancer mortality at one year. *J Clin Epidemiol.* 1988;41(1):75–82.

66. Saunders JM, McCorkle R. Social support and coping with lung cancer. *West J Nurs Res.* 1987;9(1):29–42.

67. Walker MS, Zona DM, Fisher EB. Depressive symptoms after lung cancer surgery: Their relation to coping style and social support. *Psychooncology.* 2006;15(8):684–693.

68. Courtens AM, Stevens FC, Crebolder HF, Philipsen H. Longitudinal study on quality of life and social support in cancer patients. *Cancer Nurs.* 1996;19(3):162–169.

69. Faller H, Schilling S, Lang H. Causal attribution and adaptation among lung cancer patients. *J Psychosom Res.* 1995;39(5):619–627.

70. Hann D, Baker F, Denniston M, et al. The influence of social support on depressive symptoms in cancer patients: age and gender differences. *J Psychosom Res.* 2002;52(5):279–283.

71. Hill KM, Amir Z, Muers MF, Connolly CK, Round CE. Do newly diagnosed lung cancer patients feel their concerns are being met? *Eur J Cancer Care (Engl).* 2003;12(1):35–45.

72. Downe-Wamboldt B, Butler L, Coulter L. The relationship between meaning of illness, social support, coping strategies, and quality of life for lung cancer patients and their family members. *Cancer Nurs.* 2006;29(2):111–119.

73. Meraviglia MG. The effects of spirituality on well-being of people with lung cancer. *Oncol Nurs Forum.* 2004;31(1):89–94.

74. Sarna L, Brown JK, Cooley ME, et al. Quality of life and meaning of illness of women with lung cancer. *Oncol Nurs Forum.* 2005;32(1):E9–19.

75. Anderson H, Hopwood P, Stephens RJ, et al. Gemcitabine plus best supportive care (BSC) vs BSC in inoperable non-small cell lung cancer–a randomized trial with quality of life as the primary outcome. UK NSCLC Gemcitabine Group. Non-Small Cell Lung Cancer. *Br J Cancer.* 2000;83(4):447–453.

76. Macbeth F, Stephens R. Palliative treatment for advanced non-small cell lung cancer. *Hematol Oncol Clin North Am.* 2004;18(1):115–130.

77. Medley L, Cullen M. Best supportive care versus palliative chemotherapy in nonsmall-cell lung cancer. *Curr Opin Oncol.* 2002;14(4):384–388.

78. Plunkett TA, Chrystal KF, Harper PG. Quality of life and the treatment of advanced lung cancer. *Clin Lung Cancer.* 2003;5(1):28–32.

79. Roszkowski K, Pluzanska A, Krzakowski M, et al. A multicenter, randomized, phase III study of docetaxel plus best supportive care versus best supportive care in chemotherapy-naive patients with metastatic or non-resectable localized non-small cell lung cancer (NSCLC). *Lung Cancer.* 2000;27(3):145–157.

80. Spiro SG, Rudd RM, Souhami RL, et al.; Big Lung Trial participants. Chemotherapy versus supportive care in advanced

non-small cell lung cancer: improved survival without detriment to quality of life. *Thorax.* 2004;59(10):828–836.

81. Thongprasert S, Sanguanmitra P, Juthapan W, Clinch J. Relationship between quality of life and clinical outcomes in advanced non-small cell lung cancer: best supportive care (BSC) versus BSC plus chemotherapy. *Lung Cancer.* 1999;24(1):17–24.

82. Bezjak A. Palliative therapy for lung cancer. *Semin Surg Oncol.* 2003;21(2):138–147.

83. Ganz PA, Lee JJ, Siau J. Quality of life assessment. An independent prognostic variable for survival in lung cancer. *Cancer.* 1991;67(12):3131–3135.

84. Kaasa S, Mastekaasa A, Lund E. Prognostic factors for patients with inoperable non-small cell lung cancer, limited disease. The importance of patients' subjective experience of disease and psychosocial well-being. *Radiother Oncol.* 1989;15(3):235–242.

85. Bozcuk H, Dalmis B, Samur M, Ozdogan M, Artac M, Savas B. Quality of life in patients with advanced non-small cell lung cancer. *Cancer Nurs.* 2006;29(2):104–110.

86. Fallowfield LJ, Harper P. Health-related quality of life in patients undergoing drug therapy for advanced non-small-cell lung cancer. *Lung Cancer.* 2005;48(3):365–377.

87. Langendijk JA, Aaronson NK, ten Velde GP, de Jong JM, Muller MJ, Wouters EF. Pretreatment quality of life of inoperable non-small cell lung cancer patients referred for primary radiotherapy. *Acta Oncol.* 2000;39(8):949–958.

88. Langendijk JA, ten Velde GP, Aaronson NK, de Jong JM, Muller MJ, Wouters EF. Quality of life after palliative radiotherapy in non-small cell lung cancer: a prospective study. *Int J Radiat Oncol Biol Phys.* 2000;47(1):149–155.

89. Montazeri A, Milroy R, Hole D, McEwen J, Gillis CR. How quality of life data contribute to our understanding of cancer patients' experiences? A study of patients with lung cancer. *Qual Life Res.* 2003;12(2):157–166.

90. Rummans TA, Clark MM, Sloan JA, et al. Impacting quality of life for patients with advanced cancer with a structured multidisciplinary intervention: a randomized controlled trial. *J Clin Oncol.* 2006;24(4):635–642.

91. Sarna L. Women with lung cancer: impact on quality of life. *Qual Life Res.* 1993;2(1):13–22.

92. Temel JS, Jackson VA, Billings JA, et al. Phase II study: integrated palliative care in newly diagnosed advanced non-small-cell lung cancer patients. *J Clin Oncol.* 2007;25(17):2377–2382.

93. Doorenbos AZ, Given CW, Given B, Verbitsky N. Symptom experience in the last year of life among individuals with cancer. *J Pain Symptom Manage.* 2006;32(5):403–412.

94. McCorkle R, Quint-Benoliel J. Symptom distress, current concerns and mood disturbance after diagnosis of life-threatening disease. *Soc Sci Med.* 1983;17(7):431–438.

95. Griffin JP, Koch KA, Nelson JE, Cooley ME; American College of Chest Physicians. Palliative care consultation, quality-of-life measurements, and bereavement for end-of-life care in patients with lung cancer: ACCP evidence-based clinical practice guidelines (2nd edition). *Chest.* 2007;132(3 suppl):404S–422S.

96. Kreech R, Davis L, Walsh D. Symptoms of lung cancer. *Palliat Medicine.* 1992;6:309–315.

97. Cooley ME, Short TH, Moriarty HJ. Patterns of symptom distress in adults receiving treatment for lung cancer. *J Palliat Care.* 2002;18(3):150–159.

98. Hoffman AJ, Given BA, von Eye A, Gift AG, Given CW. Relationships among pain, fatigue, insomnia, and gender in persons with lung cancer. *Oncol Nurs Forum.* 2007;34(4):785–792.

99. Lutz S, Norrell R, Bertucio C, et al. Symptom frequency and severity in patients with metastatic or locally recurrent lung cancer: a prospective study using the Lung Cancer Symptom Scale in a community hospital. *J Palliat Med.* 2001;4(2):157–165.

100. Podnos YD, Borneman TR, Koczywas M, Uman G, Ferrell BR. Symptom concerns and resource utilization in patients with lung cancer. *J Palliat Med.* 2007;10(4):899–903.

101. Tishelman C, Petersson LM, Degner LF, Sprangers MA. Symptom prevalence, intensity, and distress in patients with inoperable lung cancer in relation to time of death. *J Clin Oncol.* 2007;25(34):5381–5389.

102. Sarna L, Brecht ML. Dimensions of symptom distress in women with advanced lung cancer: a factor analysis. *Heart Lung.* 1997;26(1):23–30.

103. Tishelman C, Degner LF, Mueller B. Measuring symptom distress in patients with lung cancer. A pilot study of experienced intensity and importance of symptoms. *Cancer Nurs.* 2000;23(2):82–90.

104. Tishelman C, Degner LF, Rudman A, et al. Symptoms in patients with lung carcinoma: distinguishing distress from intensity. *Cancer.* 2005;104(9):2013–2021.

105. Kvale PA, Selecky PA, Prakash UB; American College of Chest Physicians. Palliative care in lung cancer: ACCP evidence-based clinical practice guidelines (2nd ed.). *Chest.* 2007;132(3 suppl):368S–403S.

106. Skaug K, Eide GE, Gulsvik A. Prevalence and predictors of symptoms in the terminal stage of lung cancer: A community study. *Chest.* 2007;131(2):389–394.

107. Claessens MT, Lynn J, Zhong Z, et al. Dying with lung cancer or chronic obstructive pulmonary disease: insights from SUPPORT. Study to Understand Prognoses and Preferences for Outcomes and Risks of Treatments. *J Am Geriatr Soc.* 2000;48(5 suppl):S146–S153.

108. Bruera E, Schmitz B, Pither J, Neumann CM, Hanson J. The frequency and correlates of dyspnea in patients with advanced cancer. *J Pain Symptom Manage.* 2000;19(5):357–362.

109. Dudgeon DJ, Lertzman M. Dyspnea in the advanced cancer patient. *J Pain Symptom Manage.* 1998;16(4):212–219.

110. Henoch I, Bergman B, Danielson E. Dyspnea experience and management strategies in patients with lung cancer. *Psychooncology.* 2008;17:709–715.

111. Tanaka K, Akechi T, Okuyama T, Nishiwaki Y, Uchitomi Y. Factors correlated with dyspnea in advanced lung cancer patients: organic causes and what else? *J Pain Symptom Manage.* 2002;23(6):490–500.

112. Edmonds P, Higginson I, Altmann D, Sen-Gupta G, McDonnell M. Is the presence of dyspnea a risk factor for morbidity in cancer patients? *J Pain Symptom Manage.* 2000;19(1):15–22.

113. Tanaka K, Akechi T, Okuyama T, Nishiwaki Y, Uchitomi Y. Prevalence and screening of dyspnea interfering with daily life activities in ambulatory patients with advanced lung cancer. *J Pain Symptom Manage.* 2002;23(6):484–489.

114. Hickok JT, Morrow GR, McDonald S, Bellg AJ. Frequency and correlates of fatigue in lung cancer patients receiving radiation therapy: implications for management. *J Pain Symptom Manage.* 1996;11(6):370–377.

115. Okuyama T, Tanaka K, Akechi T, et al. Fatigue in ambulatory patients with advanced lung cancer: prevalence, correlated factors, and screening. *J Pain Symptom Manage.* 2001;22(1):554–564.

116. Tanaka K, Akechi T, Okuyama T, Nishiwaki Y, Uchitomi Y. Impact of dyspnea, pain, and fatigue on daily life activities in ambulatory patients with advanced lung cancer. *J Pain Symptom Manage.* 2002;23(5):417–423.

117. Wang XS, Fairclough DL, Liao Z, et al. Longitudinal study of the relationship between chemoradiation therapy for non-small-cell lung cancer and patient symptoms. *J Clin Oncol.* 2006;24(27):4485–4491.

118. Le Guen Y, Gagnadoux F, Hureaux J, et al. Sleep disturbances and impaired daytime functioning in outpatients with newly diagnosed lung cancer. *Lung Cancer.* 2007;58(1):139–143.

119. Vena C, Parker K, Allen R, Bliwise D, Jain S, Kimble L. Sleep-wake disturbances and quality of life in patients with advanced lung cancer. *Oncol Nurs Forum.* 2006;33(4):761–769.

120. Khalid U, Spiro A, Baldwin C, et al. Symptoms and weight loss in patients with gastrointestinal and lung cancer at presentation. *Support Care Cancer.* 2007;15(1):39–46.

121. Ovesen L, Hannibal J, Mortensen EL. The interrelationship of weight loss, dietary intake, and quality of life in ambulatory patients with cancer of the lung, breast, and ovary. *Nutr Cancer.* 1993;19(2):159–167.

122. Ross PJ, Ashley S, Norton A, et al. Do patients with weight loss have a worse outcome when undergoing chemotherapy for lung cancers? *Br J Cancer.* 2004;90(10):1905–1911.

123. Sarhill N, Mahmoud F, Walsh D, et al. Evaluation of nutritional status in advanced metastatic cancer. *Support Care Cancer.* 2003;11(10):652–659.

124. Li J, Girgis A. Supportive care needs: are patients with lung cancer a neglected population? *Psychooncology.* 2006;15(6):509–516.

125. Mystakidou K, Tsilika E, Parpa E, et al. Exploring the relationships between depression, hopelessness, cognitive status, pain, and spirituality in patients with advanced cancer. *Arch Psychiatr Nurs.* 2007;21(3):150–161.

126. Murray SA, Kendall M, Boyd K, Worth A, Benton TF. Exploring the spiritual needs of people dying of lung cancer or heart failure: a prospective qualitative interview study of patients and their carers. *Palliat Med.* 2004;18(1):39–45.

127. Balboni TA, Vanderwerker LC, Block SD, et al. Religiousness and spiritual support among advanced cancer patients and associations with end-of-life treatment preferences and quality of life. *J Clin Oncol.* 2007;25(5):555–560.

128. Ferrell BR, Dow KH, Grant M. Measurement of the quality of life in cancer survivors. *Qual Life Res.* 1995;4(6):523–531.

129. Ferrell BR, Grant M, Borneman T, Juarez G, ter Veer A. Family caregiving in cancer pain management. *J Palliat Med.* 1999;2(2):185–195.

130. United States Food and Drug Administration. *Guidance for Industry Patient-Reported Outcome Measures: Use in Medical Product Development to Support Labeling Claims.* Rockville, MD: United States Food and Drug Administration; 2006.

131. Gralla RJ, Thatcher N. Quality-of-life assessment in advanced lung cancer: considerations for evaluation in patients receiving chemotherapy. *Lung Cancer.* 2004;46(suppl 2):S41–S47.

132. Eton DT, Fairclough DL, Cella D, Yount SE, Bonomi P, Johnson DH; Eastern Cooperative Oncology Group. Early change in patient-reported health during lung cancer chemotherapy predicts clinical outcomes beyond those predicted by baseline report: results from Eastern Cooperative Oncology Group Study 5592. *J Clin Oncol.* 2003;21(8):1536–1543.

133. Cella D, Herbst RS, Lynch TJ, et al. Clinically meaningful improvement in symptoms and quality of life for patients with non-small-cell lung cancer receiving gefitinib in a randomized controlled trial. *J Clin Oncol.* 2005;23(13):2946–2954.

134. Hauser CA, Stockler MR, Tattersall MH. Prognostic factors in patients with recently diagnosed incurable cancer: a systematic review. *Support Care Cancer.* 2006;14(10):999–1011.

135. Beitz J, Gnecco C, Justice R. Quality-of-life end points in cancer clinical trials: the U.S. Food and Drug Administration perspective. *J Natl Cancer Inst Monographs.* 1996;(20):7–9.

136. Gotay CC, Kawamoto CT, Bottomley A, Efficace F. The prognostic significance of patient-reported outcomes in cancer clinical trials. *J Clin Oncol.* 2008;26(8):1355–1363.

137. Aaronson NK, Ahmedzai S, Bergman B, et al. The European Organization for Research and Treatment of Cancer QLQ-C30: a quality-of-life instrument for use in international clinical trials in oncology. *J Natl Cancer Inst.* 1993;85(5):365–376.

138. Bergman B, Aaronson NK, Ahmedzai S, Kaasa S, Sullivan M. The EORTC QLQ-LC13: a modular supplement to the EORTC Core Quality of Life Questionnaire (QLQ-C30) for use in lung cancer clinical trials. EORTC Study Group on Quality of Life. *Eur J Cancer.* 1994;30A(5):635–642.

139. Pérez-Soler R, Chachoua A, Hammond LA, et al. Determinants of tumor response and survival with erlotinib in patients with non-small-cell lung cancer. *J Clin Oncol.* 2004;22(16):3238–3247.

140. Shepherd FA, Rodrigues Pereira J, Ciuleanu T, et al.; National Cancer Institute of Canada Clinical Trials Group. Erlotinib in previously treated non-small-cell lung cancer. *N Engl J Med.* 2005;353(2):123–132.

141. Cella DF, Bonomi AE, Lloyd SR, Tulsky DS, Kaplan E, Bonomi P. Reliability and validity of the Functional Assessment of Cancer Therapy-Lung (FACT-L) quality of life instrument. *Lung Cancer.* 1995;12(3):199–220.

142. Kris MG, Natale RB, Herbst RS, et al. Efficacy of gefitinib, an inhibitor of the epidermal growth factor receptor tyrosine kinase, in symptomatic patients with non-small cell lung cancer: a randomized trial. *JAMA.* 2003;290(16):2149–2158.

143. Cella D, Eton DT, Fairclough DL, et al. What is a clinically meaningful change on the Functional Assessment of Cancer Therapy-Lung (FACT-L) Questionnaire? Results from Eastern Cooperative Oncology Group (ECOG) Study 5592. *J Clin Epidemiol.* 2002;55(3):285–295.

144. Hollen PJ, Gralla RJ, Kris MG, Cox C. Quality of life during clinical trials: conceptual model for the Lung Cancer Symptom Scale (LCSS). *Support Care Cancer.* 1994;2(4):213–222.

145. Hollen PJ, Gralla RJ, Kris MG, et al. Measurement of quality of life in patients with lung cancer in multicenter trials of new therapies. Psychometric assessment of the Lung Cancer Symptom Scale. *Cancer.* 1994;73(8):2087–2098.

146. Hollen PJ, Gralla RJ, Kris MG, Potanovich LM. Quality of life assessment in individuals with lung cancer: testing the Lung Cancer Symptom Scale (LCSS). *Eur J Cancer.* 1993;29A(suppl 1):S51–S58.

147. Cella DF, Patel JD. Improving health-related quality of life in non-small-cell lung cancer with current treatment options. *Clin Lung Cancer.* 2008;9(4):206–212.

148. Sloan JA, Frost MH, Berzon R, et al.; Clinical Significance Consensus Meeting Group. The clinical significance of quality of life assessments in oncology: a summary for clinicians. *Support Care Cancer.* 2006;14(10):988–998.

26 Psychological Distress in Patients with Lung Cancer

ANDREA A. THORNTON

Psychological distress is a common and normative response to the cancer experience, with approximately one third or more of cancer patients reporting clinically significant distress over the cancer trajectory (1–3). Sadness, grief, anxiety, fear, and anger are just a few of the feelings that may accompany diagnosis, active treatment, recurrence, survivorship, and end of life. Cancer patients also face challenges in terms of the impact of cancer and its treatment on their functional abilities, body image and sexuality, financial or vocational status, and social and role changes (4). Although most cancer patients experience some level of psychological distress over the course of their illness experience, there also is significant variability in both the nature and intensity of psychological distress (3). This variability has been linked to person, environmental, and disease-related variables (1,3,5).

This chapter focuses on psychological distress in people with lung cancer. It begins, first, with a description of what is known about the nature and prevalence of psychological distress in this group of cancer patients. Second, risk factors for psychological distress that have been identified in the literature are outlined, using a framework generally guided by psychological theories of stress and coping, the work of Stanton et al. (5), and a model of adaptation provided by Schaefer and Moos (6), which focuses on event-related factors, environmental factors, personal or individual factors, and cognitive and coping processes. The chapter concludes with a discussion of the limitations of the literature and directions for future research with this population.

■ WHY STUDY LUNG CANCER?

Lung cancer is a major public health epidemic across the world. In the United States, specifically, it is the second most commonly diagnosed cancer in women and men (after breast and prostate cancer, respectively), accounting for nearly 15% of all cancer diagnoses, and it is the leading cause of cancer-related deaths (7). Although the 1-year survival rate for lung cancer has increased from approximately 35% to 41% over the past 30 years, 5-year survival for all stages combined remains low at only 15%, in large part due to the fact that most lung cancers are diagnosed at advanced stages (7). For patients with localized disease, the 5-year survival rate is higher at 50%; however, only about 16% of lung cancers are diagnosed in the early stages (7). Thus, for the overwhelming majority of lung cancer patients, the potential for long-term (i.e., >5 years) survival is low.

In addition, symptom distress is high in people with lung cancer, particularly pain, cough, dyspnea, and fatigue (8–10). Lung cancer patients also have been identified as having significant unmet supportive care needs. In one recent study, newly diagnosed lung cancer patients reported a significantly higher level of unmet supportive care needs compared to patients with other cancers, particularly in the psychological and physical/daily living domains (11). Bantum and colleagues found that the highest level of unmet need in their sample of lung cancer patients was with regard to physical/daily living needs, followed closely by psychological needs (12). In addition, even when psychological concerns are endorsed more frequently than physical symptoms, physical symptoms are more likely to be attended to by the medical team (13). Thus, this is a population that faces significant disease-related morbidity and mortality, and experiences a high level of psychological need, which may not always be identified or addressed by the health care team.

■ PREVALENCE AND NATURE OF DISTRESS IN LUNG CANCER

Given the high level of symptom burden coupled with a poor prognosis for long-term survival, it is perhaps not surprising that rates of psychological distress in lung cancer patients appear to be higher compared with other samples of people with cancer (2,14,15). To better describe the prevalence and nature of psychological distress in this population, we conducted a search of the PubMed database pairing the term *lung cancer* with *depression, anxiety, Psychological adjustment, Psychological adaptation, coping,* and *distress* with a focus on identifying recent articles (published between 1995 and the present) and quantitative studies addressing emotional distress and Psychological adjustment versus physical symptom distress, quality–of-life outcomes, or other psychiatric problems (alcohol and substance abuse, cognitive problems, etc.). We also examined the reference lists of these articles to identify additional relevant citations to include in this and other portions of our review. Table 26.1 summarizes the emotional distress prevalence data from these studies.

As shown in Table 26.1, most available data are from samples consisting entirely of or having a majority of patients with non–small cell lung cancer (NSCLC; versus small cell lung cancer; SCLC), which is the most common type of lung cancer. Again, reflecting the nature of lung cancer, which is usually diagnosed at advanced stages, patients with advanced disease comprise the majority of samples, with a few notable exceptions (16–18). However, most of the patients in these studies had fairly good performance status ratings at study entry, which was generally around the time of diagnosis or treatment initiation. Although many studies are cross-sectional, there are also several longitudinal studies that track changes in emotional distress over time, and many of the studies have relatively large sample sizes. Most patients are assessed within months of diagnosis and, for the longitudinal studies, followed over the first year after treatment. The mean age of patients in most studies is more than 60, with a few studies targeting older patients specifically (19,20). The majority of study participants are men. Data are available from groups in North America, Europe, and Japan; however, the racial or ethnic composition of the sample is often not specified. Several studies have used a clinical interview format to identify mood (i.e., depression) or anxiety disorders; however, standardized instruments also have been used such as the Beck Depression Inventory (BDI) (21), the Center for Epidemiologic Studies Depression Scale (CES-D) (22), the Profile of Mood States (23), and the Hospital Anxiety and Depression Scale (HADS) (24), with the latter being the most frequently used standardized measure of distress.

Perhaps one of the most striking features of the table is the wide variability in the level of clinically significant Psychological distress reported across the studies. On the low end, approximately 5% of patients in one study were identified as having depression 1 year following resection of NSCLC (18); on the high end, approximately 50% of newly diagnosed lung cancer patients were characterized as having borderline-severe depression and anxiety (25), or clinically significant distress (26) in two other studies. Methodological issues likely play a large role in the differences in rates across studies. First, the procedures and criteria used to establish distress vary substantially across reports. In general, studies using a clinical interview

methodology have identified lower rates of Psychological distress compared with studies that used a self-report instrument such as the CES-D (12), BDI (27), HADS (28), or distress thermometer (29). A notable exception to this is the study by Neron et al. (30), which used both the HADS as well as an interviewer-administered measure (the Montgomery-Asberg Depression Rating Scale; MADRS), and identified a higher rate of depression using the MADRS versus the HADS. Unlike the HADS, the MADRS has several somatic items, which may be attributable to disease or treatment and may confound the diagnosis of depression in cancer patients and could explain the discrepancy between outcomes using these two different assessments in this particular study. The variations in sample composition, methodology, and criteria for establishing Psychological distress (which in itself is purposefully a broad term used to capture the range of distress experienced by cancer patients and reduce stigma associated with mental health diagnoses) (31) make it difficult to form any strong conclusions regarding prevalence rates.

Indeed, the diagnosis of depressive and anxiety disorders in cancer patients can be challenging in general (32,33), and this may be even more pronounced in lung cancer patients given their relatively high rates of symptom distress. On the one hand, clinicians may underdiagnose Psychological distress for various reasons including the fact that some degree of sadness and fear is a normal and expected response to the disease, because of stigma about mental health, or due to having few resources for follow-up (33). On the other hand, use of instruments and standard psychiatric diagnostic criteria (34) that emphasize somatic symptoms of depression such as fatigue, loss of energy, appetite changes, or sleep disturbance may result in an overestimation of major depression if those symptoms are not considered within the context of the illness experience and attributed to the disease or treatment process when appropriate.

Furthermore, many patients may not be identified as having a diagnosable mood or anxiety disorder, yet may experience subsyndromal depression or clinically significant symptoms of emotional distress. For instance, in the study by Ginsburg et al. (35), rates of a current affective or anxiety disorder were low (4% and 0%, respectively, with an additional 12% of patients having an adjustment disorder); however, many patients experienced symptoms of Psychological distress and described feeling "sad," "tearful," and "low" (44%), or "frightened," "scared," and "worried" (29%) at some point since diagnosis. In addition, thoughts related to death were common (reported by 31% of patients), as was insomnia (52%), and loss of interest in activities or reduced ability to work (33%). Less frequent, but potentially significant concerns included loss of libido specific to cancer (25%), poor concentration (19%), shock (17%), suicidal ideation (13%), guilt (8%), and anger (4%). In this study, there also was a high rate

■ Table 26.1 Identifying prevalence of psychologic distress in lung cancer patients (1995—forward)

Study (Location)	% Distress	Instrument	N	Cancer Type	Stage	PS	Time Since Dx/Tx	% Female	Mean Age (Years)	% Caucasian
Cross-sectional studies										
Buchanan et al., 2009 (Scotland)	43% report medium-high anxiety	POS	170	68% NSC, 12% SC	36% of NSC III/IV; 7% of SC have ED	Md = 2	67% < 1 month post-dx	54%	69	NR
Ginsburg et al., 1995 (Canada)	4% mood disorder, 12% adjustment disorder	CI	52	71% NSC, 25% SC	63% metastatic	82% KPS ≥ 70	Md = 45 days post-dx	25%	69% b/n 50 & 70	NR
Graves et al., 2007 (USA)	62% clinically significant distress, DT M = 4.6/10	DT	333	NSC, SC	24% III/IV; 40% pre-dx	NR	NR	51%	61	94%
Hopwood & Stephens, 1995a (UK)	15–40% report moderate-severe psychologic problems	RSC	655	65% NSC	NR	78% 0,1	pre-tx	21%	66	NR
Rolke et al., 2008 (Norway)	41% severe/borderline depression; 48% severe/borderline anxiety	HADS	479	35% SC 70% NSC, 21% SC	NR 72% advanced (IIIB+)	52% 3,4 66% 0–2	pre-tx Newly dx (within 2 weeks)	37% 42%	65 68	NR% NR
Sanders et al., 2009 (USA)	37% depressed, CES-D; 38% distressed, DT	CES-D DT	109	NSC, SC	45% III/IV	NR	54 weeks	53%	67	77%
Steinberg et al., 2009 (Canada)	51% distressed, DT M = 3.64	DT, ESAS	98	89% NSC, 11% SC	56% NSC IIIB+; 82% SC ED	81% 0,1	First visit b/n dx & tx	45%	63	NR
Walker et al., 2006 (USA)	29% depressed	BDI	119	NSC	I–III	M = 0.36	Md = 7 days postsurgery	52%	59	84%
Longitudinal studies										
Akechi et al., 2001 (Japan)	52% mood disorder, 14% adjustment disorder, 3% anxiety disorder at baseline; 3% mood disorder, 16% adjustment disorder at follow-up	CI	T1 = 129; T1 & T2 = 89	NSC	Unresectable 50% stage IV	M = 1.02, 92% 0,1	T1 b/n dx & tx, T2 6-month follow-up	26%	62	0, presumed
Akechi et al., 2002 (Japan)	15% some SI (8% life not worth living; 2% desire for death; 5% suicidal ideas)	CI, HAMD	89	NSC	Unresectable 48% stage IV	59% 0,1	6-month follow-up	28%	61	0, presumed

Continued

■ Table 26.1 *Continued*

Study (Location)	% Distress	Instrument	N	Cancer Type	Stage	PS	Time Since Dx/Tx	% Female	Mean Age (Years)	% Caucasian
Akechi et al., 2006 (Japan)	Tension-anxiety and depression-dejection lessen; anger, vigor, fatigue, confusion, and total mood disturbance are constant over time	POMS	85	NSC	Unresectable 50% stage IV	98% 0,1	T1 b/n dx & tx, T2 2 months post-tx, T3 6 months post-dx	31%	61	0, presumed
Hopwood & Stephens[b], 2000 (UK)	33% depression pre-tx, 29% at follow-up; 34% anxiety pre-tx	HADS	987	47% NSC, 53% SC	NR	78% 0,1	Pre-tx and follow-up 14–35 days later (SC), or 21–56 days later (NSC)	21%	66	NR
Kurtz et al., 2002 (USA)	31–39% severely depressed	CES-D	228	87% NSC, 13% SC	46% early stage 54% late stage	NR	T1 2–6 weeks after start tx, T2 12–16 weeks, T3 26–30 weeks, T4 1 year	40%	72	NR
Montazeri et al., 1998 (Scotland)	23% severe-borderline depression & 16% severe-borderline anxiety at baseline; 44% depression & 20% anxiety at follow-up	HADS	T1 = 129; T1 & T2 = 82	NR	78% LD	89% "good PS"	T1 pre-dx, T2 3 months post-dx and completion of tx	40%	68	NR
Néron et al., 2007 (Canada)	6–20% depression by HADS over time; 41–51% by MADRS	HADS, MADRS	49	NSC	Advanced (IIIA+)	61% ≥1	1 week post-dx and 3 other times over first several weeks of starting chemotherapy	39%	Md = 63	NR
Tchekmedyian et al., 2003 (USA)	35% depression, 25% anxiety at baseline; follow-up NR	BSI	250	73% NSC, 27% SC	NR	83% 0,1	T1 pre-chemo, T2 b/n 4 and 12 weeks post-tx	29%	61	NR

Study	Findings	Measure	N	Cancer type	Stage	PS	Assessment timing	Response rate	Md age	Distress data
Turner et al., 2007 (UK)	Older comparison group: 45% depress ion pre- and 53% post-tx; 44% anxiety pre- and 38% post-tx	HADS	83	84% NSC; 8% SC	54% late stage (IIIA-IV or ED)	57% 0,1	T1 first radio-tx visit T2 M = 57 days later (post-tx)	41%	Md = 78	NR
	Younger comparison group: 47% depression pre- and 45% post-tx; 47% anxiety pre- and 48% post-tx		49	86% NSC; 12% SC	82% late stage	66% 0,1	see above	31%	Md = 60	NR
Uchitomi et al., 2000 (Japan)	15% depression within 3 months of surgery	CI	223	NSC	I, II, IIIA	99% 0,1 at presurgery	T1 1 month postsurgery, T2 3 months postsurgery	39%	63	0, presumed
Uchitomi et al., 2003 (Japan)	8% depression at 1 month, 5% at 3 months, 5% at 12 months; no significant change in rates of depression or total POMS score over time; increased anger-hostility and vigor-activity scores over time	CI, POMS	212	NSC	I, II, IIIA	99% 0,1 at presurgery	T1 1 month postsurgery, T2 3 months postsurgery, T3 12 months postsurgery	40%	62	0, presumed

[a] Patients were recruited from 2 separate palliative care trials, one for NSC, one for SC. Demographic and medical data above the line are from the larger sample of NSC patients and data below the dashed line are from the larger sample of SC patients, not all of whom completed the distress data.

[b] Patients in this study include the sample from Hopwood & Stephens, 1995, with the addition of a third sample of patients with SCLC. Data shown are from the larger sample of patients in this third sample only, not all of whom completed the distress items. Please see the prior Hopwood & Stephens entry for details about the other two samples.

BDI, Beck Depression Inventory; b/n, between; BSI, Brief Symptom Inventory; CES-D, Center for Epidemiologic Studies Depression Scale; CI, Clinical Interview; DT, Distress Thermometer; Dx, Diagnosis; ED, Extensive Disease; ESAS, Edmonton Symptom Assessment Scale; HADS, Hospital Anxiety and Depression Scale; HAMD, Hamilton Rating Scale for Depression; LD, Limited Disease; M, Mean; MADRS, Montgomery-Asberg Depression Rating Scale; Md, Median; NR, not reported; NSC, non–small cell lung cancer; POMS, Profile of Mood States; POS, Palliative Outcomes Scale; PS, performance status; RSC, Rotterdam Symptoms Checklist; SC, small cell lung cancer; Tx, Treatment.

of acceptance and optimism (38% and 25%, respectively), pointing to the importance of measuring positive, in addition to negative aspects of the cancer experience (36).

In summary, there is significant variability in the prevalence of distress across studies. The preponderance of available data address emotional distress in the weeks or months following diagnosis and treatment, and little is known about the long-term Psychological impact of lung cancer on survivors. Variability in distress rates may be attributable to multiple factors including, but not limited to, sample size and composition, assessment methodology, and criterion used to identify distress (35). Although most lung cancer patients will not be diagnosed with a formal mood, anxiety, or even adjustment disorder, many patients experience clinically significant symptoms of emotional distress that may warrant clinical attention and intervention.

■ CORRELATES OF PSYCHOLOGICAL DISTRESS

As evident in the preceding discussion, many lung cancer patients experience significant Psychological distress. However, there is also substantial variability in distress reports across studies. We turn now to examining correlates of Psychological distress in people with lung cancer. Establishing the factors that place patients at risk for distress plays a critical role in improving our ability to identify patients that may be most in need of Psychological intervention. In addition, knowledge about the predictors of adaptation may inform the development of appropriate and relevant psychosocial interventions for these patients. These correlates can be broadly categorized into the following categories: demographic variables, disease- or treatment-related variables, social contextual variables, personality and coping variables, and personal history variables, consistent with Schaefer and Moos' model of adaptation to stress (6).

Sociodemographic Variables

Gender

Several studies have examined the contribution of gender to Psychological distress in the context of lung cancer. As early as 1987, Cella et al. (37) found that women with lung cancer were at greater risk for mood disturbance compared with men. Since that time, female gender has been identified as a risk factor for distress in a few (18,28,38,39) but not all studies of lung cancer patients (17,26,29,30,32,40–43). In those studies that have identified differences in distress rates by gender, the effect is not consistent across measures and is frequently rendered nonsignificant when other variables are considered in predictive models. For instance, Hopwood and Stephens (28,39) reported greater Psychological symptoms and depression

in women compared with men with NSCLC; however, this relationship did not hold true for patients with SCLC, who generally had worse performance status. Furthermore, the difference in depression rates between the sexes nearly disappeared as performance status worsened suggesting that performance status had a stronger influence on depression than status as male or female. Similarly, Kurtz et al. (19) found an interaction between gender and radiation treatment. Thus the relationship between gender and distress after lung cancer may be complicated, and gender may be a less important predictor when other variables are included in the model. Women also tend to report higher levels of depression in the general population, which may further confuse interpretation of gender differences (34,44). Finally, as illustrated in Table 26.1, the majority of participants in most studies are men, and there may not be sufficient power to detect differences in outcome by gender.

Age

Younger cancer patients have been identified as being at greater risk for emotional distress and depression in the general cancer literature (45,46). In lung cancer patients, the data are more equivocal. Although age has not been associated with higher emotional distress in lung cancer patients in several studies (20,26,30,32,37,38), especially when other variables are included in the prediction of distress, the trend is for younger patients to be more distressed (27–29,40,41). Younger patients also showed a trend toward reporting more concerns about their cancer compared with older patients in one study (20), and reported greater interest in receiving help for their symptoms in another (29). Younger lung cancer patients may be more challenged in adapting to the stressors associated with cancer due to cancer occurring as an "off time" (i.e., earlier than is culturally expected) (47) life event. Older patients also endorse higher self-efficacy for their ability to manage the symptoms associated with their cancer which is itself associated with better emotional and physical adjustment to the illness (48).

This is not to imply, however, that the needs of older patients are secondary to those of younger patients. In fact, some data indicate that older patients are less likely to be referred for psychosocial oncology care than younger patients, even when they endorse similar levels of depressive symptoms (49). Given that cancer is generally a disease of aging and that the median age at diagnosis for lung cancer is 71 years (50), the unique issues of older patients with lung cancer who may have other comorbidities, physical and psychosocial challenges, must also be considered in comprehensive cancer care.

Ethnicity

Very few data have examined the contribution of ethnic, racial, or cultural variables to distress in people with lung cancer. In fact, as shown in Table 26.1, few studies report the ethnic or racial composition of their sample. Examination of the prevalence distress across sites suggests that depression is lower in the samples of Asian patients. However, this apparent trend could represent a methodological artifact as those studies used a clinical interview to diagnose clinical depression (vs. self-report questionnaires) or it may reflect cultural differences in the expression of emotional distress. One study found no relationship between race and distress (29). In another study that found better psychosocial adjustment in Caucasian compared with African American patients, the authors hypothesized that this effect was mediated by socioeconomic status (42).

Education

Education, which is a frequent but imperfect proxy for socioeconomic status (51), had not been consistently linked to adjustment to lung cancer. Although less education was associated with more depression 1 year after surgery in one study (18), and more helpless/hopeless coping in another (40); education was unrelated to depression 3 months after surgery in an earlier report from this group (17), nor was education related to mood disturbance 6 months after diagnosis in another report (41). Education also was not a significant correlate of distress in the study by Cella et al. (37).

Summary

The findings with regard to the influence of sociodemographic variables on emotional distress in lung cancer patients are divergent, suggesting that these are not robust predictors of emotional distress. These inconsistent results also highlight the importance of examining more complex, theoretically derived constructs in the prediction of emotional distress.

Disease-Related Variables

Cancer Type

NSCLC is more common than SCLC; thus, most studies include a greater proportion, or are solely comprised, of patients with this cancer histology. Studies that have compared both types of lung cancer patients suggest higher rates of depression (25,28,39), but not anxiety (32), in patients with SCLC versus NSCLC. However, this effect washes out once other factors including functional impairment, symptom burden, and performance status are modeled in the analyses, suggesting that the relationship may be attributed to poorer functioning and higher symptom-related distress in patients with SCLC disease (28). Thus, it appears that the *impact* of the illness on the individual's level of functioning and day-to-day life is more important in predicting emotional distress than histology per se.

Stage

The data consistently suggest that disease stage is not predictive of emotional distress in lung cancer patients (17,27,29,30). However, patients with stage II and III disease did report higher levels of a helpless/hopeless coping style in the study by Uchitomi et al., which may reflect a more accurate understanding of the meaning of their disease (40). It also should be emphasized that lung cancer is usually identified in advanced stages.

Physical Functioning and Symptoms

Several studies have confirmed that depressive symptoms and mood disturbance are higher in patients with poorer physical functioning and higher levels of symptom severity (17,28–30,37,43). Akechi's (52) group also found that declining physical function and pain were correlates of suicidal ideation in patients with lung cancer, with pain remaining significant in the multivariate model. Although performance status was not predictive of depressive symptoms in the study by Walker et al. (27), this may have been due to restricted range, patients in that investigation were early stage and had good performance status. Anxiety also seems to worsen with declining performance status and increased lung cancer symptoms, including cough, dyspnea, and hemoptysis (32). Furthermore, clinical trials aimed at improving physical symptoms, such as fatigue in lung cancer patients, may also influence measures of emotional distress such as depression and anxiety (53). Symptoms that are perceived as representative of the advancement of disease (pain, fatigue, dyspnea) may be particularly emotionally distressing to patients compared with symptoms that patients attribute to the impact of treatment (nausea, vomiting) (15).

Time Since Diagnosis or Treatment

Several of the studies described in Table 26.1 are longitudinal, and as such provide a sense of the course of Psychological distress over time. A few observations can be made from the longitudinal data. Although there is some fluctuation in rates of depression and anxiety at various observation points in most of the studies, the observation points tend to be fairly close together (i.e., within weeks or a few months of one another), and these findings are generally not statistically significant (19,20). Distress has been found to lessen over time in a few studies (32,41), remain relatively stable in some studies (28,38), and worsen over time in others (16). In addition, in some studies the direction of change depends on which measure is being evaluated (16,41).

Approximately one third to one half of patients who are identified as depressed at diagnosis remain depressed at follow-up, and about 10% to 15% of initially "nondistressed" patients develop significant distress (28,30,54).

Thus, although overall rates of distress may look similar at follow-up compared with baseline, individual patients may experience reprieve from, or develop new symptoms of, distress as their illness unfolds. In other studies, most of which are conducted with breast cancer survivors, most patients evidence high and stable, or significant improvements, in Psychological adjustment over the first year following diagnosis (1,55). Most of the patients in these studies are women with early-stage disease, unlike most patients with lung cancer. However, as will be addressed in more detail below, patients at risk for emotional distress tend to be distinguished not by demographic and medical variables, but by having fewer personal and social resources (55,56).

Summary

Of the cancer-related variables that have been evaluated in relationship to emotional distress, level of symptom burden, and the impact of the cancer on the patient's functional status are most predictive of problems in this domain. In addition, measures of symptom burden and functional status may play a key role as intervening variables that explain the relationship between other disease-related variables and emotional distress, or as moderators of these relationships (28,37,53). For example, in the study by Cella's group, performance status emerged as an important predictor of distress regardless of extent of disease (limited vs. extensive), and extent of disease was a significant predictor of emotional distress only in the context of poorer performance status. However, as these authors also point out, physical functioning variables may account for a relatively small portion of the variance themselves, and must be considered in concert with other patient variables.

Social Contextual Variables

Social resources have been shown to play an important role in adjustment to cancer (1,5,55,56). In lung cancer patients specifically, markers of social support, such as marital status (37) and presence of confidants, have generally not been found to predict emotional distress (18,40,54). However, living alone and having less support from children correlated with more Psychological distress in one study (38). Satisfaction with confidants also correlates with coping style, which has been linked to Psychological adjustment (40). In addition, psychosocial characteristics of the patient's social environment may relate to the patient's personal level of distress (32,48). Anxiety in the patient's social network has been shown to relate to the patient's personal level of anxiety, which may influence the patient's willingness to discuss their distress with significant others (32).

Whether or not social support is linked to better or worse Psychological adjustment may depend on the source and nature of support, and what other variables are modeled. For instance, Akechi et al. (54) found that most categories of confidant (including parent, neighbor, colleague, clergy) were unrelated to emotional distress; however, using one's physician as a primary confidant was associated with higher distress in the univariate, but not multivariate, model. Patients who rely on their physician as their primary source of support may be doing so because other sources of support are not available to them, placing them at significant risk for distress. Directive instrumental support, which involves family members telling a patient what to do and feel, has been linked to higher levels of depressive symptoms in patients with lung cancer (27). Social functioning was a significant predictor of depression in the study by Kurtz et al. (19), but social support was unrelated to adjustment in the study by Klemm (42).

Personal Resources

Personal Perceptions

Although personal resource variables including personality and coping factors have been frequently studied in the psychooncology literature as predictors of Psychological adjustment in other cancer populations (1,5,55), relatively few studies have examined these variables as predictors of Psychological distress in people with lung cancer.

Perceptions of low self-worth and self-esteem were associated with higher levels of anxiety in one study of lung cancer patients (32). In another study, patients with higher self-efficacy for their ability to manage specific aspects of their lung cancer, including their pain, symptoms, and functioning, reported less Psychological distress and better quality-of-life outcomes, even after controlling for medical and demographic variables (48). Psychological constructs such as self-efficacy may be targets for clinical intervention studies aimed at improving outcomes in this group of patients.

Coping

A few studies have examined the relationship between coping and adjustment to lung cancer. These studies are consistent with the broader coping and adjustment literature (5) in suggesting that the use of avoidance-based (e.g., disengagement, denial) versus approach-oriented (seeking support, problem solving, emotional expression) coping relates to poorer Psychological outcomes in lung cancer patients (27,41,43,57). In addition, coping may partly account for the observed relationship between other Psychological factors, such as the attribution one makes for one's cancer, and emotional distress, again highlighting these as important areas for future clinical research (57).

Cancer-Related Attributions

Cognitive appraisal processes play a critical role in many theories of adjustment to illness (5). With regard to lung cancer specifically, making any causal attribution for one's cancer, whether internal (i.e., related to individual factors such as smoking, eating, stress) or external (god, heredity), is related to worse Psychological adjustment (58). Distress also appears to be higher in patients who make more causal attributions for their cancer, and in those who make a psychosocial (which primarily includes inter- and intrapersonal stressors) versus nonpsychosocial attribution (57).

Any discussion of lung cancer attributions must also acknowledge the known link between tobacco smoking and lung cancer (59,60). Smoking emerges as the most frequently cited cause of lung cancer by patients [e.g., 63% (57); 44% (57,58)] particularly when patients are asked to spontaneously generate a cause of their cancer. Sell et al. (61) found that 42% of lung cancer patients, all of whom were current or former smokers, expressed guilt or regret for having smoked. Although patients frequently cite smoking as a cause of lung cancer, current or former smokers also seem to qualify the extent to which smoking may have contributed to their own cancer, which may represent an effort at mitigating self-blame for their cancer, and related emotional distress (57,58). In addition, levels of cancer-related stigma, but not general guilt and shame, are higher in lung versus breast or prostate cancer patients; and patients who blame themselves for their cancer, regardless of cancer type, report higher levels of guilt, shame, anxiety, and depression (62). Finally, a substantial minority of patients with lung cancer are never-smokers. These patients may nonetheless face the stigma associated with lung cancer and may present with unique concerns and issues.

Summary

Personal resources including coping, personality attributes, and cancer-related perceptions appear to play a significant role in adjustment to lung cancer. In addition, these theoretically based variables may be important mediators of the relationship between other categories of predictors and emotional distress as well as critical targets for intervention research with this population.

Historical Variables

A history of Psychological distress prior to one's cancer, or early on in the diagnosis and treatment process, emerges as one of the most consistent and important predictors of later adjustment problems in the setting of lung (40,41,54) as well as other types of cancer (1). This finding underscores the clinical importance of screening for distress early on in the cancer trajectory to facilitate early intervention.

Summary

Several categories of variables have been examined in relation to Psychological adjustment in people with lung cancer,

including sociodemographic, disease-related, social contextual, personal resource, and historical variables. The literature converges in suggesting that patients who are experiencing higher levels of symptom distress and poorer physical functioning have a history of emotional distress, and those who have few intra- and interpersonal resources to manage the stressors of lung cancer may be at risk for emotional distress. In addition, there is a trend toward more distress in patients who are women; however, this relationship is not always significant and gender is less predictive of distress when other factors, such as the patient's performance status, are taken into consideration. Younger patients also show a trend toward greater emotional distress as well as greater interest in supportive care interventions. Although distress lessens for many patients over time, a substantial minority of distressed patients continue to experience distress, and around 10% to 15% of previously "nondistressed" patients develop significant distress, highlighting the need for early and ongoing assessment of emotional functioning.

■ LIMITATIONS AND FUTURE DIRECTIONS

Although progress is being made in understanding the Psychological issues in lung cancer patients, the data are also limited in several respects. This chapter concludes by addressing four limitations of the existing literature and recommendations to move these areas forward.

Identification of Factors Contributing to Distress in Lung Cancer

This chapter began by noting that emotional distress appears to be higher in patients with lung cancer compared with other samples of people living with cancer. Although several reasons for this difference have been hypothesized (27,57), including the poor prognosis for long-term survival, high symptom burden, and the association between smoking and lung cancer, the relative contribution of these and other variables has not been thoroughly examined. In fact, the same variables that contribute to poor Psychological adjustment in other cancer populations are also correlated with distress in people with lung cancer, suggesting that lung cancer patients are more similar than different to other cancer patients in terms of predictors of adjustment. Lung cancer patients endorse a high level of symptom burden and poor performance status compared with other cancer patients (63), which may be predictive of greater emotional distress. Although smoking is linked to various types of cancer, as well as other health problems, it is highly related to the development of lung cancer (7,59,60). Patients who feel responsible for having contributed to their cancer appear to be at greater risk for emotional distress (62).

These factors may partly account for the higher rates of emotional distress observed in some studies of lung cancer patients; however, theory-driven investigations are needed both to (a) enhance our understanding of the pathways to distress in the context of this common cancer and (b) inform interventions aimed at alleviating suffering in these patients.

Psychosocial Intervention Research

Very little psychosocial intervention research has targeted lung cancer patients specifically, despite the documented high rates of distress in this group. There is some evidence that nursing interventions may be useful in reducing symptom distress associated with the treatment and progression of lung cancer (64,65). As noted by Ryan (66), cognitive behavioral interventions that have been shown to reduce cancer-related symptoms such as pain, nausea/vomiting, and dyspnea in other cancer populations may have the potential to play a significant role in alleviating distress in this group of patients, especially given the consistent relationship between physical symptoms and emotional distress (25,28).

Long-Term Psychological Outcomes

There is a relative paucity of data on the long-term Psychological outcomes of lung cancer survivors. Although this certainly is attributable to the nature of this disease (most patients are diagnosed with advanced disease and have low life expectancy), patients with localized disease may have a 50% 5-year survival rate, and data are needed to guide the comprehensive care of these survivors (7).

The larger cancer literature suggests that the majority of cancer survivors who remain disease-free experience a gradual reduction in cancer-related distress over time (1,55,67). However, participants in these studies are generally women diagnosed with nonmetastatic breast cancer, and results from these groups may not generalize to patients with lung cancer who are generally diagnosed with advanced disease and have a poor prognosis for long-term survival. In fact, distress may increase in lung cancer patients who are noncurative as they move further out from diagnosis and face issues related to declining health, quality of life, and their mortality. It is more likely, however, that the trajectory of distress will diverge for different groups of patients depending on multiple factors, some of which have been addressed in the literature and this review but others that have not yet been examined. In one of the few studies to examine outcomes in long-term (more than 5 years from diagnosis) NSCLC survivors, Sarna et al. (68) found that nearly a quarter of patients continued to report significant symptoms of depression and 30% reported significant anxiety. In addition, approximately 50% of participants described their illness as having made a positive impact on their life,

joining other studies reporting on benefit-finding after cancer (36,69).

Much more research is needed to understand both the negative and positive sequelae of lung cancer in the long term as well as contributors to these outcomes. Such research will be challenging to conduct, especially given that attrition may be highest in patients who are more ill and distressed (18,19,41), but is crucial to our understanding of the impact of this common cancer.

Methodological Issues

Psychosocial oncology research can be challenging to conduct, and these challenges may be amplified in patients with lung cancer. The high morbidity associated with lung cancer may limit a patient's ability to participate in clinical research and result in significant attrition due to physical symptoms, emotional distress, or death; sample selection and recruitment may be complicated, and it can be challenging to design and implement feasible, acceptable, and appropriate interventions for this diverse group. Schofield et al. (70) offer several strategies for addressing these research barriers, and highlight the importance of integrating psychosocial research with the patient's medical care, and incorporating creativity and flexibility in study design and recruitment. Future psychosocial research will also need to be responsive to the changing epidemiology of smoking, including the increased incidence in women, who may be both more susceptible to lung cancer but also may demonstrate better survival compared with men (59). Despite the potential challenges associated with conducting both basic psychosocial and clinical intervention studies with this population of cancer patients, the needs of these patients are sufficiently significant to warrant an investment of energy into such research.

■ ACKNOWLEDGMENT

The author was supported in part during the writing of this chapter by a grant from the Lance Armstrong Foundation.

■ KEY POINTS

- Lung cancer is associated with significant Psychological distress in the range of 5% to 50% of patients; however, there is also substantial variability across studies.
- Psychological distress is consistently higher in patients who are more physically symptomatic, have pre-existing emotional distress, and use avoidance-based coping. Other predictors of distress are less robust.

- Although rates of Psychological distress appear higher in patients with lung compared with other cancers, explanatory models for this difference are lacking. In general there is a need for theoretically driven research that models the contribution of multiple variables to emotional adjustment over time.
- Research aimed at developing, implementing, and testing psychosocial interventions in lung cancer patients is lacking and will be an important next step for psychosocial researchers working with this population.

■ REFERENCES

1. Glanz K, Lerman C. Psychosocial impact of breast cancer: a critical review. *Ann Behav Med.* 1992;14(3):204–212.
2. Zabora J, BrintzenhofeSzoc K, Curbow B, Hooker C, Piantadosi S. The prevalence of psychological distress by cancer site. *Psychooncology.* 2001;10(1):19–28.
3. van't Spijker A, Trijsburg RW, Duivenvoorden HJ. Psychological sequelae of cancer diagnosis: a meta-analytical review of 58 studies after 1980. *Psychosom Med.* 1997;59(3):280–293.
4. Stanton AL. Psychosocial concerns and interventions for cancer survivors. *J Clin Oncol.* 2006;24(32):5132–5137.
5. Stanton AL, Revenson TA, Tennen H. Health psychology: psychological adjustment to chronic disease. *Annu Rev Psychol.* 2007;58:565–592.
6. Schaefer JA, Moos RH. Life crises and personal growth. In: Carpenter BN, ed. *Personal Coping: Theory, Research and Application.* Westport, CT: Praeger; 1992:149–170.
7. ACS. *Cancer Facts and Figures—2009.* Atlanta, GA: Author; 2009.
8. Cooley ME, Short TH, Moriarty HJ. Symptom prevalence, distress, and change over time in adults receiving treatment for lung cancer. *Psychooncology.* 2003;12(7):694–708.
9. Podnos YD, Borneman TR, Koczywas M, Uman G, Ferrell BR. Symptom concerns and resource utilization in patients with lung cancer. *J Palliat Med.* 2007;10(4):899–903.
10. Fox SW, Lyon DE. Symptom clusters and quality of life in survivors of lung cancer. *Oncol Nurs Forum.* 2006;33(5):931–936.
11. Li J, Girgis A. Supportive care needs: are patients with lung cancer a neglected population? *Psychooncology.* 2006;15(6):509–516.
12. Sanders SL, Bantum EO, Owen JE, Thornton AA, Stanton AL. Supportive care needs in patients with lung cancer. *Psychooncology.* 2010;19(5):480–489.
13. Hill KM, Amir Z, Muers MF, Connolly CK, Round CE. Do newly diagnosed lung cancer patients feel their concerns are being met? *Eur J Cancer Care (Engl).* 2003;12(1):35–45.
14. Schag CA, Ganz PA, Wing DS, Sim MS, Lee JJ. Quality of life in adult survivors of lung, colon and prostate cancer. *Qual Life Res.* 1994;3(2):127–141.
15. Sarna L. Lung cancer. In: Holland J, ed. *Psychooncology.* New York: Oxford University Press; 1998:340–348.
16. Montazeri A, Milroy R, Hole D, McEwen J, Gillis CR. Anxiety and depression in patients with lung cancer before and after diagnosis: findings from a population in Glasgow, Scotland. *J Epidemiol Community Health.* 1998;52(3):203–204.
17. Uchitomi Y, Mikami I, Kugaya A, et al. Depression after successful treatment for nonsmall cell lung carcinoma. *Cancer.* 2000;89(5):1172–1179.
18. Uchitomi Y, Mikami I, Nagai K, Nishiwaki Y, Akechi T, Okamura H. Depression and psychological distress in patients during the year after curative resection of non-small-cell lung cancer. *J Clin Oncol.* 2003;21(1):69–77.
19. Kurtz ME, Kurtz JC, Stommel M, Given CW, Given B. Predictors of depressive symptomatology of geriatric patients with lung cancer—a longitudinal analysis. *Psychooncology.* 2002;11(1):12–22.
20. Turner NJ, Muers MF, Haward RA, Mulley GP. Psychological distress and concerns of elderly patients treated with palliative radiotherapy for lung cancer. *Psychooncology.* 2007;16(8):707–713.
21. Beck AT, Ward J. Beck depression inventory. In: Beck AT, ed. *Depression: Causes and Treatment.* Philadelphia, PA: University of Pennsylvania Press; 1972.
22. Radloff LS. The CES-D scale: a self-report depression scale for research in the general population. *Appl Psychol Meas.* 1977;1(3):385–401.
23. McNair DM, Lorr A, Droppleman L. *Manual for the Profile of Mood States.* San Diego, CA: Educational and Industrial Testing Service; 1977.
24. Zigmond AS, Snaith RP. The hospital anxiety and depression scale. *Acta Psychiatr Scand.* 1983;67(6):361–370.
25. Rolke HB, Bakke PS, Gallefoss F. Health related quality of life, mood disorders and coping abilities in an unselected sample of patients with primary lung cancer. *Respir Med.* 2008;102(10):1460–1467.
26. Steinberg T, Roseman M, Kasymjanova G, et al. Prevalence of emotional distress in newly diagnosed lung cancer patients. *Support Care Cancer.* 2009;17(12):1493–1497.
27. Walker MS, Zona DM, Fisher EB. Depressive symptoms after lung cancer surgery: Their relation to coping style and social support. *Psychooncology.* 2006;15(8):684–693.
28. Hopwood P, Stephens RJ. Depression in patients with lung cancer: prevalence and risk factors derived from quality-of-life data. *J Clin Oncol.* 2000;18(4):893–903.
29. Graves KD, Arnold SM, Love CL, Kirsh KL, Moore PG, Passik SD. Distress screening in a multidisciplinary lung cancer clinic: prevalence and predictors of clinically significant distress. *Lung Cancer.* 2007;55(2):215–224.
30. Néron S, Correa JA, Dajczman E, Kasymjanova G, Kreisman H, Small D. Screening for depressive symptoms in patients with unresectable lung cancer. *Support Care Cancer.* 2007;15(10):1207–1212.
31. NCCN Clinical Practice Guidelines in Oncology™ Distress Management (V.2.2009). 2009. http://www.nccn.org/professionals/physician_gls/PDF/distress.pdf. Accessed 8/10/2009.
32. Buchanan DD, J MacIvor F. A role for intravenous lidocaine in severe cancer-related neuropathic pain at the end-of-life. *Support Care Cancer.* 2010;18(7):899–901.
33. Berard RM, Boermeester F, Viljoen G. Depressive disorders in an out-patient oncology setting: prevalence, assessment, and management. *Psychooncology.* 1998;7(2):112–120.
34. APA. *Diagnostic and Statistical Manual of Mental Disorders.* 4th (text revision) ed. Washington, DC: Author; 2000.
35. Ginsburg ML, Quirt C, Ginsburg AD, MacKillop WJ. Psychiatric illness and psychosocial concerns of patients with newly diagnosed lung cancer. *CMAJ.* 1995;152(5):701–708.
36. Thornton AA. Perceiving benefits in the cancer experience. *J Clin Psychol Med Settings.* 2002;9(2):153–165.
37. Cella DF, Orofiamma B, Holland JC, et al. The relationship of psychological distress, extent of disease, and performance status in patients with lung cancer. *Cancer.* 1987;60(7):1661–1667.
38. Akechi T, Kugaya A, Okamura H, Nishiwaki Y, Yamawaki S, Uchitomi Y. Predictive factors for psychological distress in ambulatory lung cancer patients. *Support Care Cancer.* 1998;6(3):281–286.
39. Hopwood P, Stephens RJ. Symptoms at presentation for treatment in patients with lung cancer: implications for the evaluation of palliative treatment. The Medical Research Council (MRC) Lung Cancer Working Party. *Br J Cancer.* 1995;71(3):633–636.
40. Uchitomi Y, Akechi T, Fujimori M, Okamura M, Ooba A. Mental adjustment after surgery for non-small cell lung cancer. *Palliat Support Care.* 2003;1(1):61–70.

41. Akechi T, Okuyama T, Akizuki N, et al. Course of psychological distress and its predictors in advanced non-small cell lung cancer patients. *Psychooncology.* 2006;15(6):463–473.

42. Klemm PR. Variables influencing psychosocial adjustment in lung cancer: a preliminary study. *Oncol Nurs Forum.* 1994;21(6):1059–1062.

43. Kuo TT, Ma FC. Symptom distresses and coping strategies in patients with non-small cell lung cancer. *Cancer Nurs.* 2002;25(4):309–317.

44. Nolen-Hoeksema S. Gender differences in depression. *Curr Dir Psychol Sci.* 2001;10(5):173–176.

45. Costanzo ES, Ryff CD, Singer BH. Psychosocial adjustment among cancer survivors: findings from a national survey of health and well-being. *Health Psychol.* 2009;28(2):147–156.

46. Rodin G, Lo C, Mikulincer M, Donner A, Gagliese L, Zimmermann C. Pathways to distress: the multiple determinants of depression, hopelessness, and the desire for hastened death in metastatic cancer patients. *Soc Sci Med.* 2009;68(3):562–569.

47. Neugarten BL. Time, age, and the life cycle. *Am J Psychiatry.* 1979;136(7):887–894.

48. Porter LS, Keefe FJ, Garst J, McBride CM, Baucom D. Self-efficacy for managing pain, symptoms, and function in patients with lung cancer and their informal caregivers: associations with symptoms and distress. *Pain.* 2008;137(2):306–315.

49. Ellis J, Lin J, Walsh A, et al. Predictors of referral for specialized psychosocial oncology care in patients with metastatic cancer: the contributions of age, distress, and marital status. *J Clin Oncol.* 2009;27(5):699–705.

50. Horner MJ, Reis LAG, Krapcho M, et al., eds.; SEER Cancer Statistics Review, 1975–2006. Bethesda, MD: National Cancer Institute. http://seer.cancer.gov/csr/1975_2006/, based on November 2008 SEER data submission, posted to the SEER web site, 2009. Accessed 8/10/2009.

51. Braveman PA, Cubbin C, Egerter S, et al. Socioeconomic status in health research: one size does not fit all. *JAMA.* 2005;294(22):2879–2888.

52. Akechi T, Okamura H, Nishiwaki Y, Uchitomi Y. Predictive factors for suicidal ideation in patients with unresectable lung carcinoma. *Cancer.* 2002;95(5):1085–1093.

53. Tchekmedyian NS, Kallich J, McDermott A, Fayers P, Erder MH. The relationship between psychologic distress and cancer-related fatigue. *Cancer.* 2003;98(1):198–203.

54. Akechi T, Okamura H, Nishiwaki Y, Uchitomi Y. Psychiatric disorders and associated and predictive factors in patients with unresectable nonsmall cell lung carcinoma: a longitudinal study. *Cancer.* 2001;92(10):2609–2622.

55. Helgeson VS, Snyder P, Seltman H. Psychological and physical adjustment to breast cancer over 4 years: identifying distinct trajectories of change. *Health Psychol.* 2004;23(1):3–15.

56. Bardwell WA, Natarajan L, Dimsdale JE, et al. Objective cancer-related variables are not associated with depressive symptoms in women treated for early-stage breast cancer. *J Clin Oncol.* 2006;24(16):2420–2427.

57. Faller H, Schilling S, Lang H. Causal attribution and adaptation among lung cancer patients. *J Psychosom Res.* 1995;39(5):619–627.

58. Berckman KL, Austin JK. Causal attribution, perceived control, and adjustment in patients with lung cancer. *Oncol Nurs Forum.* 1993;20(1):23–30.

59. Olak J, Colson Y. Gender differences in lung cancer: have we really come a long way, baby? *J Thorac Cardiovasc Surg.* 2004;128(3):346–351.

60. Vineis P, Alavanja M, Buffler P, et al. Tobacco and cancer: recent epidemiological evidence. *J Natl Cancer Inst.* 2004;96(2):99–106.

61. Sell L, Devlin B, Bourke SJ, Munro NC, Corris PA, Gibson GJ. Communicating the diagnosis of lung cancer. *Respir Med.* 1993;87(1):61–63.

62. LoConte NK, Else-Quest NM, Eickhoff J, Hyde J, Schiller JH. Assessment of guilt and shame in patients with non-small-cell lung cancer compared with patients with breast and prostate cancer. *Clin Lung Cancer.* 2008;9(3):171–178.

63. Lilenbaum RC, Cashy J, Hensing TA, Young S, Cella D. Prevalence of poor performance status in lung cancer patients: implications for research. *J Thorac Oncol.* 2008;3(2):125–129.

64. McCorkle R, Benoliel JQ, Donaldson G, Georgiadou F, Moinpour C, Goodell B. A randomized clinical trial of home nursing care for lung cancer patients. *Cancer.* 1989;64(6):1375–1382.

65. Sikorskii A, Given CW, Given B, et al. Symptom management for cancer patients: a trial comparing two multimodal interventions. *J Pain Symptom Manage.* 2007;34(3):253–264.

66. Ryan LS. Psychosocial issues and lung cancer: a behavioral approach. *Semin Oncol Nurs.* 1996;12(4):318–323.

67. Compas BE, Luecken L. Psychological adjustment to breast cancer. *Curr Dir Psychol Sci.* 2002;11(3):111–114.

68. Sarna L, Padilla G, Holmes C, Tashkin D, Brecht ML, Evangelista L. Quality of life of long-term survivors of non-small-cell lung cancer. *J Clin Oncol.* 2002;20(13):2920–2929.

69. Stanton AL, Bower JE, Low CA. Posttraumatic growth after cancer. In: Calhoun LG, Tedeschi RG, eds. *Handbook of Posttraumatic Growth: Research and Practice.* Mahwah, NJ: Erlbaum; 2006:138–175.

70. Schofield P, Ugalde A, Carey M, et al. Lung cancer: challenges and solutions for supportive care intervention research. *Palliat Support Care.* 2008;6(3):281–287.

Multidisciplinary Management of Lung Cancer in the Community Setting

JONATHAN W. GOLDMAN

■ INTRODUCTION

As is well-known, lung cancer is the most common cause of cancer mortality worldwide for both men and women, causing approximately 1.2 million deaths per year. In the United States, there were an estimated 215,000 new cases of lung cancer and 162,000 deaths in 2008 (1). Because the majority of cancer care in this country is provided at nonacademic centers (2), community-based oncologists and their treatment decisions make the greatest impact on nationwide cancer outcomes.

After decades of near stasis in lung cancer care progress, we are at the dawn of a new era of personalized medicine, new treatment targets, and improved risk-to-benefit ratios. While not universal, some communities have effectively decreased smoking rates by limiting tobacco use in public areas. Lung cancer screening remains controversial, but results of a definitive randomized study are expected soon. Minimally invasive surgical techniques have been proven effective and less morbid. Radiotherapy and radiosurgery open new options for the surgically unfit due to comorbidities or extent of disease. Systemic therapies in the form of cytotoxic and targeted agents are increasingly efficacious with less toxicity.

Community-based oncologists face several challenges as they bring these advances to their patient populations. As progress accelerates, it becomes increasingly difficult to keep "up to date." Surgical expertise in new techniques may take some time to develop. While radiation oncologists have typically been quick to adopt technological advances, new machines are expensive and often require substantial capital input from hospitals or outpatient facilities. Chemotherapy options have proliferated and, in the absence of clear-cut management algorithms, decisions regarding initial and subsequent treatments are complex.

At the same time, there is pressure to move ahead of clinically proven advances. As practitioners attempt to distinguish themselves from their colleagues, there may be a temptation to utilize a therapy outside of the setting in which it has proven benefit, or to add effective treatments together even though the combination has not been studied.

Of note, the remedy for both of these challenges, being too far "behind" or "ahead" of scientific knowledge, may be one and the same. Participation in a group of cancer care providers, possibly as a tumor board or a research consortium, provides education and the opportunity to develop community-wide standards of care that are consistent with national guidelines.

Overall, the evidence suggests that the level of care provided in the community is high quality. For example, phase IV postmarketing studies of the anti-vascular endothelial growth factor antibody bevacizumab show that complication rates are lower in community practice than they were in the initial academic studies (3–7). This suggests that community oncologists quickly incorporate new treatment modalities and apply them as appropriate and with care. In fact, with less bureaucracy and greater efficiency, the community cancer clinic may be able to obtain diagnostic testing and start treatment faster. A particularly exciting development is the greater involvement of community practice sites in cancer research. The high patient volume and leaner organization of these sites allow for faster study initiation and patient accrual. Simultaneously, the opportunity to participate in clinical trials may be extended to a much greater array of patients. As a result, national rates of patient clinical trial involvement can be increased above the historic rate of 3%.

■ NONSMALL CELL LUNG CANCER: ISSUES IN COMMUNITY-BASED CARE

The annual report to the nation on the status of cancer, 1975 to 2002, published in 2005 in the *Journal of the National Cancer Institute* revealed encouraging findings. Over the last decade of that time period, lung cancer incidence decreased for men by 2% and stabilized for women (after decades of rising) (8). Lung cancer mortality decreased in men by 1.9% and increased in women slightly by 0.3%. These findings were true among nearly all racial and ethnic groups. At the same time, there was discouraging evidence that while much of contemporary cancer treatment was consistent with evidence-based guidelines, there were nevertheless geographic, racial, economic, and age-related disparities in cancer treatment. Despite the widespread availability of lung cancer treatment guidelines (9–17), a 2004 report from medical chart reviews suggested that only 52% of non–small cell lung cancer (NSCLC) patients received recommended therapy (18). A similar study of lung cancer patients with Medicare found that, among several nonmedical factors, treatment in a teaching hospital significantly increased a patient's likelihood of receiving appropriate chemotherapy (19). Another review of the Surveillance, Epidemiology, and End Results (SEER) database found that these disparities primarily affected whether or not a patient was referred to an oncologist; in contrast, among referred patients, care was mostly determined by appropriate medical factors (20). Clearly, in order to realize fully the benefits of recent breakthroughs in the understanding and treatment of lung cancer, these advances must be implemented in the care of all patients. This chapter section will review the importance of community-based care in the various subfields of NSCLC treatment: modification of risk factors, chemoprevention, screening, diagnosis, staging, and treatment. Small cell lung cancer (SCLC) will be addressed very briefly afterward. Throughout, the importance of multidisciplinary care will be emphasized.

■ RISK FACTORS

Tobacco cessation must still be the centerpiece of the public health fight against lung cancer. Tobacco use is the causative factor in greater than 85% of lung cancer, and its rise through the 20th century increased lung cancer death rates from about five cases per 100,000 people to greater than 50 cases per 100,000 (1,21). This was an increase from a rate comparable to that from pancreatic cancer to a rate greater than that from breast, colorectal, and prostate cancer combined. The physician can contribute to reducing tobacco use in several ways. Studies have shown benefit from referral to telephone hotlines and support groups, nicotine replacement, newer medications such as buproprion and varenicline, and simply doctor's admonition and encouragement. Each of these interventions improves tobacco cessation rates with a relative risk of 2 to 3 (22–24). Community-based physicians, generalists and specialists, play the greatest role in supporting their patients to quit smoking.

■ CHEMOPREVENTION

No study has shown a benefit to chemoprevention strategies. The largest such trial, following more than 18,000 subjects

randomized to placebo or β-carotene and retinol, in fact, showed a detriment from supplementation (25). Strategies currently under investigation include inhibitors of the epidermal growth factor receptor (EGFR) and cyclooxygenase-2 (COX-2) (26–29).

■ SCREENING

Lung cancer screening for patients at high risk, including former and current smokers, is a problem confronting the community practitioner more frequently than the academician. Due to the particularly high mortality of advanced-stage lung cancer, screening of high-risk populations has been under study for several decades. Chest x-ray and sputum evaluation were shown to have insufficient sensitivity and specificity and frequently diagnosed cancers that were unlikely to become clinically significant in the lifetime of the patient (30–33). A Cochrane meta-analysis of six large randomized trial and one nonrandomized trial, in fact, showed an 11% increase in lung cancer mortality associated with frequent chest x-ray screening ($P = 0.05$) (30). Lung cancer screening with low-dose computed tomography (CT) imaging was at the root of considerable recent controversy when contradictory papers were published in 2006 to 2007. The International Early Lung Cancer Action Program (I-ELCAP) was reported by Henschke et al. (34), in 2006. This revealed an exceptionally good 10-year lung cancer–specific survival of 80% among those diagnosed with lung cancer, and the great improvement over historical data was interpreted as a benefit from the screening program. The trial was widely criticized for numerous biases, including lead-time bias, length bias, overdiagnosis, and volunteer bias, not to mention alarm over the authors' financial interests as recipients of tobacco-company grants and patent-holders of the computer-aided diagnostic methods used in the study (35–37). Taken by many to confirm these concerns, Bach et al. (38) illustrated with data from the Instituto Tumori in Milan, the Mayo Clinic, and the Moffitt Cancer Center that CT screening may increase the rate of lung cancer diagnosis and treatment but might not meaningfully reduce the risk of advanced lung cancer or death from lung cancer.

This leaves the practitioner with little guidance regarding care for high-risk patients. It is hoped that the National Lung Screening Trial, run by the National Institutes of Health (NIH), will resolve these controversies. Accrual was completed in 2004 with nearly 50,000 current or former smokers at more than 30 study sites across the country (39). The trial will examine the risks and benefits of spiral CT scans compared with chest x-rays. Results are expected in 2010. Other research directions that may improve negative and positive predictive values include the addition of selective positron emission tomography (PET) scanning to

CT scans (40,41). Perhaps the most intriguing new research direction is breath analysis for cancer-associated volatile organic compounds with gas chromatography, mass spectroscopy, and sensor array technologies (42–46).

At the present time, the most appropriate approach is careful assessment of those at the highest risk of developing lung cancer. An interesting study published in *Chest* describes such an approach (47). Patients at high risk of lung cancer underwent spirometric testing; those with airflow obstruction proceeded to chest posteroanterior radiographs, thoracic CT scans, and sputum cytology. Six cancers were diagnosed in a group of 1,296 patients, at a cost per cancer found of $11,925. Of course, the possibility of overdiagnosis as seen in other trials does exist, and a controlled study of this approach with a mortality endpoint would be appropriate.

Lastly, a discussion of risk factors and screening must acknowledge a purported recent increase in lung cancers in nonsmokers. This further complicates screening strategies due to difficulties in identifying cancer risk factors among nonsmokers.

■ DIAGNOSIS AND STAGING

The diagnosis of lung cancer is made by pathologic assessment of a concerning lung mass or metastatic site. Procedures of choice to assess a lung mass include bronchoalveolar lavage for cytology, transbronchial biopsy, mediastinoscopy, CT-guided fine needle aspiration and core needle biopsy, and resection by thoracoscopy or thoracotomy. The decision between these modalities is typically driven by the location of the tumor, either central or peripheral, and whether or not radiographically enlarged lymph nodes are present. There are unlikely to be any distinctions between academic and community-based diagnostic approaches, although there may be varying access to pulmonologists, thoracic surgeons, and interventional radiologists. If there is radiographic or physical examination evidence for a metastatic site, there is general agreement that the initial biopsy should be taken from the site of possible distant disease, in that this would provide diagnostic and staging information with a single procedure.

Once a diagnosis is made, however, there is considerable controversy in both the academic and community settings regarding staging. Reviewing multiple care settings in Vermont and New Hampshire, Greenberg et al. (48) found that patients at university hospital centers underwent significantly more staging procedures and were assigned a higher stage than those in the community. Furthermore, the university patients had a better survival than the community patients, stage-for-stage, suggesting that the community patients may have been understaged. As a control, patients were also stratified by performance status; in this analysis

there was no difference in outcome between the academy and the community, suggesting that the finding was not due to a difference in quality of care between the two settings.

The most significant controversy in staging revolves around the preoperative assessment of mediastinal lymph nodes. After an early report regarding the high negative predictive value of a negative imaging study, particularly with a small peripheral lung cancer, some suggested that mediastinoscopy was not routinely required (49). The 2007 American College of Chest Physicians guidelines recommend that, given the additional benefit of PET scanning, mediastinal lymph node sampling is not required for peripheral clinical stage I tumors unless there is positive mediastinal imaging (50,51). Nevertheless, numerous centers still argue that with the present limitations of radiography, all lung cancer patients considered for definitive resection require a mediastinoscopy for histologic staging (52,53). A conservative approach is advised by Robert McKenna, Jr, MD, Chief of Thoracic Surgery at Cedars-Sinai Medical Center in Los Angeles:

> Evaluation of the mediastinum is a critical step for the treatment planning of lung cancer. Our experience with over 1000 PET scans showed a 30% false positive rate for N2 disease diagnosed by PET scan. Also, 10% of clinical T1N0 patients are found to have pathologic N2 Disease and 25% of clinical T2N0 patients have pathologic N2 disease. Therefore, patients need node biopsies to determine the true stage. We perform endobronchial ultrasound (EBUS) [with transbronchial needle aspiration] and mediastinoscopy if EBUS is negative on all patients unless they have T1N0 disease by PET/CT. For T1N0 patients we perform EBUS and, if negative, mediastinoscopy for central tumors, patients over 80 years old, and patients with poor performance status (54).

Jay M. Lee, Surgical Director of the Thoracic Oncology Program at University of California, Los Angeles, concurs that routine pathologic assessment of the mediastinal lymph nodes is appropriate due to the inaccuracy of clinical staging based on imaging studies. Nevertheless, invasive mediastinal staging may not be required for well-differentiated neuroendocrine carcinoma or bronchoalveolar carcinoma (55). A large retrospective study confirms the importance of "multimodality" staging, described as CT scanning, PET scanning, and invasive staging (56). The hazard for death is reduced by 51% if all three techniques are used compared with just CT scanning. Encouragingly, the rate of use of 2 or 3 staging modalities increased from 10.4% to 35% in just 4 years from 1998 to 2002.

While cervical mediastinoscopy remains the gold standard in invasive mediastinal staging, there is an evolving role for endoscopic methods (EUS and EBUS) with transbronchial needle aspiration (TBNA). Harrow et al. (57) presented data from 360 consecutive patients evaluated in 1995 and 1996 from four cancer centers. Patients with a nondiagnostic EUS or EBUS specimen proceeded to appropriate invasive testing, such as mediastinoscopy. TBNA had a sensitivity greater than 57% in lymph nodes greater than 10 mm, precluded additional thoracic surgery in 29% of cases, and was the sole means of cancer diagnosis in 18%. These results should be interpreted with caution because the accuracy of an endoscopic assessment of subcentimeter, metabolically inactive lymph nodes with a low likelihood of metastatic involvement needs to be further defined. As such, at the current time, Dr. Lee feels that a negative fine needle biopsy result from EUS or EBUS requires confirmation by mediastinoscopy.

Pretreatment staging procedures and imaging studies appropriate to the various clinical stages are suggested in Table 27.1.

■ TREATMENT

Referral Patterns

The first obstacle to proper treatment may be referral to a cancer specialist. In some communities, there may be a tendency not to refer lung cancer patients for treatment possibly due to misconceptions regarding its futility. A questionnaire assessment of primary care physicians in Wisconsin by Joan Schiller et al. revealed a hesitation to refer lung cancer patients compared with breast cancer patients (58). Follow-up questions suggested that practitioners mistakenly believed that chemotherapy did not improve lung cancer survival. Therefore, to improve national lung cancer outcomes, one of the projects of the community-based oncologist must be the education of local primary care providers about the significant advances in multimodality care over the last decade (58).

Cancer Care Sites

The majority of the population of the continental United States resides near cancer care specialists. In an assessment by zip code, travel times of an hour or less were estimated for 92%. For comparison, only 45% were close to a National Cancer Institute (NCI) Cancer Center and 69% were close to an academic site (59). Populations at risk for decreased geographic access to cancer care were native Americans, nonurban dwellers, and residents in the South. The association between the site of care delivery and outcome is controversial. A recent SEER data base review of Medicare patients with cancers of the lung, breast, colon/rectum, or prostate found that NCI cancer center attendees,

■ Table 27.1 Pretreatment evaluation

Clinical Stage [a]	Appropriate Imaging and Procedures	Imaging and Procedures to Consider
IA (peripheral)	CT chest with adrenals included Full body PET/CT scan PFTs Bronchoscopy ± EBUS Mediastinoscopy (may be omitted with negative mediastinal imaging)	Brain MRI[b] if headache or neurologic symptoms
IA (central)	CT chest with adrenals included Full body PET/CT scan PFTs Bronchoscopy ± EBUS Mediastinoscopy	Brain MRI[b] if headache or neurologic symptoms Bone scan (may be omitted if PET obtained)
IB, II, IIIA, or IV, M1b with solitary site	CT chest with adrenals included Full body PET/CT scan PFTs Bronchoscopy ± EBUS Mediastinoscopy Brain MRI[b]	Bone scan (may be omitted if PET obtained)
IIIB, or IV	CT chest with adrenals included Full body PET/CT scan Biopsy for pathologic confirmation of possible metastatic site Brain MRI[b]	

[a] As per Goldstraw P, Crowley J, Chansky K, et al. The IASLC Lung Cancer Staging Project: Proposals for the revision of the TNM stage groupings in the forthcoming (seventh) edition of the TNM classification of malignant tumors. *J Thorac Oncol.* 2007;2:706–714; [b] CT brain with intravenous contrast can be substituted if there is a contraindication to a brain MRI.

CT, computed tomography; EBUS, endobronchial ultrasound; MRI, magnetic resonance imaging; PET, positron emission tomography; PFTS, pulmonary function tests.

Adapted from Ref. 10.

compared with nonattendees, had improved 1- and 3-year all-cause and cancer-specific mortality rates, particular with late-stage cancers (60). This finding certainly may be open to confounders, as socioeconomic and educational status may affect cancer center attendance and have been on their own stronger predictors of cancer outcomes. For example, those with less than a high school education had two to three times the lung cancer incidence of those that were college-educated, and those earning less than $12,500 annually had 1.7 times the lung cancer incidence of those earning more than $50,000 (61).

Surgery

The association between a hospital's volume of cancer operations and its surgical outcomes has been shown in numerous tumor types including cancers of the pancreas, esophagus, colon and rectum, and prostate. This was more difficult to discern in lung cancer resections, and, in fact, several studies have found no such relationship (62). Romano and Mark (63) first demonstrated that postoperative mortality was lower at high-volume centers (greater than 24 surgeries per year) compared with low-volume centers (less than nine surgeries per year) using data from California hospitals discharge records with an adjusted odds ratio of 0.6 for pneumonectomies and for lesser resections. This corresponded to an increase in in-hospital postoperative death following pneumonectomy from 9.7% to 13.6% and following lesser resections from 3.4% to 5.2%. There was also a nonsignificant trend for improved outcomes at teaching hospitals.

These findings were confirmed by Bach et al. (64), utilizing the SEER Cancer Registries to identify patients and the Nationwide Inpatient Sample to classify the treating hospitals. Five-year survival was 44% at high-volume centers (HVC) (greater than 66 cases per year) compared with 33% at low-volume centers (LVC) (less than nine cases per year). This finding held true at both teaching and nonteaching hospitals. Although teaching hospitals were more likely to be HVC than nonteaching hospitals, regardless of the volume of procedures, the rate of survival was better among patients at teaching hospitals rather than nonteaching hospitals (42% and 34%, respectively). Hospital length of stay and complication rates were also lower at HVC. A similar study performed in Canada also found that high-volume but not hospital teaching status affected long-term death risk following lung cancer resection at a small but significant hazard ratio of 1.3 (65). A large American study using a 10-year SEER-Medicare data set quantified the effect on 5-year survival at 6%—an effect not explained by differences in adjuvant care (66).

It has been difficult to determine what factors lead to improved outcomes at high-volume centers. A large study in the *New England Journal of Medicine* comparing the effect of hospital and surgeon volume on eight different cardiovascular and cancer surgeries revealed that the odds ratio for operative death at a low-volume center was increased for lung cancer resection, but to a small degree (1.24) compared with pancreatic resections (3.61) (67). Surgeon volume per se accounted for only 24% of the effect seen in lung cancer resections. The same group then went on to assess with another Medicare cohort if there were discernible processes that accounted for improved outcomes at the high-volume centers (68). Patients treated in hospitals in the highest quintile of volume were more likely to undergo preoperative cardiac stress testing and consultation with a medical or radiation oncologist. They also had significantly longer operations and were more likely to receive perioperative invasive monitoring. However, these differences in measurable processes of care did not explain volume-related differences in operative mortality in risk-adjustment modeling.

Cheung et al. recently reviewed the experience throughout Florida, analyzing the outcomes of lung cancer surgery with curative intent by teaching facilities (TF) versus non-TF and by HVC versus LVC. They showed improved outcomes at both teaching and high-volume facilities (69). Median survival time (MST) was superior for patients treated at TF versus NTF (47.1 vs. 40.5 months, $P < 0.001$), and mortality rates at NTF were higher at 30 days (2.6% vs. 1.1%, $P < 0.001$), 90 days (6.8% vs. 3.8%, $P < 0.001$), and at 5 years (63.9% vs. 59.2%, $P = 0.005$). Similarly, MST was superior in the cohort treated at HVC versus LVC (45.1 vs. 39.8 months, $P < 0.001$), and mortality rates were higher in LVC at 30 days (2.7% vs. 1.6%, $P < 0.001$), 90 days (7.5% vs. 4.0%, $P < 0.001$), and at 5 years (63.5% vs. 59.3%, $P = 0.002$). Meguid et al. (70) attempted to isolate the effect of a facility's teaching status from its volume, and found that at teaching hospitals the odds of death for pneumonectomy and lobectomy were significantly reduced independent of surgical volume, except for at the highest hospital volume strata. These issues have led some to call for greater centralization of complex cancer surgeries to high-volume "Centers of Excellence" (71).

An issue of similar importance is a comparison of surgical outcomes for general, cardiothoracic and thoracic surgeons. Frank C. Detterbeck, Surgical Director of the Yale Thoracic Oncology Program, estimated that each subspecialty performed approximately one third of lung cancer surgeries (72). Analyzed by the surgeon's specialty, one study from the SEER database showed that the hazard of death was 11% lower for general thoracic surgeons compared with general surgeons (73). Furthermore, general thoracic surgeons more frequently used preoperative PET scanning and lymphadenectomy than either general or cardiothoracic surgeons. These results echo previous studies, which found that adjusted operative mortality rates were lowest for cardiothoracic and general thoracic surgeons (7.6% general surgeons, 5.6% cardiothoracic surgeons, 5.8% general thoracic surgeons, $P = 0.001$) (74).

Not surprisingly, this effect was partially explained by differences in hospital and surgeon volume.

Others have questioned whether the NCI-designated cancer centers have differential outcomes compared with control hospitals. Birkmeyer et al. assessed Medicare records of 63,860 elderly patients undergoing resection for lung, esophageal, gastric, pancreatic, bladder, or colon carcinoma. Patients treated at the 51 NCI cancer centers were compared with patients from 51 control hospitals with the highest volumes for each procedure (75). NCI cancer centers had lower adjusted surgical mortality rates than control hospitals for four of the six procedures, including colectomy (5.4% vs. 6.7%; $P = 0.026$), pulmonary resection (6.3% vs. 7.9%; $P = 0.010$), gastrectomy (8.0% vs. 12.2%; $P < 0.001$), and esophagectomy (7.9% vs. 10.9%; $P = 0.027$). Among patients surviving surgery, however, there were no important differences in subsequent 5-year mortality rates between NCI cancer centers and control hospitals for any of the procedures.

Perhaps the most significant recent advance in lung cancer surgery is the increased use of video-assisted thoracoscopic surgery (VATS) (76–80). VATS segmentectomy and lobectomy have been consistently found to be associated with shorter chest tube duration and hospitalization. A SEER database review showed that the odds of early death and the overall hazard of death were not different between VATS and thoracotomy (79). In contrast, a meta-analysis of published studies showed a statistically significant improvement in survival at 4 years associated with VATS (77). VATS techniques are also more frequently utilized by high-volume surgeons at high-volume hospitals (79). Some have called for standardization of terminology and procedures, increased quality assurance review, and the establishment of centers of excellence (81).

In summary, most studies have shown a small but statistically significant survival benefit to undergoing lung cancer surgery at a high-volume center with a thoracic surgeon. Some studies have also found an improvement associated with academic centers, which can be matched at the highest-volume nonacademic centers. These findings notwithstanding, there are clearly excellent surgeons at low-volume nonacademic centers; for example, one rural, single-surgeon facility reported low complication and mortality rates (2.9% and 1.2%, respectively) across a wide range of cancer surgeries (82).

Radiation Therapy

There have been few reviews of the quality of lung cancer radiation therapy in the community compared with that in an academic setting. In other arenas, however, the field of radiation oncology has been found to provide a similar quality of care at all types of sites (83,84). For example, a recently published analysis of breast cancer adjuvant radiotherapy found no statistical difference in the mean dose homogeneity index, heart and lung dose, or skin toxicities between academic and community sites (85). This may be partially due to the early implementation of national advisory guidelines (86). Others hypothesize that the rapid and widespread integration of new technologies explains the consistency of delivered radiation therapy care. Notably, intensity modulated radiation therapy (IMRT) spread quickly from its inception in the late 1990s to become widely available less than 10 years later. An early 2003 study by questionnaire found that one third of respondents utilized IMRT (87). Reflecting the high cost of entry to the field, IMRT capabilities were present in 15% of single physician practices, but in 44% of practices with greater than four physicians. A follow-up study 2 years later showed that the rate of IMRT use had more than doubled to 73% (88). A recent review of the field assessed the state-of-the-art and identified concerns and caveats for practitioners (89).

Lung cancer–specific radiotherapy patterns of care studies have demonstrated similar treatment algorithms across the various types of institutions (90). Nevertheless, there are certain patient subpopulations seen more frequently at community than academic sites, such as those with older age, more comorbidities, and lower performance status. Medical Director of Radiation Therapy at Saint John's Health Center in Santa Monica, Robert Wollman, MD, reviewed the lung cancer experience at his facility:

> In my experience, community radiation oncologists deal more often with an older population with greater comorbidity. Patients are very often inadequately staged with mediastinoscopy. Non-standard chemotherapy protocols are used more often. The departments are smaller which means more time for one-on-one patient to MD, nurse, or therapist interaction. Many departments are single machine departments which means technological upgrades are often lagging. However, doctors seem to work more closely with one another in the multi-disciplinary setting outside of academia (91).

Lisa Chaiken, MD, also in the Saint John's Radiation Oncology Department, concurred:

> There is now, more than ever, a push to multidisciplinary care. Upfront mediastinoscopy and careful staging before treatment are helping to get more patients appropriately to surgery or definitive chemotherapy and radiation. More and more, this is happening in the community setting and I don't think there is a gap between community and academic treatment if there is a well trained thoracic surgeon on board (92).

As will be discussed below, multidisciplinary communication and coordination is a most effective method of ensuring the provision of the highest level of care.

Within the field of lung cancer radiotherapy, there are certain areas of significant controversy. Treatment of stage III NSCLC is particularly contentious. Most guidelines suggest that resection in high-functioning patients is reasonable for stage IIIA but not for IIIB (13), with the exception of superior sulcus or other T4N0–1 tumors (93–95). Nevertheless, there are community-specific standards that may be more or less aggressive, possibly due to the surgeon's preference. A recently reported trial by Albain et al. (96) showed equivalent overall survival for stage IIIA patient whether they underwent resection following chemoradiotherapy or not; progression-free survival was higher with surgery but so were treatment-related deaths.

As mentioned by Dr. Wollman the chemotherapeutic regimen used concurrently with radiation may differ between the academic and community settings. Although anecdotal, it does appear that cisplatin and etoposide (as per the Southwest Oncology Group trial 9019) is used most frequently in university settings, as it is the regimen with the most evidence for efficacy (97). In community sites, however, there has been a rapid movement to newer regimens such as pemetrexed with either cisplatin or carboplatin. Although this was found to be safe in a phase I study (98), efficacy is unknown while trials such as PROCLAIM and Cancer and Leukemia Group B (CALGB) study 30407 are underway (99). It may be rational to switch pemetrexed for etoposide in the treatment of nonsquamous NSCLC because it appears to be more active in the metastatic setting. However, the appropriateness of using an unproven regimen, particularly in a potentially curative setting, is a matter of debate and certainly would require appropriate discussions with the patient.

Increasingly, stereotactic body radiosurgery (SBRT) is used for early-stage cancers in patients who are poor surgical candidates (80). The Radiation Therapy Oncology Group has recently adopted quality assurance guidelines (100). Nevertheless, the difficulty of implementing a radiosurgery program has been well documented (101). As Michael Steinberg, MD, Chair of the UCLA Radiation Oncology department cautions, "SBRT can be treacherous for facilities without experience and significant medical physics support"(102).

Chemotherapeutics

Regarding chemotherapeutics for metastatic disease, "ground zero" may be marked by the 2002 publication from Schiller et al. (103) of the Eastern Cooperative Oncology Group's comparison of four platinum-based chemotherapy regimens from 1996 to 1999. None of the regimens was more efficacious than another, and the outcome was equally discouraging with each: a response rate of 19%, a median survival of 7.9 months, a 1-year survival rate of 33%, and a 2-year survival rate of 11%. In the following 10 years, randomized phase III trials have approached and surpassed a 12-month median survival. The understanding of histologic, genetic, and protein expression determinants of treatment responses has ushered in the age of targeted treatment.

Because there have been very few published comparisons of medical oncology in community or academic institutions, I have relied primarily on a Patterns of Care report edited by Love and Miller (104). This was based on a survey completed in October 2008 by 100 randomly selected community-based oncologists and 25 clinical investigators who specialized in lung cancer management. Although it is a small sample set, it is instructive. (It is acknowledged that not all the clinical investigators were academics, but the majority were.) While it shows that medical oncologists in both settings have similar approaches toward adjuvant and metastatic chemotherapy, employing newer cytotoxic and biologic agents when possible, there are some differences in agents used. In general, there is a different weighing of the risks and benefits. For example community-based oncologists tend to use more carboplatin-based regimens and academic oncologists more cisplatin-based; presumably, this is because the former believe that carboplatin is better tolerated and easier to deliver and the latter believe cisplatin to be more efficacious. Below is a review of several of the latest developments in NSCLC care, and how these various approaches are applied in academic and community settings.

Adjuvant Chemotherapy

Adjuvant chemotherapy for resectable stage II–III NSCLC (and possibly stage IB) is one of the great advances of the past decade. Adjuvant therapy offers the thoracic medical oncologist a rare opportunity—to cure a patient. Cisplatin-based chemotherapy likely provides a 5-to-10% absolute long-term survival advantage. The initial evidence came from a 1995 meta-analysis showing detriment from alkylating agents but a benefit from cisplatin-based regimens (105). Four larger trials—International Adjuvant Lung Cancer Trial (IALT), JBR.10, Adjuvant Navelbine International Trialist Association, and CALGB 9633—have shown a benefit to adjuvant platinum doublets, although the improvement in the CALGB lost statistical significance at the second evaluation (106–109). Of note, that study was the only one of the four to use carboplatin-based doublet therapy instead of cisplatin.

The LACE meta-analysis included 4,584 patients from the five largest trials of cisplatin-based adjuvant therapy (that were conducted after the 1995 meta-analysis) and showed an overall hazard ratio (HR) of death of 0.89 (95% confidence interval [CI] 0.82–0.96; $P = 0.005$), corresponding to a 5-year absolute survival benefit of 5.4% from chemotherapy (110). The benefit varied with stage, with an HR of 0.83 for stages II and III (CI did not cross unity), 0.93 for stage IB (not significant), and 1.40 for stage IA. The data were not sufficient to identify which secondary agent was most efficacious, but most of the patients were treated with vinorelbine. The most recent updated datasets come from IALT, presented at the American Society of Clinical Oncology (ASCO) Annual Meeting

2008, and JBR.10, presented at ASCO 2009 (111,112). Both show a diminished survival benefit at reanalysis, with IALT maintaining only borderline-significance and JBR.10 retaining significance. The IALT data suggests a late, noncancer-related death increase in the chemotherapy arm, and a JBR.10 subset analysis raises the possibility that the chemotherapy benefit may be confined to lymph node–positive patients.

The effect of adjuvant chemotherapy on quality of life (QOL) has also been evaluated. Subjects in the JBR.10 trial randomized to receive chemotherapy reported a transient impact on QOL at 3 months, marked by increased fatigue, anorexia, nausea, vomiting, and hair loss (113). By 9 months, QOL returned to baseline except for persistent sensory neuropathy and hearing loss. This effect was further quantified in a quality-adjusted time without symptoms or toxicity (Q-TWiST) analysis showing that, despite chemotherapy toxicity, adjuvant therapy provided increased quality-adjusted survival (114).

The 2008 Patterns of Care report suggests some differences in how these findings are applied in the community and academic settings (acknowledging that the JBR.10 update occurred after the questionnaire was completed). Regarding whether or not a 60-year-old with good performance status and a node-negative NSCLC should in general receive adjuvant chemotherapy, community oncologists are more likely to treat. For a 3-cm tumor, 32% of community oncologists versus 8% of academic investigators would recommend adjuvant chemotherapy. For a 5-cm tumor, the respective percentages are 76% and 60% (104). This suggests, surprisingly, that community oncologists may be overly aggressive for smaller cancers, while clinical investigators may be too timid for larger ones. In contrast, there was near-complete agreement that most resected lymph node–positive tumors should be treated with adjuvant chemotherapy.

There are also significant differences in the specific chemotherapy regimen applied. Community oncologists use carboplatin and cisplatin to an approximately equal extent, while their academic peers treat with cisplatin three times as often as with carboplatin (104). Accordingly, in the community, carboplatin with paclitaxel is the most common adjuvant regimen, while in academia, almost 75% treat with cisplatin and one of vinorelbine, docetaxel, or gemcitabine. In general, it is clear that the majority of evidence supporting adjuvant chemotherapy is with cisplatin-based treatment, but that in certain populations it is difficult to deliver. In the JBR.10 trial, only 48% of subjects completed all four cycles of cisplatin and vinorelbine (115), and possibly the community patients may have more comorbidities or be less tolerant of treatment toxicities. Other controversies in adjuvant treatment that will not be addressed here include the use of radiation therapy in addition to chemotherapy, consolidation chemotherapy after definitive radiotherapy and the use of an EGFR tyrosine kinase inhibitor in the adjuvant setting.

Treatment options for NSCLC by stage are summarized in Table 27.2.

Chemotherapy for Advanced Disease

In the advanced setting, perhaps the most significant recent advance is the identification of the histology-dependence of pemetrexed activity. In a seminal paper by Scagliotti et al. (116) overall survival for cisplatin and pemetrexed was noninferior to cisplatin and gemcitabine (both with a median survival of 10.3 months); however, in a preplanned subset analysis by histology, overall survival was statistically superior for the pemetrexed regimen in patients with adenocarcinoma (12.6 vs. 10.9 months) and large-cell carcinoma histology (10.4 vs. 6.7 months), and inferior in patients with squamous cell histology (9.4 vs. 10.8 months). These results were initially reported at the ASCO Annual Meeting in 2008, shortly before the Patterns of Care questionnaire. Its results suggest that the data were incorporated into practice quickly among academic doctors, in that physicians in this setting utilized pemetrexed in their first-line metastatic regimen for nonsquamous cancers 52% of the time. In contrast, this regimen was used in the community 10% of the time, perhaps because physicians in this setting preferred to use the three-agent regimen, carboplatin, paclitaxel, and bevacizumab. Figure 27.1 demonstrates the reported use of several first-line chemotherapy regimens in academic and community settings.

Targeted therapies

The other significant contribution to the rapid evolution of metastatic NSCLC care is the development of targeted therapies, specifically bevacizumab, cetuximab, erlotinib, and gefitinib. As reported by Sandler et al. (117) in 2006, the addition of bevacizumab to carboplatin and paclitaxel was associated with an improved median survival from 10.3 to 12.3 months (HR for death, 0.79; $P = 0.003$). Median progression-free survival and response rates were also improved, at the cost of more clinically significant bleeding (4.4% vs. 0.7%) and 15 treatment-related deaths. The issue of pulmonary hemorrhage was of particular concern. However, several postmarketing reports confirmed that bevacizumab was being used safely in community practice, even as its application was broadened to allow its use in the setting of treated brain metastases and of therapeutic anticoagulation (3–7). As demonstrated in the Patterns of Care report from Love and Miller, there was a difference in the chemotherapy backbone for bevacizumab in the community and academic settings. In the community, in the vast majority of cases, it was used following phase III trial evidence, in combination with carboplatin and paclitaxel. In contrast, the clinical trialists

■ **Table 27.2** Treatment options for non–small cell lung cancer by stage

Stage[a]	Preferred Management Options	Other Management Options to Consider
IA (peripheral)	Lobectomy (with LN sampling if not previously performed).	For nonoperative candidates, local ablation (SBRT preferred over RFA or cryotherapy).
IA (central), IB, IIA or IIB	Lobectomy or pneumonectomy depending on anatomic location, with LN sampling. Adjuvant chemotherapy for stage II (and possibly large stage IB).	For nonoperative candidates: SBRT, RFA, or cryotherapy may or may not be feasible due to location. Chemoradiotherapy (concurrent preferred).
IIIA	Lobectomy or pneumonectomy depending on anatomic location, LN sampling, and neoadjuvant or adjuvant chemoradiotherapy.	Primary chemoradiotherapy (concurrent preferred), with or without consolidation chemotherapy.
IIIB	Primary chemoradiotherapy (concurrent preferred), with or without consolidation chemotherapy.	Lobectomy or pneumonectomy depending on anatomic location, LN sampling, and neoadjuvant or adjuvant chemoradiotherapy.
IV, M1b with solitary site	Lobectomy or pneumonectomy depending on anatomic location, with LN sampling. Concurrent or sequential metastatectomy of a single adrenal, brain, or liver lesion. Adjuvant chemotherapy.	Palliative systemic therapy. Palliative radiotherapy.
Other Stage IV	Palliative systemic therapy.	Palliative radiotherapy for symptomatic sites including painful bone and brachial plexus lesions, high-risk spine or hip lesions, and pulmonary lesions causing obstruction.

[a] As per Goldstraw P, Crowley J, Chansky K, et al. The IASLC Lung Cancer Staging Project: Proposals for the revision of the TNM stage groupings in the forthcoming (seventh) edition of the TNM classification of malignant tumors. *J Thorac Oncol.* 2007;2:706–714.

LN, lymph node; RFA, radio-frequency ablation; SBRT, stereotactic body radiotherapy.

Adapted from Ref. 10.

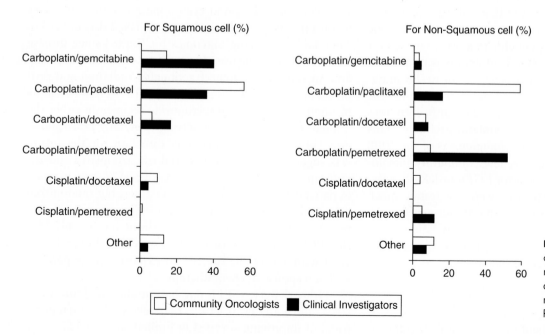

FIGURE 27.1 Reported use of doublet chemotherapy regimens (alone or with a biologic agent) in academic and community settings. Adapted From Ref. 104.

gave bevacizumab often in combination with carboplatin and an alternative agent, such as pemetrexed, docetaxel, or gemcitabine. Although there is phase II data for safety in the pemetrexed regimen, there is no efficacy data as of yet (118,119).

The second monoclonal antibody to show efficacy in the treatment of NSCLC was cetuximab, which targets the extracellular domain of EGFR. Four randomized phase II and III trials have been reported, all showing an increase in survival with the addition of the biologic agent, although only the results from the FLEX trial were statistically significant (120–123). The FLEX trial regimen—cetuximab, cisplatin, and vinorelbine given on a 3-week cycle—has been infrequently employed in the United States due to its cumbersome schedule of weekly visits, concern regarding a relatively small survival benefit (1.2 months at the mean), and the surprising lack of a progression-free survival benefit on the trial.

First reported in the laboratory just 12 years ago, erlotinib and gefitinib target the tyrosine kinase activity of EGFR (124). It was not until 2004 that Lynch et al. (125) associated treatment responsiveness with activating mutations in the EGFR gene. Phase III trial proof of efficacy came the following year with the publication of BR.21, showing a 2-month overall survival benefit from the use of erlotinib compared with placebo in previously treated NSCLC (126). QOL was also found to be improved by treatment (127). Follow-up publications have elucidated the role of EGFR mutations and gene amplification in tumor sensitivity and KRAS mutations in tumor resistance (128,129). The most intriguing recent development was the release of progression-free survival data from the IPASS trial, comparing first-line gefitinib with carboplatin and paclitaxel; these showed that among Asian light- or nonsmokers, gefitinib was superior to the cytotoxic regimen (130). Particularly enlightening was that the best predictor of a benefit to EGFR-inhibition was not any clinical characteristic but the presence of an EGFR mutation. Furthermore, in patients who were negative for the mutation, progression-free survival was significantly longer among those who received carboplatin-paclitaxel. This finding should become practice changing. As of the 2008 Patterns of Care questionnaire, few community oncologists had tested NSCLC tumors for EGFR or KRAS mutations, and academic investigators were not testing much more frequently (104). It is hoped that tumor genetic testing will become a common practice. Identification of the proper population to receive a targeted treatment is the sine qua non of personalized medicine.

Maintenance Therapy

A contemporary development of uncertain importance is the reporting of several studies of maintenance therapy following first-line treatment (131–134). These data are relatively recent and there is little information regarding how these findings are being applied in practice. Although the results include statistically significant prolongations in progression-free and/or overall survival, some question whether or not they represent a new paradigm (135).

Delivery of Chemotherapy

There are large SEER-Medicare database studies revealing possible inequities in the delivery of chemotherapy. Although chemotherapy has been proven to extend survival for unresectable lung cancer patients, it is used in only a third of those who are eligible (136). Reasons for this are many, but not all are medically pertinent. Persons older than 75 years, females, and African Americans were significantly less likely to receive chemotherapy. In order to extend the benefits of modern lung cancer care to the entire U.S. population, barriers to care will have to be addressed. If the current first-, second-, and third-line regimens, with each of their known associated increases in survival, are applied to just two thirds of the population, this could be calculated to improve overall median survival by 70%—an amount that would make front page news if it were due to a new drug. Gandara et al. (137) recently synthesized the state-of-the-art treatment options for advanced NSCLC; their proposal is summarized in Figure 27.2.

■ SMALL CELL LUNG CANCER (SCLC): A BRIEF REVIEW OF ISSUES IN COMMUNITY CARE

Despite early excitement regarding the radio- and chemo-sensitivity of SCLC, and even hope for a cure, progress toward that goal has been slow in the last 2 decades (138). That said, improving outcomes for limited-stage disease were seen due to the use of concurrent chemoradiotherapy and, in some cases, hyperfractionated radiation and prophylactic cranial irradiation (PCI) (139–142). Attempts to improve on a platinum/etoposide regimen in either the limited- or extensive-stage settings generally failed, however (143–145). One intriguing direction for the future was suggested by a phase II trial of carboplatin and irinotecan, which showed an impressive 65% response rate in patients with known brain metastases, but randomized data in this subset are lacking (146). The most significant recent advance was the finding by Slotman et al. (147,148) that PCI improved both the disease-free and overall survival with acceptable toxicity in extensive-stage patients with a response to chemotherapy.

Other than two SEER database studies, by Jänne et al. (142), and Lally et al. (139), that reviewed the temporal trend of improving survival in limited-stage SCLC, there are very few patterns of care reports in the United States, and therefore, it is difficult to compare academic and

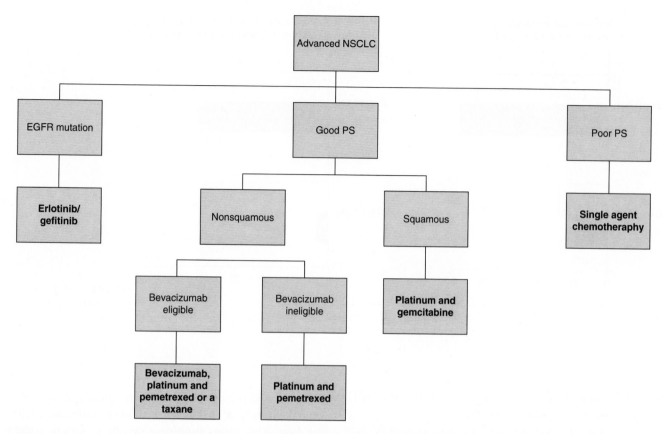

FIGURE 27.2 First-line treatment algorithm for advanced non–small cell lung cancer. From Ref. 137.

community treatment. An analysis of clinical practice in Turkey revealed great variation in diagnostic testing and treatment strategies for limited- and extensive-stage SCLC, but as many as 71% of limited-stage patients received PCI when appropriate (149). An American study from SEER records revealed that of a total of 7,995 patients with limited-stage SCLC diagnosed between 1988 and 1997, 670 were identified as having received PCI as a component of their first course of therapy; however, there were not sufficient data to show who had achieved a complete response, and therefore, it was unknown how many of the 7,995 patients were appropriate for PCI according to contemporary guidelines (150).

In the small Patterns of Care questionnaire by Love and Miller, there was general agreement in practice patterns among clinical investigators and community oncologists (104). Regarding the first-line therapy for extensive-stage SCLC, at both types of treatment sites approximately 40% of physicians choose cisplatin/etoposide and 60% carboplatin/etoposide. For second-line, 48% of clinical investigators treat with topotecan and 36% with irinotecan, while 66% of community oncologists select topotecan, 10% irinotecan, and 9% an unspecified regimen. Nearly all physicians recommend PCI for 60-year-old patients with limited-stage SCLC with a good treatment response, while there is hesitation to treat an 80-year-old patient in the same circumstance.

In contrast, there is not quite the same use of PCI for extensive-stage patients; 84% of clinical investigators and 61% of community oncologists advise PCI in this setting. This may represent a short delay in the community to incorporate the impressive results of the PCI trial reported by Slotman et al. the year prior. This data regarding PCI use is summarized in Figure 27.3.

■ NOVEL TREATMENT APPROACHES: CLINICAL TRIALS IN THE COMMUNITY SETTING

Clinical trials—which are essential for improving patient care and outcomes—have traditionally been solely within the purview of the academic community. However, there are several characteristics of community-based care that make it an ideal site for at least certain types of clinical trials. Firstly, the majority of American patients are treated in the community, and opening investigations in this setting could expand the population available for accrual by fivefold. Secondly, the leaner bureaucracy of community oncology offices may speed study initiation processes. With the advent of private institutional review boards that evaluate protocols in weeks instead of months, a community-based study can enroll patients approximately

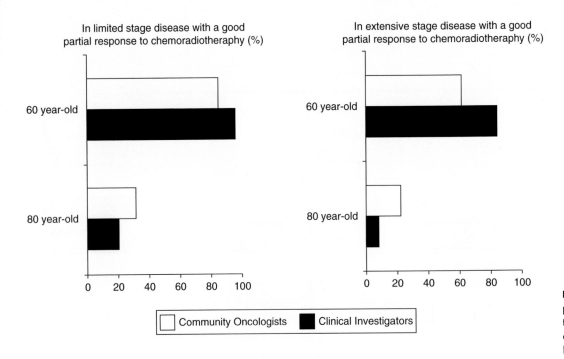

FIGURE 27.3 Use of prophylactic cranial irradiation for small cell lung cancer patients. (Adapted from Ref. 104.)

1 month after contracts are signed, instead of the 6 to 12 months common in most universities.

Community-based clinical oncology research was initially promoted by the National Cancer Act of 1971 (151). The Cooperative Group Outreach Program, initiated in 1978, allowed community hospitals to enroll to cooperative group trials. Soon thereafter, in 1982, the NCI founded the Community Clinical Oncology Program (CCOP) as a federation of community oncologist, academic investigators, and the NCI. Currently there are 61 CCOP affiliates nationwide, including more than 4,000 community physicians.

The first 5 years of the CCOP experience was reviewed by Frelick, showing significant improvement in clinical trial accrual while at the same time promoting the practice of the state-of-the-art cancer management found in the research protocols (152). Other articles also supported the claim that CCOP participation elevated the level of care, even for off-protocol treatment (153–155). Regarding accrual, a follow-up report showed ongoing improvements, with CCOPs contributing approximately one third of patients placed on investigational protocols (156). In the field of head and neck cancer, the percentage of patients enrolled on trial at a CCOP center in Wilmington, Delaware was increased from the national average of 2.5% to an impressive 24% (155). A 2009 review by Lyss and Lilenbaum (157) of cooperative group NSCLC trials revealed that from 12% to 62% of subjects were accrued from a CCOP.

In recent years, private oncology practices have initiated research programs outside of the cooperative groups. My practice, Premiere Oncology in Santa Monica, was founded in 2004. We conduct more than 30 phase I and II clinical trials annually, place approximately 40% of our patients on

protocols, and present our findings frequently at the ASCO Annual Meeting as well as other national conferences (158). The four other most prominent private programs nationally are The Sarah Cannon Cancer Center, U.S. Oncology, The START Center for Cancer Care and The Translational Genomics Research Institute (TGen). Sarah Cannon is composed of nine medical facilities in Tennessee and southern Kentucky; with this large clinical practice, the institution began conducting phase I clinical trials in 1997 and formed the Sarah Cannon Research Institute in 2004 (159). Founded in 1999, and composed of over 75 sites and more than 1,000 physicians, U.S. Oncology moved into cancer research in 2002 and participated in or ran many pivotal phase I, II, and III trials (160). START was formed in 1997, focused on phase I cancer research, and recently became an international organization with a branch in Madrid (161). TGen, launched in 2002, also specializes in phase I trials, and performs some phase II and III studies as well. All of these practices have in common a marriage of community cancer care and oncology research at the highest level, allowing the two arenas to strengthen each other. Clinical trials can be run efficiently with high accrual rates, so that cutting-edge experimental therapy is offered to a wide population and patients receive exceptional care on- and off-protocol.

■ MULTIMODALITY LUNG CANCER CARE

Clearly, the development of multidisciplinary lung cancer practices is central to accelerating clinical research, raising the standards of clinical care, and improving outcomes for our patients. Reviewing the establishment of a successful community lung cancer program at Hoag Hospital in Newport Beach, Fischel and Dillman (2) identify a multidisciplinary approach as critical to clinical and research excellence. Encompassed in this concept are eight guidelines, enumerated in Table 27.3, that improve physician services and patient flow through the diagnostic and treatment process. The establishment of a multidisciplinary lung cancer program at the Frederick Memorial Hospital in Maryland also was found to facilitate the coordination of care and improve patient satisfaction (162).

A similar article by Petrelli and Grusenmeyer (163) outlines a statewide program in Delaware. In 2002, the Helen F. Graham Cancer Center was opened as a centralized and highly coordinated comprehensive cancer care facility. Multidisciplinary disease site centers were established, accrual to CCOP/NIH studies doubled to 13% and translational research programs such as a tissue procurement center were initiated. Of course, centralizing care could be difficult for previously established care settings and treatment patterns. To address these issues in Delaware, a weekly videoconferencing program was later initiated (164). Among four community hospitals, all cases were prospectively presented. ASCO and the National Comprehensive *Cancer* Network guidelines were followed in 92% of cases, and clinical trial accrual increased as well. A similar multi-institution partnership in Georgia also improved research participation and the provision of care in a predominantly rural population (165). These successful initiatives from multiple states and demographics demonstrate the research and clinical benefits that derive from the establishment of community-based multidisciplinary programs. It is hoped that they are a sign of what is to come.

■ CLOSING THOUGHTS

The task of improving lung cancer outcomes can be broken down to two primary issues: (a) improving accrual to clinical trials, thus improving our understanding of pathophysiology and novel treatment approaches, and (b) applying our hard-won knowledge to the treatment of the largest possible population. The difficulty of enrolling lung cancer patients to protocols is well documented in several studies, as is the potential benefit of establishing multidisciplinary teams, which increase physician and patient investment in clinical trials (166,167). Furthermore, the adoption of proven novel treatment paradigms is highest among physicians who participate in such trials (168). These factors taken together indicate that the establishment of community-based multidisciplinary care, with its focus on clinical trial participation and up-to-date treatment decisions, provides the means to better outcomes for our lung cancer patients.

■ KEY POINTS

- Community-based lung cancer care dramatically impacts national cancer outcomes.
- Community-based physicians, generalists, and specialists, play the greatest role in supporting their patients to quit smoking.
- Proper radiographic and pathologic staging is critical to optimal management.
- There is an association between better surgical outcomes and surgeon and hospital patient volume. Teaching hospitals also do tend to have better outcomes, but these can be matched at nonteaching facilities with high volume. New, less invasive surgical techniques have reduced morbidity and recovery times.
- Radiation therapy is remarkably consistent across treatment sites. New chemoradiotherapy regimens are under study.
- Systemic therapy for non–small cell lung cancer has undergone a revolution in the last 10 years with the development of adjuvant therapy, new targeted agents, and new histologic, genetic, and protein expression predictors of treatment responses.
- Treatment of small cell lung cancer has changed comparatively less, but the important role of prophylactic cranial irradiation has been demonstrated.

■ Table 27.3 Eight characteristics of a successful community lung cancer program

(1)   A weekly multidisciplinary lung cancer case conference with medical doctor representatives from medical oncology, thoracic surgery, pulmonary medicine, radiology, radiation oncology, and nuclear medicine who discuss patient presentation, test results, treatment history, and plans for therapy.

(2)   Thoracic surgeons skilled in minimally invasive video-assisted thoracoscopic surgery.

(3)   Nurse navigator/coordinators to help patients through the process from detection to recovery and provide a personal bond that greatly improves patient satisfaction.

(4)   Utilization of treatment guidelines for patient-specific treatment strategies.

(5)   Formal continuing medical education.

(6)   An emphasis on early detection that includes consideration of CT screening of former smokers.

(7)   A cancer center that allows for many services to be offered at a single location for patient convenience and to promote interdisciplinary care.

(8)   Access to research protocols.

CT, computed tomography.

Adapted From Ref. 2.

- Community practices, with their large patient populations and leaner bureaucracies, are often ideal sites for clinical research.
- Multimodality care is crucial to elevating the level of clinical care and improving accrual to clinical trials.

■ REFERENCES

1. Jemal A, Siegel R, Ward E, et al. Cancer statistics, 2008. *CA Cancer J Clin.* 2008;58(2):71–96.

2. Fischel RJ, Dillman RO. Developing an effective lung cancer program in a community hospital setting. *Clin Lung Cancer.* 2009;10(4):239–243.

3. Hirsh V. Emerging safety data for bevacizumab in advanced non–small-cell lung cancer. *Clinical Lung Cancer.* 2008;9:S62–S70.

4. Lynch T, Jaganzeb M, Kosty M, et al. Safety of bevacizumab (BV) combined with chemotherapy (CTX) in patients (pts) with non-small cell lung cancer (NSCLC): interim results from the ARIES Lung observational cohort study (OCS) [abstract O-9006]. *European CanCer Organisation/European Society for Medical Oncology.* 2009.

5. Dansin E, Tsai CM, Pavlakis N, et al. Safety and efficacy of first-line bevacizumab-based therapy in advanced non-small cell lung cancer (NSCLC): results of the SAiL study (MO19390) [abstract P-9168]. http://ex2.excerptamedica.com/CIW-09ecco/index.cfm?fuseaction=CIS2002&hoofdnav=Abstracts&conten=abs.details&what=AUTHOR&searchtext=garrido&topicselected=*&selection=ABSTRACT&qryStartRowDetail=1 Accessed October 7, 2009.

6. Garrido P, Thatcher N, Crino L, et al. Safety and efficacy of first-line bevacizumab (Bv) plus chemotherapy in elderly patients (pts) with advanced or recurrent non-squamous non-small cell lung cancer (NSCLC): SAiL (MO19390) [abstract P-9170]. http://ex2.excerptamedica.com/CIW-09ecco/index.cfm?fuseaction=CIS2002&hoofdnav=Abstracts&content=abs.details&what=AUTHOR&searchtext=garrido&topicselected=*&selection=ABSTRACT&qryStartRowDetail=2 Accessed October 7, 2009.

7. Tsai C, Griesinger F, Crino L, et al. Low incidence of grade 3 bleeding events and low discontinuation rates associated with first-line bevacizumab (Bev) in patients with advanced NSCLC: data from the SAiL (MO19390) study [abstract P-9171]. http://ex2.excerptamedica.com/CIW-09ecco/index.cfm?fuseaction=CIS2002&hoofdnav=Abstracts&content=abs.details&what=AUTHOR&searchtext=garrido&topicselected=*&selection=ABSTRACT&qryStartRowDetail=3 Accessed October 7, 2009.

8. Edwards BK, Brown ML, Wingo PA, et al. Annual report to the nation on the status of cancer, 1975–2002, featuring population-based trends in cancer treatment. *J Natl Cancer Inst.* 2005;97(19):1407–1427.

9. Pfister DG, Johnson DH, Azzoli CG, et al.; American Society of Clinical Oncology. American Society of Clinical Oncology treatment of unresectable non-small-cell lung cancer guideline: update 2003. *J Clin Oncol.* 2004;22(2):330–353.

10. NCCN – Evidence-based cancer guidelines, oncology drug compendium, oncology continuing medical education. http://www.nccn.org/index.asp Accessed October 4, 2009.

11. Vokes EE. Optimal therapy for unresectable stage III non-small-cell lung cancer. *J Clin Oncol.* 2005;23(25):5853–5855.

12. Scott WJ, Howington J, Feigenberg S, Movsas B, Pisters K; American College of Chest Physicians. Treatment of non-small cell lung cancer stage I and stage II: ACCP evidence-based clinical practice guidelines (2nd edition). *Chest.* 2007;132(3 suppl): 234S–242S.

13. Jett JR, Schild SE, Keith RL, Kesler KA; American College of Chest Physicians. Treatment of non-small cell lung cancer, stage IIIB: ACCP evidence-based clinical practice guidelines (2nd edItion). *Chest.* 2007;132(3 suppl):266S–276S.

14. Socinski MA, Crowell R, Hensing TE, et al.; American College of Chest Physicians. Treatment of non-small cell lung cancer, stage IV: ACCP evidence-based clinical practice guidelines (2nd edition). *Chest.* 2007;132(3 suppl):277S–289S.

15. Robinson LA, Ruckdeschel JC, Wagner H Jr, Stevens CW; American College of Chest Physicians. Treatment of non-small cell lung cancer-stage IIIA: ACCP evidence-based clinical practice guidelines (2nd edition). *Chest.* 2007;132(3 suppl): 243S–265S.

16. Bordoni R. Consensus conference: multimodality management of early- and intermediate-stage non-small cell lung cancer. *Oncologist.* 2008;13(9):945–953.

17. Evans WK, Graham ID, Cameron D, Mackay JA, Brouwers M. Practitioner feedback on lung cancer practice guidelines in Ontario. *J Thorac Oncol.* 2006;1(1):10–18.

18. Potosky AL, Saxman S, Wallace RB, Lynch CF. Population variations in the initial treatment of non-small-cell lung cancer. *J Clin Oncol.* 2004;22(16):3261–3268.

19. Earle CC, Venditti LN, Neumann PJ, et al. Who gets chemotherapy for metastatic lung cancer? *Chest.* 2000;117(5):1239–1246.

20. Earle CC, Neumann PJ, Gelber RD, Weinstein MC, Weeks JC. Impact of referral patterns on the use of chemotherapy for lung cancer. *J Clin Oncol.* 2002;20(7):1786–1792.

21. Alberg AJ, Ford JG, Samet JM; American College of Chest Physicians. Epidemiology of lung cancer: ACCP evidence-based clinical practice guidelines (2nd edition). *Chest.* 2007;132(3 suppl):29S–55S.

22. Office of the Surgeon General (OSG). Treating tobacco use and dependence – quick reference guide. http://www.surgeongeneral.gov/tobacco/ Accessed September 27, 2009.

23. Hughes J, Stead L, Lancaster T. Antidepressants for smoking cessation. *Cochrane Database Syst Rev.* 2004;(4):CD000031.

24. Rigotti NA. Clinical practice. Treatment of tobacco use and dependence. *N Engl J Med.* 2002;346(7):506–512.

25. Omenn GS, Goodman GE, Thornquist MD, et al. Effects of a combination of beta carotene and vitamin A on lung cancer and cardiovascular disease. *N Engl J Med.* 1996;334(18): 1150–1155.

26. Hirsch FR, Lippman SM. Advances in the biology of lung cancer chemoprevention. *J Clin Oncol.* 2005;23(14):3186–3197.

27. Keith RL. Chemoprevention of lung cancer. *Proc Am Thorac Soc.* 2009;6(2):187–193.

28. Winterhalder RC, Hirsch FR, Kotantoulas GK, Franklin WA, Bunn PA Jr. Chemoprevention of lung cancer–from biology to clinical reality. *Ann Oncol.* 2004;15(2):185–196.

29. Khuri FR. Primary and secondary prevention of non-small-cell lung cancer: the SPORE Trials of Lung Cancer Prevention. *Clin Lung Cancer.* 2003;5(suppl 1):S36–S40.

30. Manser RL, Irving LB, Stone C, Byrnes G, Abramson M, Campbell D. Screening for lung cancer. *Cochrane Database Syst Rev.* 2004;(1):CD001991.

31. Kubík AK, Parkin DM, Zatloukal P. Czech Study on Lung Cancer Screening: post-trial follow-up of lung cancer deaths up to year 15 since enrollment. *Cancer.* 2000;89(11 suppl):2363–2368.

32. Marcus PM, Bergstralh EJ, Fagerstrom RM, et al. Lung cancer mortality in the Mayo Lung Project: impact of extended follow-up. *J Natl Cancer Inst.* 2000;92(16):1308–1316.

33. Flehinger BJ, Kimmel M, Polyak T, Melamed MR. Screening for lung cancer. The Mayo Lung Project revisited. *Cancer.* 1993;72(5):1573–1580.

34. Henschke CI, Yankelevitz DF, Libby DM, Pasmantier MW, Smith JP, Miettinen OS; International Early Lung Cancer Action Program Investigators. Survival of patients with stage I lung cancer detected on CT screening. *N Engl J Med.* 2006;355(17):1763–1771.

35. Goldberg P. Tobacco company Liggett gave $3.6 million to Henschke for CT screening research. *The Cancer Letter* (March 25, 2008).

36. Moy B. Medical integrity up in smoke? Conflicts of interest and the lung cancer screening controversy. *Oncologist.* 2008;13(5):474–476.

37. Publisher's note. Recently, concerns were raised regarding the possible nondisclosure of pertinent financial interests on the part of 2 scientists who were authors on 5 articles concerning lung cancer screening in the journals Cancer and Cancer Cytopathology from 2001 through 2007. *Cancer.* 2008;112(10):2329–2330.

38. Bach PB, Jett JR, Pastorino U, Tockman MS, Swensen SJ, Begg CB. Computed tomography screening and lung cancer outcomes. *JAMA.* 2007;297(9):953–961.

39. What is NLST? – National Cancer Institute. http://www.cancer.gov/nlst/what-is-nlst Accessed September 25, 2009.

40. Bastarrika G, García-Velloso MJ, Lozano MD, et al. Early lung cancer detection using spiral computed tomography and positron emission tomography. *Am J Respir Crit Care Med.* 2005;171(12):1378–1383.

41. Pastorino U, Bellomi M, Landoni C, et al. Early lung-cancer detection with spiral CT and positron emission tomography in heavy smokers: 2-year results. *Lancet.* 2003;362(9384):593–597.

42. Horváth I, Lázár Z, Gyulai N, Kollai M, Losonczy G. Exhaled biomarkers in lung cancer. *Eur Respir J.* 2009;34(1):261–275.

43. Poli D, Carbognani P, Corradi M, et al. Exhaled volatile organic compounds in patients with non-small cell lung cancer: cross sectional and nested short-term follow-up study. *Respir Res.* 2005;6:71.

44. Machado RF, Laskowski D, Deffenderfer O, et al. Detection of lung cancer by sensor array analyses of exhaled breath. *Am J Respir Crit Care Med.* 2005;171(11):1286–1291.

45. Phillips M, Gleeson K, Hughes JM, et al. Volatile organic compounds in breath as markers of lung cancer: a cross-sectional study. *Lancet.* 1999;353(9168):1930–1933.

46. Phillips M, Cataneo RN, Cummin AR, et al. Detection of lung cancer with volatile markers in the breath. *Chest.* 2003;123(6):2115–2123.

47. Bechtel JJ, Kelley WA, Coons TA, Klein MG, Slagel DD, Petty TL. Lung cancer detection in patients with airflow obstruction identified in a primary care outpatient practice. *Chest.* 2005;127(4):1140–1145.

48. Greenberg ER, Baron JA, Dain BJ, Freeman DH Jr, Yates JW, Korson R. Cancer staging may have different meanings in academic and community hospitals. *J Clin Epidemiol.* 1991;44(6):505–512.

49. Thermann M, Bluemm R, Schroeder U, Wassmuth E, Dohmann R. Efficacy and benefit of mediastinal computed tomography as a selection method for mediastinoscopy. *Ann Thorac Surg.* 1989;48(4):565–567.

50. Detterbeck FC, Jantz MA, Wallace M, Vansteenkiste J, Silvestri GA; American College of Chest Physicians. Invasive mediastinal staging of lung cancer: ACCP evidence-based clinical practice guidelines (2nd edition). *Chest.* 2007;132(3 suppl):202S–220S.

51. Lee BE, Redwine J, Foster C, et al. Mediastinoscopy might not be necessary in patients with non-small cell lung cancer with mediastinal lymph nodes having a maximum standardized uptake value of less than 5.3. *J Thorac Cardiovasc Surg.* 2008;135(3):615–619.

52. Groth SS, Whitson BA, Maddaus MA. Radiographic staging of mediastinal lymph nodes in non-small cell lung cancer patients. *Thorac Surg Clin.* 2008;18(4):349–361.

53. Whitson BA, Groth SS, Maddaus MA. Recommendations for optimal use of imaging studies to clinically stage mediastinal lymph nodes in non-small-cell lung cancer patients. *Lung Cancer.* 2008;61(2):177–185.

54. Robert McKenna, Jr., M.D., Chief of Thoracic Surgery at Cedars-Sinai Medical Center, Los Angeles. Personal Communication. 2009.

55. Jay Moon Lee, MD., Surgical Director of the Thoracic Oncology Program at University of California, Los Angeles. Personal Communication. 2009.

56. Farjah F, Flum DR, Ramsey SD, Heagerty PJ, Symons RG, Wood DE. Multi-modality mediastinal staging for lung cancer among medicare beneficiaries. *J Thorac Oncol.* 2009;4(3):355–363.

57. Harrow EM, Abi-Saleh W, Blum J, et al. The utility of transbronchial needle aspiration in the staging of bronchogenic carcinoma. *Am J Respir Crit Care Med.* 2000;161(2 Pt 1):601–607.

58. Wassenaar TR, Eickhoff JC, Jarzemsky DR, Smith SS, Larson ML, Schiller JH. Differences in primary care clinicians' approach to non-small cell lung cancer patients compared with breast cancer. *J Thorac Oncol.* 2007;2(8):722–728.

59. Onega T, Duell EJ, Shi X, Wang D, Demidenko E, Goodman D. Geographic access to cancer care in the U.S. *Cancer.* 2008;112(4):909–918.

60. Onega T, Duell EJ, Shi X, Demidenko E, Gottlieb D, Goodman DC. Influence of NCI cancer center attendance on mortality in lung, breast, colorectal, and prostate cancer patients. *Med Care Res Rev.* 2009;66(5):542–560.

61. Clegg LX, Reichman ME, Miller BA, et al. Impact of socioeconomic status on cancer incidence and stage at diagnosis: selected findings from the surveillance, epidemiology, and end results: National Longitudinal Mortality Study. *Cancer Causes Control.* 2009;20(4):417–435.

62. Begg CB, Cramer LD, Hoskins WJ, Brennan MF. Impact of hospital volume on operative mortality for major cancer surgery. *JAMA.* 1998;280(20):1747–1751.

63. Romano PS, Mark DH. Patient and hospital characteristics related to in-hospital mortality after lung cancer resection. *Chest.* 1992;101(5):1332–1337.

64. Bach PB, Cramer LD, Schrag D, Downey RJ, Gelfand SE, Begg CB. The influence of hospital volume on survival after resection for lung cancer. *N Engl J Med.* 2001;345(3):181–188.

65. Simunovic M, Rempel E, Thériault ME, et al. Influence of hospital characteristics on operative death and survival of patients after major cancer surgery in Ontario. *Can J Surg.* 2006;49(4):251–258.

66. Birkmeyer JD, Sun Y, Wong SL, Stukel TA. Hospital volume and late survival after cancer surgery. *Ann Surg.* 2007;245(5):777–783.

67. Birkmeyer JD, Stukel TA, Siewers AE, Goodney PP, Wennberg DE, Lucas FL. Surgeon volume and operative mortality in the United States. *N Engl J Med.* 2003;349(22):2117–2127.

68. Birkmeyer JD, Sun Y, Goldfaden A, Birkmeyer NJ, Stukel TA. Volume and process of care in high-risk cancer surgery. *Cancer.* 2006;106(11):2476–2481.

69. Cheung MC, Hamilton K, Sherman R, et al. Impact of teaching facility status and high-volume centers on outcomes for lung cancer resection: an examination of 13,469 surgical patients. *Ann Surg Oncol.* 2009;16(1):3–13.

70. Meguid RA, Brooke BS, Chang DC, Sherwood JT, Brock MV, Yang SC. Are surgical outcomes for lung cancer resections improved at teaching hospitals? *Ann Thorac Surg.* 2008;85(3):1015–24; discussion 1024.

71. Birkmeyer JD. Improving outcomes with lung cancer surgery: selective referral or quality improvement? *Ann Surg Oncol.* 2009;16(1):1–2.

72. Love N, Detterbeck F. Lung cancer update 3 | 2009. http://www.lungcancerupdate.com/medonc/2009/3/ Accessed October 10, 2009.

73. Farjah F, Flum DR, Varghese TK Jr, Symons RG, Wood DE. Surgeon specialty and long-term survival after pulmonary resection for lung cancer. *Ann Thorac Surg.* 2009;87(4):995–1004; discussion 1005.

74. Goodney PP, Lucas FL, Stukel TA, Birkmeyer JD. Surgeon specialty and operative mortality with lung resection. *Ann Surg.* 2005;241(1):179–184.

75. Birkmeyer NJ, Goodney PP, Stukel TA, Hillner BE, Birkmeyer JD. Do cancer centers designated by the National Cancer Institute have better surgical outcomes? *Cancer.* 2005;103(3):435–441.

76. Shaw JP, Dembitzer FR, Wisnivesky JP, et al. Video-assisted thoracoscopic lobectomy: state of the art and future directions. *Ann Thorac Surg.* 2008;85(2):S705–S709.

77. Whitson BA, Groth SS, Duval SJ, Swanson SJ, Maddaus MA. Surgery for early-stage non-small cell lung cancer: a systematic review of the video-assisted thoracoscopic surgery versus thoracotomy approaches to lobectomy. *Ann Thorac Surg.* 2008;86(6):2008–16; discussion 2016.

78. Manser R, Wright G, Hart D, Byrnes G, Campbell DA. Surgery for early stage non-small cell lung cancer. *Cochrane Database Syst Rev.* 2005;(1):CD004699.

79. Farjah F, Wood DE, Mulligan MS, et al. Safety and efficacy of video-assisted versus conventional lung resection for lung cancer. *J Thorac Cardiovasc Surg.* 2009;137(6):1415–1421.

80. Pennathur A, Abbas G, Christie N, Landreneau R, Luketich JD. Video assisted thoracoscopic surgery and lobectomy, sublobar resection, radiofrequency ablation, and stereotactic radiosurgery: advances and controversies in the management of early stage non-small cell lung cancer. *Curr Opin Pulm Med.* 2007;13(4):267–270.

81. Chin CS, Swanson SJ. Video-assisted thoracic surgery lobectomy: centers of excellence or excellence of centers? *Thorac Surg Clin.* 2008;18(3):263–268.

82. Sariego J. Surgical oncology in the community hospital: can it be done safely? *South Med J.* 2007;100(11):1091–1094.

83. Chuba PJ, Moughan J, Forman JD, Owen J, Hanks G. The 1989 patterns of care study for prostate cancer: five-year outcomes. *Int J Radiat Oncol Biol Phys.* 2001;50(2):325–334.

84. Smitt MC, Stouffer N, Owen JB, Hoppe RT, Hanks GE. Results of the 1988–1989 Patterns of Care Study process survey for Hodgkin's disease. *Int J Radiat Oncol Biol Phys.* 1999;43(2):335–339.

85. Bhatnagar AK, Beriwal S, Heron DE, et al. Initial outcomes analysis for large multicenter integrated cancer network implementation of intensity modulated radiation therapy for breast cancer. *Breast J.* 2009;15(5):468–474.

86. Hanks GE, Kramer S. Quality assurance in radiation therapy: clinical and physical aspects. Consensus of best current management: the starting point for clinical quality assessment. *Int J Radiat Oncol Biol Phys.* 1984;10(suppl 1):87–97.

87. Mell LK, Roeske JC, Mundt AJ. A survey of intensity-modulated radiation therapy use in the United States. *Cancer.* 2003;98(1):204–211.

88. Mell LK, Mehrotra AK, Mundt AJ. Intensity-modulated radiation therapy use in the U.S., 2004. *Cancer.* 2005;104(6):1296–1303.

89. Sanghani M, Mignano J. Intensity modulated radiation therapy: a review of current practice and future directions. *Technol Cancer Res Treat.* 2006;5(5):447–450.

90. Movsas B, Moughan J, Komaki R, et al. Radiotherapy patterns of care study in lung carcinoma. *J Clin Oncol.* 2003;21(24):4553–4559.

91. Robert Wollman, M.D., Medical Director of Radiation Therapy, Saint John's Health Center, Santa Monica. Personal Communication. 2009.

92. Lisa M. Chaiken, M.D., Radiation Oncology, Saint John's Medical Center, Santa Monica. Personal Communication. 2009.

93. Rusch VW, Giroux DJ, Kraut MJ, et al. Induction chemoradiation and surgical resection for superior sulcus non-small-cell lung carcinomas: long-term results of Southwest Oncology Group Trial 9416 (Intergroup Trial 0160). *J Clin Oncol.* 2007;25(3):313–318.

94. Demir A, Sayar A, Kocaturk CI, et al. Surgical treatment of superior sulcus tumors: results and prognostic factors. *Thorac Cardiovasc Surg.* 2009;57(2):96–101.

95. Vandenbroucke E, De Ryck F, Surmont V, van Meerbeeck JP. What is the role for surgery in patients with stage III non-small cell lung cancer? *Curr Opin Pulm Med.* 2009;15(4):295–302.

96. Albain KS, Swann RS, Rusch VW, et al. Radiotherapy plus chemotherapy with or without surgical resection for stage III non-small-cell lung cancer: a phase III randomised controlled trial. *Lancet.* 2009;374(9687):379–386.

97. Albain KS, Crowley JJ, Turrisi AT 3rd, et al. Concurrent cisplatin, etoposide, and chest radiotherapy in pathologic stage IIIB non-small-cell lung cancer: a Southwest Oncology Group phase II study, SWOG 9019. *J Clin Oncol.* 2002;20(16):3454–3460.

98. Seiwert TY, Connell PP, Mauer AM, et al. A phase I study of pemetrexed, carboplatin, and concurrent radiotherapy in patients with locally advanced or metastatic non-small cell lung or esophageal cancer. *Clin Cancer Res.* 2007;13(2 Pt 1):515–522.

99. Vokes EE, Senan S, Treat JA, Iscoe NA. PROCLAIM: A phase III study of pemetrexed, cisplatin, and radiation therapy followed by consolidation pemetrexed versus etoposide, cisplatin, and radiation therapy followed by consolidation cytotoxic chemotherapy of choice in locally advanced stage III non-small-cell lung cancer of other than predominantly squamous cell histology. *Clin Lung Cancer.* 2009;10(3):193–198.

100. Shaw E, Kline R, Gillin M, et al. Radiation Therapy Oncology Group: radiosurgery quality assurance guidelines. *Int J Radiat Oncol Biol Phys.* 1993;27(5):1231–1239.

101. Dahele M, Pearson S, Purdie T, et al. Practical considerations arising from the implementation of lung stereotactic body radiation therapy (SBRT) at a comprehensive cancer center. *J Thorac Oncol.* 2008;3(11):1332–1341.

102. Michael Steinberg, MD, Chair of Radiation Oncology, University of California, Los Angeles. Personal Communication. 2009.

103. Schiller JH, Harrington D, Belani CP, et al.; Eastern Cooperative Oncology Group. Comparison of four chemotherapy regimens for advanced non-small-cell lung cancer. *N Engl J Med.* 2002;346(2):92–98.

104. Love N, Miller VA. *Patterns of Care: Lung Cancer,* 2008; Issue 1, | Research To Practice. http://researchtopractice.com/browse-tumor-types/lung-cancer/poc-lce/2/1 Accessed October 6, 2009.

105. Chemotherapy in non-small cell lung cancer: a meta-analysis using updated data on individual patients from 52 randomised clinical trials. Non-small Cell Lung Cancer Collaborative Group. *BMJ.* 1995;311(7010):899–909.

106. Douillard JY, Rosell R, De Lena M, et al. Adjuvant vinorelbine plus cisplatin versus observation in patients with completely resected stage IB-IIIA non-small-cell lung cancer (Adjuvant Navelbine International Trialist Association [ANITA]): a randomised controlled trial. *Lancet Oncol.* 2006;7(9):719–727.

107. Arriagada R, Bergman B, Dunant A, Le Chevalier T, Pignon JP, Vansteenkiste J; International Adjuvant Lung Cancer Trial Collaborative Group. Cisplatin-based adjuvant chemotherapy in patients with completely resected non-small-cell lung cancer. *N Engl J Med.* 2004;350(4):351–360.

108. Winton T, Livingston R, Johnson D, et al.; National Cancer Institute of Canada Clinical Trials Group; National Cancer Institute of the United States Intergroup JBR.10 Trial Investigators. Vinorelbine plus cisplatin vs. observation in resected non-small-cell lung cancer. *N Engl J Med.* 2005;352(25):2589–2597.

109. Strauss GM, Herndon JE 2nd, Maddaus MA, et al. Adjuvant paclitaxel plus carboplatin compared with observation in stage IB non-small-cell lung cancer: CALGB 9633 with the Cancer and Leukemia Group B, Radiation Therapy Oncology Group, and North Central Cancer Treatment Group Study Groups. *J Clin Oncol.* 2008;26(31):5043–5051.

110. Pignon JP, Tribodet H, Scagliotti GV, et al.; LACE Collaborative Group. Lung adjuvant cisplatin evaluation: a pooled analysis by the LACE Collaborative Group. *J Clin Oncol.* 2008;26(21):3552–3559.

111. Le Chevalier T, Dunant A, Bergman B, et al. Long-term results of the International Adjuvant Lung Cancer Trial (IALT) evaluating adjuvant cisplatin-based chemotherapy in resected non-small cell lung cancer (NSCLC) [abstract 7507]. *J Clin Oncol.* 2008;26(May 20 suppl).

112. Vincent MD, Butts C, Seymour L, et al. Updated survival analysis of JBR.10: A randomized phase III trial of vinorelbine/cisplatin

versus observation in completely resected stage IB and II non-small cell lung cancer (NSCLC) [abstract 7501]. *J Clin Oncol.* 2009;27:15s(suppl).

113. Bezjak A, Lee CW, Ding K, et al. Quality-of-life outcomes for adjuvant chemotherapy in early-stage non-small-cell lung cancer: results from a randomized trial, JBR.10. *J Clin Oncol.* 2008;26(31):5052–5059.

114. Jang RW, Le Maître A, Ding K, et al. Quality-adjusted time without symptoms or toxicity analysis of adjuvant chemotherapy in non-small-cell lung cancer: an analysis of the National Cancer Institute of Canada Clinical Trials Group JBR.10 trial. *J Clin Oncol.* 2009;27(26):4268–4273.

115. Alam N, Shepherd FA, Winton T, et al. Compliance with postoperative adjuvant chemotherapy in non-small cell lung cancer. An analysis of National Cancer Institute of Canada and intergroup trial JBR.10 and a review of the literature. *Lung Cancer.* 2005;47(3):385–394.

116. Scagliotti GV, Parikh P, von Pawel J, et al. Phase III study comparing cisplatin plus gemcitabine with cisplatin plus pemetrexed in chemotherapy-naive patients with advanced-stage non-small-cell lung cancer. *J Clin Oncol.* 2008;26(21):3543–3551.

117. Sandler A, Gray R, Perry MC, et al. Paclitaxel-carboplatin alone or with bevacizumab for non-small-cell lung cancer. *N Engl J Med.* 2006;355(24):2542–2550.

118. Patel JD, Hensing TA, Rademaker A, et al. Phase II study of pemetrexed and carboplatin plus bevacizumab with maintenance pemetrexed and bevacizumab as first-line therapy for nonsquamous non-small-cell lung cancer. *J Clin Oncol.* 2009;27(20):3284–3289.

119. Patel JD, Bonomi P, Socinski MA, et al. Treatment rationale and study design for the pointbreak study: a randomized, open-label phase III study of pemetrexed/carboplatin/bevacizumab followed by maintenance pemetrexed/bevacizumab versus paclitaxel/carboplatin/bevacizumab followed by maintenance bevacizumab in patients with stage IIIB or IV nonsquamous non-small-cell lung cancer. *Clin Lung Cancer.* 2009;10(4):252–256.

120. Butts CA, Bodkin D, Middleman EL, et al. Randomized phase II study of gemcitabine plus cisplatin or carboplatin [corrected], with or without cetuximab, as first-line therapy for patients with advanced or metastatic non small-cell lung cancer. *J Clin Oncol.* 2007;25(36):5777–5784.

121. Rosell R, Robinet G, Szczesna A, et al. Randomized phase II study of cetuximab plus cisplatin/vinorelbine compared with cisplatin/vinorelbine alone as first-line therapy in EGFR-expressing advanced non-small-cell lung cancer. *Ann Oncol.* 2008;19(2):362–369.

122. Lynch T, Patel T, Dreisbach L. A randomized mulitcenter phase III study of cetuximab (Erbitux) in combination with Taxane/Carboplatin versus Taxane/Carboplatin alone as first-line treatment for patients with advanced/metastatic non-small cell lung cancer (NSCLC) [abstract B3–03]. *J Thorac Oncol.* 2007;2(suppl 4):S340.

123. Pirker R, Pereira JR, Szczesna A, et al.; FLEX Study Team. Cetuximab plus chemotherapy in patients with advanced non-small-cell lung cancer (FLEX): an open-label randomised phase III trial. *Lancet.* 2009;373(9674):1525–1531.

124. Moyer JD, Barbacci EG, Iwata KK, et al. Induction of apoptosis and cell cycle arrest by CP-358,774, an inhibitor of epidermal growth factor receptor tyrosine kinase. *Cancer Res.* 1997;57(21):4838–4848.

125. Lynch TJ, Bell DW, Sordella R, et al. Activating mutations in the epidermal growth factor receptor underlying responsiveness of non-small-cell lung cancer to gefitinib. *N Engl J Med.* 2004;350(21):2129–2139.

126. Shepherd FA, Rodrigues Pereira J, Ciuleanu T, et al.; National Cancer Institute of Canada Clinical Trials Group. Erlotinib in previously treated non-small-cell lung cancer. *N Engl J Med.* 2005;353(2):123–132.

127. Bezjak A, Tu D, Seymour L, et al.; National Cancer Institute of Canada Clinical Trials Group Study BR.21. Symptom improvement in lung cancer patients treated with erlotinib: quality of life analysis of the National Cancer Institute of Canada Clinical Trials Group Study BR.21. *J Clin Oncol.* 2006;24(24):3831–3837.

128. Tsao MS, Sakurada A, Cutz JC, et al. Erlotinib in lung cancer - molecular and clinical predictors of outcome. *N Engl J Med.* 2005;353(2):133–144.

129. Zhu CQ, da Cunha Santos G, Ding K, et al.; National Cancer Institute of Canada Clinical Trials Group Study BR.21. Role of KRAS and EGFR as biomarkers of response to erlotinib in National Cancer Institute of Canada Clinical Trials Group Study BR.21. *J Clin Oncol.* 2008;26(26):4268–4275.

130. Mok TS, Wu YL, Thongprasert S, et al. Gefitinib or carboplatin-paclitaxel in pulmonary adenocarcinoma. *N Engl J Med.* 2009;361(10):947–957.

131. Belani C. Maintenance pemetrexed (Pem) plus best supportive care (BSC) versus placebo (Plac) plus BSC: A randomized phase III study in advanced non-small cell lung cancer (NSCLC) [abstract CRA8000]. *J Clin Oncol.* 2009;27:18s(suppl).

132. Cappuzzo F. SATURN: A double-blind, randomized, phase III study of maintenance erlotinib versus placebo following non-progression with first-line platinum-based chemotherapy in patients with advanced NSCLC [abstract 8001]. *J Clin Oncol* 2009;27:15s.

133. Miller VA. A randomized, double-blind, placebo-controlled, phase IIIb trial (ATLAS) comparing bevacizumab (B) therapy with or without erlotinib (E) after completion of chemotherapy with B for first-line treatment of locally advanced, recurrent, or metastatic non-small cell lung cancer (NSCLC) [abstract LBA8002]. *J Clin Oncol.* 2009;27:18s(suppl).

134. Casal J. Erlotinib as maintenance therapy after concurrent chemoradiotherapy in patients (p) with stage III non-small cell lung cancer (NSCLC): A Galician Lung Cancer Group phase II study [abstract 7537]. *J Clin Oncol* 2009;27:15s(suppl).

135. Hanna N. Discussion: maintenance therapy for NSCLC: is this a new paradigm? 2009.

136. Ramsey SD, Howlader N, Etzioni RD, Donato B. Chemotherapy use, outcomes, and costs for older persons with advanced non-small-cell lung cancer: evidence from surveillance, epidemiology and end results-Medicare. *J Clin Oncol.* 2004;22(24):4971–4978.

137. Gandara DR, Mack PC, Li T, Lara PN Jr, Herbst RS. Evolving treatment algorithms for advanced non-small-cell lung cancer: 2009 looking toward 2012. *Clin Lung Cancer.* 2009;10(6):392–394.

138. Lally BE, Urbanic JJ, Blackstock AW, Miller AA, Perry MC. Small cell lung cancer: have we made any progress over the last 25 years? *Oncologist.* 2007;12(9):1096–1104.

139. Lally BE, Geiger AM, Urbanic JJ, et al. Trends in the outcomes for patients with limited stage small cell lung cancer: An analysis of the Surveillance, Epidemiology, and End Results database. *Lung Cancer.* 2009;64(2):226–231.

140. Gregor A, Cull A, Stephens RJ, et al. Prophylactic cranial irradiation is indicated following complete response to induction therapy in small cell lung cancer: results of a multicentre randomised trial. United Kingdom Coordinating Committee for Cancer Research (UKCCCR) and the European Organization for Research and Treatment of Cancer (EORTC). *Eur J Cancer.* 1997;33(11):1752–1758.

141. Turrisi AT 3rd, Kim K, Blum R, et al. Twice-daily compared with once-daily thoracic radiotherapy in limited small-cell lung cancer treated concurrently with cisplatin and etoposide. *N Engl J Med.* 1999;340(4):265–271.

142. Jänne PA, Freidlin B, Saxman S, et al. Twenty-five years of clinical research for patients with limited-stage small cell lung carcinoma in North America. *Cancer.* 2002;95(7):1528–1538.

143. Socinski MA, Smit EF, Lorigan P, et al. Phase III study of pemetrexed plus carboplatin compared with etoposide plus carboplatin

in chemotherapy-naive patients with extensive-stage small-cell lung cancer. *J Clin Oncol.* 2009;27(28):4787–4792.

144. Lara PN Jr, Natale R, Crowley J, et al. Phase III trial of irinotecan/cisplatin compared with etoposide/cisplatin in extensive-stage small-cell lung cancer: clinical and pharmacogenomic results from SWOG S0124. *J Clin Oncol.* 2009;27(15):2530–2535.

145. Hanna N, Bunn PA Jr, Langer C, et al. Randomized phase III trial comparing irinotecan/cisplatin with etoposide/cisplatin in patients with previously untreated extensive-stage disease small-cell lung cancer. *J Clin Oncol.* 2006;24(13):2038–2043.

146. Chen G, Huynh M, Fehrenbacher L, et al. Phase II trial of irinotecan and carboplatin for extensive or relapsed small-cell lung cancer. *J Clin Oncol.* 2009;27(9):1401–1404.

147. Slotman BJ, Mauer ME, Bottomley A, et al. Prophylactic cranial irradiation in extensive disease small-cell lung cancer: short-term health-related quality of life and patient reported symptoms: results of an international Phase III randomized controlled trial by the EORTC Radiation Oncology and Lung Cancer Groups. *J Clin Oncol.* 2009;27(1):78–84.

148. Slotman B, Faivre-Finn C, Kramer G, et al.; EORTC Radiation Oncology Group and Lung Cancer Group. Prophylactic cranial irradiation in extensive small-cell lung cancer. *N Engl J Med.* 2007;357(7):664–672.

149. Demiral AN, Alicikus ZA, Isil Ugur V, et al. Patterns of care for lung cancer in radiation oncology departments of Turkey. *Int J Radiat Oncol Biol Phys.* 2008;72(5):1530–1537.

150. Patel S, Macdonald OK, Suntharalingam M. Evaluation of the use of prophylactic cranial irradiation in small cell lung cancer. *Cancer.* 2009;115(4):842–850.

151. Jean-Pierre P, Mustian K, Kohli S, Roscoe JA, Hickok JT, Morrow GR. Community-based clinical oncology research trials for cancer-related fatigue. *J Support Oncol.* 2006;4(10):511–516.

152. Frelick RW. The Community Clinical Oncology Program (CCOP) story: review of community oncologists' experiences with clinical research trials in cancer with an emphasis on the CCOP of the National Cancer Institute between 1982 and 1987. *J Clin Oncol.* 1994;12(8):1718–1723.

153. McFall SL, Warnecke RB, Kaluzny AD, Ford L. Practice setting and physician influences on judgments of colon cancer treatment by community physicians. *Health Serv Res.* 1996;31(1):5–19.

154. McFall SL, Warnecke RB, Kaluzny AD, Aitken M, Ford L. Physician and practice characteristics associated with judgments about breast cancer treatment. *Med Care.* 1994;32(2):106–117.

155. Witt RL, Frelick RW. Head and neck cancer care at a community-based teaching hospital. *Head Neck.* 2005;27(7):613–615.

156. Cobau CD. Clinical trials in the community. The community clinical oncology program experience. *Cancer.* 1994;74(9 suppl):2694–2700.

157. Lyss AP, Lilenbaum RC. Accrual to National Cancer Institute-sponsored non-small-cell lung cancer trials: insights and contributions from the CCOP program. *Clin Lung Cancer.* 2009;10(6):410–413.

158. Premiere Oncology – Home. http://www.premiereoncology.com/po/ Accessed October 11, 2009.

159. Oncology Focus Dec08. http://www.sarahcannonresearch.com/CustomPage.asp?guidCustomContentID=1063E44F-7E82-430-E-B4F2-CAE56AE3B423 Accessed October 11, 2009.

160. US Oncology Research. http://www.usoncology.com/portal/page/portal/PubWeb/2CancerCareNetwork/03USOncologyResearch Accessed October 11, 2009.

161. START – South Texas Accelerated Research Therapeutics. http://www.startthecure.com/index.html Accessed October 11, 2009.

162. Seek A, Hogle WP. Modeling a better way: navigating the health-care system for patients with lung cancer. *Clin J Oncol Nurs.* 2007;11(1):81–85.

163. Petrelli NJ, Grusenmeyer PA. Establishing the multidisciplinary care of patients with cancer in the state of Delaware. *Cancer.* 2004;101(2):220–225.

164. Dickson-Witmer D, Petrelli NJ, Witmer DR, et al. A statewide community cancer center videoconferencing program. *Ann Surg Oncol.* 2008;15(11):3058–3064.

165. Goodman M, Almon L, Bayakly R, et al. Cancer outcomes research in a rural area: a multi-institution partnership model. *J Community Health.* 2009;34(1):23–32.

166. Spiro SG, Gower NH, Evans MT, Facchini FM, Rudd RM. Recruitment of patients with lung cancer into a randomised clinical trial: experience at two centres. On behalf of the Big Lung Trial Steering Committee. *Thorax.* 2000;55(6):463–465.

167. Curran WJ Jr, Schiller JH, Wolkin AC, Comis RL; Scientific Leadership Council in Lung Cancer of the Coalition of Cancer Cooperative Groups. Addressing the current challenges of non-small-cell lung cancer clinical trial accrual. *Clin Lung Cancer.* 2008;9(4):222–226.

168. Stephens R, Gibson D. The impact of clinical trials on the treatment of lung cancer. *Clin Oncol (R Coll Radiol).* 1993;5(4):211–219.

28 Future Directions in the Multidisciplinary Care of Patients with Lung Cancer

PAUL A. BUNN

ROBERT C. DOEBELE

YORK E. MILLER

NIR PELED

ALI MUSANI

KAVITA GARG

WILBUR FRANKLIN

FRED R. HIRSCH

JOHN D. MITCHELL

MICHAEL WEYANT

D. ROSS CAMIDGE

LAURIE GASPAR

BRIAN KAVANAGH

T. J. PUGH

JESSICA FLAGIELLO

ANA B. OTON

■ INTRODUCTION

Lung cancer is the leading cause of cancer death in the United States and in the world (1). The majority of patients present with disease that has spread to mediastinal lymph nodes or distant organs for whom a single modality of therapy is neither curative nor optimal. Lung cancer is a very heterogenous disease with four major histologic types and many subclassifications (2,3). There are many known mutations within each histologic class, and, increasingly, therapies for specific mutations are becoming standard (4,5). There are many reasons why multidisciplinary teams will play an increasingly important role in the treatment of lung cancer. First, new methods for early detection, for biopsy of peripheral lung lesions, and for endobronchial ultrasound (EBUS)–guided node fine-needle aspirations will create an increasing role for pulmonologists and radiologists in diagnosis and staging. Second, new imaging techniques will lead to an increased role for radiologists in early diagnosis and staging. Third, the importance of histologic typing and subtyping and analysis of molecular markers will increase the importance of the pathologist on the team. Fourth, multimodality therapy will continue to be used in the majority of patients stressing the roles of surgical, radiation, and medical oncology. Finally, as patients live longer, the role for individuals involved in supportive care will increase.

■ PULMONOLOGISTS

The majority of patients with lung cancer have advanced stages at diagnosis emphasizing the need for early detection. While there are no established modalities for early detection and screening, many tests are under investigation. Pulmonologists will need to apply existing and new risk models to select those individuals who are at highest risk to undergo these procedures. Such risk models include the Bach model and the Liverpool Lung Project Risk Models (6,7), but others will be developed and may include analysis of genes identified by genome-wide screening analysis (8).

As the incidence of lung cancer in never-smokers increases, as the frequency of peripheral adenocarcinomas increases, and as small nodules are detected on computed tomography (CT) scans, advanced bronchoscopic techniques for diagnosis include "navigational bronchoscopy" described in detail elsewhere in the book. The goal is to be able to reach distal pulmonary nodules and to biopsy these nodules through these advanced procedures. In addition to screening efforts, increasing numbers of high-risk individuals are receiving CT scans for other indications. Between 20% and 50% of these will reveal noncalcified pulmonary nodules. A recent publication has demonstrated that 1% of high-risk subjects who underwent a CT of the chest for screening purposes had a major thoracic surgical procedure (mediastinoscopy, video assisted thoracoscopy, or thoracotomy) for benign disorders. One third of the major thoracic surgical procedures resulted in a benign diagnosis (9). The advanced bronchoscopic techniques also involve EBUS with fine-needle aspiration of lymph nodes (10–12). This procedure may allow for both diagnosis and staging if the mediastinal or contralateral hilar nodes are positive for tumor involvement.

There are no proven chemoprevention agents but such an approach is critical for former smokers who make up approximately 50% of newly diagnosed patients in the United States. Chemoprevention studies with high-dose vitamin A and derivatives such as 13-cis retinoic acid as well as vitamin E and its derivates were not shown to be useful in reducing lung cancer incidence (13). There was some evidence that there was an increase in the incidence of lung cancer in smokers who received the high-dose vitamin therapy. A trial of selenium supplementation recently failed to produce any reduction in the development of second primary lung cancers. However, a large prospective randomized phase II trial of the prostacyclin analog, iloprost, showed that it could improve dysplasia and abnormal bronchial histologies (14). A phase III trial with a lung cancer endpoint is being planned for iloprost. The COX-2 inhibitor, celecoxib, has been tested in phase II chemoprevention trials, showing a reduction in the Ki67 labeling index with an increase in the expression of nuclear survivin in the bronchial epithelium (15). Larger studies of celecoxib in chemoprevention are underway. Thus, the future will bring an increased need for multidisciplinary teams for new prevention strategies.

■ RADIOLOGISTS

Thoracic radiologists are an essential part of the multidisciplinary lung cancer team to assist in diagnosis and staging and to assess response to therapy. Volumetric software programs can now accurately assess tumor volume and this has important implications for determining which pulmonary nodules require resection, observation, or no further follow-up. Volumetric scanning may also play an increasing role in assessing response to therapy in clinical trials.

For small nodules thin-section CT helps in their characterization. Nodules with ground-glass attenuation, mixed density nodules, or nodules with air bronchogram are consistent with adenocarcinoma. Ground-glass density nodules predict an early-stage or preinvasive adenocarcinoma (atypical adenomatous hyperplasia or bronchioloalveolar cell carcinoma or carcinoma in situ) (16). These nodules are typically fluorodeoxyglucose–positron emission tomography (FDG-PET) negative. These early cancers often correlate with epidermal growth factor receptor (EGFR) mutations, whereas the more aggressive type nodules demonstrating predominantly solid components with spiculation or cavitations often correspond to *KRAS* mutations. and shorter doubling times. Follow-up of these predominantly ground-glass

density nodules is not yet well defined but given their slow growth, annual CT scans for lesions smaller than 8 to 10 mm appears reasonable. Minimally invasive surgery is indicated if they grow in size or change in attenuation. It is debated if routine lymph node dissection is indicated at the time of surgery for these nodules because typically they are not associated with nodal metastases (17).

Radiologists can perform CT-guided biopsy of pulmonary lesions that provide adequate material for molecular analysis. In the era of selection of patients for personalized therapies where molecular analyses are crucial, tumor biopsies—not fine-needle aspirates—may be required for the molecular analyses,

Currently both anatomical and functional imaging are used to monitor treatment response to anticancer agents. Historically, response evaluation criteria in solid tumors (RECIST) has been used to measure tumor size (18,19). CT is the most commonly used and reproducible method to measure target lesions selected for response assessment. Although anatomic measurements are the standard for characterizing treatment response, there are several factors that contribute to variability in uni- or bidimensional measure of response assessment. Technical factors known to influence tumor size and anatomic response assessment include slice thickness, the axial plane on which the lesion is visible when measured, the use and timing of intravenous contrast administration, and the measurement techniques used (electronic caliper vs. automated techniques, etc.). Patient-related factors such as the state of respiration during scan acquisition and tumor margin also influence response assessment (20). Reader variability is a well known cause of measurement error in anatomic response assessment (21). It is therefore important to have consistent techniques and interpretations of baseline and follow-up scans.

Limitations of RECIST have encouraged volumetric approaches to the anatomic measure of response assessment (22). The rational for volumetric approaches is multifactorial. First, cancers grow and regress irregularly in three dimensions. Measurements obtained in the axial plane fail to account for growth or regression in longitudinal axis. Various volumetric measurements incorporate changes in all dimensions. Secondly, changes in volume are less subject to either reader error or interscan variations. The much greater magnitude of volumetric changes is less prone to measurement error than changes in diameter, particularly if the lesions are irregularly shaped. Various computer-aided diagnosis systems for nodule detection, and other software programs to do volumetric measurements of tumors, are being tested.

■ PATHOLOGISTS

Pathologists are playing an increasingly important role in the team management of patients with lung cancer. It has been appreciated for many years that small cell lung cancers (SCLCs) should be distinguished from the non–small cell histologies because the natural history and therapies are different. Previous studies suggested that the three major non–small cell histologies did not need to be distinguished for therapeutic purposes as outcomes following surgery, chemotherapy, and chemoradiotherapy were not different by histology (23). As a result, as many as one third of non–small cell lung cancers (NSCLC) have recently been described as NSCLC–not otherwise specified (NOS). Several recent studies have highlighted the importance of accurate histologic interpretations of lung cytology and histology specimens because the activity of new drugs such as pemetrexed or the toxicity of other new drugs (e.g., bevacizumab) are dependent on histology.

Increasing data suggests that the frequency of mutations and amplifications in several dominant oncogenes is related to histology. For example, *KRAS*, *BRAF*, and *EGFR* mutations are far more common in adenocarcinomas than in squamous cell carcinomas (4). In addition, the *EML4/anaplastic lymphoma kinase (ALK)* fusion gene occurs almost exclusively in adenocarcinomas (24). In the determination of which molecular tests to order, histology may play a major role in selection. The use of predictive markers for therapy selection was recently reviewed by Coate et al. (25).

Pathologists are involved in the preparation of materials for molecular testing and selection of the type of tests to order. Mutations in *KRAS* and *EGFR* are frequently tested and can be determined by a variety of techniques including direct sequencing and polymerase chain reaction (PCR)–based amplification techniques. For most molecular analysis, at least 10 unstained slides with microdissection or a punch selection of a tumor area in the formalin-fixed paraffin-embedded tissue are required. Ensuring that the DNA is extracted from the tumor tissue is critical and performed by pathologists. The direct sequencing techniques are less sensitive than other techniques but are subject to fewer false positive results. It is important for the physicians involved in patient care to work with the pathologists in selecting the appropriate tests and also to understand the limitations of different molecular tests (e.g., the possibility of false negatives when testing for *EGFR* mutations). In cases where there is insufficient material for molecular testing, the clinician must determine the importance and risks of rebiopsy.

THORACIC SURGEONS

Thoracic surgeons play a critical role in the cure of patients with early-stage lung cancer and in the palliation of patients with symptomatic metastatic lesions. At present pathologic stage is the only prognostic variable

that is used in the selection of patients for postoperative adjuvant therapy with radiation therapy and/or chemotherapy. It is likely that surgical tissues will be used for analyses of gene signatures that will predict not only the chance of relapses (26) but also the predictive likelihood that a therapy will prolong progression-free and overall survival (OS). Surgeons will be involved in the collection of tissue and the interpretation of the results. The surgical therapy of patients with NSCLC is discussed in other chapters.

SURGERY IN SCLC

Patients with SCLC may also benefit from surgical resection (27,28). The revised International Association for the Study of Lung Cancer staging system demonstrates the utility of the TNM system for SCLC (29). Patients with T1N0, T2N0, and T1N1 disease, usually followed by systemic chemotherapy, had good 5-year-survival results with this approach (29).

RADIATION ONCOLOGY

Radiation oncologists are involved in the pretreatment staging and the treatment of patients with lung cancer. In the preoperative staging of early lung cancer, it is extremely important for radiation oncologists to be involved in decisions regarding "medical" and technical operability and to ensure that the appropriate CT and CT/PET scans are available for radiation treatment planning.

RADIATION WITH CURATIVE INTENT IN EARLY STAGE NSCLC

Stereotactic body radiation therapy (SBRT) is an appropriate treatment option for patients with localized lesions (T1N0, T2N0) who are medically inoperable or who decline surgery (31,32). Small peripheral lesions are easier to treat than central tumors but some central tumors may be treated (32). The techniques and results with SBRT for these lesions are described elsewhere in this book. Stereotactic radiotherapy is also a treatment option for patients with metastatic pulmonary nodules (33).

Conventional chest radiotherapy is used in medically inoperable patients whose disease cannot be treated with SBRT. Five-year-survival rates may not be as high as reported with surgical resection but these patients have many more comorbid conditions. Systemic chemotherapy given concurrently can also be considered in these patients.

Meta-analyses have shown that concurrent chemo-therapy and radiotherapy are superior to their sequential application. However, the role of additional chemotherapy after the concurrent chemotherapy is more uncertain and is discussed in other chapters.

The South West Oncology Group (SWOG) also conducted a randomized trial evaluating the value of gefitinib given after the SWOG regimen of etoposide/cisplatin and concurrent radiation therapy followed by docetaxel (34). Surprisingly, the progression-free survival (PFS) and OS favored placebo over gefitinib. The differences could not be explained by an increased rate of death from toxicity in the gefitinib-treated patients. Because of these unanticipated results, gefitinib and erlotinib should not be used in this setting outside of a clinical trial.

■ MEDICAL ONCOLOGY

Medical oncologists frequently become the primary care physicians for patients with lung cancer. Therefore, it is critical that they understand the staging and pathologic classification systems, the natural history, and the potential role of each therapeutic modality alone and in combination. Medical oncologists must also be prepared to handle the frequent comorbid conditions of lung cancer patients. Referral of patients to specialists in palliative care is an important role for the medical oncologists.

Medical oncologists are routinely responsible for prescribing and administering the systemic therapy for patients who present with stage IV disease and those who have distant relapse after surgery for stage I–IIIA disease or after chemotherapy plus radiotherapy for stage III disease. Medical Oncologists must be involved in the early treatment planning of patients with resectable disease to plan for neoadjuvant or adjuvant chemotherapy as discussed in other chapters.

Recent studies of novel targeted therapies using biomarkers to assess the molecular expression of certain oncogenes are changing the paradigm for the selection of therapy and for the relationships between medical oncologists and pathologists and other lung cancer team members. Investigators initially showed that the EGFR tyrosine kinase inhibitor (TKI), erlotinib, improved survival in unselected NSCLC patients in the 2nd/3rd line setting (35). It was subsequently shown that patients with activating mutations in the EGFR gene were associated with higher response rates (36). Further, patients of Asian ethnicity, adenocarcinoma histology, and light- or never-smoking status were more likely to have activating EGFR mutations and more likely to respond to EGFR TKI's (37). These data led to randomized phase II and III trials comparing gefitinib or erlotinib to multiagent chemotherapy in the first-line setting (5,38–40). In the IPASS trial, Asian

patients with advanced adenocarcinoma of the lung and never- or light-smoking status were randomized to receive oral gefitinib or the combination of intravenous carboplatin and paclitaxel (5). In patients with an EGFR mutation, gefitinib produced a higher response rate, a longer PFS, superior quality of life, and less toxicity compared to patients treated with combination chemotherapy. Survival was slightly better in the gefitinib-treated group with EGFR mutations but the differences were not significant because chemotherapy-treated patients who crossed over to gefitinib also had a good outcome. In contrast, chemotherapy was superior to gefitinib in patients without activating patients with respect to response rates and PFS. OS also favored chemotherapy in this group although the differences were not statistically significant. Thus, the molecularly defined patients with activating EGFR mutations should clearly receive first-line EGFR TKI. Other similar trials in Japan and Korea that were limited to patients with EGFR mutations showed similar results (39,40). These results appear to be true for erlotinib as well as gefitinib and for Caucasians as well as Asians as a large phase II study of erlotinib in European patients with activating EGFR mutations showed high response rates (~75%) and long PFS (>12 mo) with first-line erlotinib (36,40).

Four large randomized trials comparing chemotherapy alone to chemotherapy plus erlotinib or gefitinib showed no advantage for the combination (41–44). In fact, outcomes were slightly worse in the combination arm during the period of induction therapy. This was likely due to the arrest of cells in the G1 phase of the cell cycle by the EGFR TKIs. This cell cycle–related antagonist effect could be avoided in preclinical in vitro studies by intercalating erlotinib and docetaxel (45). This approach was tested in a randomized phase II study comparing erlotinib alone to erlotinib alternating with paclitaxel/carboplatin in chemonaive, advanced NSCLC patients who were EGFR positive by immunohistochemistry and/or fluorescence in situ hybridization (FISH) (46). The study was conducted in the United States and the United Kingdom. In patients with EGFR mutations, erlotinib alone was superior to the intercalated combined therapy in overall response rate, PFS, and OS indicating frank antagonism between the combined therapies. In patients without EGFR mutations, the chemotherapy arm was superior in efficacy. These data also indicate that results in Caucasians are the same as Asians and that a single agent TKI is the treatment of choice for patients with activating EGFR mutations irrespective of clinical features.

In 2007 Soda et al. reported that the ALK oncogene could be activated in lung cancer patients by fusion with other genes such as EML4 on the same chromosome (46), and ALK could act a "driver" mutation similar to EGFR mutations in other NSCLCs. Subsequent studies showed that EML4/ALK fusions were more common in adenocarcinomas and in never-smokers (24,47). ALK gene fusions can be detected using FISH probes, using ALK specific antibodies, or using PCR techniques. Although it is not clear which of these is best, clinical trial selection has been based on FISH testing. Once again, coordination between pathologists and clinicians is critical. An ALK inhibitor termed crizotinib (PF-02341066) was studied in a phase I trial. Because an NSCLC patient with an *EML4/ALK* fusion gene had an excellent response to this therapy an expanded cohort was added in which 82 patients with advanced NSCLC whose tumors harbored an *EML4/ALK* fusion gene were treated with crizotinib (48). Objective responses were documented in 52 of these 82 patients and 78/82 had some tumor shrinkage. These exciting results have led to phase II and III trials of crizotinib in this patient population. These studies emphasize the importance of the lung cancer multidisciplinary team in caring for lung cancer patients. The patients tumor must be obtained by biopsy from a team member, prepared for genetic analysis by the pathologist, and the therapeutic implication assessed by the medical oncologist!

■ PALLIATIVE CARE

Because the 5-year-survival rate for lung cancer is only about 15%, nearly 85% of patients will eventually die from their disease. Most of these patients will develop metastatic disease after recurrence following curative therapies or present with metastatic disease at the time of diagnosis. Symptoms referable to the disease will be present in 90% or more of patients with metastatic disease. The most frequent symptoms are cough, dyspnea, chest pain, and hemoptysis from the primary tumors. Symptoms may also be caused by metastatic disease such as brain, bone, and liver metastases and from paraneoplastic syndromes such as venous and arterial emboli, hypercalcemia, hypernatremia, Cushing's syndrome, and weight loss. Once treatment has been instituted, symptoms may be induced by any of the therapeutic modalities including surgery, radiotherapy, and chemotherapy. Each of these symptoms must be addressed by the team caring for lung cancer patients. A recent study from Boston demonstrated that early intervention by a palliative care team could improve both quality of life and survival (49).

■ REFERENCES

1. Jemal A, Siegel R, Ward E, Hao Y, Xu J, Thun MJ. Cancer statistics, 2009. *CA Cancer J Clin.* 2009;59(4):225–249.

2. Beasley MB, Brambilla E, Travis WD. The 2004 World Health Organization classification of lung tumors. *Semin Roentgenol.* 2005;40(2):90–97.

3. Motoi N, Szoke J, Riely GJ, et al. Lung adenocarcinoma: modification of the 2004 WHO mixed subtype to include the major histologic subtype suggests correlations between papillary and micropapillary adenocarcinoma subtypes, EGFR mutations and gene expression analysis. *Am J Surg Pathol.* 2008;32(6):810–827.

4. Ding L, Getz G, Wheeler DA, et al. Somatic mutations affect key pathways in lung adenocarcinoma. *Nature.* 2008;455(7216):1069–1075.

5. Mok TS, Wu YL, Thongprasert S, et al. Gefitinib or carboplatin-paclitaxel in pulmonary adenocarcinoma. *N Engl J Med.* 2009;361(10):947–957.

6. Cronin KA, Gail MH, Zou Z, Bach PB, Virtamo J, Albanes D. Validation of a model of lung cancer risk prediction among smokers. *J Natl Cancer Inst.* 2006;98(9):637–640.

7. Raji OY, Agbaje OF, Duffy SW, Cassidy A, Field JK. Incorporation of a genetic factor into an epidemiologic model for prediction of individual risk of lung cancer: the Liverpool Lung Project. *Cancer Prev Res (Phila Pa).* 2010;3(5):664–669.

8. Cassidy A, Myles JP, Liloglou T, Duffy SW, Field JK. Defining high-risk individuals in a population-based molecular-epidemiological study of lung cancer. *Int J Oncol.* 2006;28(5):1295–1301.

9. Wilson DO, Weissfeld JL, Fuhrman CR, et al. The Pittsburgh Lung Screening Study (PLuSS): outcomes within 3 years of a first computed tomography scan. *Am J Respir Crit Care Med.* 2008;178(9):956–961.

10. Ernst A, Eberhardt R, Krasnik M, Herth FJ. Efficacy of endobronchial ultrasound-guided transbronchial needle aspiration of hilar lymph nodes for diagnosing and staging cancer. *J Thorac Oncol.* 2009;4(8):947–950.

11. Navani N, Spiro SG, Janes SM. EBUS-TBNA for the mediastinal staging of non-small cell lung cancer. *J Thorac Oncol.* 2009;4(6):776; author reply 776–776; author reply 777.

12. Tournoy KG, De Ryck F, Vanwalleghem LR, et al. Endoscopic ultrasound reduces surgical mediastinal staging in lung cancer: a randomized trial. *Am J Respir Crit Care Med.* 2008;177(5):531–535.

13. Hecht SS, Kassie F, Hatsukami DK. Chemoprevention of lung carcinogenesis in addicted smokers and ex-smokers. *Nat Rev Cancer.* 2009;9(7):476–488.

14. Keith RL, Miller YE, Jackson MK, et al. Update on the use of oral iloprost for the chemoprevention of lung cancer. 12th World Conference on Lung Cancer, September 2–6, 2007, Seoul, South Korea. *J Thorac Oncol.* 2007;2(8 suppl 4):S330–S331.

15. Mao JT, Cui X, Reckamp K, et al. Chemoprevention strategies with cyclooxygenase-2 inhibitors for lung cancer. *Clin Lung Cancer.* 2005;7(1):30–39.

16. Gandara DR, Aberle D, Lau D, et al. Radiographic imaging of bronchioloalveolar carcinoma: screening, patterns of presentation and response assessment. *J Thorac Oncol.* 2006;1(9 suppl):S20–S26.

17. Sakao et al Ann. Thor. Surg 83:209–214, 2007

18. James K, Eisenhauer E, Christian M, Terenziani M, Vena D, Muldal A, et al. Measuring response in solid tumors: Unidimensional versus bidimensional measurement. *J Natl Cancer Inst.* 1999;91:523–528.

19. Jaffe CC. Measures of response: RECIST, WHO, and new alternatives. *J Clin Oncol.* 2006;24(20):3245–3251.

20. Petrou M, Quint LE, Nan B, Baker LH. Pulmonary nodule volumetric measurement variability as a function of CT slice thickness and nodule morphology. *AJR Am J Roentgenol.* 2007;188(2):306–312.

21. Kostis WJ, Yankelevitz DF, Reeves AP, Fluture SC, Henschke CI. Small pulmonary nodules: reproducibility of three-dimensional volumetric measurement and estimation of time to follow-up CT. *Radiology.* 2004;231(2):446–452.

22. Buckler AJ, Mulshine JL, Gottlieb R, Zhao B, Mozley PD, Schwartz L. The use of volumetric CT as an imaging biomarker in lung cancer. *Acad Radiol.* 2010;17:100–106.

23. Rossi G, Pelosi G, Graziano P, Barbareschi M, Papotti M. A reevaluation of the clinical significance of histological subtyping of non–small-cell lung carcinoma: diagnostic algorithms in the era of personalized treatments. *Int J Surg Pathol.* 2009;17(3):206–218.

24. Shaw AT, Yeap BY, Mino-Kenudson M, et al. Clinical features and outcome of patients with non-small-cell lung cancer who harbor EML4-ALK. *J Clin Oncol.* 2009;27(26):4247–4253.

25. Coate LE, John T, Tsao MS, Shepherd FA. Molecular predictive and prognostic markers in non-small-cell lung cancer. *Lancet Oncol.* 2009;10(10):1001–1010.

26. Potti A, Mukherjee S, Petersen R, et al. A genomic strategy to refine prognosis in early-stage non-small-cell lung cancer. *N Engl J Med.* 2006;355(6):570–580.

27. Waddell TK, Shepherd FA. Should aggressive surgery ever be part of the management of small cell lung cancer? *Thorac Surg Clin.* 2004;14(2):271–281.

28. Lim E, Belcher E, Yap YK, Nicholson AG, Goldstraw P. The role of surgery in the treatment of limited disease small cell lung cancer: time to reevaluate. *J Thorac Oncol.* 2008;3(11):1267–1271.

29. Vallières E, Shepherd FA, Crowley J, et al.; International Association for the Study of Lung Cancer International Staging Committee and Participating Institutions. The IASLC Lung Cancer Staging Project: proposals regarding the relevance of TNM in the pathologic staging of small cell lung cancer in the forthcoming (seventh) edition of the TNM classification for lung cancer. *J Thorac Oncol.* 2009;4(9):1049–1059.

30. Baumann P, Nyman J, Hoyer M, et al. Outcome in a prospective phase II trial of medically inoperable stage I non-small-cell lung cancer patients treated with stereotactic body radiotherapy. *J Clin Oncol.* 2009;27(20):3290–3296.

31. Fakiris AJ, McGarry RC, Yiannoutsos CT, et al. Stereotactic body radiation therapy for early-stage non-small-cell lung carcinoma: four-year results of a prospective phase II study. *Int J Radiat Oncol Biol Phys.* 2009;75(3):677–682.

32. Song SY, Choi W, Shin SS, et al. Fractionated stereotactic body radiation therapy for medically inoperable stage I lung cancer adjacent to central large bronchus. *Lung Cancer.* 2009;66(1):89–93.

33. Rusthoven KE, Kavanagh BD, Burri SH, et al. Multi-institutional phase I/II trial of stereotactic body radiation therapy for lung metastases. *J Clin Oncol.* 2009;27(10):1579–1584.

34. Kelly K, Chansky K, Gaspar LE, et al. Phase III trial of maintenance gefitinib or placebo after concurrent chemoradiotherapy and docetaxel consolidation in inoperable stage III non-small-cell lung cancer: SWOG S0023. *J Clin Oncol.* 2008;26(15):2450–2456.

35. Shepherd FA, Rodrigues Pereira J, Ciuleanu T, et al.; National Cancer Institute of Canada Clinical Trials Group. Erlotinib in previously treated non-small-cell lung cancer. *N Engl J Med.* 2005;353(2):123–132.

36. Rosell R, Moran T, Queralt C, et al.; Spanish Lung Cancer Group. Screening for epidermal growth factor receptor mutations in lung cancer. *N Engl J Med.* 2009;361(10):958–967.

37. Hung JJ, Jeng WJ, Hsu WH, Liu JS, Wu YC. EGFR mutations in non-small-cell lung cancer. *Lancet Oncol.* 2010;11(5):412–3; author reply 413.

38. Mitsudomi T, Morita S, Yatabe Y, et al.; West Japan Oncology Group. Gefitinib versus cisplatin plus docetaxel in patients with non-small-cell lung cancer harbouring mutations of the epidermal growth factor receptor (WJTOG3405): an open label, randomised phase 3 trial. *Lancet Oncol.* 2010;11(2):121–128.

39. Maemondo M, Inoue A, Kobayashi K, et al.; North-East Japan Study Group. Gefitinib or chemotherapy for non-small-cell lung cancer with mutated EGFR. *N Engl J Med.* 2010;362(25):2380–2388.

40. Lee JS, Park J, Kim SW, et al. A randomized phase III study of gefitinib (IRESSA® versus standard chemotherapy (gemcitabine plus cisplatin) as a first-line treatment for never-smokers with advanced or metastatic adenocarcinoma of the lung. *J Thorac Oncol.* 2009;4:S283.

41. Giaccone G, Herbst RS, Manegold C, et al. Gefitinib in combination with gemcitabine and cisplatin in advanced non-small-cell lung cancer: a phase III trial–INTACT 1. *J Clin Oncol.* 2004;22(5):777–784.

42. Herbst RS, Giaccone G, Schiller JH, et al. Gefitinib in combination with paclitaxel and carboplatin in advanced non-small-cell lung cancer: a phase III trial–INTACT 2. *J Clin Oncol.* 2004;22(5):785–794.

43. Gatzemeier U, Pluzanska A, Szczesna A, et al. Phase III study of erlotinib in combination with cisplatin and gemcitabine in advanced non-small-cell lung cancer: the Tarceva Lung Cancer Investigation Trial. *J Clin Oncol.* 2007;25(12):1545–1552.

44. Herbst RS, Prager D, Hermann R, et al.; TRIBUTE Investigator Group. TRIBUTE: a phase III trial of erlotinib hydrochloride (OSI-774) combined with carboplatin and paclitaxel chemotherapy in advanced non-small-cell lung cancer. *J Clin Oncol.* 2005;23(25):5892–5899.

45. Gandara D, Davie AM, Gautschi O, et al. Epidermal growth factor receptor inhibitors plus chemotherapy in non-small-cell lung cancer: biologic rationale for combination strategies. *Clin Lung Cancer.* 2007;8(suppl 2):S61–S67.

46. Hirsch FR, Dziadziuszko R, Kabbinavar, F, et al. Randomized phase II study of erlotinib (E) or intercalated E with carboplatin/paclitaxel (C/P) in chemo-naive advanced NSCLC: Biomarker status correlates with clinical benefit. Proceedings of the 2009 Annual Meeting, May 29–June 2, 2009, Orlando, FL [abstract 8026]. *Proc Am Soc Clin Oncol.* 2009;27:15S(May 20 suppl).

47. Soda M, Choi YL, Enomito M, et al. Identification of the transforming EML4/ALK fusion gene in non-small cell lung cancer. *Nature.* 2007;448;561–566.

48. Bang Y, Kwak EL, Shaw AT, et al. Clinical activity of the oral ALK inhibitor PF-02341066 in ALK-positive patients with non-small cell lung cancer (NSCLC) [abstract 3]. *J Clin Oncol.* 2010;28:946s.

49. Temel JS, Greer JA, Mizikansky A, et al: Early palliative care for patients with metastatic non-small cell lung cancer. New Engl J Med. 2010; 363(8): 733–742.

Index

Note: Page numbers followed by "*f*" and "*t*" refer to figures and tables, respectively.

Abraxas protein, 271
Acute respiratory distress
        syndrome (ARDS), 99
Additional tumor nodule(s), 45
Adenocarcinoma, 1, 21–22, 24–26, 26*f*
    pathogenesis, 27–28
    pathologic and molecular
        characteristics of, 22*t*
    smokers and never-smokers
        comparison of, 27*f*
        molecular characteristics
            comparison of, 27*t*
Adenosquamous carcinoma, 1, 22
Adjuvant chemotherapy, 106, 123–125,
        133, 139, 341–342
    versus induction chemotherapy,
        127–128
    for N2, 146
    phase III trials of, 124*t*
    surgical management
        following, 145–146
Adjuvant Lung Project Italy (ALPI), 123
Adjuvant Navelbine International
        Trialist Association (ANITA)
        trial, 124, 342
Adjuvant therapy, 3, 263
    for NSCLC, 279–280
Adrenal metastasectomy, 176*t*
Adrenal metastasis, 84, 176*t*
    isolated, 175
Adrenocorticotropic hormone
        (ACTH), 111
Adriamycin, 239, 271
Advanced non-small cell lung cancer, 4,
        32, 185, 186, 187, 188, 190, 199,
        243, 280–281
    first-line treatment algorithm for, 345*f*
Age and distress, 328
Akt, 252
ALK oncogene, 356
Alpha-Tocopherol, Beta-Carotene
        Cancer Prevention Study (ATBC),
        62, 63, 64
Altered fractionation, 152–154
American College of Chest Physicians
        (ACCP) guidelines, 3, 7, 169, 337
American College of Surgeons Oncology
        Group, 3, 142
Amifostine, 207

Amrubicin, 118–119
Anaplastic lymphoma kinase
        (ALK) fusion, 271
Ancillary diagnostic
        immunohistochemistry, 23–24
Anisotropic analytic algorithm
        (AAA), 221
Antiangiogenic agents, 271
Antiangiogenic therapies, 243
    and EGFR-targeting therapy,
        combining, 255
    monoclonal antibodies, 243–245
    small molecule tyrosine kinase
        inhibitors, 245–247
Anti-Bcl-2 family protein inhibitors, 120
Anti-Lung Cancer Association (ALCA)
        study, 55, 58
Aortic resections, 163–164
APC gene, 25, 26, 32
ATM gene, 26
Atrial resection, 164
Atypical adenomatous hyperplasia
        (AAH), 21, 27
AVAiL trial, 189, 244, 271, 285
5'-Aza-2'-deoxycytidine, 32

B7.1 (CD80) vaccine, 5, 301–302
BCRP1, 29
BEC2, 305
Beck Depression Inventory (BDI), 324
Belagenpumatucel, 5, 299–300
β-carotene studies, 64
Bevacizumab, 4, 128, 187, 188, 189,
        190, 243–245, 248, 255, 285,
        342, 344
Bexarotene, 257
BIBW 2992, 189, 201, 252
Big Lung Trial (BLT), 123
Biomarker-Integrated Approaches
        of Targeted Therapy for Lung
        Cancer Elimination clinical trial
        program, 257
BMS-099 (Bristol-Myers Squibb-099)
        study, 189, 269
Bone metastasis, 8, 84, 176
Bortezomib, 202
Brachytherapy, 3, 4, 96, 239–240

BRAF mutation, 1, 24, 355
Brain metastasis, 29, 84
    isolated, 174–175
    prophylactic cranial irradiation
        in, 213
Brain MRI, 2, 84
BRCA1, 192, 271
Brinkman Index, 76
British Columbia Cancer Agency
        (BCCA) registry, 286
Bronchial margins, 95
Bronchioloalveolar cancer, 1
Bronchioloalveolar carcinoma
        (BAC), 21, 22, 169
Bronchioloalveolar stems cells
        (BASCs), 29
Bronchoplastic procedures, 98, 99
Bronchopulmonary carcinoids, 46–47
Bronchoscopic treatment, indications
        for, 235, 236
Bronchoscopy, 7
    flexible, 235–236
    indications for, 236
    rigid, 235

CALGB 9633, 130, 341
CALGB 30610, 115
CALGB 39801, 155, 184
Cancer and Leukemia Group B
        (CALGB) trial, 114, 115, 125,
        154, 155, 158, 184, 212, 280
Cancer care sites, 338–339
Carboplatin, 155, 156, 158, 184,
        185, 246, 247, 250, 251,
        254–255, 267, 269, 280, 282,
        283, 342, 344
Carcinoid tumors, 23
Carcinoma in situ (CIS), 19–21
Cardiopulmonary bypass (CPB), 163
    need for, 164
Cardiopulmonary exercise tests
        (CPETs), 92
Care coordination, 9–10
CARET study, 63, 65
Carinal resection, 99–100, 161
CAV (cyclophosphamide, doxorubicin,
        vincristine), 113, 117

CD133, 29
CD24, 29
CD29, 29
CD31, 29
CD34, 29
CD44, 29
CD326, 29
CDH13 gene, 25, 32
CDK4 gene, 32
CDKN2A gene, 26
cDNA microarray, 32–33
Cediranib, 189
Celecoxib, 64, 68, 254, 256, 354
Center for Epidemiologic Studies
    Depression Scale (CES-D), 324
Central airway disease, signs and
    symptoms of, 236
Central nervous system (CNS), 84
Cervical mediastinoscopy, 92, 92*f*,
    141, 337
Cetuximab, 5, 158, 184, 187, 189, 201,
    247, 255, 269, 285, 342, 344
  in neoadjuvant setting, 249
  with radiation, 248–249
Charlson Comorbidity Index (CCI), 278
Chemoradiation, 5, 97, 113, 114, 134,
    155, 184, 280
Chemotherapeutics, 117, 239, 341–344
Chemotherapy, 33–34, 114, 158, 264
  adjuvant, 106, 123–125, 341–343
    for N2, 146
  for advanced disease, 281–284, 342
  concurrent chemotherapy with
    radiation, 154
  consolidation, 156–157
  delivery of, 344
  doublet chemotherapy, 185, 198
  for ES-SCLC management, 117
  induction, 125–127
    for N2, 143–144
  for LS-SCLC management, 114
  neoadjuvant, 133
  postoperative, 133
  sequential chemotherapy followed by
    radiation, 154
Chest radiography, 73
Chest X-ray, randomized controlled
    trials of, 53–55
Chronic obstructive pulmonary disease
    (COPD), 65
Chronic post-thoracotomy pain
    (CPTP), 314
Circulating tumor cells (CTCs), 300
Cisplatin, 34, 155, 156, 185, 205, 211,
    212, 245, 248, 265, 270, 279,
    280, 282, 285, 286, 287, 341,
    342, 344, 342
Cisplatin-based chemotherapy, 114, 154,
    155, 156, 157, 183, 185, 341
City of Hope quality of life model
    (COH-QOL) model, 317
Classification of lung cancer, 19, 29

Class III β-tubulin, 270
Clinical target volume, 219
Clinical tumor volume, 206, 208, 209
Clinicians, roles and responsibilities
    of, 11*t*
Community-based care, issues
    in, 335–336
Community-based clinical oncology
    research, 346
Community-based lung cancer, 5
Community lung cancer program,
    characteristics of, 346, 347*t*
Comparative genomic hybridization
    (CGH), 31
Computed tomography (CT), 2, 55,
    73–74, 83, 168, 354
Concurrent chemotherapy with
    radiation, 154–156
Concurrent modality therapy, 154, 155
Conformality index, 221
Conformal radiotherapy, 205
  dose and fractionation, 211–212
  dose escalation, 212
  intensity-modulated radiation therapy
    (IMRT)7, 205–210
  new directions, 214
  prophylactic cranial
    irradiation, 213–214
  radiation volume, 213
  in recurrent/persistent NSCLC
    retreatment, 210
  for small cell lung cancer (SCLC), 211
  timing of, 211
Consolidation chemotherapy, 156–157
  for small cell lung cancer, 211
Continuous hyperfractionated
    accelerated radiotherapy
    (CHART), 153
Conventional fractionated radiation
    therapy (CFRT), 217, 218
CONVERT trial, 115
Core needle biopsies (CNB), 21, 31
CP-751, 871, 252
CT-guided transthoracic needle
    biopsy, 8
CT screening. *See* low-dose
    helical CT screening
Curative resection, 3
CyberKnife, 209, 219, 226
Cyclooxygenase (COX)-2
    inhibitors, 254, 256
Cyclooxygenase, 68
Cyclophilin B (CypB), 304
Cyclophosphamide, 205, 211, 212
Cyclophosphamide, doxorubicin, and
    cisplatin (CAP), 187
Cyclophosphamide, epirubicin,
    vincristine (CEV) arm, 114
Cytokeratin 5 (*CK5*), 23
Cytokeratin 6 (*CK6*), 23
Cytokeratin 7 (*CK7*), 23
Cytotoxic lymphocytes (CTL), 301, 304

Detection and Screening of Early
    Lung Cancer by Novel Imaging
    Technology and Molecular
    Assays (DANTE), 61
Dexosome vaccine, 303
Diagnosis, of lung cancer, 7–9
Diffuse idiopathic pulmonary
    neuroendocrine cell hyperplasia
    (DIPENECH), 21
2′,2′-Difluorodeoxycytidine, 265
Dihydrofolate reductase, 265
Disease-free survival (DFS), 124
Disease-related variables, 329–330
  cancer type, 329
  physical functioning and symptoms, 329
  stage, 329
  time since diagnosis/
    treatment, 329–330
Distress in lung cancer, prevalence and
    nature of, 323–328
DNA copy number profiles, 31–32
Docetaxel, 156, 184, 186, 197–201,
    246, 250, 251, 254, 264, 271,
    281, 282, 344
Doxorubicin, 211
DUSP6 gene, 32
Dysplastic squamous lesions, 21

Early Lung Cancer Action Project
    (ELCAP), 55, 58
Early-phase clinical trial designs, 66–67
Early-stage lung cancer, 55, 61, 123,
    157, 295–296
  symptoms and quality of
    life in, 313–315
Early stage NSCLC, radiation with
    curative intent in, 355–356
Echinoderm microtubule-associated
    protein like-4 (EML4), 271
ECOG 4599 trial, 188, 243–244, 245
Education and distress, 329
EGFR FISH, 248, 268–269, 270
EGFR gene, 26, 183, 249, 263,
    266–269, 344
EGFR-inhibition-related rash (EIRR)
    rating scale has, 248
EGFR mutations, 1, 5, 24, 25,
    27–28, 29, 35, 129, 189, 190,
    191, 355, 356
EGFR-TKI therapy, 191, 266, 270
EGFR tyrosine-kinase inhibitors, 197
EML-ALK fusion, 254
EML4-ALK fusion gene, 1, 24,
    271–272, 357
Endobronchial biopsy, 7
Endobronchial brachytherapy, 239–240
Endobronchial treatment, of lung
    cancer, 4
Endobronchial ultrasound
    (EBUS), 7, 92, 92*f*, 93

Enzastaurin, 202
EPHA3 gene, 26
EPHA5 gene, 26
Epidermal growth factor (EGF)
        vaccine, 302–303
Epidermal growth factor
        receptor (EGFR), 128, 187,
        189, 197, 200, 263, 302
    EGFR inhibitors, 266, 269
        and COX-2 inhibitors, 256
        and mTOR inhibitors, 256
    EGFR-targeting therapies, 247
        and antiangiogenic therapy, 255
        and COX-2 inhibitors, 256
        dual inhibition of, 255–256
        monoclonal antibodies, 247–249
        small molecule tyrosine kinase
            inhibitors, 249–251
    protein expression, 269
Epigenetics, 32
Epothilone B, 200
ERBB3 gene, 32
ERBB4 gene, 26
ErbB family, of protein, 247, 247*f*,
        251, 256
Erlotinib, 189, 190, 199, 249–250,
        255–256, 257, 268, 269, 284,
        285, 342
Esophageal involvement, in
        T4 invasion, 164
Ethnicity and distress, 328–329
Etoposide, 155, 156, 211, 212, 253,
        271, 286, 287, 341
European Organization for
        Research and Treatment of
        Cancer (EORTC) study, 3, 134,
        154, 166
EUROSCAN study, 63
Evaluation of lung cancer patient, 7
    care coordination, 9–10
    diagnosis and staging, of
        lung cancer, 7–9
    lung nodule clinics, 10
    multidisciplinary clinic, 10
    physician and hospital volume, 10–14
    thoracic tumor board, 10
    timeliness of care, 14–15, 14*t*
ExacTrac positioning, 219–220
Excision repair cross-complementation
        group 1 (ERCC1), 2, 34, 128,
        191, 264
Exhaled breath condensate (EBC), 62
Extensive disease (ED) stage, 79, 80*f*
Extensive-stage SCLC (ESLC), 115
    chemotherapy, 117
    novel therapeutics, 118–120
    prophylactic cranial
        irradiation in, 118
    relapsed disease, 118
External-beam radiation
        therapy, 240
"Extracapsular disease", 139

FDG-PET, see Fluorodeoxyglucose–
        positron emission tomography
FGFR4 gene, 26
Fine needle aspirates (FNA), 21, 31
FLEX (First line Erbitux in Lung
        Cancer) study, 269
Flexible bronchoscope, 235–236
FLEX trial regimen, 344
Fluorescence in situ hybridization
        (FISH), 24, 248
    in EGFR gene detection, 268–269
Fluorine-18-fluorodeoxyglucose
        (FDG), 75
Fluorodeoxyglucose–positron emission
        tomography (FDG-PET), 1, 2, 75,
        76, 77*f*, 79*f*, 83, 218, 227
    nodule avidity to, 78
    in post-SBRT surveillance, 227
5-Fluorouracil (5-FU), 266
Folkmann, Judah, 243
Formalin-fixed paraffin embedded
        (FFPE) tissues, 31
Fucosyl GM1, 305
Functional subunits (FSUs), 218

α-Galactosylceramide (αGalCer), 5, 301
α(1,3)-Galactosyltransferase (agal)
        epitopes, 303–304
Ganglioside GD3, 305
Gas chromatography–mass
        spectrometry (GC-MS), 62
Gefitinib, 5, 156, 189, 245, 250–251,
        252, 255, 256, 266, 269, 270,
        284–285, 342
Gemcitabine, 158, 254, 264, 265, 281,
        282, 342, 344
Gene-expression (mRNA)
        profiles, 32–33
Glycinamide ribonucleotide
        formyltransferase, 265
GNAS gene, 26
Go-no go" decision, 64
Grade 3 esophagitis, 114
Granulocyte-macrophage colony-
        stimulating factor (GM-CSF)
        gene, 300
Gross tumor volume (GTV), 205, 208,
        209, 219
Ground glass opacities", 21
GVAX vaccine, 300–301

Hammar classification, 47, 47*f*
Hedgehog (Hh) pathway inhibitors, 120
Helical CT screening, low-dose. *See*
        low-dose helical CT screening
Hematoxylin and eosin (H&E)-stained
        biopsy samples, 23
HER2 gene mutations, 24, 25, 201

Heterogeneous nuclear
        ribonucleoprotein (hnRNP), 61
High-dose-rate brachytherapy (HDR),
        239, 240
High-risk cohorts, identification of, 65
Hilar nodes, 7
Histone deacetylase (HDAC)
        inhibitors, 254
Histopathologic abnormalities, of lung
        cancer precursor lesions, 20*t*
Historical perspective, on lung
        chemoprevention clinical trials
    lessons learned, 64
    phase III clinical trials, 62–64
Historical variables, 331
HKI-272, 251–252
Hoosier Oncology group (HOG), 156
Hospital Anxiety and Depression
        Scale (HADS), 324
Human telomerase reverse
        transcriptase (hTERT), 303
Hyperfractionated accelerated radiation
        therapy (HART), 153–154
Hyperfractionating radiotherapy, 114
Hyperfractionation, 153
Hypofractionated dosages, 4

IALT (International Adjuvant Lung
        Cancer Trial), 264
IASLC database, 43
IASLC lymph node map, 47
IASLC recommendations, external
        validation of, 48
IDM-2101, 5, 301
IFN-γ production, 304
Ifosfamide, 197
Ikeda, Shigeto, 236
Imaging in lung cancer, 2–3, 73
    non-small cell lung cancer, 80
        metastasis (M stage),
            evaluation of, 83–84
        nodal metastasis (N stage),
            evaluation of, 83
        tumor status (T stage), 80–83
    small cell lung cancer (SCLC), 79–80
    solitary pulmonary nodule (SPN), 76
        imaging guided percutaneous
            needle biopsy, 78–79
        location, 77
        morphology, 77
        size, 76–77
        tissue-specific and metabolic
            characteristics, 77–78
    techniques
        chest radiography, 73
        computed tomography (CT), 73–74
        magnetic resonance imaging
            (MRI), 74–75
        positron emission tomography
            (PET), 75–76

Imaging tests, 8*t*
IMC-A12, 252
Immunohistochemistry (IHC)
    analysis, 23
Induction chemoradiotherapy, 133
Induction chemotherapy, 125–127
    versus adjuvant
        chemotherapy, 127–128
    phase III trials of, 126*t*
Induction chemotherapy, 184
INHBA gene, 26
In-room stereoscopic x-ray imaging
    device, 209
Insulin-like growth factor 1 receptor
    (IGF-1R) targeting therapies, 252
Insulin-like growth factor receptor
    inhibition, 270–271
INT01159 trial, 123
Intensity-modulated proton therapy
    (IMPT), 208, 214
INTEREST trial, 197, 268–269
Intermediate endpoints, 65–66
Internal target volume (ITV), 208, 209
International Adjuvant Lung Cancer
    Trial (IALT), 124, 341–342
International Association for the Study
    of Lung Cancer (IASLC), 140
International Early Lung Cancer Action
    Project (I-ELCAP), 55, 61
International Staging Committee
    (ISC), 43
International Union against Cancer
    (UICC), 1
Intraepithelial neoplasia" (IEN), 66
INT trial, 3
Invasive mediastinal staging, 7
Ipsilateral different lobe nodules,
    170–172
Ipsilobar satellite nodule, 169
Iressa-Pan Asian Study (IPASS), 189,
    191
Iressa Survival Evaluation in Lung
    Cancer (ISEL) study, 251
Iridium-192, 239
Irinotecan, 253, 287, 344, 345
Isolated distant metastases, 173
    general series of surgery in patients
        with, 173–174
    isolated adrenal metastasis, 175
    isolated brain metastasis, 174–175
Isotretinoin, 63
Italian ChEST trial, 127

JBR.10, 342

Kaplan-Meier survival curves, 106*f*
Karnofsky performance status
    (KPS), 278
KDR gene, 26

Killian, Gustave, 235
KRAS gene, 32, 34, 269–270
KRAS mutation, 1, 2, 24, 25, 26,
    344, 355

L523S vaccine, 302
LACE meta-analysis, 341
Lambert-Eaton myasthenic
    syndrome, 112
Lapatinib, 201–202
Large cell carcinoma (LCC), 22
Large cell neuroendocrine carcinomas
    (LCNEC), 22, 23
Laser capture microdissection
    (LCM), 31
Laser resection, 237–238
Late-stage lung cancer, symptoms and
    quality of life in, 315–316
L-BLP-25 vaccine, 5, 301
LCK gene, 32
Lead-time bias, 60
Length-biased sampling, 60
Limited disease stage, 79
Limited-stage SCLC
    (LS-SCLC), 112, 113
    chemotherapy, 114
    key clinical trials in, 115
    prophylactic cranial
        irradiation in, 115
    radiation therapy, 114–115
Linear quadratic (LQ) model, 218
Lineberger Comprehensive Cancer
    Center (LCCC) trial 9719, 283
5-Lipoxygenase (5-LO), 68
Liver metastasis, 84
    SBRT for, 226
Lobectomy, 3, 97
    versus wedge resection, 107
Locally advanced and metastatic
    NSCLC, surgery for, 3–4
Lomustine, 205
Lonafarnib, 34
Loss of heterozygosity (LOH), 26
Low-dose helical CT
    (LDCT) screening
    issues in, 55–60
        lead-time bias, 60
        length-biased sampling, 60
        mortality, of lung cancer, 61
        overdiagnosis, 60–61
        randomized controlled
            trials of, 59*t*, 61
        single-arm studies of helical CT, 55
Low dose-rate brachytherapy
    (LDR), 240
LRP1B gene, 26
LTK gene, 26
Lung Adjuvant Cisplatin Analysis
    (LACE), 279
Lung Adjuvant Cisplatin
    Evaluation, 4, 125

Lung cancer disparities
    advanced disease, 295
    early-stage disease, 295–296
    tobacco, 296
Lung nodule clinics, 10
Lung Screening Study (LSS), 61
LUX-Lung 2 trial, 252
Lymph node station, anatomic
    definitions for, 49*t*

MAGE-3 protein, 303
MAGE-3 vaccines, 5
Magnetic resonance imaging
    (MRI), 2, 74–75, 81
MAGRIT study, 128
Maintenance therapy, 344
MALDI-TOF proteomic analyses, 255
Malignant lung cancer tumors, 21
    carcinoid tumors, 23
    non-small cell lung carcinoma, 21
        adenocarcinoma, 21–22
        adenosquamous carcinoma, 22
        large cell carcinoma (LCC), 22
        sarcomatoid carcinomas, 22–23
        squamous cell carcinoma, 22
        small cell lung carcinoma (SCLC), 23
Malignant pleural involvement, 172–173
Mammalian target of rapamycin
    (mTOR) inhibitors, 252–253
    and EGFR inhibitors, 256
Matrix-assisted laser
    desorption/ionization
    (MALDI) proteomics, 256
Matrix-assisted laser desorption/
    ionization time-of-flight
    mass spectrometry
    (MALDI-TOF MS), 33
Maximumtolerated dose
    (MTD), 114, 115
M descriptors, 46
MDM2 gene, 32
Mediastinal assessment, for staging and
    treatment planning, 92–94
Mediastinal lymph node, 7–8, 141
    assessment, during surgical
        resection, 141
Mediastinoscopy, 8
Mediastinum, management of, 100
Medical oncology, 356–357
    roles and responsibilities, 11*t*
Medical unresectability, 152
Melanoma-associated antigen E-3
    vaccine, 303
Metagene array model, ", 263
Metastasis (M stage)
    evaluation of, 83
        adrenal metastasis, 84
        bone metastasis, 84
        brain metastasis, 84
        liver metastasis, 84
        progression to, 29

Metastatic NSCLC, 223, 226
  patients with, 4
MiR-21, 24
MiR-34a, 29
MiR-38, 24
MiRNA profiles, 24, 33
Mitomycin, ifosfamide, and
      cisplatin (MIC), 186
Mitomycin, lomustine, and
      methotrexate (MCM), 187
MMD gene, 32
Molecular abnormalities of lung cancer
      precursor lesions, 20*t*
Molecular-analysis directed
      individual treatment (MADeIT)
      algorithm, 191
Molecular characteristics of
      tumors, 24
  non-small cell lung cancer, 24
      adenocarcinoma, 24–26
      squamous cell carcinoma, 26
  small cell lung cancer (SCLC), 26
Molecular profiling, of lung cancer, 30*f*
Monoclonal antibodies, 243–245,
      247–249, 285
Montgomery-Asberg Depression Rating
      Scale (MADRS), 324
Mortality, of lung cancer, 61
mTOR. *See* Mammalian target of
      rapamycin (mTOR) inhibitors
Mucin (MUC)-1, 301
Multidisciplinary approach to palliative
      and symptom management of
      disease, 313
  early stage, 313–315
  late-stage lung cancer, 315–316
  palliative care, defining, 313
  symptoms and QOL, assessing,
      317–318
Multidisciplinary care of
      lung cancer patients
  future directions in, 353
      pulmonologists, 353–354
      radiologists, 354
      pathologist, 354–355
      thoracic surgeons, 355
      SCLC, surgery in, 355
      radiation oncology, 355
      radiation with curative intent in
        early stage NSCLC, 355–356
      medical oncology, 356–357
      palliative care, 357
Multidisciplinary clinic, 10
Multidisciplinary management, of lung
      cancer, 335
  chemoprevention, 336
  diagnosis and staging, 337–338
  multimodality lung cancer care,
      346–347
  nonsmall cell lung cancer (NSCLC),
      335–336
  novel treatment approaches, 345–346
  risk factors, 336

screening, 336–337
  small cell lung cancer
      (SCLC), 344–345
  treatment, 338
      cancer care sites, 338–339
      chemotherapeutics, 341–344
      pretreatment evaluation, 338*t*
      radiation therapy, 340–341
      referral patterns, 338
      surgery, 339–340
Multifocal lung cancer (MFLC), 169
Multimodality lung cancer
      care, 5, 346–347
Multimodality therapy, 164–168
Multiple primary lung cancer (MPLC),
      168, 169–170, 171, 171*t*
MutS homolog 2 (MSH2)
      protein, 264
MYC gene, 32

N2 disease, 133, 141
  adjuvant chemotherapy for, 146
  induction chemotherapy for, 143–145
  radiotherapy for, 144–145
  single modality surgical
      management of, 143
N2 potentially resectable disease, 3
N3 disease, 168
N3 patients, 4
NATCH trial, 127
National Lung Screening Trial
      (NLST), 61, 336
Navigational bronchoscopy, 1, 2
Nd:YAG. *See* Neodynium:yttrium
      aluminum garnet (Nd:YAG)
N descriptors, 45
Neisseria meningitides, 302
Neoadjuvant therapy, 133, 161, 278
  for patients with T4$_{Inv}$ or
      N3 disease, 167*t*
Neodynium:yttrium aluminum garnet
      (Nd:YAG) laser, 237
NeuGcGM3, 304, 305
New lung cancer staging system, 2
NF1 gene, 26
NKX2-1 gene, 25, 32
Nodal metastasis (N stage),
      evaluation of, 83
Non-small cell lung cancer (NSCLC), 2,
      3, 4, 5, 21, 24, 73, 80, 183, 299
  adenocarcinoma, 21–22, 24–26
  adenosquamous carcinoma, 22
  adjuvant therapy for, 279–280
  advanced disease
      biologic therapy for, 284–285
      chemotherapy for, 281–284
  biomarkers in, 263–264
  community-based care,
      issues in, 335–336
  intensity-modulated radiation therapy
      (IMRT) for, 205–210

large cell carcinoma (LCC), 22
locally advanced NSCLC, 3–4,
      280–281
  metastatic, 3–4
  molecular profiling of, 29
      DNA copy number profiles, 31–32
      epigenetics, 32
      gene-expression (mRNA)
        profiles, 32–33
      miRNA profiles, 33
      proteomic profiles, 33
      tissue considerations, 30–31
  nodal metastasis (N stage),
      evaluation of, 83
  pathogenesis of, 26
      adenocarcinoma pathogenesis, 27–28
      progenitors and stem cells, 28–29
      SCC pathogenesis, 28
  predictive markers of, 33
      chemotherapy resistance
        markers, 33–34
      targeted therapy, 34–35
  radiation therapy alone
      for, 285–286
  sarcomatoid carcinomas, 22–23
  and small cell lung carcinoma (SCLC)
      molecular differences between, 25*t*
  squamous cell carcinoma, 22, 26
  stage IIIA, 3
  surgery for, 278
      in octogenarians, 278–279
  symptoms and quality of life in,
      313–315
  treatment options for, 343*t*
  tumor status (T stage), 80–83
  vaccine development
      α(1,3)-galactosyltransferase,
        303–304
      α-galactosylceramide, 301
      1E10 vaccine, 304–305
      B7.1 vaccine, 301–302
      belagenpumatucel, 299–300
      cyclophilin B, 304
      dendritic cell vaccines, 304
      dexosome vaccine, 303
      epidermal growth factor vaccine,
        302–303
      GVAX, 300–301
      IDM-2101, 301
      L523S vaccine, 302
      L-BLP-25, 301
      melanoma-associated antigen E-3
        vaccine, 303
      transcriptase catalytic subunit
        antigen vaccine, 303
North Central Cancer
      Treatment Group (NCCTG)
      trial 94-24-52, 280
Novalis radiosurgery system, 219
N-propionylation (NP-polySA), 306
NRAS gene, 26
NTRK1 gene, 26
NTRK3 gene, 26

Obstructive airway lesions, 4
Oct4, 29
Octogenarians with NSCLC,
        surgery in, 278–279
Older adults, lung cancer in, 277
    non-small cell lung cancer (NSCLC)
        adjuvant therapy for, 279–280
        advanced disease, biologic
            therapy for, 284–285
        advanced disease, chemotherapy
            for, 281–284
        locally advanced NSCLC, 280–281
        radiation therapy alone
            for, 285–286
        surgery for, 278–279
    palliative care, 287
    small cell lung cancer (SCLC)
        extensive disease, 286–287
        limited disease (LD), 286
    treatment, general considerations
        in, 277–278
1E10 vaccine, 304–305
OSI-774–203 protocol, 267
Overdiagnosis
    evidence against, 61
    evidence in support of, 60–61

p16^Ink4, 24, 25
p16^INK4a methylation, 26, 28
p63, 23, 24
Paclitaxel, 34, 155, 158, 246, 254, 264,
        267, 269, 271, 282, 283, 342
Paclitaxel poliglumex, 200
PAK3 gene, 26
Palliation, 4
Palliative care, 6, 313
    in older adults, 287
    roles and responsibilities, 11*t*
    surgery in, 107–108
Pancoast tumor, 97, 98*f*
Pan-DR epitope (PADRE), 301
Pan-HER inhibitors, 251–252
Papanicolaou-stained cytology
        samples, 23
Parenchymal margins, 95
Pathologic disease stage, 21
Pathologist, 354–355
Pathology, of lung cancer, 1–2, 19
    ancillary diagnostic
        immunohistochemistry, 23–24
    malignant lung cancer tumors, 21
        carcinoid tumors, 23
        non-small cell lung carcinoma
            (NSCLC), 21–23
        small cell lung carcinoma
            (SCLC), 23
    metastasis, progression to, 29
    molecular characteristics of, 24
        non-small cell lung cancer
            (NSCLC), 24–26
        small cell lung cancer (SCLC), 26

NSCLC, molecular profiling of, 29
    DNA copy number profiles, 31–32
    epigenetics, 32
    gene-expression (mRNA)
        profiles, 32–33
    miRNA profiles, 33
    proteomic profiles, 33
    tissue considerations, 30–31
NSCLC, pathogenesis of, 26
    adenocarcinoma pathogenesis, 27–28
    progenitors and stem cells, 28–29
    SCC pathogenesis, 28
NSCLC, predictive markers of, 33
    chemotherapy resistance
        markers, 33–34
    targeted therapy, 34–35
premalignant lesions, 19
    atypical adenomatous hyperplasia
        (AAH), 21
    diffuse idiopathic pulmonary
        neuroendocrine cell hyperplasia
        (DIPENECH), 21
    squamous dysplasia/carcinoma in
        situ, 19–21
Patient-reported outcomes
        (PROs), 313, 317–318
Patupilone, 200
Pazopanib, 247
PDGFRA gene, 26
Pemetrexed, 158, 184, 185, 186, 187,
        197–199, 246, 264–265, 266,
        342, 344
Percutaneous needle biopsy
        (PCNB), 2, 78
Personalized medicine, role of, 263
    biomarkers in NSCLC, prognostic
        association of, 263–264
    novel directions
        ALM4-ALK fusion, 271–272
        antiangiogenic agents, 271
        BRCA1 in lung cancer, 271
        Class III β-tubulin, 270
        gene expression, 271
        insulin-like growth factor receptor
            inhibition, 270–271
        serum proteomics as a predictor of
            clinical benefit, 270
    tailoring chemotherapy by
        biomarkers
        EGFR gene copy number, 268–269
        EGFR gene mutation, 266–268
        EGFR protein expression, 269
        EGFR-related therapies, 266
        ERCC1, 264
        KRAS gene mutation, 269–270
        RRM1, 364–265
        thymidylate synthase, 265–266
Personal resource variables
    cancer-related attributions, 330–331
    coping, 330
    personal perceptions, 330
Pertuzumab, 256
PET-CT, 93, 107, 208, 209, 214

Phase III lung chemoprevention
        trials, 62–64, 63*t*
Phorylated *EGFR* (p-*EGFR*), 29
Phosphatidylinositol 3-kinase
        (PI3K), 29, 68, 252
Phospho-Akt, 251
Photodynamic therapy
        (PDT), 238–239, 241
Physician and hospital volume, 10–14
Physicians, roles and
        responsibilities of, 11*t*
Planning target volume
        (PTV), 206, 208, 209
Platinum-based adjuvant therapy, 3
Platinum-based doublet, 4, 33
Platinum/etoposide
        regimen, 117, 118, 344
Platinum-sensitivity, 118
Pleural dissemination, 45, 46
Pleurodesis, 108
Pneumonectomy, 3, 97, 98, 145
Pneumothorax, 58
Polymerase chain reaction (PCR)
        analysis, 32, 265, 285
Polysialic acid (PolySA), 305–306
Positron emission tomography
        (PET), 2, 7, 75–76, 113, 213
    with 2-fluoro-2-deoxyglucose
        (FDG-PET), 221
Posterolateral thoracotomy, 94, 99
Postoperative radiotherapy (PORT),
        123, 133, 134, 141
Post-thoracotomy pain syndrome, 314
Premalignant lesions, 19
    atypical adenomatous hyperplasia
        (AAH), 21
    diffuse idiopathic pulmonary
        neuroendocrine cell hyperplasia
        (DIPENECH), 21
    squamous dysplasia/carcinoma
        in situ, 19–21
Preoperative pulmonary lung
        function assessment, 91–92
Pretreatment evaluation, 338*t*
Prevascular/periaortic lymph nodes, 7
Prevention of lung cancer, 2, 62
    current approaches, 64
        early-phase clinical trial
            designs, 66–67
        high-risk cohorts,
            identification of, 65
        intermediate endpoints, 65–66
        target identification, 64–65
    historical perspective
        lessons learned, 64
        phase III clinical trials, 62–64
    ongoing studies and new directions,
        67–68
Primary care and specialist
        physicians, roles and
        responsibilities of, 11*t*
Primary care provider
    roles and responsibilities, 11*t*

Profile of Mood States, 324
Progenitors and stem cells, 28–29
Progression-free survival (PFS), 123, 134, 184, 189, 200, 201, 246, 251, 267, 344
Prophylactic cranial irradiation (PCI), 107, 113, 157, 213–214, 286
Prostacyclin (PGI$_2$), 68
Protein kinase B (AKT), phosphorylation of, 266
Proteomic pattern analysis, 33
Proteomic profiles, 33
p-S6 expression, 29
Psychologic distress, in lung cancer patients, 323
  correlates of, 328
    disease-related variables, 329–330
    historical variables, 331
    personal resources, 330–331
    social contextual variables, 330
    sociodemographic variables, 328–329
  limitations and future directions, 331
    factors contributing to distress, identification of, 331–332
    long-term psychologic outcomes, 332
    methodological issues, 332
    psychosocial intervention research, 332
  lung cancer study, importance of, 323
  prevalence and nature of, 323–328
Psychosocial care, in lung cancer, 6
Psychosocial intervention research, 332
PT1N0M0 tumors, 45
PT2N0M0 tumors, 45
PTPRD gene, 26
Pulmonary medicine
  roles and responsibilities, 11t
Pulmonary resection in elderly, 100
Pulmonologists, 353–354

Quality of life (QOL), 3, 6, 313
  adjuvant chemotherapy effect on, 342
  assessment, 317–318
  in early stage, 313–315
  in late stage, 315–316

Racial disparities, in lung cancer, 293
  advanced disease, 295
  early-stage disease, 295–296
  racial disparities model, 293–294
  socioeconomic status, 294–295
  tobacco, 296
Radiation-induced lung injury, 58, 227
Radiation oncology, 355
  roles and responsibilities, 11t
Radiation therapy, 146–147, 340–341
  for NSCLC, 285–286
  for unresectable stage III NSCLC, 152

Radiation Therapy Oncology Group (RTOG) 115, 152, 153t
Radiofrequency ablation (RFA), 217
Radiologic techniques, 2
Radiologists, 354
Radiology, 11t
Radiotherapy, for lung cancer, 4
Randomized controlled trials
  of CT, 61
  of PET, 9t
RAP80 (receptor-associated protein 80), 130, 271
RARβ gene, 25, 32
RASSF1A gene, 32
RASSF1 gene, 32
RB1 gene, 26
Real-time tracking, 209, 219
Recurrent NSCLC, 226–227
Referral patterns, 338
Resection extent, in surgical techniques, 94–100
  carinal resection, 99–100
  lobectomy, 97
  pneumonectomy, 97
  segmentectomy, 96–97
  sleeve resections, 97–99, 100f
  tumor margins, adequacy of, 95
    bronchial margins, 95
    parenchymal margins, 95
  wedge resection, 95–96
Respiratory gating, 209
Respiratory tumor motion, 208
Response evaluation criteria in solid tumors (RECIST), 354
13-cis-Retinoic acid (13cRA), 63
Reverse phase protein arrays (RPPA), 33
Ribonucleotide reductase M1 (RRM1), 2, 34, 191
Rigid bronchoscopy, 4, 235
Robotic lobectomy, 97, 98f
Rofecoxib, 64
RRM1 (ribonucleotide reductase subunit M1), 264–265
RTOG 0241, 212
RTOG 83–11, 153
RTOG 9712, 212
RUNX3 gene, 32

S0124 trial, 117
Sarah Cannon Cancer Center, 346
Sarcomatoid carcinomas, 22–23
Screening, of lung cancer, 2, 53
  chest X-ray and sputum cytology, randomized controlled trials of, 53–55
  low-dose helical CT screening
    issues in, 55–60
    lead-time bias, 60
    length-biased sampling, 60
    mortality, of lung cancer, 61
    overdiagnosis, 60–61

randomized controlled trials of CT, 61
  single-arm studies of helical CT, 55
Second primary lung cancer, 169
Segmentectomy, 96–97
Sequential/maintenance therapy, 185–186, 186t
Serum proteomics, 270
Siemens Primaotom, 219
Single-nucleotide polymorphism (SNP) arrays, 31
Single-photon emission computed tomography (SPECT), 92
Single versus multistation disease, 142–143
Sleeve lobectomy, 3
Sleeve resections, 97–99, 100f
Small cell lung cancer (SCLC), 3, 5, 23, 26, 46, 79–80, 80f, 105–108, 111, 344–345, 355
  conformal radiotherapy for, 211
  early-stage SCLC, role of surgery for, 113
  extensive disease, 286–287
  extensive-stage SCLC (ESLC), 115
    chemotherapy, 117
    novel therapeutics, 118–120
    prophylactic cranial irradiation in, 118
    relapsed disease, 118
  limited disease (LD), 286
  limited-stage SCLC (LS-SCLC), 113
    chemotherapy, 114
    key clinical trials in, 115
    prophylactic cranial irradiation in, 115
    radiation therapy, 114–115
  management, future of
    amrubicin, 118–119
    anti-Bcl-2 family protein inhibitors, 119–120
    Hedgehog (Hh) pathway inhibitors, 120
  and non-small cell lung carcinoma (NSCLC)
    molecular differences between, 25t
  pathology and clinical presentation, 111–112
  refractory SCLC, 118
  staging
    and evaluation, 112–113
    and prognosis, 113t
  surgical treatment of, 3, 105, 107–108, 355
    future directions, 108
    historical perspective, 105
    lobectomy versus wedge resection, 107
    surgery and preoperative evaluation, indications for, 105–107
    surgical palliative care, role of

Small cell lung cancer(SCLC)—(*Continued*)
  vaccine development
    BEC2, 305
    fucosyl GM1, 305
    polySA, 305–306
    Wilm's tumor gene, 306
Small molecule tyrosine kinase
    inhibitors, 245
  erlotinib, 249–250
  gefitinib, 250–251
  pazopanib, 247
  sorafenib, 245–246
  sunitinib, 245
  vandetanib, 246
Smoking, 331
  cessation, 2
Snap-freezing of fresh tissue, 31
Social contextual variables, 330
Sociodemographic variables
  age, 328
  education, 329
  ethnicity, 328–329
  gender, 328
Socioeconomic status
    (SES), 294–295
Solitary pulmonary nodule (SPN), 76
  imaging guided percutaneous
    needle biopsy, 78–79
  location, 77
  morphology, 77
  size, 76–77
  tissue-specific and metabolic
    characteristics, 77–78
Sorafenib, 189, 190, 201, 245–246,
    255, 257
Southwest Oncology Group
    (SWOG), 126, 356
Southwest Oncology Group
    (SWOG) 9019 trial, 184
Specialist physicians, roles and
    responsibilities of, 11*t*
Special patient considerations, 190–191
Spinal metastasis, SBRT for, 226
Spiritual challenges, 316
Sputum analysis, 2, 61
Sputum cytology, randomized
    controlled trials of, 53–55
Squamous cell carcinoma
    (SCC), 22, 26
  pathogenesis, 28
  pathologic and molecular
    characteristics of, 22*t*
Squamous dysplasia/carcinoma
    in situ, 19–21
Stage grouping, 46
Stage I NSCLC
  SBRT for, 221–223, 224*t*–225*t*
Stage III NSCLC, 151
  classification, 151
    bulky stage, 151
    nonbulky stage, 151
  consolidation chemotherapy, 156–157
  future directions

    chemotherapy, 158
    radiation, 158
  management, overview of, 152
  prophylactic cranial irradiation, 157
  treatment
    altered fractionation, 152–154
    concurrent chemotherapy with
      radiation, 154–156
    radiation alone, 152
    sequential chemotherapy followed
      by radiation, 154
  unresectable disease,
    definition of, 151
Stage III A lung cancer,
    patients with, 3
Stage IIIA–N2 NSCLC, 133
  analytical bias, 136
  causation bias, 135–136
  comparison bias, 136
  efficacy bias, presumption of, 136
  exploratory subgroup
    analysis bias, 137
  historical bias, 134
  induction chemotherapy followed by
    surgery/radiotherapy, 134
  prognostic factor bias, 136
  reporting bias, 136
  selection bias, 137
  treatment of, 133
Stage IIIA NSCLC, 139
  definition, 140
  mediastinal lymph node
    assessment, 141
    during surgical resection, 141
  N2 disease, 141
    adjuvant chemotherapy for, 146
    induction chemotherapy
      for, 143–145
    radiotherapy for, 144–145
    single modality surgical
      management of, 143
  radiation therapy, 146–147
  single versus multistation
    disease, 142–143
  staging guidelines, 140
  surgical management, 145–146
  surgical role in, 3
  T3N1 tumors, 140–141
Stage IIIB and IV NSCLC, 197
  docetaxel, 197
  EGFR TKIs, 199–200
  erlotinib, 199
  gefitinib, 199
  new drugs in recurrent advanced
    NSCLC, 200
    chemotherapy agents, 200
    targeted agents, 200–202
  pemetrexed, 197–199
  perspectives, 202
Stage IIIB/IV NSCLC, primary therapy
    for, 183
  combined modality approach, 183
    chemotherapy doublets, 185

    duration of therapy, 185
    molecular-targeted agents, 188–190
Staging, in lung cancer, 2, 7–9, 43
  controversial points, 48–50
  external validation, of IASLC
    recommendations, 48
  IASLC database, 43
  results and recommendations
    bronchopulmonary carcinoids,
      46–47
    IASLC lymph node map, 47
    M descriptors, 46
    N descriptors, 45
    small cell lung cancer, 46
    stage grouping, 46
    T descriptors, 45
    visceral pleura invasion, 47
Standardized uptake values (SUV), 75,
    227
START Center for Cancer Care, 346
STAT1 gene, 32
Stereotactic body radiation therapy
    (SBRT), 217, 355
  clinical outcomes
    early-stage (stage I) NSCLC, 221–
      223, 224*t*–225*t*
    metastatic NSCLC, 223–226
    recurrent NSCLC, 226–227
  historical development, 217–218
  radiobiology of, 218
  selection of patients for, 221
  technical aspects, 218
    immobilization and respiratory
      motion control, 219
    physics and dosimetry, 220–221
    target delineation, 218–219
    treatment devices, 219–220
  toxicities, 227–228
  treatment response, evaluation of, 227
Stereotactic body radiosurgery, 341
Stereotactic radiosurgery (SRS), 217
STK11 gene, 26
Subcarinal nodes, 7
Sunitinib, 201, 245
Surgery, 339–340
Surgery and preoperative evaluation,
    indications for, 105–107
Surgical management, of lung cancer,
    91, 145–146
  mediastinal assessment, 92–94
  mediastinum, management of, 100
  preoperative pulmonary lung function
    assessment, 91–92
  pulmonary resection in elderly, 100
  techniques, 94
    resection, extent of, 94–100
    thoracic cavity, approaches to, 94
Surgical palliative care, in SCLC,
    107–108
Surgical resection, 3, 4
Surgical role, in small cell lung cancer, 3
Surgical treatment of lung cancer, 3
Surgical unresectability, 152

Surveillance, Epidemiology, and
	End Results (SEER)
	registries, 43, 46, 278
Surveillance bronchoscopy, 238
Suspicious lung lesions,
	patients with, 1
SVC resections, 163
Symptom distress, 323, 324
Systemic therapy, in lung cancer, 4–5

T1N0 SCLC tumors, 106
T1–T2N0 SCLC, 106
T2aN1M0 tumors, 46
T2bN0M0 tumors, 46
T3N1 tumors, 140–141
	surgical resection of, 3
T4 invasion
	additional tumor nodules
		general approach, 168–169
		ipsilateral different lobe
			nodules, 170–172
		ipsilobar satellite nodule, 169
		multiple primary lung cancer
			(MPLC), 169–170
	carinal resection, 161–163
	esophageal involvement, 164
	great vessel and cardiac
		invasion, 163, 163t
		aortic resections, 163–164
		atrial resection, 164
		CPB, need for, 164
		SVC resections, 163
	isolated distant metastases, 173
		general series of surgery in patients
			with, 173–174
		isolated adrenal metastasis, 175
		isolated brain metastasis, 174–175
	malignant pleural
		involvement, 172–173
	multimodality therapy, 164–168
	with N2 nodes, 164
	N3 disease, 168
	surgery for heterogeneous
		cohort of, 165t
	vertebral body involvement, 164
T4M0 tumors, 46
T4N0-N1M0 tumors, 46
T790M mutation, 266
Tailoring chemotherapy by biomarkers
	EGFR gene copy number, 268–269
	EGFR gene mutation, 266–268
	EGFR protein expression, 269
	EGFR-related therapies, 266
	ERCC1, 264
	KRAS gene mutation, 269–270
	RRM1, 364–265
	thymidylate synthase, 265–266
Targeted pathways, in NSCLC and
	SCLC, 243
	antiangiogenic therapies, 243
		monoclonal antibodies, 243–245

small molecule tyrosine kinase
	inhibitors, 245–247
cyclooxygenase-2 inhibitors, 254
EGFR-targeting therapies, 247
	monoclonal antibodies, 247–249
	small molecule tyrosine kinase
		inhibitors, 249–251
future directions, 257
histone deacetylase (HDAC)
	inhibitors, 254
insulin-like growth factor 1
	receptor–targeting therapies, 252
mammalian target of rapamycin
	(mTOR) inhibitors, 252–253
pan-HER inhibitors, 251–252
rational combinations, 254
	antiangiogenic and EGFR-targeting
		therapy, 255
	EGFR, dual inhibition of, 255–256
	EGFR and COX-2 inhibitors, 256
	EGFR and mTOR inhibitors, 256
Targeted therapies, 19, 342–344
Target identification, 64–65
Taxane, 247
T descriptors
	additional tumor nodule(s) and
		pleural dissemination, 45
	tumor size, 45
Technetium 99m-methylene
	diphosphate (Tc-99m-MDP)
	scintigraphy, 84
TERT gene, 32
TGF-β2, 299
TGF-β "blockade.", 300
Thoracic cavity, approaches to, 94
Thoracic irradiation, 113, 114
Thoracic surgeons, 355
Thoracic surgery
	roles and responsibilities, 11t
Thoracic tumor board, 10
3D-CRT, 205, 207, 210
Thymidylate synthase (TS), 265–266
	overexpression, 2
Timeliness of care, 14–15, 14t
Tissue sampling, 8t
TITF1, 32
TNM classification and staging
	system, 46–47, 50
TNM descriptors, definitions for, 44t
Tobacco, 65, 296, 336
TomoTherapy HiArt System, 219, 220
Topotecan, 118, 271, 345
TP53, 24, 26, 29, 34
TP533 mutations, 24, 26, 34
Tracheobronchial cancers,
	treatment of, 235
	airway stent insertion, 238
	brachytherapy, 239–240
	bronchoscopic intervention,
		results of, 240–241
	bronchoscopic treatment, indications
		for, 236
	laser resection, 237–238

photodynamic therapy, 238–239
rigid and flexible
	bronchoscopy, 235–236
Tracheobronchial stents, 238
Transbronchial needle aspiration biopsy
	(TBNA), 7, 141, 337
Transcriptase catalytic subunit antigen
	vaccine, 303
Treatment of lung cancer, 5–6, 299
	bronchoscopic treatment, indications
		for, 235, 236
	cancer care sites, 338–339
	chemotherapeutics, 341–344
	endobronchial treatment, 4
	first-line treatment algorithm, 345f
	NSCLC vaccine development
1E10 vaccine, 304–305
	α(1,3)-galactosyltransferase, 303–304
	α-galactosylceramide, 301
	B7.1 vaccine, 301–302
	belagenpumatucel, 299–300
	cyclophilin B, 304
	dexosome vaccine, 303
	epidermal growth factor vaccine,
		302–303
	GVAX, 300–301
	IDM-2101, 301
	L523S vaccine, 302
	L-BLP-25, 301
	melanoma-associated antigen E-3
		vaccine, 303
	NSCLC dendritic
		cell vaccines, 304
	transcriptase catalytic subunit
		antigen vaccine, 303
pretreatment evaluation, 338t
radiation therapy, 340–341
referral patterns, 338
SCLC vaccine development
	BEC2, 305
	fucosyl GM1, 305
	polySA, 305–306
	Wilm's tumor gene, 306
small cell lung cancer (SCLC),
	surgical treatment of, 3, 105,
	107–108, 355
	future directions, 108
	historical perspective, 105
	lobectomy versus wedge
		resection, 107
	surgery and preoperative evaluation,
		indications for, 105–107
	surgical palliative care, role of
in select populations, 5–6
surgical treatment, 3, 339–340
tracheobronchial cancers, see
	Tracheobronchial cancers,
	treatment of
TRIBUTE (Tarceva Responses in
	Conjunction with Taxol and
	Carboplatin) phase III trial, 269
TTF-1, 23, 25, 32
TTF-1 IHC expression, 23

Tumor, node, metastases
       (TNM) staging system, 21, 43,
       44*t*, 112
Tumor margins, adequacy of, 95
   bronchial margins, 95
   parenchymal margins, 95
Tumor protein 53 (*TP533*), 34
Tumor size, 45
Tumor status (T stage), 80–83
Tumor suppressor gene (TSG), 19, 24,
       26, 32
Tyrosine kinase inhibitors
       (TKIs), 24, 35, 189

Universal survival
       curve (USC), 218
Unresectable stage III
       NSCLC, 152
   medical unresectability, 152
   surgical unresectability, 152

Vandetanib, 200–201, 246, 257
Vascular endothelial growth factor
       (VEGF), 285
   inhibitor, 128
   ligands, 243, 244*f*
Vascular endothelial growth factor
       receptor (VEGFR)-2, 200, 201
Vascular endothelial growth factor
       receptor (VEGFR) system, 271
VeriStrat, 270
Vertebral body involvement, in T4
       invasion, 164
VGFA gene, 32
Video-assisted thoracic surgery (VATS),
       279, 94, 95, 95*f*, 97, 340
Vinblastine, 154, 155, 174, 280
Vinca alkaloids, 270
Vindesine, 155, 187, 205, 211
Vinorelbine, 197, 245, 248, 250, 264,
       270, 279, 281, 282, 284, 344
Vinflunine, 200
Visceral pleura invasion, 47

V-Ki-ras2 Kirsten rat sarcoma
       viral oncogene homolog
       (*KRAS*), 34
Volume and outcome, relationship
       between, 12–13*t*
VP-16, 212

Wedge resection, 95–96
Whole brain radiation, 174–175, 245
Whole-brain radiotherapy, 250
Wilm's tumor gene (WT1), 306

XLC38A3 gene, 26

Zileuton, 254
ZMYND10 gene, 26